Medical Radiology

Diagnostic Imaging

Series Editors

Albert L. Baert
Maximilian F. Reiser
Hedvig Hricak
Michael Knauth

Editorial Board

Andy Adam, London
Fred Avni, Brussels
Richard L. Baron, Chicago
Carlo Bartolozzi, Pisa
George S. Bisset, Durham
A. Mark Davies, Birmingham
William P. Dillon, San Francisco
D. David Dershaw, New York
Sam Sanjiv Gambhir, Stanford
Nicolas Grenier, Bordeaux
Gertraud Heinz-Peer, Vienna
Robert Hermans, Leuven
Hans-Ulrich Kauczor, Heidelberg
Theresa McLoud, Boston
Konstantin Nikolaou, Munich
Caroline Reinhold, Montreal
Donald Resnick, San Diego
Rüdiger Schulz-Wendtland, Erlangen
Stephen Solomon, New York
Richard D. White, Columbus

For further volumes:
http://www.springer.com/series/4354

Patrice Taourel
Editors

CT of the Acute Abdomen

Foreword by
Albert L. Baert

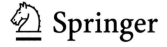

Springer

Editor
Prof. Dr. Patrice Taourel
Imagerie Médicale
Hôpital Lapeyronie
avenue du Doyen Gaston Giraud 371
34295 Montpellier CX 5
France
e-mail: p-taourel@chu-montpellier.fr

ISSN 0942-5373
ISBN 978-3-540-89231-1   e-ISBN 978-3-540-89232-8
DOI 10.1007/978-3-540-89232-8
Springer Heidelberg Dordrecht London New York

Library of Congress Control Number: 2011935932

© Springer-Verlag Berlin Heidelberg 2011
This work is subject to copyright. All rights are reserved, whether the whole or part of the material is concerned, specifically the rights of translation, reprinting, reuse of illustrations, recitation, broadcasting, reproduction on microfilm or in any other way, and storage in data banks. Duplication of this publication or parts thereof is permitted only under the provisions of the German Copyright Law of September 9, 1965, in its current version, and permission for use must always be obtained from Springer. Violations are liable to prosecution under the German Copyright Law.
The use of general descriptive names, registered names, trademarks, etc. in this publication does not imply, even in the absence of a specific statement, that such names are exempt from the relevant protective laws and regulations and therefore free for general use.
Product liability: The publishers cannot guarantee the accuracy of any information about dosage and application contained in this book. In every individual case the user must check such information by consulting the relevant literature.

Cover design: eStudio Calamar S.L.

Printed on acid-free paper

Springer is part of Springer Science+Business Media (www.springer.com)

Foreword

Radiological imaging plays a key role in the correct differential diagnosis and the decision-making for medical or surgical treatment of acute abdominal conditions.

For many decades and until the advent of CT, standard radiography was the main imaging tool to guide clinicians towards the correct management of the patients. Notwithstanding the sophisticated rules and guidelines that were invented and developed over the years by many highly talented radiologists, for the Optimal interpretation of the standard radiogram of the abdomen; the important limitations of this diagnostic tool, which could mostly provide only indirect evidence for the cause or the site of the lesions, remained painfully evident in our daily practice.

The introduction of CT, especially the multislice technology and the multi-planar reconstructions, have opened immense new opportunities and possibilities for the rapid and exact diagnosis as well as for the evaluation of the extent of lesions in the patient with an acute abdominal condition and has profoundly changed the diagnostic approach of these patients.

This volume offers a comprehensive and detailed description of the optimal use of CT in acute abdomen and of the wide range of its clinical applications in this large group of patients. The text is supported by numerous, high-quality images, well-chosen to illustrate the key-CT findings in a Broad Spectrum of traumatic and non-traumatic acute abdomen.

I am indebted to the editor, P. Taourel, an internationally well known abdominal radiologist, with a long experience in abdominal CT for his out-standing editorial coordination and for his personal contributions to this work. I am also very grateful for the high-level contributions from a large group of other recognised experts in the field.

This excellent volume will greatly appeal to not only the general, abdominal as well as emergency radiologists but also to gastroenterologists and abdominal surgeons, who will find this book a great help for the better management of their patients.

I am convinced that it will meet great interest of the readership for our series: Medical Radiology.

Albert L. Baert

Contents

Part I   Epidemiological Data and Clinical Findings

Epidemiology of Acute Abdominal Pain in Adults in the Emergency Department Setting 3
Mustapha Sebbane, Richard Dumont, Riad Jreige,
and Jean-Jacques Eledjam

Epidemiology of Abdominal Trauma 15
Françoise Guillon

Part II   Elementary CT Findings

Key CT Findings 31
Eric Delabrousse

Part III   CT Techniques

Volume CT of Acute Abdomen: Acquisition and Reconstruction Techniques 65
Samuel Mérigeaud, Ingrid Millet, Fernanda Curros-Doyon,
and Patrice Taourel

Part IV   CT Diagnosis in Non Traumatic Abdomen

Acute Liver Disease 83
Valérie Vilgrain and François Durand

Biliary Emergencies 93
Yves Menu, Julien Cazejust, Ana Ruiz, Louisa Azizi, and Lionel Arrivé

Acute Splenic Disease 115
Eric Delabrousse

Acute Pancreatitis 125
Catherine Ridereau-Zins and Christophe Aubé

Acute Appendicitis 143
Samuel Mérigeaud, Ingrid Millet, and Patrice Taourel

Ischemia (Acute Mesenteric Ischemia and Ischemic Colitis) 183
Stefania Romano and Luigia Romano

Diverticulitis 199
Jean-Michel Bruel and Patrice Taourel

Nonischemic Colitis 221
Philippe Soyer, Mourad Boudiaf, Youcef Guerrache, Christine Hoeffel,
Xavier Dray, and Patrice Taourel

Acute Gastritis and Enteritis 239
Denis Régent, Valerie Croisé-Laurent, Julien Mathias, Aurélia Fairise,
Hélène Ropion-Michaux, and Clément Proust

Bowel Obstruction 273
Patrice Taourel, Denis Hoa, and Jean-Michel Bruel

Bowel Perforations 309
Patrice Taourel, Joseph Pujol, and Emma Pages-Bouic

Acute Gastrointestinal Bleeding 329
Benoit Paul Gallix

Intra- and Retroperitoneal Hemorrhages 343
Philippe Otal, Julien Auriol, Marie-Charlotte Delchier,
Marie-Agnès Marachet, and Hervé Rousseau

Urological Emergencies 359
Patrice Taourel and Rodolphe Thuret

Gynecologic Emergencies 377
Patrice Taourel, Fernanda Curros Doyon, and Ingrid Millet

Acute Diseases Related to Intra-abdominal Fat in Adults 393
Etienne Danse

Acute Disease of the Abdominal Wall 399
Catherine Cyteval

**Complications of Abdominal Surgery (Abdominal, Urologic
and Gynecologic Emergencies)** 409
Marc Zins and Isabelle Boulay-Coletta

Part V CT Diagnosis in Traumatic Abdomen

Abdominal Trauma 421
Ingrid Millet and Patrice Taourel

Index 465

Part I

Epidemiological Data and Clinical Findings

Epidemiology of Acute Abdominal Pain in Adults in the Emergency Department Setting

Mustapha Sebbane, Richard Dumont, Riad Jreige, and Jean-Jacques Eledjam

Contents

1	**Introduction**	3
2	**Acute Abdominal Pain Based on Age**	4
2.1	Clinical Presentation of Abdominal Pain Based on Age	4
2.2	Etiology of Abdominal Pain Based on Age	5
3	**Abdominal Pain Based on Gender**	7
4	**Abdominal Pain Based on Pain Location**	7
4.1	Surgical Abdominal Pain	7
4.2	Nonsurgical Abdominal Pain	8
5	**Abdominal Pain Based on Pain Features**	9
6	**Population at Risk of Severity**	9
6.1	Abdominal Pain in the Seropositive Patient	10
7	**Abdominal Pain Based on Severity Signs**	10
7.1	Two Disorders Must Be Primarily Considered Because of the Risk of Sudden Death	10
7.2	Causes Associated with Risks of Severity	10
8	**General Management**	11
9	**Conclusion**	11
	References	12

M. Sebbane (✉) · R. Dumont · R. Jreige · J.-J. Eledjam
Service des Urgences, Hôpital Lapeyronie,
371 avenue du Doyen Gaston Giraud,
34295 Montpellier, France
e-mail: m-sebbane@chu-montpellier.fr

Abstract

Managing acute abdominal pain is a great challenge for the emergency physician. The diagnostic approach for acute abdominal pain is one of the most difficult for a physician. This is primarily due to the large extent of the clinical manifestations for abdominal pain, as well as to the subjectivity of the patient's feelings when it comes to clearly expressing the symptoms. Accurate measurement of the prevalence of the origin of acute abdominal pain is difficult. The cause of these pains is indeed wide-ranging, including very different clinical situations, extending from a viral gastroenteritis to abdominal aneurysm complications, through nonspecific abdominal pain.

1 Introduction

Acute abdominal pain classically refers to pain projecting onto the abdomen that has evolved for less than 1 week at the time of consultation. It can reflect intra-abdominal conditions, including gastrointestinal (GI), urogenital, or vascular disorders, as well as a symptom revealing extra-abdominal conditions, including cardiac, pulmonary, endocrinal, or metabolic disorders.

It is one of the most frequent reasons for admission of an adult to the emergency department, ranging from 4 to 10% of all admissions. Physical examination, especially the interview, remains one of the key elements of the diagnostic approach for acute abdominal pain conditions. However, the success of physical examination to accurately diagnose the cause

P. Taourel (ed.), *CT of the Acute Abdomen,* Medical Radiology. Diagnostic Imaging,
DOI: 10.1007/174_2010_135, © Springer-Verlag Berlin Heidelberg 2011

is no greater than 50%. Physical examination along with simple laboratory tests improve the diagnosis accuracy in 60% of cases (Nagurney et al. 2003), because of the highly variable cause and clinical pattern with age, sex, type, and location of pain or severity signs. With the population aging, reasoning by range of ages becomes a determining element in the diagnostic approach. With the variable prevalence of the different diagnoses, the older the patient, the more organic and surgical the condition.

These orientating epidemiologic elements will allow the diagnostic strategy to be improved in most patients. However, radiologic explorations, including ultrasonography and tomodensitometry, may be necessary to confirm the diagnosis (Stoker et al. 2009; de Dombal 1979).

A totally standardized and articulated management, essentially based on the physical examination along with, when required, additional laboratory and morphological tests, will support or allow one to rule out a diagnosis, with the aim to optimize the intervention delays, and facilitate the patient's orientation.

Abdominal emergency can be defined as a condition to be medically or surgically treated within 6 h. It represents about 40% of all emergency surgical operations. Overacute abdominal emergency or life-threatening emergency only concerns 1% of acute abdominal pain cases in the emergency setting.

Acute abdominal pain is a source of anxiety, and is often associated with emotional stress suffered either by the patient or by the patient's relatives, which could interfere with an objective evaluation. To help the decision-making, management must be simple and obey a predefined algorithm. If the digestive surgeon's evaluation is frequently sought, then the emergency physician often faces challenging decision-making when it comes to orientating the patient, especially for discharging the patient from hospital. The emergency physician must resolve the reason for the admission. He therefore has to work out an appropriate cognitive approach, to differentiate overacute from acute or subacute abdominal pain. He must seek criteria which will ensure he can assess the level of emergency. From that time on, immediately after the initial clinical examination, the decision strategy should set up the patient's clinical course, to the first minute, hour, and 24 h, and eventually prevent mid-term and long-term complications.

Table 1 Causes of main acute abdominal disorders and their prevalence (Bouillot and Bresler 2004)

Cause of acute abdominal pain	Prevalence (%)
Nonspecific	34.8
Cholecystitis	6.1
Appendicitis	7.5
Intestinal obstruction	6.7
Renal or ureteric colic	11
Acute pancreatitis	4.3
Diverticular disease	3.8
Hernia	3.4
Gynecologic disorder	6.1
Other diagnoses	6

2 Acute Abdominal Pain Based on Age

2.1 Clinical Presentation of Abdominal Pain Based on Age

Clinical presentation varies with age. Patients over 50 years old account for about a quarter of emergency admissions. The clinical presentation of acute abdominal pain in patients over 50 years old may differ from that of younger patients (Ahmed et al. 2005; Samaras et al. 2010; Laurell et al. 2006). The most common causes of abdominal conditions and their prevalence are reported in Table 1.

The risk of misdiagnoses and delay in diagnosis can be detrimental. Specific diagnostic challenges are encountered in the elderly, especially in patients over 75 years old. Besides an often, long medical history, and heavy medication, these patients present with nonspecific symptoms, and a certain delay between the onset of symptoms and admission. Often a wider range of differential diagnoses must be considered (Marco et al. 1998). The most common causes of abdominal conditions and their prevalence in the elderly are reported in Tables 2 and 3.

Potential challenges to the clinical assessment in the elderly are history taking and clinical assessment. They include altered mentation from fever or electrolyte abnormalities, cognitive impairment, decreased mentation from drugs (e.g., opiates, benzodiazepines) dementia, hearing difficulties, intoxication, language barriers, psychiatric disorders, the

Table 2 Causes of abdominal conditions and their prevalence based on age (adapted from de Dombal 1994)

Cause of acute abdominal pain	Prevalence (%)	
	Age less than 50 years	Age more than 50 years
Nonspecific	40	16
Cholecystitis	6	21
Appendicitis	32	15
Intestinal obstruction	2	12
Acute pancreatitis	2	7
Complicated diverticular disease	<0.1	6
Cancer	<0.1	4
Hernia	<0.1	3
Vasculary cause	<0.1	2

Table 3 Causes of abdominal conditions and their prevalence in patients over 75 years old (adapted from Bugliosi et al. 1990)

Cause of acute abdominal pain	Prevalence (%)
Nonspecific	23
Cholecystitis	12
Appendicitis	4
Intestinal obstruction	14
Gastritis	8
Acute pancreatitis	2
Complicated diverticular disease	6
Hollow viscus perforation	7
Ureteric colic	4
Urinary causes	6
Constipation	2
Extra digestive origin	9

absence of fever despite a serious bacterial infection or surgical condition, the absence of leukocytosis despite a surgical condition, altered pain perception from chronic pain medications, coexistent disease, 4 times higher likelihood of hypothermic response with a significant intra-abdominal process, lower likelihood of localized tenderness despite a focal surgical condition, reduced rebound and guarding from decreased abdominal wall musculature, suppressed tachycardia from medications, and intrinsic cardiac disease (Lyon and Clark 2006).

The so-called nonspecific abdominal pain mostly affects the young adult, gastric and pancreatobiliary disorders are encountered in patients aged about 40–60 years, whereas ischemic or tumoral conditions mostly affect the elderly (Tables 2, 3).

Proper knowledge of the prevalence of the main abdominal pain conditions based on the patient's age will improve management efficiency (de Dombal 1994).

2.2 Etiology of Abdominal Pain Based on Age

2.2.1 Cholecystitis

Biliary tract disorders, including cholecystitis requiring surgical treatment, represent one third of all acute abdominal pains in persons over 55 years old (de Dombal 1994; Huffman and Schenker 2010). A significant number of elderly patients do not present with typical signs of cholecystitis. The Murphy sign is found in half of cases, and with less accuracy than in younger patients. A retrospective study of patients over 65 years old presenting with acute cholecystitis concluded that over 60% of them did not have back or flank pain, 5% had no pain at all, over 40% did not experience nausea, more than half were afebrile, and 41% had a normal white blood cell count. Thirteen percent of patients had no abnormal liver function test findings (Parker et al. 1997).

Complications of acute cholecystitis, including cholangitis, gallbladder perforation, emphysematous cholecystitis, and biliary peritonitis, are frequent, more likely affecting the population over 65 years old.

2.2.2 Acute Appendicitis

Generalized pain, with extended duration, along with abdominal distension, contracture, decreased air-fluid noises, and the presence of a mass at palpation are classic findings in the elderly, likely due to a longer delay to presentation. Fever is a poor prognosis factor for acute appendicitis in the elderly, as only 23% of patients with acute appendicitis had a body temperature greater than 37.7°C. A band cell count greater than 6% and right lower quadrant pain were highly associated with pathologically proven appendicitis (positive predictive values of 100 and 90%, respectively). It is essential to have a high degree of suspicion to recognize acute appendicitis in an afebrile elderly patient who has abdominal pain, a mildly elevated white cell count, and a band cell count in the upper limits of normal. Ultrasonography may be of no use in a number of patients. Tomodensitometry contributes greatly to the diagnosis and should be highly considered (Rao et al. 1998; Raman et al. 2008).

Appendectomy accounts for 40% of all abdominal surgical operations in France. For most patients, the diagnosis is easy. Nevertheless, 20–30% of patients have an atypical clinical presentation and about 15–45% of patients who underwent appendectomy do not show any histopathology findings of appendiceal inflammation. Numerous appendicitises are diagnosed at the complicated appendicitis stage, including perforated appendicitis, plastron and appendiceal abscess, leading to an increased postoperative morbidity rate. A recently published retrospective analysis of 1,003 adults with acute appendicitis found a rate of perforated appendicitis as high as 23.8% (Howell et al. 2010; Boomer et al. 2010).

2.2.3 Acute Pancreatitis

The mortality rate of acute pancreatitis is increased in the elderly, as compared with the general population, with rates of 20–25% and 8–10%, respectively. The usual risk factors include alcoholism, biliary disease, infections, hypertriglyceridemia, and carbon monoxide exposure. A biliary lithiasis origin is found in 65–75% of cases. The utility of pancreatic laboratory tests, such as serum amylase or lipase levels, in aiding the diagnosis with regard to their sensitivity and specificity is similar to that for the general population (Vissers et al. 1999). Advanced age is a poor prognosis factor in acute pancreatitis patients (Ross and Forsmark 2001).

2.2.4 Gastric Ulcers and Complications

The absence of abdominal pain is found in about one third of patients over 60 years old with peptic ulcer (Hilton et al. 2001). Complications such as digestive hemorrhage or perforation are often the primary clinical presentations.

2.2.5 Intestinal Obstruction

Intestinal obstructions are the most frequent surgical emergencies, accounting for up to 20% of all emergency admissions to a surgery department. The causes are variable, but small bowel obstruction by adhesions from previous surgery is by far the leading cause (60%). Other, less frequent causes include malignancy (20%), hernia (10%), and GI tract inflammatory disorders (5%).

Three possible pathologic processes are involved. In adhesive small bowel obstruction, either complete or partial, there is no intestinal stress, the risk of parietal gangrene is low, and the chances of recovery after GI content has been suctioned are high. Obstruction by strangulation may be caused by tight stricture or by volvulus if the rotation of the bowel loop around the mesenteric axis is more than 180°. In both cases, obstruction is often complete, rarely cedes, and the risk of parietal gangrene is high, especially in volvulus. (Bass et al. 1997; Hayanga et al. 2005). This has led to the non actual dogma for emergency management of all acute obstructions by postoperative adhesions. In the setting of complete obstruction, the risk of strangulation is 20–40%.

Colonic obstructions are 5 times less frequent than small bowel obstructions. Accurate determination of the site and cause is required for proper therapeutic management. Common causes, in descending order of frequency, include primary malignant tumors (53%), volvulus (17%), diverticular disease (12%), and metastasis (6%). Other, miscellaneous causes (12%) include stenosis, hernia, fecaloma, pseudo-obstruction, adhesion, and undetermined cause .

Colonic volvulus is a twisting of the colon by more than 180° around its mesocolic axis. The sigmoid colon is involved in 76.2% of cases, the cecum in 21.7%, the transverse colon in 1.9%, and left flexure in 0.2%.

2.2.6 Diverticular Disease of the Colon and Sigmoid Volvulus of the Elderly

The incidence of diverticular disease increases with age to affect two thirds of persons over 90 years old, in contrast to 5% of the general population (Stollman and Raskin 2004; Sheth et al. 2008). Common risk factors include a tendency for constipation, a nonadapted diet, and reduced autonomy. In elderly persons, the obstructive syndrome is frequently related to a sigmoid volvulus, the most common type of colonic volvulus (75–80% of cases). Laxative use, sedatives, anticholinergics, and antiparkinsonian medicines predispose patients to a volvulus. Chronic distention, elongation, and increased mobility of the colon allow parts of the colon to twist on itself.

2.2.7 Abdominal Aortic Aneurysms

In emergency conditions, management of abdominal aortic aneurysms (AAA) is associated with a high mortality. The challenge is to screen patients early before any complication occurs or at an early stage of pain onset, which could correspond to the beginning of fissuration. AAA are usually infrarenal in origin and commonly extend into the iliac arteries. Most are diagnosed on routine examination or as an incidental finding on an imaging study.

Patients at highest risk for AAA are older men who use tobacco and have hypertension, peripheral vascular disease, and a family history of AAA. Smoking is the strongest independent risk factor; 90% of patients with AAA have used tobacco (Powell and Greenhalgh 2003; Sakalihasan et al. 2005; Kent et al. 2010). In 2005, the US Preventive Services Task Force recommended one-time screening by ultrasonography for AAA in all men between 65 and 75 years of age with a history of smoking tobacco (Fleming et al. 2005). Very recently, a genomic variant conferring susceptibility to AAA has been identified, within DAB2IP, which encodes an inhibitor of cell growth and survival (Gretarsdottir et al. 2010).

3 Abdominal Pain Based on Gender

Analysis of the background and comorbidities may allow the etiologic diagnosis to be better orientated. Gastric ulcer, alcoholic pancreatitis, and ureteric colic more often affect men, whereas biliary disorders, urinary tract infections, and strangulated hernia more often affect women. Women of childbearing age must be differentiated from other women, as it is a severity factor and management has to be codified.

According to a US observational study evaluating the influence of gender on the clinical outcome in the elderly presenting to the emergency department with abdominal pain, men had a much higher mortality rate within 3 months than women (19 vs. 1%, respectively), despite a similar predicted mortality rate and emergency department evaluation (Gardner et al. 2010).

Men and women presenting with abdominal pain differ in the short-term prognosis (within 3 months). Proper knowledge of the prevalence of the main abdominal pain conditions based on gender will improve management efficiency. It is therefore common to distinguish them on the basis of gender (Table 4).

Table 4 Main causes of acute abdominal pain based on gender and their prevalence (adapted from Bouillot and Bresler 2004)

Cause of pain	Prevalence (%)	
	Men	Women
Appendicitis	30	23
Nonspecific	21.7	25.3
Obstruction	7.8	8.9
Cholecystitis	7.7	12.4
Perforated ulcer	6.5	1.6
Pancreatitis	5.2	1.8
Other diagnoses	5.1	3.4
Renal colic	4.9	1.9
Ulcer onset	4	0.8
Salpingitis	–	4.5
Ectopic pregnancy	–	3.1
Ovarian cyst	–	2.8
Peritonitis	2.5	2.1
Strangulated hernia	2.3	3.7
Sigmoiditis	2.1	2
Urinary tract infection	0.2	2.7

4 Abdominal Pain Based on Pain Location

4.1 Surgical Abdominal Pain

The leading orientating elements are the clinical ones. In more than 70% of cases, accurate diagnosis and further examination, when necessary, can be made upon localization of pain into the nine quadrants.

In localized peritoneal syndrome, characterized by the clinical findings guarding, contracture, rebound tenderness, or exacerbation of pain when coughing or moving, the localization of pain along with clinical findings is the main etiologic orientation for appendicitis, or gallbladder and sigmoid causes (Broder et al. 2010).

The classic pathognomonic characteristics of those signs for the diagnosis of appendicitis or peritonitis are questioned by the literature data (Paulson et al. 2003; Bennett et al. 1994; Wagner et al. 1996; McCartan et al. 2010). The Murphy sign, defined as pain in the right hypochondrium associated with pain on inhibition of inspiration, is very frequently observed in biliary lithiasis. The Murphy sign is valuable in diagnosing acute cholecystitis, with reported sensitivity of 97% and a predictive positive value of 93% (Trowbridge et al. 2003). Obstructive syndrome must be differentiated in either bowel or colonic obstruction. Physical examination is sometimes poorly contributive. In the absence of specific clinical or laboratory findings, hospitalization for follow-up or imaging [computed tomography (CT) or ultrasonography] can be ordered to allow the diagnosis to be refined and a decision for medical or surgical orientation to be made.

Some pain features are more frequently encountered in severe or surgical conditions. The likelihood that pain is related to a surgical condition is greater if the pain is violent, recent (less than 48 h duration), or constant; if it is localized; if it is the first sign, and notably if it occurs before vomiting; if age is advanced; or if there is any history of surgery or peritoneal signs at physical examination.

The frequency of surgery and the prevalence of the most common causes are reported in Table 5. The data are only indicative and may differ with patient regional recruiting and management (Jordan 1980).

Table 5 Most frequent causes of emergency visits and surgery for abdominal pain (adapted from Jordan 1980)

Disorders	Prevalence (%)	Surgical treatment (%)
Gastroenteritis	6.9	–
Pelvic inflammatory condition	6.7	1.5
Genitourinary infection	5.2	–
Renal colic	4.3	–
Appendicitis	4.3	36.9
Cholecystitis	3.7	6.2
Intestinal obstruction	2.5	35.2
Constipation	2.3	–
Ulcer	2.0	8
Dysmenorrhea, pregnancy, ectopic pregnancy, ovarian cyst	1–2	–
Acute pancreatitis	<1	2.1
Aortic aneurysm	<1	–
Abscess	–	4.4
Perforated colon	–	1.1
Others	20	–
Undetermined	40	–

4.2 Nonsurgical Abdominal Pain

Abdominal pain can be the symptom of a medical condition. In such medical conditions, knowledge of the clinical background and history is essential. These medical conditions are numerous, and the following list is not exhaustive.

Diffuse pain in a drug-addicted patient may indicate a withdrawal syndrome. This diagnosis may be only retained when other concomitant detoxification signs are present, including bilateral mydriasis, sweating, and agitation.

Homozygous individuals with sickle cell anemia often have vasoocclusive crisis with attacks of abdominal pain, although rarely isolated. Other causes of abdominal pain should be systematically investigated. Urgent analgesia is needed in these patients, as pain also sustains sickle cell formation (Ahmed et al. 2005).

The presence of feverish symptoms and vaginal fluids must be investigated in the context of a young woman with pain in the right hypochondrium that is exacerbated by movement such as coughing or walking. Ultrasonography typically displays perihepatic adhesions. In the context of Fitz–Hugg–Curtis syndrome, laboratory testing of a vaginal fluid sample identifies chlamydial infection, to be treated with appropriate antibiotherapy.

Pain in either hypochondrium must also lead to lung examination, with fever and respiratory signs such as coughing as orientating elements in the search for pulmonary diseases of the inferior lobe. Lung X-ray findings may appear normal (radioclinical delay), and a scanner may be valuable. Age, coronary risk factors, and epigastric pain help rule out a myocardial infarction, most often inferior.

Abdominal pain in the upper region along with vomiting can be specific of metabolic emergencies, including acidoketosis in the diabetic patient, hyperkalemia and hypokalemia, and adrenal insufficiency. Rare causes of nonsurgical abdominal pain include acute porphyria, shingles, and others causes of neuropathic pain.

More frequently, abdominal pain develops in an infectious context associated with diarrhea-type digestive disorders, as in diarrheas of viral, bacterial,

Epidemiology of Acute Abdominal Pain in Adults

Table 6 Some pain features and related diagnosis orientations (adapted from Wind et al. 2007)

Features of pain	Diagnostic orientations
Pain aggravated by coughing, movement	Peritonis, appendicitis
Pain radiating to either shoulder	Hemoperitoneum
Pain radiating right shoulder	Hepatobiliary disease
Pain radiating to genital organs	Kidney disease: renal colic and pyelonephritis
Pain radiating to lumbar fossa	Urologic disease, retrocecal appendicitis, adnexal disease in women
Transfixiant pain radiating to the back	Pancreatic disease
Pain relieved by gas	Abdominal aortic aneurysm, colonic disease (irritable bowel syndrome)
Pain relieved by food	Gastric disease (gastritis, ulcer)
Pain with agitation	Renal colic, small bowel obstruction by strangulation, adnexal torsion
Pain with initial shock	Severe acute pancreatitis, mesenteric infarction, ruptured abdominal aortic aneurysm

or parasitic origin. In addition, there is the whole group of inflammatory bowel diseases, in which the onset or exacerbation of pain must systematically lead to investigation of abscess or perforation-type surgical complications.

5 Abdominal Pain Based on Pain Features

Synthesis of the clinical elements resulting from a thorough clinical interview and physical examination would increase the decision-making performance by up to 10%. Proper knowledge of a few pain features would allow better understanding and avoidance of pitfalls (Table 6).

A true *visceral pain* can be caused by distention of a viscus, ischemia, or inflammation limited to the viscus, and transmitted through the autonomic nervous system. When the patient can localize it, it is felt on the median line (epigastrium, umbilicus, or hypogastrium).

A *parietal pain* occurs when the parietal peritoneum is stimulated by an inflammation and is transmitted through the central nervous system. It is generally better localized by the patient, and mostly perceived over the organ involved. Nevertheless, subphrenic inflammation, such as an abscess or hemoperitoneum, by stimulating the diaphragm is frequently referred to the posterior shoulder area. Two successive pain patterns, with initial pain in the umbilicus or epigastrium followed by pain in the right iliac fossa, is typical of appendicitis (Table 6).

The rapidity of pain onset may guide the pathologic mechanisms:

- A *sharp pain* (within a few seconds), initially at its maximum, that forces the patient to stop any activity may reveal a perforation, embolism, or a rupture (tubar pregnancy, aneurysm, etc.).
- A *rapidly progressing pain* that reaches its maximum over a few hours may suggest an obstacle, ischemia, or torsion.
- A *progressing pain* that gradually develops over days and remains bearable may suggest an inflammatory focus, an obstruction, or a tumor.

Some pain modulating factors may help narrow the etiopathologic mechanism. Those situations mobilizing the visceral mass, such as walking, coughing, deep inhalation, and depression of the abdominal wall, may worsen the pain resulting from an intra-abdominal inflammatory focus. In such situations, rest will decrease the pain.

Similarly, evolution of the pain intensity over time may be very informative. Cramping pain is intermittent pain of variable duration, often bearable, essentially arising from inflammatory foci. Intense persistent pain is typical of ischemia or visceral distention.

Painful colic paroxysms reveal the contraction of the smooth muscles against an obstacle.

6 Population at Risk of Severity

Three populations of patients deserve particular attention because of the likelihood of misdiagnosis pertaining to their situation: the *elderly*, *women of childbearing age*, and the *immunocompromised*.

In the former two, modulations in both the immune system and abdominal muscles as well as peritoneum hyperreactivity may mask the peritoneal signs till late in the disease evolution.

Both acquired immunosuppression (as in HIV infection, hemodialysis patients with kidney failure, etc.) and induced immunosuppression (as in patients treated with corticoid or other immunosuppressive drugs, or in patients who have undergone transplants) are sources of frequent misdiagnoses.

A wide variety of opportunistic infections, including cytomegalovirus infection, cryptosporidiosis, *Mycobacterium avium-intracellulare*, and neoplasms with atypical presentation, including non-Hodgkin lymphoma, undifferentiated carcinoma, or Kaposi sarcoma, are likely to occur. Immunosuppressive states are often associated with nociceptive reflexivity disorders of the peritoneum. They are often of asthenic types, and clinical presentations can be subtle.

6.1 Abdominal Pain in the Seropositive Patient

Around 15% of seropositive patients present with severe abdominal pain that can be associated with reduced patient survival. Causes include HIV-independent pathologic conditions and opportunistic affections, with reported frequencies of 18 and 65%, respectively (Parente et al. 1994).

A cytomegalovirus colitis can be exacerbated by hemorrhage or perforation. A withdrawal syndrome may be investigated in a seropositive patient with drug addiction. A certain number of antiretroviral drug side effects, such as renal colic secondary to indinavir (Crixivan®) intake or acute pancreatitis secondary to didanosine (Videx®) intake, must be investigated (Hill and Balkin 2009).

7 Abdominal Pain Based on Severity Signs

Considering the poor specificity and sensitivity of the clinical signs, the physical examination should be done at least twice, within the course of emergency management, to improve the diagnostic performance. A first step allows stratification of patients on the

basis of their belonging to any population at risk [elderly (50 years or older), women of childbearing age, and immunocompromised patients (HIV)]. The presence of fever, coronaropathy risk factors, and history of chronic alcoholism must also be considered. Diabetes and obesity have been identified as risk factors. Other severity risk factors must be systematically investigated, including hypotension or the existence or onset of organ dysfunction highlighting a tissue distress: the type of pain, the onset of pain prior to vomiting, a continuous and persisting pain evolving over less than 48 h, the lack of history of similar pain, and a history of abdominal surgery. Considering the likelihood of misdiagnosis in these groups, a more rigorous approach must be undertaken, and the decision to hospitalize the patient must be made if there is the least doubt.

7.1 Two Disorders Must Be Primarily Considered Because of the Risk of Sudden Death

- *Hemoretroperitoneum and Hemoperitoneum*: AAA, ruptured ectopic pregnancy, splenic rupture, or other intra-abdominal vascular rupture. A hemoretroperitoneum seen in its early course is often not associated with hemodynamic instability, which corresponds to a progressive retroperitoneal fissuration of a posterior aneurysm.
- *Acute coronary syndrome with ST elevation, often of inferior localization*: intense epigastralgia-type pain.

7.2 Causes Associated with Risks of Severity

Pain is most often diffuse, with serious signs of general involvement in the first line (or associated). This diagnosis of overacute abdominal emergency is made by physical examination (hypotension, confusion, respiratory distress, anuria, hemorrhage, etc.) as well as laboratory findings (dehydration, anemia, metabolic acidosis, and renal failure). Depending on the context and abdomen evaluation, the etiologic diagnosis may sometimes be evident, leading to immediate surgery, or can be easily confirmed by ultrasonography or CT emergency evaluation. The main causes include a ruptured ectopic pregnancy, or another cause of hemoperitoneum, ruptured aneurysm, obstruction, and peritonitis, seen late or within a fragile background (elderly, immunocompromised patient), mesenteric ischemia or bowel necrosis, and acute necrotic hemorrhagic pancreatitis. Such diagnoses require immediate resuscitation procedures, and for most conditions, a surgical intervention with uncertain results depending on the patient's initial state, delays in decision-making, and the quality of the initial resuscitation.

8 General Management

Pain management must be in the first line of treatment, immediately after the initial clinical assessment. It is well recognized that the earlier the administration, the more efficient the analgesic treatment. Withholding administration of narcotic analgesia in patients with acute abdominal pain for fear of masking disease is not justified (McHale and LoVecchio 2001). Nevertheless, the release of pain with analgesia must not be an argument against the patient's hospitalization. The diagnosis of nonspecific or undetermined acute abdominal pain is most commonly made, with the diagnosis of irritable bowel syndrome being made in 37% of diagnoses in women and 19% in men (Heaton 2000). Although the patient's age, localization of pain, and the accompanying signs must guide the diagnosis orientation, these elements are informal. It is especially fundamental not to limit the diagnosis hypotheses, only relying on pain localization (Heaton 2000). Certain features are more frequently observed in severe or surgical conditions. The chance that pain is related to a surgical condition is greater when pain is violent, recent (less than 48 h), or constant, when it is localized, when it is the first sign, notably when it occurs before vomiting, when the patient's age is advanced, when there is a history of surgery, or when there are peritoneal signs at physical examination. Hospitalization is judged necessary in 18–42% of adults, reaching up to 75% in the elderly (Lyon and Clark 2006). Only a minority (about 15%) of patients presenting with abdominal pain require a surgical treatment (similar to the proportion in numerous conditions), with the diagnosis remaining undetermined in about 40% of patients. In such situations, complementary examinations, and most often imaging studies, are necessary to confirm the clinically suspected diagnosis.

In real conditions, the local organization may guide the choice between the preferred and consecutive examinations. If plain radiography is not very helpful, then ultrasonography and CT may play a major role. Hence, ultrasonography is the first examination for evaluating a suspected hepatobiliary or gynecologic disease. In women, full bladder pelvic examination is performed because of the high frequency of obstetric or gynecologic diseases. When necessary, pelvic studies are complemented by endovaginal examination.

Abdominal CT has a diagnosis sensitivity of 90%, as compared with that of the clinical evaluation (76%). It has a marked effect on abdominal pain management, modulating the initial treatment management in up to 27% of patients (Siewert et al. 1997; Stoker et al. 2009).

Laboratory testing is much less contributive, although it can aid in planning the patient's going back home.

Only 10% of patients would benefit from a short follow-up, and 80–90% can be discharged from hospital. A doubtful diagnosis justifies the need for an evolutive protocolized follow-up, eventually conducted in the emergency department, including monitoring by repeated clinical evaluation, laboratory testing, and imaging studies, as well as consultation with a specialist within 12–24 h. Lastly, a young patient with acute abdominal pain, presenting spontaneously, with no digestive history or with a history evoking a functional colopathy, who belongs to a low-risk population, with physical examination findings within normal limits, and whose pain has regressed spontaneously or after symptomatic treatment may not benefit from complementary investigations. The emergency physician will take good care of the patient's immediate and final outcome.

9 Conclusion

In acute abdominal pain, the clinical examination remains one of the key elements of the diagnostic approach. The symptoms often differ with age and background, may be atypical in their presentation, and the diagnosis may be uncertain. However, knowledge of the epidemiologic elements allows one to improve the diagnostic orientation and the evaluation of severity. The indication of the morphological investigations has to be discussed, and results have to be confronted with clinical findings.

The use of ultrasonography or CT must be highly considered, as it has substantially modified the diagnostic approach for acute abdominal pain urgent conditions. CT imaging allows us to adjust numerous diagnoses, and to more rapidly treat patients, thereby decreasing the morbidity related to delays in diagnosis and the cost of treatment.

References

Ahmed S, Shahid RK, Russo LA (2005) Unusual causes of abdominal pain: sickle cell anemia. Best Pract Res Clin Gastroenterol 19(2):297–310

Bass KN, Jones B, Bulkley GB (1997) Current management of small-bowel obstruction. Adv Surg 31:1–34

Bennett DH, Tambeur LJ, Campbell WB (1994) Use of coughing test to diagnose peritonitis. BMJ 308(6940):1336

Boomer L, Freeman J, Landrito E, Feliz A (2010) Perforation in adults with acute appendicitis linked to insurance status, not ethnicity. J Surg Res 163(2):221–224

Bouillot JL, Bresler L (2004) Abdomens aigus: prise en charge diagnostique. 106° Congrès de l'AFC, Arnette

Broder JS, Hollingsworth CL, Miller CM, Meyer JL, Paulson EK (2010) Prospective double-blinded study of abdominal-pelvic computed tomography guided by the region of tenderness: estimation of detection of acute pathology and radiation exposure reduction. Ann Emerg Med 56(2):126–134

Bugliosi TF, Meloy TD, Vukov LF (1990) Acute abdominal pain in the elderly. Ann Emerg Med 19(12):1383–1386

de Dombal FT (1979) Acute abdominal pain—an O.M.G.E. survey. Scand J Gastroenterol Suppl 56:29–43

de Dombal FT (1994) Acute abdominal pain in the elderly. J Clin Gastroenterol 19(4):331–335

Fleming C, Whitlock EP, Beil TL, Lederle FA (2005) Screening for abdominal aortic aneurysm: a best-evidence systematic review for the U.S. Preventive Services Task Force. Ann Intern Med 142(3):203–211

Gardner RL, Almeida R, Maselli JH, Auerbach A (2010) Does gender influence emergency department management and outcomes in geriatric abdominal pain? J Emerg Med 39(3):275

Gretarsdottir S, Baas AF, Thorleifsson G, Holm H, den Heijer M, de Vries JP, Kranendonk SE, Zeebregts CJ, van Sterkenburg SM, Geelkerken RH, van Rij AM, Williams MJ, Boll AP, Kostic JP, Jonasdottir A, Jonasdottir A, Walters GB, Masson G, Sulem P, Saemundsdottir J, Mouy M, Magnusson KP, Tromp G, Elmore JR, Sakalihasan N, Limet R, Defraigne JO, Ferrell RE, Ronkainen A, Ruigrok YM, Wijmenga C, Grobbee DE, Shah SH, Granger CB, Quyyumi AA, Vaccarino V, Patel RS, Zafari AM, Levey AI, Austin H, Girelli D, Pignatti PF, Olivieri O, Martinelli N, Malerba G, Trabetti E, Becker LC, Becker DM, Reilly MP, Rader DJ, Mueller T, Dieplinger B, Haltmayer M, Urbonavicius S, Lindblad B, Gottsater A, Gaetani E, Pola R, Wells P, Rodger M, Forgie M, Langlois N, Corral J, Vicente V, Fontcuberta J, Espana F, Grarup N, Jorgensen T, Witte DR, Hansen T, Pedersen O, Aben KK, de Graaf J, Holewijn S, Folkersen L, Franco-Cereceda A, Eriksson P, Collier DA, Stefansson H, Steinthorsdottir V, Rafnar T, Valdimarsson EM, Magnadottir HB, Sveinbjornsdottir S, Olafsson I, Magnusson MK, Palmason R, Haraldsdottir V, Andersen K, Onundarson PT, Thorgeirsson G, Kiemeney LA, Powell JT, Carey DJ, Kuivaniemi H, Lindholt JS, Jones GT, Kong A, Blankensteijn JD, Matthiasson SE, Thorsteinsdottir U, Stefansson K (2010) Genome-wide association study identifies a sequence variant within the DAB2IP gene conferring susceptibility to abdominal aortic aneurysm. Nat Genet 42(8):692–697

Hayanga AJ, Bass-Wilkins K, Bulkley GB (2005) Current management of small-bowel obstruction. Adv Surg 39:1–33

Heaton KW (2000) Diagnosis of acute non-specific abdominal pain. Lancet 355(9215):1644

Hill A, Balkin A (2009) Risk factors for gastrointestinal adverse events in HIV treated and untreated patients. AIDS Rev 11(1):30–38

Hilton D, Iman N, Burke GJ, Moore A, O'Mara G, Signorini D, Lyons D, Banerjee AK, Clinch D (2001) Absence of abdominal pain in older persons with endoscopic ulcers: a prospective study. Am J Gastroenterol 96(2):380–384

Howell JM, Eddy OL, Lukens TW, Thiessen ME, Weingart SD, Decker WW (2010) Clinical policy: critical issues in the evaluation and management of emergency department patients with suspected appendicitis. Ann Emerg Med 55(1):71–116

Huffman JL, Schenker S (2010) Acute acalculous cholecystitis: a review. Clin Gastroenterol Hepatol 8(1):15–22

Jordan GL Jr (1980) The acute abdomen. Adv Surg 14:259–315

Kent KC, Zwolak RM, Egorova NN, Riles TS, Manganaro A, Moskowitz AJ, Gelijns AC, Greco G (2010) Analysis of risk factors for abdominal aortic aneurysm in a cohort of more than 3 million individuals. J Vasc Surg 52(3):539–548

Laurell H, Hansson LE, Gunnarsson U (2006) Acute abdominal pain among elderly patients. Gerontology 52(6):339–344

Lyon C, Clark DC (2006) Diagnosis of acute abdominal pain in older patients. Am Fam Phys 74(9):1537–1544

Marco CA, Schoenfeld CN, Keyl PM, Menkes ED, Doehring MC (1998) Abdominal pain in geriatric emergency patients: variables associated with adverse outcomes. Acad Emerg Med 5(12):1163–1168

McCartan DP, Fleming FJ, Grace PA (2010) The management of right iliac fossa pain—is timing everything? Surgeon 8(4):211–217

McHale PM, LoVecchio F (2001) Narcotic analgesia in the acute abdomen–a review of prospective trials. Eur J Emerg Med 8(2):131–136

Nagurney JT, Brown DFM, Chang Y, Sane S, Wang AC, Weiner JB (2003) Use of diagnostic testing in the emergency department for patients presenting with non-traumatic abdominal pain. J Emerg Med 25(4):363

Parente F, Cernuschi M, Antinori S, Lazzarin A, Moroni M, Fasan M, Rizzardini G, Rovati V, Morandi E, Molteni P et al (1994) Severe abdominal pain in patients with AIDS: frequency, clinical aspects, causes, and outcome. Scand J Gastroenterol 29(6):511–515

Parker LJ, Vukov LF, Wollan PC (1997) Emergency department evaluation of geriatric patients with acute cholecystitis. Acad Emerg Med 4(1):51–55

Paulson EK, Kalady MF, Pappas TN (2003) Clinical practice. Suspected appendicitis appendicitis. N Engl J Med 348(3):236–242

Powell JT, Greenhalgh RM (2003) Clinical practice. Small abdominal aortic aneurysms. N Engl J Med 348(19):1895–1901

Raman SS, Osuagwu FC, Kadell B, Cryer H, Sayre J, Lu DS (2008) Effect of CT on false positive diagnosis of appendicitis and perforation. N Engl J Med 358(9):972–973

Rao PM, Rhea JT, Novelline RA, Mostafavi AA, McCabe CJ (1998) Effect of computed tomography of the appendix on treatment of patients and use of hospital resources. N Engl J Med 338(3):141–146

Ross SO, Forsmark CE (2001) Pancreatic and biliary disorders in the elderly. Gastroenterol Clin North Am 30(2):531–545

Sakalihasan N, Limet R, Defawe OD (2005) Abdominal aortic aneurysm. Lancet 365(9470):1577–1589

Samaras N, Chevalley T, Samaras D, Gold G (2010) Older patients in the emergency department: a review. Ann Emerg Med 56(3):261–269

Sheth AA, Longo W, Floch MH (2008) Diverticular disease and diverticulitis. Am J Gastroenterol 103(6):1550–1556

Siewert B, Raptopoulos V, Mueller MF, Rosen MP, Steer M (1997) Impact of CT on diagnosis and management of acute abdomen in patients initially treated without surgery. AJR Am J Roentgenol 168(1):173–178

Stoker J, van Randen A, Lameris W, Boermeester MA (2009) Imaging patients with acute abdominal pain. Radiology 253(1):31–46

Stollman N, Raskin JB (2004) Diverticular disease of the colon. Lancet 363(9409):631–639

Trowbridge RL, Rutkowski NK, Shojania KG (2003) Does this patient have acute cholecystitis? JAMA 289(1):80–86

Vissers RJ, Abu-Laban RB, McHugh DF (1999) Amylase and lipase in the emergency department evaluation of acute pancreatitis. J Emerg Med 17(6):1027–1037

Wagner JM, McKinney WP, Carpenter JL (1996) Does this patient have appendicitis? JAMA 276(19):1589–1594

Wind P, Malamut G, Cuénod C-A, Bénichou J (2007) Stratégie des explorations des douleurs abdominales. Médecine d'Urgence, 25–050-A20 edn. Elsevier Masson, Paris

Epidemiology of Abdominal Trauma

Françoise Guillon

Contents

1 Introduction 15

2 Epidemiology 16
2.1 General Traumatology 16
2.2 Abdominal Traumas 17

3 Specificities by Organs 23
3.1 Spleen 23
3.2 Liver 24
3.3 Gastrointestinal Tract 25
3.4 Pancreas 25

4 Conclusion 26

References 26

Abstract

Traumas are a major health care concern owing to their frequency and potential seriousness because they occur in relatively young subjects. Mortality rates of abdominal traumas are estimated to range between 10 and 30%. Hemorrhagic shock is considered to be a therapeutic emergency when it occurs following abdominal traumas. Over the past 30 years, computed tomodensitometry has become the reference examination for the initial management and the follow-up of patients with abdominal traumas. At the same time, the surgical indications have decreased in favor of an "armed surveillance", including a combination of reanimation procedures, surgical interventions, and interventional radiology procedures.

1 Introduction

Traumas are a major health care concern owing to their frequency and potential seriousness because they occur in relatively young subjects. Mortality rates of abdominal traumas are estimated to range between 10 and 30%. Hemorrhagic shock is considered to be a therapeutic emergency when it occurs following abdominal traumas. Over the past 30 years, computed tomodensitometry (CT) has become the reference examination for the initial management and the follow-up of patients with abdominal traumas. At the same time, the surgical indications have decreased in favor of an "armed surveillance", including a combination of reanimation procedures, surgical interventions, and interventional radiology procedures.

F. Guillon (✉)
Service de Chirurgie Digestive A,
Hôpital ST ELOI,
80 avenue Augustin fliche,
34295 Montpellier Cedex 5, France
e-mail: f-guillon@chu-montpellier.fr

P. Taourel (ed.), *CT of the Acute Abdomen*, Medical Radiology. Diagnostic Imaging,
DOI: 10.1007/174_2010_137, © Springer-Verlag Berlin Heidelberg 2011

2 Epidemiology

2.1 General Traumatology

Traumas are the third most frequent cause of death in the general population, after cardiovascular disease and cancer. In the subgroup of adult patients under 40 years of age, traumas are the main cause of death (Tentillier and Masson 2000).

In the USA, the number of trauma victims is estimated at 57 million each year, resulting in two million hospitalizations and 150,000 deaths (Elliott and Rodriguez 1996).

In an industrialized country such as France, the incidence of traumas related to daily life accidents is 7.5 for 100 inhabitants, and the incidence of traumas due to public road accidents is 0.3 for 100 inhabitants (Tentillier and Masson 2000). Although the mortality due to public road accidents has been decreasing over the past few years, in France, more than 40,000 subjects were hospitalized for severe traumas in 2006, with 4,709 accident-related deaths (Traffic Accident Statistics 2006) (Table 1).

In public road accidents, the car is the main cause of death (Table 2); however, among subjects under 20 years of age, two-wheeled vehicles are the main cause of death.

Rates of chronic alcohol abuse are estimated at 50–60% among trauma victims (Jenkins 2000). Acute alcoholic intoxication is responsible for 10% of all accidents, and, notably, for 50% of all accident-related deaths. Studies conducted in North America have revealed that 40% of injured patients test positive for one or more illegal drugs (Soderstrom et al. 1988; Sloan et al. 1989; Jurkovich et al. 1992). A population case–control study was conducted in France from October 2001 to September 2003 on 10,748 car drivers involved in a fatal car accident, with known blood alcohol and drug levels. This study revealed that driving after using cannabis significantly increased the risk of a driver being involved in a car accident in a dose-dependent manner (odds ratio 3.32; 95% confidence interval 2.63–4.18), although in France the fraction of car accidents attributable to cannabis use is significantly lower than that due to positive blood alcohol levels (2.5% vs. 28.6%) (Laumon et al. 2005).

The economic burden of trauma is significant: it is estimated that trauma mortality is responsible for 26% of lost years of life (first cause), and for more than half of the number of lost productive life years (Tentillier and Masson 2000). In the USA, acute health care costs due to trauma were evaluated at 16 billion dollars in 1992, and the costs stemming from follow-up care, disabilities, and tax deficits were estimated at 150 billion dollars (Elliott and Rodriguez 1996).

Following a traffic accident or a fall, it is estimated that abdominal trauma is seen in 7–20% of hospitalized patients (Cayten 1984). In Quebec, Bergeron et al. (2007) found a 16% rate of thoracic or abdominal trauma in a population of 16,430 patients hospitalized for blunt trauma [Abbreviated Injury Score (AIS) 2 or greater].

In traumatology, a trimodal distribution of death is noted: 50% of deaths are estimated to occur at the scene of the accident, mainly due to severe vessel lesions and cerebral injuries. Approximately 30% of deaths take place within the first 24 h, secondary to hemorrhagic shock or severe cranial trauma. Finally, 20% of deaths occur in the following days or weeks, due to infections or multiple organ failure (MOF) (Trunkey 1991; ATLS 1994).

Although hemorrhagic shock constitutes the major therapeutic challenge in the management of the patient during the first hours following an abdominal trauma, mortality may vary owing to a variety of factors:

- The cause of the abdominal lesion, with a mortality rate estimated to range from 10 to 30% for abdominal contusions, from 5 to 15% for injuries caused by firearms, and from 1 to 2% for cold-weapon injuries (Cayten 1984).
- The type of organ involved, the severity of the lesion, and the number of intra-abdominal organs affected, with mortality rates estimated at 6% for isolated liver traumas, 15% for three-organ involvement, and 50 and 70% for four- and five-organ involvement, respectively (Carretier et al. 1991).
- The coexistence of extra-abdominal lesions. The most commonly accepted definition of a polytraumatized patient is that of a severely injured patient presenting with two or more traumatic lesions, with at least one being life-threatening. This concept of polytraumatism is an independent prognostic factor of mortality.
- The patient's age and medical history.

Epidemiology of Abdominal Trauma

Table 1 Evolution of morbidity/mortality in public road accidents (Traffic Accident Statistics, France)

	2000	2002	2004	2006
Physical injury	121,223	105,470	85,390	80,309
Slightly injured (not hospitalized)	134,710	113,748	91,292	61,463
Seriously injured (hospitalized on day 6)	27,407	24,091	17,435	40,662
Dead on day 30	8,079	7,741	5,593	4,709

Table 2 Distribution of transportation means involved in road accident mortality in 2006 (Traffic Accident Statistics)

	Frequency of involvement (%)
Car	55.8
Pedestrians	11.4
Motorcycle	16.3
Moped	6.7
Bicycle	3.8
Heavy truck	1.8
Others (commercial vehicle, public transport, tractor, etc.)	4.2

Table 3 Causes of preventable deaths (from Kreis et al. 1986)

Preventable causes of death	Number (percentage)
Decision for surgery not taken	25 (48)
Time lapse before surgery too long	21 (40)
Resuscitation error	5 (10)
Undiagnosed lesion	4 (8)

The total exceeds 100% as several causes may coexist in the same patient.

surgical intervention or delay in the surgical decision-making process (Kreis et al. 1986) (Table 3).

- The rapidity and the quality of the patient's diagnostic and therapeutic management. Several studies have investigated the causes of death in the field of traumatology, with a subgroup analysis of evitable deaths. Shackford et al. (1993) performed a chronological analysis of 623 cases of trauma-induced death to determine whether death could have been avoided by an optimal environment. This evaluation was based on the severity of lesions, the moment of death, the principal cause of death, and factors contributing to death. The evaluation was carried out according to the chronology of events: accident prevention, discovery of the injured person, pre-hospital management, occurrence of secondary lesions, and medical and paramedical errors. From the study results, it appears that three quarters of all deaths could have been prevented, which, in North America, would have resulted in a gain of 20,817 life years and 9,255 productivity years. Although, in most cases, trauma prevention would have saved the patient's life, 151 deaths were accounted for by a management error during the hospital phase.

In a study involving 246 polytraumatized patients who eventually died, the major cause of avoidable death during the hospital phase was the lack of

2.2 Abdominal Traumas

Abdominal traumas are defined as traumas involving the area between the diaphragm above and the pelvis below. They are classified into two types: blunt traumas or abdominal contusions, and penetrating traumas or abdominal wounds.

2.2.1 Blunt Traumas

In Europe, blunt abdominal traumas have always been more common, representing approximately 80% of all abdominal traumas. In three quarters of the cases, a traffic road accident is responsible for the trauma, and the abdominal trauma involves a polytraumatized patient (Lorgeron et al. 1983; Orliaguet and Cohen 1991). Falls represent the second most common cause of abdominal contusions (Cayten 1984). They are mainly due to suicide attempts with defenestration (two thirds of cases), work-related accidents, and sport accidents. Other causes associated with crushing (work accidents, fights) are less common.

In the USA, although penetrating traumas due to firearms or cold weapons were the main cause of hepatic lesions during the period between 1945 and 1975, blunt traumas are presently the principal etiological causes of liver and spleen lesions (Richardson 2005).

2.2.2 Penetrating Traumas

Penetrating traumas or abdominal wounds represent 20% of abdominal traumas, with a cold weapon as an injuring agent in two thirds of cases. Firearms of different calibers are used in the other cases.

2.2.3 Lesionel Mechanisms and Organ Lesions

Blunt Traumas

Following abdominal contusions, the intra-abdominal lesions depend on both the physical features of the initial mechanism and the organ affected, such as its anatomical relations, solid or hollow feature, fixed or mobile status, and whether it is in a state of repletion. Different mechanisms may be individualized when considering blunt traumas, but they are mostly associated in the case of traffic road accidents or falls:

- Direct shock responsible for compression crushing of the organs between the external force and the posterior plane. The standard example is the crushing of the pancreatic isthmus against vertebral body L1 by the steering wheel.
- A brutal increase in intra-abdominal pressure may lead to organ rupture away from the site of impact. This is the predominant mechanism involved in the traumatic rupture of the diaphragm.
- A sudden horizontal deceleration (brutal collision of a vehicle moving at great speed) or vertical deceleration (fall from a high place) causes stretching of the fixing structures of organs such as the vascular pedicles, bracketing areas, and ligaments. This mechanism may cause lesions of the organ itself at the insertion areas, but may also damage the vascular pedicles, leading to hemorrhages or ischemia. The rupture of sushepatic veins following a sagittal fracture of the hepatic dome is a standard example of this mechanism (Fingerhut and Trunkey 2000).
- Tangent forces on the abdominal wall may result in a separation of superficial layers, with vascular involvement. In the case of concomitantly increased intra-abdominal pressure, the muscular aponeurotic wall may split, without any cutaneous lesions (Balkan et al. 1999).

Following blunt abdominal traumas, the lesions involve mainly solid organs, particularly the spleen and the liver, and may cause a hemoperitoneum (McAnena et al. 1990) (Table 4).

Table 4 Incidence of organ lesions in the case of abdominal contusions (from McAnena et al. 1990)

Organs	Incidence (%)
Spleen	46
Liver	33
Mesentery	10
Kidney–bladder	9
Small intestine	8
Colon	7
Duodenum–pancreas	5
Vessels	4
Stomach	2
Gallbladder	2

Table 5 Incidence of organ lesions in the case of open abdominal traumas (from Nicholas et al. 2003)

Organs	Percentage of patients with organ lesions
Small intestine	48
Colon	36.4
Liver	34.4
Spleen	9.2
Stomach	17.6
Kidney	14
Bladder	6.4
Rectum	5.2
Duodenum–pancreas	7.2
Vessels	30
Diaphragm	22.8

Penetrating Traumas

The penetrating feature of an abdominal wound is based on a break in the parietal peritoneal wall. Should this occur, the injuring agent may cause damage to any intra-abdominal organ. Cold weapons are responsible for direct lesions of the organs involved, whereas firearms cause damage not only to the trajectory of the projectile but also at a distance, depending on the caliber and type of projectile used. Thus, a distinction is made between small-caliber arms with slow kinetics (.22 Long Rifle; 6.35 mm) and high-caliber arms with rapid kinetics (9–11.43 mm, military weapons). The importance of the attrition chamber depends on both the characteristic features of the projectile (speed, mass, and instability) and those of the tissues shot through (Pailler et al. 1990). Identifying the entrance and exit orifices allows the physician to reconstitute the projectile's trajectory, enabling him or her to target the organs that are potentially involved, whether intra-abdominal or in other parts of the body (thoracic, retroperitoneal, or pelvic).

Penetrating abdominal traumas cause major damage to hollow organs. A US study conducted between 1997 and 2001 on 250 patients injured by either firearms (two thirds) or cold weapons (one third) found a lesion of the small intestine in half of the patients. This is the organ most commonly involved, followed by the colon (Nicholas et al. 2003) (Table 5).

Lesion Classification

The following different mechanisms may cause various organ lesions: intraparenchymal hematomas or subcapsular hematomas, fractures, channel lesions, vessel lesions, or parietal lesions. For each organ, there are descriptive lesion schemes classifying lesions according to their degree of severity. The most common classification system in international publications is that of the American Association for the Surgery of Trauma (AAST) (Moore et al. 1990).

In 2008, an analysis based on US trauma registry data involving 54,148 registered patients with a lesion code for spleen, liver, and kidney, of which 35,897 patients presented with an isolated solid organ lesion, validated the correlation between lesion severity established using the AAST classification and the patient outcomes. In the case of an isolated solid organ lesion, the evaluation parameters (mortality, duration of hospital stay, length of intensive care unit stay, specific intervention rate, and hospital costs) significantly increased with the lesion grade (Tinkoff et al. 2008).

2.2.4 Management of Abdominal Traumas

Physiopathology

For abdominal traumas, hemorrhagic shock and MOF are the principal causes of mortality. Hemorrhagic shock refers to acute tissue hypoperfusion caused by a decrease in circulating blood volume, resulting in an imbalance between oxygen supply and cellular oxygen needs (Duranteau 1995). Prolonged hypoperfusion is associated with anaerobic cellular metabolism, causing lactic acid production. The degree and particularly the persistence of the negative oxygen balance are major risk factors for acute respiratory distress syndrome and MOF (Rixen and Siegel 2000). Clinical and biological signs, reflecting decompensated shock, may be observed: hypothermia, acidosis, and coagulation disorders. These three elements work together and reinforce each other, rapidly leading to a vicious cycle, which may be fatal for the patient ("bloody vicious cycle") (Moore et al. 1998) (Fig. 1).

Hypothermia, defined by a temperature below 35°C, may be accounted for by hemorrhagic shock or by multiple other causes occurring in a polytraumatized patient (meteorological conditions at the accident site, freeing of the victim, vascular filling, laparotomy, etc.). Hypothermia has proven to be an independent risk factor of morbidity and mortality (Gentilello et al. 1997). Acidosis is defined by a pH below 7.36. The degree of acidosis and the clearance of lactates have also been shown to be independent prognostic factors of morbidity and mortality (Burch et al. 1997). Hypothermia and acidosis, along with hemodilution and coagulation factor consumption caused by the hemorrhage, reinforce each other, resulting in the development of acute posttraumatic coagulopathy (Eddy et al. 2000).

In this context, from a therapeutic viewpoint, the first-line emergency treatment consists of performing surgical hemostasis, in association with the correction of metabolic disorders, hypothermia, and coagulopathy. Abbreviated laparotomy is a necessary response to these physiological and clinical observations.

MOF may be described as an autodestructive process during which circulating factors have a deleterious impact on organs that were not affected by the initial aggression. It is associated with the progressive development of multiple organ deficiencies, resulting in the patient's death in 30–70% of cases (Carlet 1993). The factor time is of paramount importance in the initial patient management, so as to prevent the development of snowballing events comprising inflammatory responses associated with decompensated hemorrhagic shock. The second line of treatment consists of establishing an early diagnosis and initiating therapy for secondary complications such as infections, which may be a second risk factor for MOF (Fig. 2).

Evolution of Management

Over the past 30 years, the therapeutic strategies for blunt abdominal traumas have progressed toward a

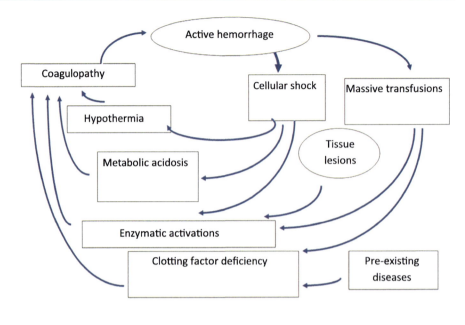

Fig. 1 The bloody vicious cycle

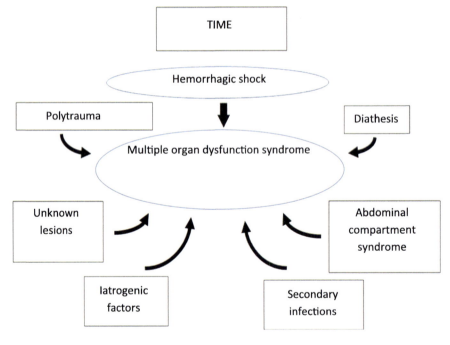

Fig. 2 Origin of the multiple organ dysfunction syndrome (MOF)

decrease in surgical indications, based on both the diagnostic reliability of the CT scan and the therapeutic possibilities of interventional radiology. Currently, 70–80% of splenic traumas and 80–90% of hepatic traumas are treated nonsurgically. Our better understanding of the pathophysiological changes of hemorrhagic shock has allowed us to further develop reanimation, surgical, and interventional radiology procedures, as illustrated by the standard concept of abbreviated laparotomy in the case of hepatic trauma.

Potential lesion progression requires frequent and complete evaluations of the injured patient's status, particularly at the early stages, with continuous adaptations of diagnostic and therapeutic measures. Repeated imaging is an essential part of patient management.

Severity Evaluation and Prognostic Index

The evaluation of lesion severity is a necessary step in all the treatment phases in order to optimize therapeutic and diagnostic orientations and choices. This evaluation must be initiated during the prehospital phase. The Vittel criteria, which pertain to the severity of the lesion, are an objective and simple tool for grading trauma patients. They are based on the analysis of the elements surrounding the accident and take into account information relating to physiological parameters, lesion, reanimation, and patient history. The presence of a single criterion is sufficient to characterize the severity of the trauma, except for the terrain, which must be evaluated on a case-by-case basis. Among the criteria, some are considered serious because they are associated with very high mortality: systolic arterial pressure below 65 mmHg (mortality 65%), Glasgow Coma Scale score of 3 (mortality 62%), and O_2 saturation below 80% or not measurable (mortality 76%) (Riou et al. 2002) (Table 6).

Besides this classification index, there are prognostic indices that allow us to statistically predict the likelihood of survival, risks of sequelae, and the length of hospital stay. The most commonly used index is the Injury Severity Score (ISS), which takes into account the anatomical region, the organ involved, the severity of the lesion, as well as the lesion's penetrating feature (or not), but does not consider the terrain or physiological parameters. This score is based on the description of the lesions by means of the AIS (Baker et al. 1974), which provides for each organ an estimation of the lesion severity using a six-point scale as follows: 1 for minor lesion; 2 for moderate lesion; 3 for severe, non-life-threatening lesion; 4 for severe, life-threatening lesion; 5 for critical lesion with uncertain survival; 6 for non-viable lesion. The ISS takes into account the seriousness of all lesions in a polytraumatized patient. An ISS greater than 16 usually defines a set of serious traumatic lesions; if the ISS is above 25, the patient's vital prognosis is involved; with an ISS ranging from 40 to 75, the patient's survival is uncertain. Likewise, the physiological impact of the trauma may also be a source of seriousness. The Revised Trauma Score (RTS) is a simple means that allows this impact to be evaluated at the accident site or upon admission to the hospital (Moreau et al. 1985; Champion et al. 1989). This evaluation takes into account the most negative

Table 6 Vittel criteria

Five assessment steps	Severity criteria
1. Psychological variables	Glasgow Coma Scale score below 13
	Systolic blood pressure below 90 mmHg, O_2 saturation below 90%
2. Kinetic variables	Occupant ejection
	Other passenger dead in the same vehicle
	Fall more than 6 m
	Victim thrown out of the vehicle or crushed
	Overall assessment (vehicle deformity, estimated speed, absence of helmet, absence of safety belt)
	Blast
3. Anatomical lesions	Penetrating trauma of the head, neck, thorax, abdomen, pelvis, arm, or thigh
	Flail chest
	Severe burn, smoke inhalation
	Pelvic fracture
	Suspicion of medullary injury
	Amputation at the level of the wrist, ankle, or above
	Acute limb ischemia
4. Prehospital resuscitation	Assisted ventilation
	Vascular filling with more than 1,000 mL of colloids
	Catecholamines
	Inflated medical antishock trousers
5. Diathesis (to be assessed)	Age more than 65 years
	Cardiac or coronary insufficiency
	Respiratory insufficiency
	Pregnancy (2nd and 3rd trimesters)
	Blood crasis disorders

values of the Glasgow Coma Scale, systolic arterial pressure, and respiratory frequency (appendices). An RTS of less than 10 requires that the patient be admitted to an intensive care unit, without giving any indications on the length of hospitalization. The combination of ISS, RTS, and the patient's age (more or less than 55 years) is used to compute the probability of survival and the quality of the patient's management by a medical facility (TRISS method). Finally, the standard resuscitation scores (IGS II and

Simplified Acute Physiology Score: SAPS II) (Bach and Frey 1971) are also widely used for trauma patients admitted for resuscitation. A trauma patient with an IGS II score greater than 30 is considered to present a significant vital risk.

The Principles of Initial Management

Any injured patient with abdominal trauma must be considered, a priori, as being a polytraumatized patient and should thus benefit from systematic and full treatment. Priority must be given to accurate diagnosis and treatment of immediately life threatening lesions. The goal of resuscitation is to restore and maintain optimal tissue oxygenation and perfusion by means of an adapted ventilation and volemic expansion, while preventing hypothermia. The next diagnostic and therapeutic measures depend on the resuscitation-induced hemodynamic responses.

If hemodynamic instability persists, the diagnosis of active intracavitary hemorrhage must be considered. At this stage, focused assessment with sonography for trauma (FAST) ultrasonography in the shock resuscitation unit may guide the diagnosis toward intrathoracic, intraperitoneal, or pelvic hemorrhages. In this case, a strict collaboration between surgeons, resuscitation physicians, and radiologists is necessary to direct the patient to the operation room or to the interventional radiology unit without any further delay, in order for the required hemostatic gestures (surgical measures and/or arterial embolization) to be performed immediately.

In this setting of decompensated hemorrhagic shock, abbreviated laparotomy may be a particularly adapted surgical response. Its primary goal is to achieve rapid control of all hemorrhagic sources in order to interrupt the vicious cycle of hemorrhages. Surgical hemostatic interventions include vascular ligatures, total splenectomy, and "packings".

Controlling bacterial contamination is based on simple closure of openings in the digestive tract using clips or ligatures. At this stage, there is no indication to reestablish digestive continuity or to create stomas.

Parietal closure is restricted to simple skin closure or laparostomy, and the injured patient is left in the care of the resuscitation team for the control of physiological functions and the correction of metabolic disorders. It is at this stage that an arterial embolization may be performed, relatively early on, in order to complete the surgical intervention.

A secondary laparotomy is performed 36 h later, with the goal of performing reconstruction interventions, proceeding to the ablation of packing, completing surgical exploration, and carrying out the full parietal closure.

Abdominal compartment syndrome is a complication that must be checked in the case of an abbreviated laparotomy with packing. Should this complication occur, resumption of intraperitoneal or retroperitoneal hemorrhages must be considered. This syndrome is characterized by a significant increase in intra-abdominal pressure, resulting in a decrease of both cardiac output and thoracic compliance, along with an alteration of renal function. The diagnosis of this syndrome is based on the evolution of intravesical pressure measurements, which allows physicians to direct the patient to emergency surgical decompression via a laparotomy, as deemed necessary.

If the injured patient has a hemodynamic status that is stable or has been stabilized by resuscitation measures, complete and precise lesion screening must be performed, which is based on an abdominal CT scan, the reference examination which has become indispensable in managing polytraumatized patients. Its diagnostic accuracy has led to the development of various nonsurgical strategies for solid organ lesions.

The entire set of aforementioned data is instrumental in establishing decision algorithms (Figs. 3, 4). For blunt abdominal traumas, the strategy is systematized, whereas it is still being debated for penetrating abdominal traumas.

For open abdominal traumas, however, there is consensus on a certain number of rules. Immediate laparotomy is necessary in the case of noncontrolled hemorrhagic shock, flow of digestive fluid, or apparent peritoneal signs. Immediate laparotomy is also routinely performed in the case of a firearm wound affecting the anterolateral abdominal wall. Under these conditions, visceral lesions are present in 80% of cases (Cayten 1984). For cold-weapon wounds, the standard strategy included a laparotomy for every diagnosis of peritoneal rupture. Because it was later shown that 30% of these procedures turned out to be unnecessary, a more pragmatic attitude was taken, consisting of a repeated examination for hemorrhage or peritonitis signs before deciding on a surgical intervention. For some authors, performing a laparoscopy would represent an alternative to simple clinical surveillance. For all penetrating traumas, a CT

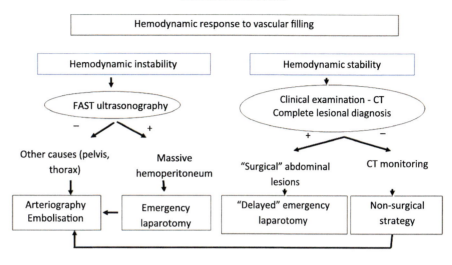

Fig. 3 Therapeutic strategy in the case of trauma

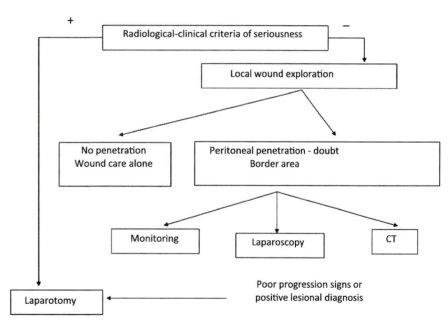

Fig. 4 Therapeutic strategy in the case of penetrating abdominal trauma

scan may be useful in the decision-making process when physicians are confronted with wounds involving borderline regions (thorax, retroperitoneum).

3 Specificities by Organs

3.1 Spleen

The spleen is the most commonly injured organ in blunt abdominal traumas. The current trend toward nonoperative management of splenic traumas is largely accounted for by the identification of immune functions that are specific to the spleen and the risk of fulminant infections following splenectomy. Only hemodynamic instability requires laparotomy, with total splenectomy carried out in most cases. On the basis of data in the American National Trauma Data Bank, the analysis of 23,532 cases of splenic contusions which occurred in 565 trauma centers over 5 years (1999–2004) revealed a 90% rate of initial nonoperative management, associated with an 80% success rate

Table 7 Efficacy of spleen embolization in abdominal traumas

Series	Number of patients	Preservation of spleen (%)	Morbidity (%)	Mortality (%)
Ekeh et al. (2005)	15	100	27	0
Haan et al. (2004)	143	87	16	0
Gaarder et al. (2006)	27	88	7	0
Bessoud et al. (2007)	37	97	3	0
Brugère et al. (2008)	22	91	27	0
Total	244	93	16	0

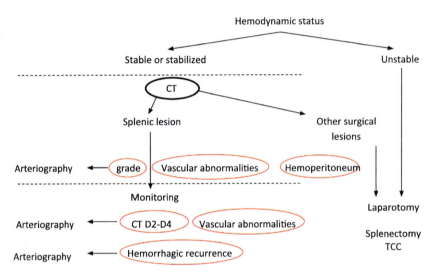

Fig. 5 Place of arteriography in the management of splenic traumas

(Smith et al. 2008). Identified factors of therapeutic success in the case of surgical abstention included hemodynamic stability, ISS below 15, Glasgow Coma Scale score above 12, lower than grade IV splenic lesion, and minor hemoperitoneum (perisplenic).

Splenic artery embolization is an additional therapeutic option among nonoperative strategies, which would result in an increased splenic preservation rate. Its therapeutic value is recognized in the clinical practice guidelines of the Eastern Association for the Surgery of Trauma (EAST; Eastern Association for the Surgery of Trauma 2003) and has been demonstrated in several published series (Table 7).

Morbidity arises from major complications and/or complications specific to embolization (persistent splenic hemorrhage, splenic infarction, abscess, and renal insufficiency).

However, the utilization level of splenic artery embolization in the decision-making algorithm for splenic traumas remains to be seen (Moore et al. 2008). One level corresponds to the prevention of secondary splenic hemorrhage. In this case, arteriography with embolization should be performed when the initial CT scan or systematic imaging examination during the first week following the trauma reveals grade III or higher lesions or vascular abnormalities. The other level corresponds to the treatment of subacute or chronic hemorrhages in a patient who is stable or has been stabilized during initial management or the monitoring period. Figure 5 summarizes the potential value of arteriography with embolization in the management of splenic traumas.

3.2 Liver

Liver traumas mainly occur in the case of blunt abdominal traumas and represent the primary cause of death in these injuries. Poor prognosis of blunt liver traumas is predominantly attributable to the hemorrhagic nature of liver lesions, and to a lesser extent to their anatomical severity. Mortality rates have considerably decreased, from 25% in the 1970s, to a current rate 10–15%, with only 20–25% of cases being directly related to liver lesions (Malhotra et al. 2000; Richardson et al. 2000). Currently, nonoperative management of liver traumas is chosen as first-line therapy in more than 80% of cases, including initial accurate CT assessment and hepatic artery embolization for hemorrhagic lesion management.

This initial surgical abstention should not delay a secondary indication for laparotomy or laparoscopy if, during repeated monitoring, there is any suspicion of intra-abdominal surgical lesions, such as a hollow organ rupture. Surgical techniques for the treatment of active hemorrhagic liver lesions are currently conservative: safety procedures such as liver packing and abbreviated laparotomy are preferred over standard hepatic surgery procedures, such as vascular clamping and hepatic resection. Nonoperative management requires effective and early cooperation between the surgeon, the resuscitation physician, and the interventional radiologist (Létoublon and Arvieux 2003).

3.3 Gastrointestinal Tract

The incidence of gastrointestinal tract lesions is predominant in penetrating abdominal traumas. A study involving 85,643 injured subjects with abdominal contusion revealed a 2.9% incidence rate of small intestine lesions and a 0.7% incidence rate of lesions with perforation. This low rate contrasts with a 29% morbidity rate and a 15% mortality rate. Even in the case of an isolated small intestine wound, the mortality remains high, with an estimated 6% death rate. The major prognostic factor is the time delay until surgical intervention, with a rate multiplied by a factor of 4 if this period exceeds 24 h (Fakhry et al. 2003). The incidence rate of colic lesions caused by blunt trauma is only 0.3%, although this condition is associated with a 36% morbidity rate and 19% mortality rate. The presence of a colic lesion is an independent risk factor for longer hospital stay and higher morbidity (Williams et al. 2003). The incidence of digestive tract lesions is particularly significant in the case of penetrating abdominal traumas.

The detection at clinical examination of a seat belt mark on the abdominal wall is associated with a 2.4 times higher risk of small intestine wound and, more generally, with a 8 times higher risk of intra-abdominal lesions.

Early diagnosis and treatment of the intestinal lesions are thus essential prognostic factors. Initial clinical examination is difficult and unreliable as abdominal wall traumas are often associated with other traumas in a polytrauma context. Likewise, a CT scan is not always conclusive. In the EAST study, no pneumoperitoneum was visualized on the initial CT scan in 75% of the small intestine rupture cases, with CT scan findings considered "normal" in 13% of patients (Fakhry et al. 2003). Thus, CT examination must be repeated within the 12–24 h following the initial trauma.

Surgical management of small intestine wounds is straightforward and generally based on sutures and immediate resection–anastomoses. Surgical treatment of colic wounds is more controversial owing to the risk of sepsis and postoperative fistulae. A meta-analysis performed in 2003 based on five controlled randomized studies was in favor of immediate reconstructive surgery in the case of penetrating colon traumas (Nelson and Singer 2003). However, a strategy of avoiding immediately reestablishing digestive continuity must be considered under the following conditions: significant stercoral contamination, a more than 24 h delay prior to the surgical intervention, and prolonged hemorrhagic shock, as well as the presence of several abdominal lesions.

3.4 Pancreas

In the case of abdominal traumas, pancreatic lesions are rare, but their diagnosis is far from easy. Clinical examination is difficult owing to the organ's retroperitoneal location. The diagnosis of pancreatic lesions should be considered in the case of abdominal traumas caused by bicycle handlebars or compression of the driver of a motor vehicle against the steering wheel. An increase in lipase levels upon repeated measurements presents a diagnostic value after the third hour following the accident (Takishima et al. 1997). The diagnosis of pancreatic lesions is essentially based on CT scan results; however, there is a 40% rate of false-negative test results if the scan is performed within the first 12 h after the accident.

The two main specific risk factors of pancreatic traumas are pancreatic duct lesions and delayed diagnosis of these lesions (more than 24 h) (Bach and Frey

1971; Heitsch et al. 1976; Bradley et al. 1998). Their diagnosis is currently based on retrograde cholangio-pancreatography. The value of pancreatography using nuclear magnetic resonance for pancreatic duct screening still needs to be defined (Nirula et al. 1999; Fulcher et al. 2000). The management of these lesions depends on the integrity of the Wirsung channel, the degree of parenchymal involvement, and the exact location of the lesion. Should the diagnosis of channel rupture be confirmed, the preferred strategy consists of surgical intervention, such as simple external drainage or distal pancreatic resection.

4   Conclusion

The management of abdominal traumas represents a triple challenge:

- A therapeutic challenge due to the immediate seriousness of hemorrhages, which may be highly reversible among young adults, who are the most exposed to this risk, from an epidemiological point of view
- An organizational challenge, as this requires the implementation of a patient care chain, starting at the accident site and involving different health care teams and facilities
- A human challenge, as the care chain is unable to function without any effective, early, and continuing cooperation between the different actors

References

ATLS (1994) Cours avancé de réanimation des poly-traumatisés. In: Manuel de l'étudiant. Comité de Trauma-tologie, American College of Surgeons

Bach RD, Frey CF (1971) Diagnosis and treatment of pancreatic trauma. Am J Surg 121:20–29

Baker SP, O'Neill B, Haddon W Jr, Long WB (1974) The injury severity score: a method for describing patients with multiple injuries and evaluating emergency care. J Trauma 14:187–196

Balkan M, Kosk O, Guleç B et al (1999) Traumatic lumbar hernia due to seat belt injury: case report. J Trauma 47:154–155

Bergeron E, Lavoie A, Belcaid A et al (2007) Surgical management of blunt thoracic and abdominal injuries in Quebec: a limited volume. J Trauma 62:1421–1426

Bessoud B, Duchosal MA, Siegrist CA, Schlegel S, Doenz F, Calmes JM et al (2007) Proximal splenic artery embolization

for blunt splenic injury: clinical, immunologic, and ultra-sound-Doppler follow-up. J Trauma 62:1481–1486

Bradley EL, Young PR, Chang MC et al (1998) Diagnosis and initial management of blunt trauma pancreatic: guidelines from a multiinstitutional review. Ann Surg 227:861–869

Brugère C, Arvieux C, Dubuisson V, Guillon F, Sengel C, Bricault I et al (2008) L'embolisation précoce dans le traitement non opératoire des traumatismesspléniques fer-més : étude rétrospective multicentrique. J Chir (Paris) 145:126–132

Burch JM, Denton JR, Noble RD (1997) Physiologic rationale for abbreviated laparotomy. Surg Clin North Am 77:779–782

Carlet J (1993) Physiopathologie du syndrome de défaillance multiviscérale. In: Anesthésie et réanimation; conférences d'actualisation. Masson, Paris

Carretier M, Rouffineau J, Houssin D (1991) Traumatismes du foie. In: Pathologie chirurgicale, vol II. Chirurgie digestive et thoracique. Masson, Paris, pp 419–429

Cayten CG (1984) Abdominal trauma. Emerg Med Clin North Am 2:799–821

Champion HR, Sacco WJ, Copes WS, Gann DS, Gennarelli TA, Flanagan ME (1989) A revision of the Trauma Score. J Trauma 29:623–629

Duranteau J (1995) Choc hémorragique. In: Anesthésie réan-imation chirurgicale. Flammarion, Paris

Eastern Association for the Surgery of Trauma (2003) Practice management guidelines for the non operative management of blunt injury of the liver and spleen

Eddy VA, Morris JA, Cullinane DC (2000) Hypothermia, coagulopathy and acidosis. Surg Clin North Am 80:845–853

Ekeh AP, McCarthy MC, Woods RJ, Haley E (2005) Complications arising from splenic embolization after blunt splenic trauma. Am J Surg 189:335–339

Elliott DC, Rodriguez A (1996) Cost effectiveness in trauma care. Surg Clin North Am 76:47–62

Fakhry SM et al (2003) Blunt small bowel injury: analysis from 275 557 trauma admissions. J Trauma 54:295–306

Fingerhut A, Trunkey D (2000) Surgical management of liver injuries in adults. Current indications and pitfalls of operative and non-operative policies: a review. Eur J Surg 166:676–686

Fulcher AS, Turner MA, Yelon JA et al (2000) Magnetic resonance cholangiopancreatography (MRCP) in the assess-ment of pancreatic duct trauma and its sequelae: preliminary findings. J Trauma 48(6):1001–1007

Gaarder C, Dormagen JB, Eken T, Skaga NO, Klow NE, Pillgram-Larsen J et al (2006) Nonoperative management of splenic injuries: improved results with angioembolization. J Trauma 61:192–198

Gentilello LM, Jurkowitch GJ, Stark MS et al (1997) Is hypothermia in the victim of major trauma protective or harmful? A randomized, prospective study? Ann Surg 226:439–449

Haan JM, Biffl W, Knudson MM, Davis KA, Oka T, Majercik S et al (2004) Splenic embolization revisited: a multicenter review. J Trauma 56:542–547

Heitsch RC, Knutson CO, Fulton RL et al (1976) Delineation of critical factors in the treatment of pancreatic trauma. Surgery 80:523–529

Jenkins DH (2000) Substance abuse and withdrawal in the intensive care unit. Contemporary issues. Surg Clin North Am 80:1033–1053

Jurkovich GJ, Rivara FP, Gurney JG et al (1992) Effects of alcohol intoxication on the initial assessment of trauma patients. Ann Emerg Med 21:704–708

Kreis DJ, Plasencia G, Augenstein D et al (1986) Preventable trauma deaths: Dade County, Florida. J Trauma 26:649–654

Létoublon C, Arvieux C (2003). Traumatismes fermés du foie. Principes de technique et de tactique chirurgicales. Encycl Méd Chir (Elsevier), Techniques chirurgicales - Appareil digestif, 40–785

Lorgeron P, Parmentier G, Katz A et al (1983) L'abdomen du polytraumatisé: étude comparative portant sur 225 polytraumatisés avec et sans lésions abdominales. Incidence des complications abdominales. J Chir 120:85–93

Malhotra AK, Fabian TC, Croce MA, Gavin TJ, Kudsk KA, Minard G et al (2000) Blunt hepatic injury: a paradigm shift from operative to nonoperative management in the 1990s. Ann Surg 231:804–813

McAnena OJ, Moore EE, Marx JA (1990) Initial evaluation of the patient with blunt abdominal trauma. Abdominal trauma. Surg Clin North Am 70:495–515

Moore EE, Cogbill TH, Malangoni MA et al (1990) Organ injury scaling. Surg Clin North Am 75:293–300

Moore EE, Burch J, Franciose R et al (1998) Staged physiologic restoration and damage control surgery. World J Surg 22:1184–1191

Moore FA, Davis JW, Moore EE et al (2008) Western Trauma Association (WTA) critical decisions in trauma: management of blunt splenic trauma. J Trauma 65:1007–1011

Moreau M, Gainer PS, Champion H, Sacco WJ (1985) Application of the trauma score in the prehospital setting. Ann Emerg Med 14:1049–1054

Nelson R, Singer M (2003) Primary repair for penetrating colon injuries. Cochrane Database Syst Rev 3:CD002247

Nicholas JM, Rix EP, Easley KA et al (2003) Changing patterns in the management of penetrating abdominal trauma: the more things change, the more they stay the same. J Trauma 55:1095–1110

Nirula R, Velmahos GC, Demetriades D (1999) Magnetic resonance cholangiopancreatography in pancreatic trauma: a new diagnostic modality? J Trauma 47:585–587

Orliaguet G, Cohen S (1991) Traumatismes abdominaux. In: Carli P, Riou B (eds) Urgences médico chirurgicales de l'adulte. Arnette, Paris, pp 495–503

Pailler JL, Brissiaud JC, Jancovici R, Vicq P (1990) Contusions et plaies de l'abdomen. Encycl Méd Chir (Paris), estomac intestin, 9007 A

Richardson JD (2005) Changes in the management of injuries to the liver and spleen. J Am Coll Surg 200:5

Richardson DJ, Franklin GA, Lukan JK, Carrillo EH, Spain DA, Miller FB et al (2000) Evolution in the management of hepatic trauma: a 25-year perspective. Ann Surg 232:324–330

Riou B, Thicoïpé M, Atain-Kouadio P et al (2002) Comment évaluer la gravité? In: SAMU de France (ed) Actualités en réanimation préhospitalière: le traumatisé grave. SFEM, Paris, pp 115–128

Rixen D, Siegel JH (2000) Metabolic correlates of oxygen debit predict posttrauma early acute respiratory distress syndrome and the delayed cytokine response. J Trauma 49:392–403

Shackford SR, Mackersie RC, Holbrook TL et al (1993) The epidemiology of traumatic death. A population-based analysis. Arch Surg 128:571–575

Sloan EP, Zalenski RJ, Smith RF et al (1989) Toxicology screening in urban trauma patients: drug prevalence and its relationship to trauma severity and management. J Trauma 29:1647–1653

Smith J, Armen S, Cook CH, Martin LC (2008) Blunt splenic injury: have we watched long enough? J Trauma 64:656–665

Soderstrom CA, Trifillis AL, Shankar BS, Clark WE, Cowley RA (1988) Marijuana and alcohol use among 1023 trauma patients. A prospective study. Arch Surg 123:733–737

Statistiques de l'accidentalité routière ONISR (2006)

Takishima T, Sugimoto K, Hirata M et al (1997) Serum amylase level on admission in the diagnosis of blunt injury to the pancreas: its significance and limitations. Ann Surg 226:70–76

Tentillier E, Masson F (2000) In: Beydon L, Carli P, Riou B (eds) Epidemiologie des traumatismes, traumatismes graves. Arnette, Paris, pp 1–15

Tinkoff G, Esposito TJ, Reed J et al (2008) American Association for the Surgery of Trauma Organ Injury Scale I: spleen, liver and kidney, validation based on the National Trauma Data Bank. J Am Coll Surg 207(5)

Trunkey DD (1991) Initial treatment of patients with extensive trauma. New Engl J Med 324:1259–1263

Williams MD, Watts D, Fakhry S (2003) Colon injury after blunt abdominal trauma: results of the EAST multi-institutional Hollow Viscus Injury Study. J Trauma 55:906–912

Laumon B, Gadegbeku B, Martin JL, Biecheler MB, SAM Group (2005) Cannabis intoxication and fatal road crashes in France: population based case-control study. BMJ 331(7529):1371

Part II

Elementary CT Findings

Key CT Findings

Eric Delabrousse

Contents

1	**Introduction**	32
2	**Accordion Sign**	33
2.1	Features	33
2.2	Significance	33
2.3	Causes	33
3	**Beak Sign**	33
3.1	Features	33
3.2	Significance	33
3.3	Diagnosis	34
4	**Bowel Halo Sign**	34
4.1	Features	34
4.2	Significance	34
4.3	Causes	35
5	**Coffee Bean Sign**	35
5.1	Features	35
5.2	Significance	35
5.3	Cause	36
6	**Collar Sign**	36
6.1	Features	36
6.2	Significance	36
6.3	Cause	36
7	**Comb Sign**	36
7.1	Features	36
7.2	Significance	37
7.3	Causes	37
8	**Contrast Material Extravasation**	37
8.1	Features	37
8.2	Significance	37
8.3	Causes	37

9	**Dependent Viscera Sign**	38
9.1	Features	38
9.2	Significance	38
9.3	Cause	38
10	**Disproportionate Fat Stranding Sign**	38
10.1	Features	38
10.2	Significance	38
10.3	Causes	39
11	**Draped Aorta Sign**	39
11.1	Features	39
11.2	Significance	39
11.3	Cause	40
12	**Fat Halo Sign**	40
12.1	Features	40
12.2	Significance	40
12.3	Causes	41
13	**Fat Notch Sign**	41
13.1	Features	41
13.2	Significance	41
13.3	Diagnosis	41
14	**Flat Vena Cava Sign**	42
14.1	Features	42
14.2	Significance	42
14.3	Causes	42
15	**Hemoperitoneum**	42
15.1	Features	42
15.2	Significance	42
15.3	Causes	43
16	**Hemoretroperitoneum**	43
16.1	Features	43
16.2	Significance	43
16.3	Causes	43
17	**High-Attenuating Crescent Sign**	44
17.1	Features	44
17.2	Significance	44
17.3	Cause	44
18	**Misty Mesentery**	44
18.1	Features	44

E. Delabrousse (✉)
Service de Imagerie Digestive et Génito-urinaire,
CHU Besançon, Hôpital Jean Minjoz,
3, Boulevard Fleming, 25030 Besançon, France
e-mail: edelabrousse@chu-besancon.fr

P. Taourel (ed.), *CT of the Acute Abdomen,* Medical Radiology. Diagnostic Imaging,
DOI: 10.1007/174_2010_92, © Springer-Verlag Berlin Heidelberg 2011

18.2	Significance	44
18.3	Causes	44
19	**Mosaic Pattern**	45
19.1	Features	45
19.2	Significance	45
19.3	Causes	46
20	**Northern Exposure Sign**	46
20.1	Features	46
20.2	Significance	46
20.3	Cause	46
21	**Periportal Collar Sign**	47
21.1	Features	47
21.2	Significance	47
21.3	Causes	47
22	**Pneumatosis Intestinalis**	48
22.1	Features	48
22.2	Significance	48
22.3	Causes	48
23	**Pneumobilia**	48
23.1	Features	48
23.2	Significance	48
23.3	Causes	49
24	**Pneumoperitoneum**	49
24.1	Features	49
24.2	Significance	49
24.3	Causes	50
25	**Pneumoretroperitoneum**	50
25.1	Features	50
25.2	Significance	50
25.3	Causes	50
26	**Portomesenteric Venous Gas**	51
26.1	Features	51
26.2	Significance	51
26.3	Causes	51
27	**Round Belly Sign**	51
27.1	Features	51
27.2	Significance	52
27.3	Cause	52
28	**Sentinel Clot Sign**	52
28.1	Features	52
28.2	Significance	52
28.3	Cause	53
29	**Small Bowel Feces Sign**	53
29.1	Features	53
29.2	Significance	53
29.3	Cause	53
30	**Spoke Wheel Sign**	54
30.1	Features	54
30.2	Significance	54
30.3	Cause	54

31	**String of Pearls Sign**	54
31.1	Features	54
31.2	Significance	54
31.3	Cause	55
32	**Tissue Rim Sign**	55
32.1	Features	55
32.2	Significance	55
32.3	Cause	55
33	**Whirl Sign**	56
33.1	Features	56
33.2	Significance	56
33.3	Causes	56
References		56

Abstract

The CT semiology of acute abdomen is extremely rich and is based on the analysis of the organs of the abdominal cavity. Defined criteria, such as the morphological aspect of organs, spontaneous attenuation of the tissues, enhancement of parenchyma after intravenous contrast material injection, and location of the organs within the abdominal cavity, are the basis of this analysis. It is also very important to look for some key CT findings which correspond to acute modifications of the normal feature and are often specific. Thus, a meticulous analysis of the CT scans and good knowledge of these key CT findings may allow accurate CT diagnosis in acute abdomen.

1 Introduction

The CT semiology of acute abdomen is extremely rich and is based on the analysis of the organs of the abdominal cavity. Defined criteria, such as the morphological aspect of organs, spontaneous attenuation of the tissues, enhancement of parenchyma after intravenous contrast material injection, and location of the organs within the abdominal cavity, are the basis of this analysis. It is also very important to look for some key CT findings which correspond to acute modifications of the normal feature and are often specific. Thus, a meticulous analysis of the CT scans and good knowledge of these key CT findings may allow accurate CT diagnosis in acute abdomen.

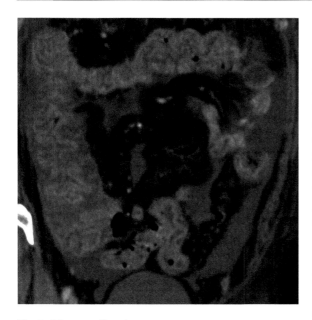

Fig. 1 The accordion sign

2 Accordion Sign

2.1 Features

The accordion sign is a finding that may be seen on CT scans in patients who have received oral contrast material. It was originally defined as alternating edematous haustral folds separated by transverse mucosal ridges filled with oral contrast material simulating the appearance of an accordion (Fishman et al. 1991; O'Sullivan 1998) (Fig. 1).

2.2 Significance

The lower soft-tissue attenuation component of the accordion sign represents marked thickening of the haustral folds due to transmural edema. Small amounts of oral contrast material may become trapped within the crevices between these thickened haustral folds. The bands of alternating lower and higher attenuation have been likened to the appearance of an accordion (Fishman et al. 1991). This appearance may be variable depending on the degree of edema of the haustral folds and the amount of contrast material trapped between the folds (O'Sullivan 1998).

2.3 Causes

2.3.1 Pseudomembranous Colitis

The accordion sign was described first as a finding indicative of pseudomembranous colitis (Fishman et al. 1991). In this case, the high-attenuating oral contrast material is trapped between thickened edematous folds and pseudomembranes in the colonic mucosa. The degree of colonic wall thickening caused by the pseudomembranes and edematous tissues that develop in this condition has been suggested as the reason for the sign's specificity (Ros et al. 1996).

2.3.2 Other Colitides

For some authors, the accordion sign is indicative of severe colonic edema or inflammation, but has no cause-related specificity. It may be related to infectious, inflammatory, or ischemic conditions, and it may even be present in patients with edema secondary to cirrhosis (Macari et al. 1999). Although they were not specifically identified as the accordion sign, massive colonic wall thickening and a similar colonic mucosal pattern have been documented in many CT reports of colitis from other causes (Balthazar et al. 1985; Macari et al. 1999). When the accordion sign is identified in CT studies, it should be viewed as a sign indicative of severe colonic edema of uncertain cause. Correlation with the clinical and laboratory results should be performed to determine the exact cause.

3 Beak Sign

3.1 Features

The beak sign may be seen as a fusiform tapering of the bowel at the site of the obstruction (Fig. 2).

3.2 Significance

At the transition zone of a mechanical small bowel obstruction, a beak sign corresponds to extrinsic compression of the bowel loop.

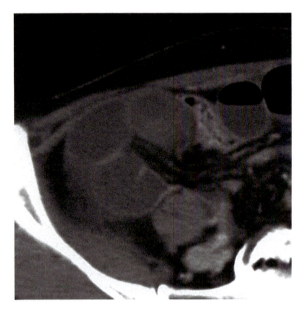

Fig. 2 The beak sign

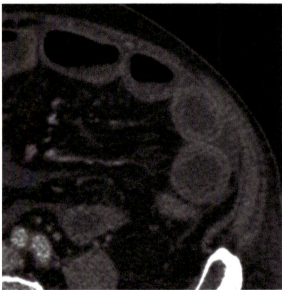

Fig. 3 The bowel halo sign

3.3 Diagnosis

3.3.1 Adhesive Small Bowel Obstruction

Adhesions themselves cannot be identified by CT. Recognition of a beak sign at the transition zone of small bowel obstruction is highly suggestive of adhesions as the cause for the occlusion (Ha et al. 1993).

3.3.2 Small Bowel Volvulus

In small bowel obstruction, a double beak sign associated with a whirl sign is a CT finding of small bowel volvulus (Balthazar et al. 1992).

3.3.3 Cecal Volvulus

A beak sign and a whirl sign are demonstrated on CT scans in cecal volvulus (Delabrousse et al. 2007).

3.3.4 Sigmoid Volvulus

A beak sign and a double beak sign may be seen in organoaxial sigmoid volvulus and mesentericoaxial sigmoid volvulus, respectively (Bernard et al. 2010).

3.3.5 Closed Loop Obstruction Due to Hernia

The double beak sign is also present in closed loop obstruction secondary to external and internal hernia (Yen et al. 2005).

4 Bowel Halo Sign

4.1 Features

The bowel halo sign is defined by stratification within a thickened bowel wall that consists of either two rings (double halo)—an inner gray attenuation ring surrounded by an outer higher-attenuation ring—or three rings (target sign)—an inner and an outer ring of high attenuation, and a middle ring of lower attenuation (gray attenuation) (Wittenberg et al. 2002). The bowel halo sign is best visualized during the portal venous phase of intravenous contrast material enhancement (Macari and Balthazar 2001) (Fig. 3).

4.2 Significance

A double halo is composed of a higher-attenuation outer annular ring, corresponding to the muscularis propria, surrounding a second ring of gray attenuation (0–10 HU), which is believed to be edema. In the target sign, the inner and outer rings of high attenuation are regarded as the bowel mucosa and the muscularis propria, respectively, whereas the middle ring of gray attenuation represents edema and can be assumed to be located in the submucosa (Macari and

Balthazar 2001). The higher attenuation of the inner and outer rings is assumed to be the consequence of preferential enhancement corresponding to hyperemia.

4.3 Causes

4.3.1 Crohn Disease
The double halo sign was first reported by Frager et al. (1983) in patients with Crohn disease.

4.3.2 Bowel Ischemia
The bowel halo sign (double halo or target sign) may also be present in bowel ischemia (Taourel et al. 1996).

4.3.3 Ulcerative Colitis
The bowel halo sign was initially described with ulcerative colitis (Gore et al. 1996).

4.3.4 Infectious Enterocolitis
The target sign is also a well-known CT feature in infectious enterocolitis, particularly in pseudomembranous colitis (Kawamoto et al. 1999).

4.3.5 Lupus Erythematosus
CT of the abdomen in patients with lupus erythematosus who have abdominal vasculitis shows ascites and thickening of the bowel walls, with a double halo or a target sign (Ko et al. 1997; Horton et al. 2000).

4.3.6 Intestinal Hematoma
Initially, CT should be performed without contrast material, as this may mask the presence of intramural hemorrhage. The findings consist of a thickening of the wall greater than 1 cm, with partial reduction to total obstruction of the passage, and hyperdensity, ranging from 50 to 80 HU depending on the time elapsed between the onset of the event and the examination. The target sign is better demonstrated on contrast-enhanced CT scans (Sorbello et al. 2007).

4.3.7 Portal Hypertension
The bowel halo sign has also been reported as a CT feature of cirrhosis and portal hypertension (Ormsby et al. 2007).

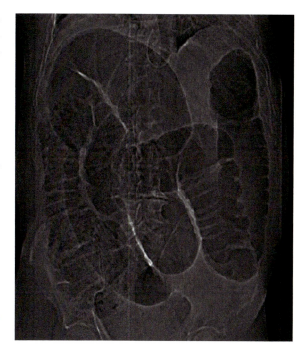

Fig. 4 The coffee bean sign

5 Coffee Bean Sign

5.1 Features

The coffee bean sign is a finding that may be diagnosed on CT scout views. It was originally defined on supine abdominal radiographs as an area of hyperlucency that resembles the shape of a coffee bean (Messmer 1994) (Fig. 4).

5.2 Significance

As the closed loop of the sigmoid colon distends with gas, apposition of the medial walls of the dilated bowel forms the cleft of the coffee bean, whereas the lateral walls of the dilated bowel form the outer walls of the bean (Feldman 2000). Since the volvulus is located at the sigmoid colon, the coffee bean arises from the pelvis and may occupy the entire abdomen. Its apex often extends above the T10 vertebral level and can lie to the left or right of the midline (Young et al. 1978; Burrel et al. 1994). Other terms for this sign include the kidney bean sign and the bent inner tube sign (Kerry et al. 1971; Ballantyne 1982).

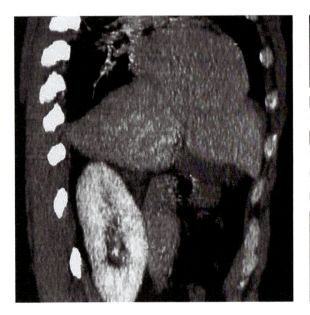

Fig. 5 The collar sign

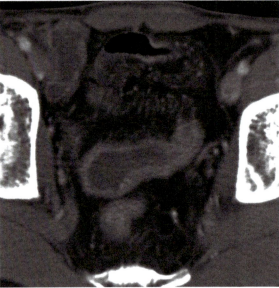

Fig. 6 The comb sign

5.3 Cause

5.3.1 Sigmoid Volvulus

Initially described as an indication of a closed loop in small bowel obstruction (Riger 1944; Mellins and Riger 1954), the coffee bean sign commonly applies to the appearance of a closed loop obstruction of the sigmoid colon (Feldman 2000). Up to 80% of the time, sigmoid volvulus can be diagnosed by viewing the CT scout view alone (id. to the supine abdominal radiograph) (Jones and Fazio 1989). The absence of rectal gas may also contribute to the diagnosis (Messmer 1994).

6 Collar Sign

6.1 Features

The collar sign is defined as a waistlike low-attenuation rim of the diaphragm around the herniated organ (Iochum et al. 2002). On the right side, it can appear as a focal indentation of the liver, a subtle sign easily overlooked on axial images. The collar sign is better seen on sagittal and coronal multi-planar reformatted images (Larici et al. 2002) (Fig. 5).

6.2 Significance

The collar sign corresponds to constriction of the herniated hollow viscus at the site of the diaphragmatic tear.

6.3 Cause

6.3.1 Diaphragmatic Rupture

The collar sign is a valuable CT sign for the diagnosis of blunt diaphragmatic rupture. The collar sign has been reported to have 63% sensitivity and 100% specificity as a sign of diaphragmatic rupture with helical CT (Killen et al. 1999). Other studies have reported a lower incidence of 27–36% for this feature (Demos et al. 1989; Murray et al. 1996).

7 Comb Sign

7.1 Features

The comb sign is defined on contrast-enhanced CT scans as multiple tubular, tortuous opacities on the mesenteric side of the ileum that are aligned as the teeth of a comb (Madureira 2004) (Fig. 6).

7.2 Significance

The arteries that supply the small bowel branch off within the mesentery as a series of intestinal arteries interconnected by arcades. The terminal branches (or vasa recta) are tall and widely spaced in the jejunum and are short and more closely arranged in the ileum (Stallard et al. 1994). When CT depicts hypervascularity of the mesentery with vascular dilatation, tortuosity, and wide spacing of the vasa recta, the comb sign is produced. This is attributed to the increased flow and fibrofatty proliferation in the mesentery of the affected bowel (Meyers and McGuire 1995).

7.3 Causes

7.3.1 Crohn Disease

Hypervascularity of the mesentery with vascular dilatation, tortuosity, and prominence of the vasa recta, which together produce the comb sign, should suggest Crohn disease first (Madureira 2004). It has been reported that the presence of prominent perienteric vasculature seen on CT in patients with Crohn disease suggests that the disease is clinically active, advanced, and extensive (Lee et al. 2002). Moreover, in patients presenting with clinical symptoms for the first time, the comb sign should raise the possibility of the diagnosis of Crohn disease.

7.3.2 Other Small Bowel Diseases

The comb sign is not absolutely pathognomonic for Crohn disease as it has also been reported in cases of lupus mesenteric vasculitis (Ko et al. 1997; Byun et al. 1999), polyarteritis nodosa, Henoch–Schönlein syndrome, microscopic polyangiitis, Behçet syndrome, mesenteric thromboembolism, and strangulated small bowel obstruction (Rha et al. 2000; Jeong et al. 1997; Ha et al. 1998; Kim et al. 2001; Balthazar et al. 1992). The clinical history, distribution of the disease, and associated findings are useful in the differential diagnosis of these diseases.

8 Contrast Material Extravasation

8.1 Features

Contrast material extravasation is defined by the presence of an area of focal or diffuse high-attenuation

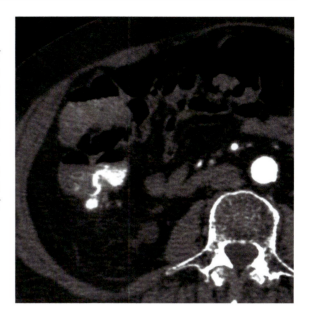

Fig. 7 Contrast material extravasation

isodense structures compared with major adjacent arterial structures that is surrounded by high-attenuation fluid representing hematoma. It may be seen in an organ (Fig. 7) or in the intraperitoneal and retroperitoneal spaces.

8.2 Significance

Contrast material extravasation corresponds to active arterial bleeding (more than 1 mL/min).

8.3 Causes

8.3.1 Blunt Trauma

Contrast-enhanced helical CT has been reported to be the gold standard imaging modality to visualize arterial extravasation after blunt abdominal trauma (Yao et al. 2002).

8.3.2 Gastrointestinal Bleeding

Contrast material extravasation is an accurate CT finding for detection and localization of bleeding sites in patients with acute massive gastrointestinal bleeding (Yoon et al. 2006) (Fig. 7).

8.3.3 Spontaneous Spleen Rupture

Extravasation of contrast material from the spleen has also been reported in the case of spontaneous splenic rupture (Aoyagi et al. 2009).

8.3.4 Intra-abdominal Hemorrhagic Tumors

In intra-abdominal tumors, the presence of contrast material extravasation on CT scans allows the accurate diagnosis and has a direct impact on clinical decision making (Furlan et al. 2009).

9 Dependent Viscera Sign

9.1 Features

The dependent viscera sign is diagnosed on CT scans in the thoracoabdominal area. The viscera (i.e., bowel or solid organ) are positioned against the posterior ribs, with obliteration of the posterior costophrenic recess (Cantwell 2006) (Fig. 8).

9.2 Significance

When blunt diaphragmatic rupture occurs, the absence of posterior support by the diaphragm allows viscera to fall against the posterior ribs to a dependent position. On the right side, the upper third of the liver typically does not abut the posterior chest wall when the diaphragm is intact. On the left side, the stomach and bowel lie anterior to the spleen and generally do not abut the posterior left ribs when the diaphragm is intact. Therefore, the dependent viscera sign is said to be present on the right side if the upper third of the liver abuts the posterior ribs and to be present on the left side if the stomach or bowel abuts the posterior ribs or lies posterior to the spleen (Bergin et al. 2001).

9.3 Cause

9.3.1 Diaphragmatic Rupture

The dependent viscera sign is a valuable CT sign that dramatically increases the CT diagnosis of blunt diaphragmatic rupture. In a study published in 2001, Bergin et al. (2001) reported this CT sign to be present in 90% of patients with blunt diaphragmatic rupture. In their series, the dependent viscera sign was up to 100% sensitive as a sign of diaphragmatic rupture and 83% sensitive for right-sided injury

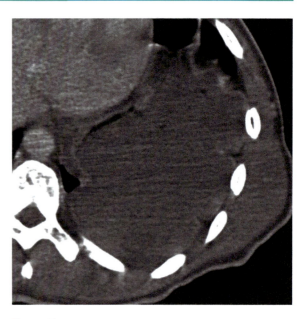

Fig. 8 The dependent viscera sign

(Bergin et al. 2001). The dependent viscera sign is not, however, a reliable indicator of diaphragmatic injury in penetrating trauma, owing to the small size and variable position of the defect (Larici et al. 2002).

10 Disproportionate Fat Stranding Sign

10.1 Features

The disproportionate fat stranding sign is defined on CT scans by stranding that is more severe than expected for the degree of bowel wall thickening present (Pereira et al. 2004) (Fig. 9).

10.2 Significance

Most acute inflammatory diseases of the gastrointestinal tract, including infectious, inflammatory, traumatic, and ischemic disorders, are centered in the bowel wall. For these diseases, the degree of bowel wall thickening typically exceeds the degree of associated fat stranding. However, in a few acute diseases of the gastrointestinal tract, the pathologic process is characteristically centered in the mesentery adjacent to the bowel wall rather than in the bowel wall itself. In these diseases, a positive disproportionate fat stranding sign is diagnosed (Pereira et al. 2004).

10.3 Causes

10.3.1 Acute Diverticulitis

Diverticulitis occurs when the neck of a diverticulum becomes occluded, resulting in inflammation, erosion, and microperforation. Microperforation results in pericolonic inflammation that is typically more severe than the inflammation of the colon itself. On CT, the most common finding in acute diverticitis is paracolic fat stranding. This fat stranding is characteristically disproportionate to the relatively mild, focal colonic wall thickening.

10.3.2 Acute Appendicitis

Direct visualization of a dilated fluid-filled appendix is the most specific CT finding of appendicitis (Rao et al. 1997; Benjaminov et al. 2002). However, other indirect CT signs are often useful. In acute appendicitis, periappendicular fat stranding remains typically mild to moderate, but it may be severe. The finding of severe fat stranding in the right lower quadrant, even in the absence of substantial appendicular, cecal, or ileal thickening, has been reported to be useful in the diagnosis of appendicitis (Checkoff et al. 2002).

10.3.3 Epiploic Appendagitis

Epiploic appendages are normally invisible on CT scans. CT findings of epiploic appendagitis are usually diagnostic (Torres et al. 1994; Rao et al. 1997). A paracolonic oval fatty mass representing the inflamed or infarcted appendage, surrounded by a well-circumscribed hyperattenuated rim and a very important paracolonic fat stranding, is a pathognomonic feature. These paracolonic inflammatory changes are typically disproportionately more severe than the mild local reactive thickening of the adjacent colonic wall.

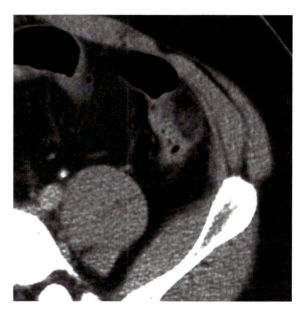

Fig. 9 Disproportionate fat stranding

10.3.4 Segmental Omental Infarction

On CT scans, segmental omental infarction, which is secondary to thrombosis of omental veins, appears as a large high-attenuation fatty mass centered in the omentum (Puylaert 1992; Van Bresla Vriesman et al. 1999). Reactive bowel wall thickening may occur, but the inflammatory process in the omentum is disproportionately more severe.

11 Draped Aorta Sign

11.1 Features

The draped aorta sign is a CT finding that corresponds to close application to the spine and lateral draping of the aneurysm around the vertebral body (Halliday and Al-Kutoubi 1996) (Fig. 10).

11.2 Significance

It is believed that the path of least resistance for extravasated blood from a leaking abdominal aneurysm is into the psoas muscle and, after a subsequent breach of the psoas fascia, into the posterior pararenal space (Hopper et al. 1985). Most cases of leak,

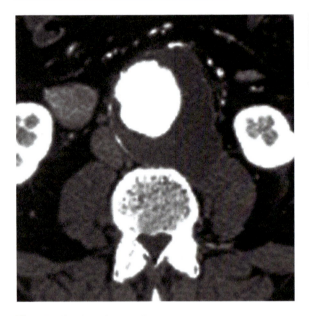

Fig. 10 The draped aorta sign

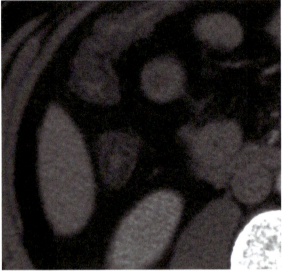

Fig. 11 The fat halo sign

therefore, show some posterior periaortic hemorrhage (Gale et al. 1986) and, in cases of massive hemorrhage, the posterior pararenal, and perirenal compartments are the most frequently involved sites (Morehouse et al. 1992; White et al. 1992; Siegel and Cohan 1994). The draped aorta sign on CT scans represents an early stage in this sequence where hemorrhage is contained anteriorly by the confluence of the anterior renal fascia and the root of the dorsal mesentery and is starting to pass posteriorly toward the psoas muscle (Halliday and Al-Kutoubi 1996).

11.3 Cause

11.3.1 Contained Leak of Aortic Aneurysm

Although a large leak may be easily identified by CT, a smaller, contained leak may be difficult to diagnose with confidence (Gale et al. 1986). It is important that such cases are identified since clinical features may be misleading, and although the condition of a patient with a contained leak may remain stable for months or even years (Rosenthal et al. 1986; Nakagawa et al. 1990), massive hemorrhage may occur at any time. On CT images, the draped aorta sign is highly indicative of deficiency of the aortic wall and a contained leak (Halliday and Al-Kutoubi 1996).

12 Fat Halo Sign

12.1 Features

The fat halo sign is a CT finding that is defined by the presence of a thickened bowel wall demonstrating three layers: an inner and an outer layer of soft-tissue attenuation, between which lies a third layer of fatty attenuation (-10 to -50 HU) (Wittenberg et al. 2002; Ahualli 2007) (Fig. 11).

12.2 Significance

The inner layer of soft-tissue attenuation represents the bowel mucosa, whereas the layer of negative attenuation results from widening and fatty infiltration of the submucosa. The outer soft-tissue attenuation layer represents the muscularis propria and serosa (Philpotts et al. 1994; Gore et al. 1996). The fat halo sign may be depicted on CT scans obtained without intravenous contrast material because of the marked differences in tissue attenuation. However, the different layers of attenuation can also be appreciated during the portal venous phase of contrast enhancement (Macari and Balthazar 2001).

12.3 Causes

12.3.1 Ulcerative Colitis
The fat halo sign has been described as typically appearing in patients with inflammatory bowel disease (Jones et al. 1986; Gore et al. 1996). In ulcerative colitis, this sign occurs only in the large bowel. The fat halo sign is present in 60% of patients with ulcerative colitis (Philpotts et al. 1994).

12.3.2 Crohn Disease
When the fat halo sign is seen in both the small and the large bowel, it is considered evidence of Crohn disease. However, the fat halo sign is seen in less than 10% of patients with Crohn disease (Philpotts et al. 1994).

12.3.3 Graft-Versus-Host Disease
Graft-versus-host disease has been reported as an acute condition that may cause the fat halo sign (Muldowney et al. 1995).

12.3.4 Chronic Radiation Enteritis
The presence of fat within the submucosal layer of the small bowel is a finding which may be demonstrated in patients who have had radiation therapy (Chen et al. 2003).

12.3.5 Chronic Enteritis After Cytoreductive Therapy
The fat halo sign has also been reported as a consequence of cytoreductive therapy (Muldowney et al. 1995).

12.3.6 Normal Variant
Intramural fat may exist in both the distal ileum and the colon as a normal variant in patients without symptoms of gastrointestinal disease or a history of gastrointestinal disease. The normal intramural fat layer is generally thinner than the fat layer seen with inflammatory intestinal disease. Harisingjhani et al. (2003) noted such a normal appearance in 21% of 100 patients with no history of inflammatory bowel disease.

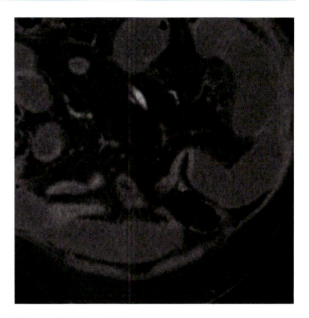

Fig. 12 The fat notch sign

13 Fat Notch Sign

13.1 Features
The fat notch sign is a newly described CT sign which is defined by the presence of a lateral fat notch on the bowel wall at the transition zone in small bowel obstruction (Delabrousse et al. 2009) (Fig. 12).

13.2 Significance
In adhesive small bowel obstruction, the fat notch sign corresponds to lateral extrinsic compression of the bowel made by a band at the transition zone (Delabrousse et al. 2009).

13.3 Diagnosis

13.3.1 Small Bowel Obstruction Due to Adhesive Bands
Although adhesive bands themselves cannot be identified by CT, recognition of CT findings suggestive of an extraluminal band compressing the bowel at the transition zone, which is the natural place to look for clues to the cause of small bowel obstruction

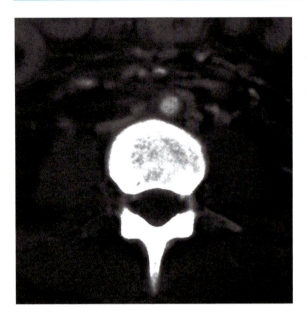

Fig. 13 The flat vena cava sign

(Ha et al. 1993), could enhance the radiologist's ability to diagnose small bowel obstruction from adhesive bands (Petrovic et al. 2006). In simple small bowel obstruction, a dedicated search for a fat notch sign allows good sensitivity (61%) and excellent specificity (100%) for the diagnosis of adhesive bands (Delabrousse et al. 2009).

14 Flat Vena Cava Sign

14.1 Features

The flat vena cava sign on CT was first defined as flattening of the inferior vena cava on at least three contiguous 1-cm images (Jeffrey and Federle 1988). Eisenstat et al. (2002) defined a flattened inferior vena cava by a maximal transverse-to-maximal anteroposterior diameter of 3:1 or more, whereas Mirvis et al. (1994) defined a flattened vena cava as less than 9 mm in the maximal anteroposterior dimension at the level of the renal veins (Fig. 13).

14.2 Significance

In blunt trauma, the collapse of the inferior vena cava in patients with hypovolemia is most likely due to decreased venous return. In some cases, the demonstration of the collapsed inferior vena cava may precede the clinical detection of shock (Jeffrey and Federle 1988). A flat vena cava sign in association with decreased caliber of the aorta, marked diffuse fluid-filled bowel distention, moderate to large fluid peritoneal collections, and abnormally intense enhancement of the bowel wall, kidneys, and pancreas has also been reported to define the hypoperfusion complex in children (Taylor et al. 1987). In clinical practice, the presence of a collapsed inferior vena cava in blunt trauma may be considered evidence of significant hypovolemia from major blood loss and should prompt careful hemodynamic and central venous pressure monitoring.

In contrast to patients with blunt trauma, a flattened vena cava may be seen in normovolemic and normotensive adult patients. Several explanations may be proposed: a normal variation, especially in elderly women, or a change in the vessel tone or connective tissues within the caval wall that occurs with aging; a redistribution of blood volume that does not manifest itself as clinical hypovolemia; and variation in caval shape and volume with ventilation, intra-abdominal pressure, and position of the patient (Eisenstat et al. 2002).

14.3 Causes

14.3.1 Hypovolemia from Blood Loss
The presence of a flat vena cava sign is an important CT sign of hypovolemia from major blood loss (Jeffrey and Federle 1988).

14.3.2 Inferior Vena Cava Variation
The presence of a flat vena cava sign is commonly seen in women and in older patients (Eisenstat et al. 2002).

15 Hemoperitoneum

15.1 Features

Hemoperitoneum is defined by the presence of a high-attenuating fluid (35–60 HU) within the peritoneal cavity. However, its attenuation may vary, and its appearance often depends on the age, extent, and location of the hemorrhage (Lubner et al. 2007) (Fig. 14).

15.2 Significance

The presence of hemoperitoneum corresponds to intraperitoneal bleeding.

Key CT Findings

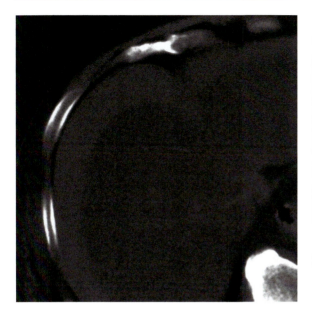

Fig. 14 Hemoperitoneum

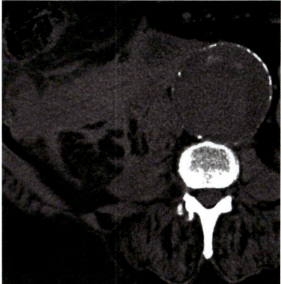

Fig. 15 Hemoretroperitoneum

15.3 Causes

15.3.1 Blunt Abdominal Trauma
Liver (Shanmuganathan and Mirvis 1998), spleen (Becker et al. 1994), bowel, and mesentery (Breen et al. 1997) are the more affected sites in blunt abdominal trauma.

15.3.2 Ectopic Pregnancy
Ruptured tubal pregnancy should be the first diagnosis to be searched for in a young female patient with pelvic pain and massive hemoperitoneum on CT scans (Coulier et al. 2008).

15.3.3 Intraabdominal Hemorrhagic Tumors
Ruptured hepatocellular carcinoma (Choi 2001) and adenoma are tumors responsible for intra-abdominal bleeding.

15.3.4 Spontaneous Spleen Rupture
Spontaneous splenic rupture is rare and in most cases occurs in a spleen affected by hematologic, neoplastic, or infectious disease or as a complication of pancreatic pseudocyst (Torricelli et al. 2001).

15.3.5 Ruptured Splenic Artery Aneurysm
This acute condition is often secondary to pancreatitis (Brunet and Greenberg 1991).

16 Hemoretroperitoneum

16.1 Features
Hemoretroperitoneum is defined by the presence of a high-attenuating fluid (35–60 HU) within the retroperitoneal space (Fig. 15).

16.2 Significance
The presence of hemoretroperitoneum corresponds to retroperitoneal bleeding.

16.3 Causes

16.3.1 Rupture of an Abdominal Aortic Aneurysm
Abdominal aortic aneurysm rupture is the most common cause of retroperitoneal hemorrhage (Schwartz et al. 2007).

16.3.2 Blunt Retroperitoneal Trauma
In blunt retroperitoneal trauma, injuries to the pancreas (Venkatesh and Wan 2008), kidneys (Harris et al. 2001), and vertebrae may lead to important retroperitoneal hemorrhage or hematoma.

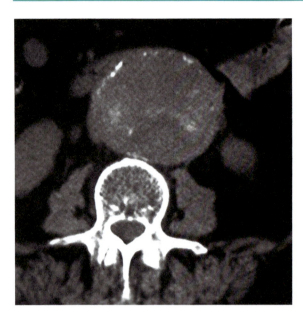

Fig. 16 The high-attenuating crescent sign

16.3.3 Spontaneous Retroperitoneal Hemorrhage

The main condition corresponding to spontaneous retroperitoneal hemorrhage is iliopsoas muscle hematoma in patients undergoing anticoagulant therapy (Lenchick et al. 1994).

16.3.4 Necrotizing Pancreatitis

Retroperitoneal hemorrhage is a rare but life-threatening complication of severe acute pancreatitis (Stroud et al. 1981).

17 High-Attenuating Crescent Sign

17.1 Features

On unenhanced CT scans, the criterion for a positive high-attenuating crescent sign is the presence of a crescent-shaped peripheral area with higher attenuation than that of the true abdominal aortic lumen but with lower attenuation than that of mural calcification. On contrast-enhanced CT scans, the criterion is the presence of a crescent-shaped area with higher attenuation than that of adjacent psoas muscle (Mehard et al. 1994; Arita et al. 1997; Fig. 16).

17.2 Significance

The peripheral high-attenuating crescent sign is due to acute hematoma within the abdominal aneurysm wall or within adjacent mural thrombus (Mehard et al. 1994; Arita et al. 1997).

17.3 Cause

17.3.1 Impending Abdominal Aortic Rupture Aneurysm

In patients without CT evidence of frank aneurysm leak, the high-attenuating crescent sign has a statistically significant correlation with the presence of pain, large aneurysm size, and complicated aneurysms (Mehard et al. 1994). Thus, the high-attenuating crescent sign should be regarded as a sign of impending abdominal aortic rupture, particularly in patients with pain.

18 Misty Mesentery

18.1 Features

The misty mesentery is defined by the CT appearance of mesenteric fat infiltrated with soft-tissue density (Mindelzun et al. 1996) (Fig. 17).

18.2 Significance

Normal mesenteric fat is similar in density (-100 to -160 HU) to the fat in subcutaneous and retroperitoneal spaces. The misty mesentery is defined by a mean density of the mesenteric fat that increases to -40 to -60 HU secondary to infiltration of the mesentery by fluid or cells. Depending on the nature and extent of the infiltration, mesenteric vessels may be either completely or partially effaced. A clue to mesenteric disease is often revealed along the visceral peritoneum as the edge of the mesentery becomes accentuated against the surrounding fat (Mindelzun et al. 1996).

18.3 Causes

18.3.1 Mesenteric Edema

Mesenteric edema may be secondary to many causes (Seo et al. 2003), including hypoalbuminemia,

Key CT Findings

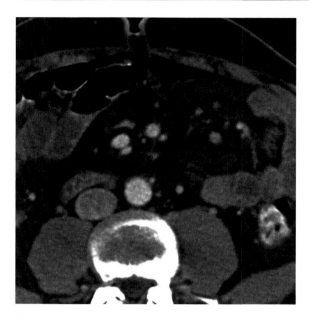

Fig. 17 The misty mesentery

cirrhosis, nephrosis, heart failure, tricuspid disease, constrictive pericarditis, portal hypertension, portal vein thrombosis, mesenteric artery and vein thrombosis, vasculitis, Budd–Chiari syndrome, inferior vena cava obstruction, and trauma (Silverman et al. 1987; Nghiem et al. 1993).

18.3.2 Lymphedema
Lymphedema of the mesentery may result from causes such as congenital anomalies, inflammation, neoplasm, surgery, and radiation therapy. In all of these, fluid permeates from the lymphatic channels into the interstitium of the mesentery (Browse et al. 1992).

18.3.3 Inflammation
Acute pancreatitis is the typical inflammatory process associated with infiltration of the small bowel mesentery. Other focal inflammatory diseases such as acute appendicitis and diverticulitis may also cause infiltration of the adjacent mesenteries.

18.3.4 Hemorrhage
Blood dissecting into the mesentery may originate from mesenteric vessels. Acute hemorrhage is characterized by its classically high (40–60 HU) CT numbers (Nghiem et al. 1993).

18.3.5 Neoplasms
Non-Hodgkin lymphoma is the most common cause of an isolated misty mesentery (Karaosmanoglu et al. 2009).

18.3.6 Idiopathic Causes
Mesenteric panniculitis (liposclerotic or retractile) is a frequent cause of misty mesentery (Horton et al. 2003). Diagnosis should be suggested on CT scans by radiating bands of soft-tissue density that surround the central vessels without displacing them. Typically, a halo of normal fat surrounds the vessels in the mesentery. Non-Hodgkin lymphoma remains the most difficult differential diagnosis.

19 Mosaic Pattern

19.1 Features

The mosaic pattern corresponds to an inhomogeneous, mottled reticulated-mosaic pattern of parenchymal contrast enhancement of the liver (Gore et al. 1994) (Fig. 18).

19.2 Significance

The mosaic pattern is an accurate CT sign for passive hepatic congestion. It is presumably due to impaired venous outflow leading to altered hepatic hemodynamics and hepatic parenchymal distortion (Gore et al. 1994). Linear and curvilinear regions of poor enhancement may be due to delayed enhancement in the regions of small and medium-sized hepatic veins. Larger patchy regions of poor or delayed enhancement in the periphery of the liver are probably due to a tendency of blood flow to be more stagnant in these regions in patients with hepatic venous hypertension. This stagnant blood most highly affects inflow from the hepatic arterial and portal venous circulations (Holley et al. 1989).

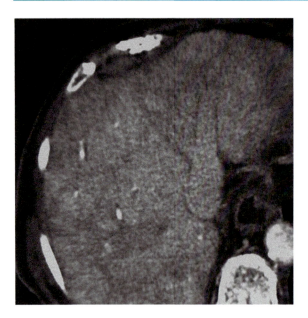

Fig. 18 The mosaic pattern

19.3 Causes

19.3.1 Congestive Heart Failure

In congestive heart failure, the mosaic pattern is due to the elevated central venous pressures which are directly transmitted from the right atrium to the inferior vena cava and the hepatic veins (De Las Heras and Pages 2001). The liver becomes tensely swollen as the hepatic sinusoids dilate and engorge to accommodate the backflow of blood.

19.3.2 Constrictive Pericarditis

Owing to rapid elevation of central venous pressure, constrictive pericarditis leads to a dilated inferior vena cava, dilated hepatic veins, ascites, mesenteric soft-tissue stranding, and mottled-mosaic enhancement of hepatic parenchyma (Johnson et al. 2008).

20 Northern Exposure Sign

20.1 Features

The northern exposure sign is a finding that may be demonstrated on CT scout views and on CT scans (Levsky et al. 2010). It was originally defined on supine abdominal radiographs as a dilated sigmoid colon that ascends cephalad to the transverse colon (Javors et al. 1999) (Fig. 19).

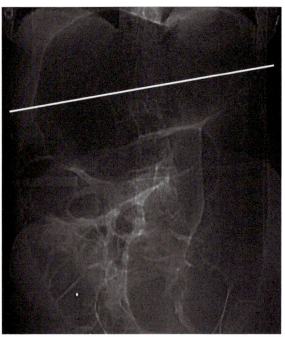

Fig. 19 The northern exposure sign

20.2 Significance

Intraluminal gas always seeks the least dependent colonic location. When the patient is supine, intraluminal gas tends to accumulate in the transverse colon, the most ventral segment of the large bowel. The transverse colon crosses the midline, with its suspending mesentery separating the greater peritoneal cavity into supramesocolic and inframesocolic hemispheres (Meyers 1994). Thus, the transverse colon may be considered the equator of the abdomen. In this schema, the sigmoid colon is normally confined to the southern hemisphere, caudad to the transverse colon. When the apex of the sigmoid colon migrates cephalad (or north) to the transverse colon, as in cases of sigmoid volvulus, this sign is termed the northern exposure sign (Javors et al. 1999).

20.3 Cause

20.3.1 Sigmoid Volvulus

The northern exposure sign is based on the anatomic and physiologic relationships of the sigmoid colon to the other portions of the bowels rather than on vertebral landmarks or the location of other

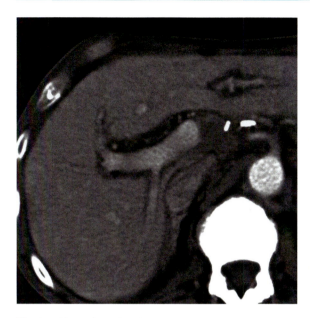

Fig. 20 The periportal collar sign

viscera. According to Javors et al. (1999), the elevation of the distended sigmoid colon above the transverse colon is a valuable discriminator of sigmoid volvulus from the other causes of large bowel dilatation. Using conventional radiography, they demonstrated the northern exposure sign as a sensitive (88%) and very specific (100%) sign for sigmoid volvulus.

21 Periportal Collar Sign

21.1 Features

The periportal collar sign (or periportal halo sign) corresponds to regions with a relatively low attenuation value approaching that of water paralleling central or peripheral branches of the portal vein on CT scans (Koslin et al. 1988; Shanmuganathan et al. 1993) (Fig. 20).

21.2 Significance

Periportal edema, which is usually attributed to dilatation of lymphatic channels and accumulation of lymph due to obstruction of normal hepatic drainage, may cause this sign in patients with congestive heart failure and secondary liver congestion, hepatitis, or enlarged lymph nodes or tumors in the porta hepatis (Marineck et al. 1986). A periportal halo, attributed either to tracking of hemorrhaged blood along the course of the portal veins (Macrander et al. 1989) or to elevated venous pressure (Shanmuganathan et al. 1993), has been described in patients with hepatic injury. This sign can also be seen in recipients of liver transplants or bone marrow transplants.

21.3 Causes

21.3.1 Blunt Hepatic Trauma
The periportal low attenuation is frequently seen on CT scans of trauma patients, particularly when diffuse and peripheral, and most likely represents distension of periportal lymphatic vessels and lymphedema associated with elevated central venous pressure produced by vigorous intravenous fluid administration (Shanmuganathan et al. 1993). Dissection of hemorrhage along the portal tracts associated with hepatic injury may contribute to focal regions of periportal low density at the site of injury.

21.3.2 Cardiac Failure
In cardiac failure, elevated central venous pressure is assumed to be the cause of the periportal collar sign (Lawson et al. 1993).

21.3.3 Acute Hepatitis
The periportal collar sign may be seen in the preicteric phase of hepatitis, due to liver congestion (Lawson et al. 1993).

21.3.4 Non-Hodgkin Lymphoma
In non-Hodgkin lymphoma, enlarged lymph nodes present in the porta hepatis may obstruct lymphatic drainage and cause a periportal collar sign (Karcaaltincaba et al. 2007).

21.3.5 Liver Transplants
The periportal collar sign is seen more commonly in patients with recently transplanted allografts. The presence of a central or peripheral collar on CT is not reliable CT evidence of acute allograft rejection (Wechsler et al. 1987; Stevens et al. 1991).

Fig. 21 a "Bubblelike" pneumatosis intestinalis; b "bandlike" pneumatosis intestinalis

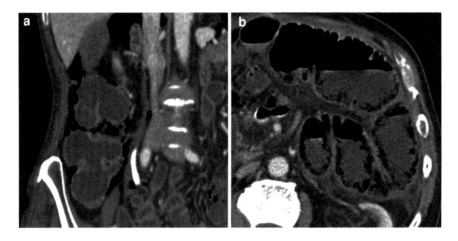

22 Pneumatosis Intestinalis

22.1 Features

Pneumatosis intestinalis is defined as the presence of gas in the bowel wall (Knechtle et al. 1990). It is classified as "bubblelike" if it consists only or mainly of isolated bubbles of air in the bowel wall, whereas it is classified as "bandlike" if it consists of continuous bands of air in the affected bowel wall (Wiesner et al. 2001; Soyer et al. 2008) (Fig. 21).

22.2 Significance

Two basic mechanical features characterize most cases of pneumatosis intestinalis: mucosal injury, the most important and prevalent feature, and increased intraluminal pressure. Moreover, gas-forming organisms invading the bowel wall may also produce pneumatosis intestinalis.

22.3 Causes

22.3.1 Pneumatosis Cystoides Coli
"Bubblelike" pneumatosis intestinalis consists of cystic collections of air, usually located in the colon. It is generally a benign condition that may remain stable for years but may be complicated by obstruction or bleeding. Its cause is unknown, but its frequent association with emphysema suggests that air may dissect through the mediastinum tissues to enter the bowel mesentery and subserosal spaces (Marshak et al. 1977).

22.3.2 Gastrointestinal Disorders
"Bandlike" pneumatosis intestinalis, on the other hand, is characterized by linear or circumferential air in any part of the gastrointestinal tract and is associated with many clinical conditions, such as bowel obstruction (Merlin et al. 2008), ischemic bowel (Keyting et al. 1961), blunt bowel trauma (Furuya et al. 2002), gastrointestinal endoscopy (Meyers et al. 1977), bacterial or fungal enteritis (Kleinman et al. 1980), and cancer cytoreductive therapy (Rha et al. 2000).

Patients manifesting symptoms or signs of acute abdomen merit an aggressive surgical approach. Associated acidosis suggests necrotic bowel and portends a grave prognosis.

23 Pneumobilia

23.1 Features

Pneumobilia is defined in the liver by the presence of multiple tubular branching air images ($-1,000$ HU) on CT scans. Air is usually central in the liver (as opposed to portal venous gas, which is peripheral) (Fig. 22).

23.2 Significance

Air in the biliary tree may come either from the intestinal tract or from gas-forming infections of the bile ducts. Nonsurgical causes of pneumobilia are

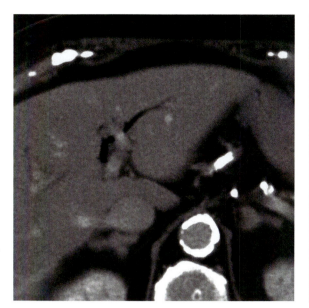

Fig. 22 Pneumobilia

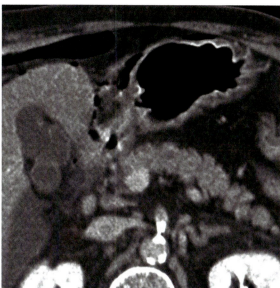

Fig. 23 Pneumoperitoneum

uncommon and are usually indicative of serious disease.

23.3 Causes

23.3.1 Iatrogenic

Pneumobilia is most commonly seen in patients following surgery in which a biliary-enteric anastomosis has been created or a sphincterotomy has been performed (Sherman and Tran 2006).

23.3.2 Gallstone Ileus

Gallstone ileus is a rare complication of recurrent gallstone cholecystitis and is defined by small bowel obstruction due to an ectopic gallstone. In gallstone ileus, the gallstone reaches the intestinal tract by creation of a cholecystoduodenal fistula (Shimono et al. 1998). This fistula between the duodenum and the gallbladder usually leads to the presence of air within the biliary tract (Delabrousse et al. 2000). Bouveret syndrome is defined by a duodenal impaction of the ectopic gallstone (Brennan et al. 2004).

23.3.3 Recurrent Pyogenic Cholangitis

Pneumobilia may be seen in recurrent pyogenic cholangitis due to gas-forming organisms (Afagh and Pancu 2004).

23.3.4 Emphysematous Cholecystitis

Emphysematous cholecystitis is an acute infection of the gallbladder wall caused by gas-forming organisms. Gas may occur in the wall and the lumen of the gallbladder. Pneumobilia is a rare but possible CT sign of emphysematous cholecystitis (Van Dyck et al. 2001).

23.3.5 Incompetence of the Sphincter of Oddi

Transient pneumobilia has been attributed to incompetence of the sphincter of Oddi (Shariatzadeh and Bolivar 1973), particularly when duodenal air pressure increases.

24 Pneumoperitoneum

24.1 Features

Pneumoperitoneum is defined by the presence of air out of the gastrointestinal tract (Baker 1996) (Fig. 23).

24.2 Significance

In an acute condition, pneumoperitoneum is often a sign of intestinal perforation. Periportal free air on CT scans has been reported to be specific of upper gastrointestinal tract perforation (Cho et al. 2009).

24.3 Causes

24.3.1 Gastrointestinal Perforation
When pneumoperitoneum is diagnosed in a nontraumatic patient, gastrointestinal perforation due to gastric or duodenal ulcer, sigmoid diverticulitis, bowel ischemia, toxic megacolon, or a foreign body must be looked for (Ghekiere et al. 2007).

24.3.2 Gastrointestinal Anastomosis Leakage
Perianastomotic loculated fluid containing air is the only feature statistically more frequently seen with gastrointestinal anastomosis leakage (Power et al. 2007).

24.3.3 Blunt Abdominal Trauma with Gastrointestinal Injury
The initial and follow-up CT scans are reported to detect extraluminal air in 58 and 92% of cases, respectively. The chance of detecting extraluminal air increases as time elapses (Saku et al. 2006).

24.3.4 Penetrating Peritoneal Trauma
Unlike pneumoperitoneum seen on plain films, pneumoperitoneum detected on CT scans is not pathognomonic of bowel perforation (Kane et al. 1991), and an associated pneumothorax may be considered as a possible cause.

24.3.5 Iatrogenic Perforation
Gastrointestinal perforation may occur during bowel endoscopy (Eisenbach et al. 2008), bowel surgery, or colonic enema (Chong et al. 1987).

24.3.6 Spontaneous Pneumoperitoneum
The more common sites of origin of spontaneous peritoneum are intrathoracic sites, and the genital organs in women (Madura et al. 1982).

25 Pneumoretroperitoneum

25.1 Features

Pneumoretroperitoneum is defined by the presence of free air (−1,000 HU) within the retroperitoneal space. Most often, air is seen surrounding the kidneys, and overlying the contour of the iliopsoas muscles (Fig. 24).

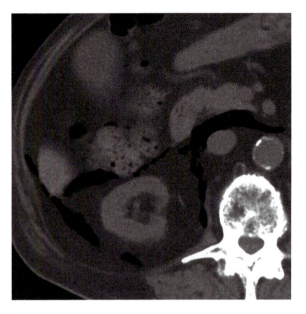

Fig. 24 Pneumoretroperitoneum

25.2 Significance

Free air can accumulate in the retroperitoneal space after perforation of a retroperitoneal bowel segment, or air can spread below the diaphragm from a pneumomediastinum (Daly et al. 2008).

25.3 Causes

25.3.1 Duodenal Perforation
Duodenal perforation may be secondary to peptic ulcer (Pun and Firkin 2004), leukemia (Chao et al. 1999), a penetrating foreign body (Maniatis et al. 2000), and duodenal trauma (Yagan et al. 2009).

25.3.2 Rectal Perforation
Perforation is mainly due to iatrogenic causes (endoscopy, surgery, biopsy) (Miyatani and Yashida 2007) and rectal trauma (foreign body) (Waraich et al. 2007).

25.3.3 Spread of Pneumomediastinum
Air tracks along the great vessels (aorta and inferior vena cava) through the diaphragm into the pararenal spaces (Perrone et al. 2005).

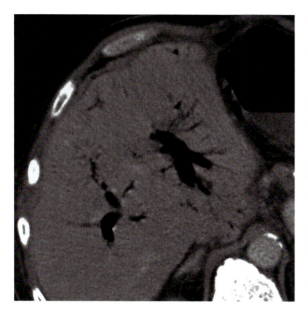

Fig. 25 Portomesenteric venous gas

26 Portomesenteric Venous Gas

26.1 Features

Portomesenteric venous gas is defined as the presence of gas (−1,000 HU) in the portomesenteric venous circulation (Wiesner et al. 2001). In the liver, the more peripheral position of the tubular air images (extending to within 2 cm of the liver capsule) will help to differentiate them from pneumobilia, which is situated more centrally (Fig. 25).

26.2 Significance

Portomesenteric venous gas may occur after damage to the wall of gastrointestinal tract caused by infection and inflammation, but also secondary to ulceration or overdistention (Sebastia et al. 2000). Besides, portomesenteric venous gas may occur without pneumatosis intestinalis in many other conditions.

26.3 Causes

26.3.1 Bowel Ischemia
Portomesenteric venous gas is an impressive, but uncommon, CT finding that most commonly develops because of bowel ischemia (Schulze et al. 1995). In bowel ischemia, the presence of portomesenteric venous gas on CT is associated with a mortality rate of 56% (Wiesner et al. 2001).

26.3.2 Ulcerative Colitis
Portal venous gas may be a benign finding in cases of stable ulcerative colitis.

26.3.3 Gastric Ulcer
Few cases of portal venous gas from peptic gastric ulcer have been reported (Liebman et al. 1978).

26.3.4 Bowel Obstruction
Hepatic portal venous gas and small bowel obstruction with no signs of intestinal gangrene after appendicectomy have been reported by Tsai et al. (2000).

26.3.5 Necrotizing Pancreatitis
Acute necrotizing pancreatitis is a rare cause of hepatic portal venous gas (Wu and Wang 2009).

26.3.6 Complicated Acute Diverticulitis
Sigmoid diverticulitis complicated by a colovenous fistula, pylephlebitis, or a perisigmoid abscess is a rare cause of hepatic portal venous gas (Haak et al. 1990; Heye et al. 2002).

26.3.7 Blunt Abdominal Trauma
Blunt abdominal trauma may lead to portal venous gas. The gas is caused by a sudden increase in the intra-abdominal pressure with concomitant mucosal disruption, which thus forces intraluminal gas into the portal circulation in blunt trauma patients (Furuya et al. 2002).

26.3.8 Iatrogenic
Barium enema (Stein et al. 1983), colonoscopy, a nasogastric intubation, and liver transplantation are classic causes of portomesenteric venous gas in adults.

27 Round Belly Sign

27.1 Features

The positive round belly sign is defined by an increased ratio of anteroposterior-to-transverse abdominal diameter > 0.80. This ratio is measured at

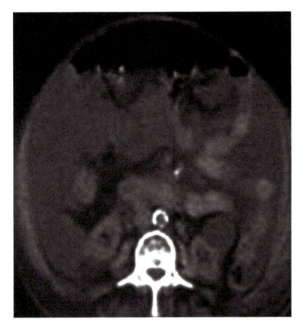

Fig. 26 The round belly sign

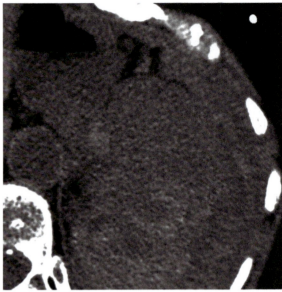

Fig. 27 The sentinel clot sign

the level where the left renal vein crosses the aorta, not including the subcutaneous fat (Pickhardt et al. 1999) (Fig. 26).

27.2 Significance

The round belly sign corresponds to massive abdominal distention secondary to increased intra-abdominal pressure.

27.3 Cause

27.3.1 Abdominal Compartment Syndrome

The round appearance of the abdomen on axial CT scans in patients with abdominal compartment syndrome correlates well with the massive abdominal distention on physical examination. Pickhardt et al. (1999) reported a cutoff value of 0.80 (the round belly sign) with 100% sensitivity and 94% specificity for the diagnosis of abdominal compartment syndrome. For other authors, more than an absolute value for this ratio, the occurrence of an acute increase, without any explanation for it, such as the development of ascites or a bowel obstruction, may give additional support for the diagnosis of abdominal compartment syndrome (Zissin 2000; Laffargue et al. 2002; Patel et al. 2007).

28 Sentinel Clot Sign

28.1 Features

On unenhanced CT scans, the sentinel clot sign is defined by the presence of a focal high-density collection having a mean CT number greater than 60 HU when measured by computed region of interest cursor readout. If region of interest measurements are unavailable, the presence of a focal heterogeneous collection that is visibly more dense than hemoperitoneum is accepted as evidence of a sentinel clot sign (Orwig and Federle 1989) (Fig. 27).

28.2 Significance

The sentinel clot sign corresponds to a localized intra-abdominal blood clot. The sentinel clot sign is assigned a relationship to an adjacent solid or

Key CT Findings

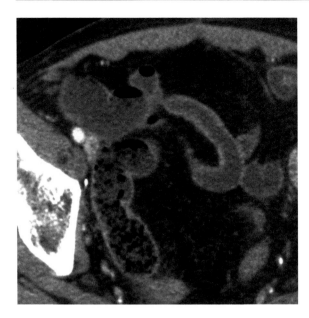

Fig. 28 The small bowel feces sign

hollow viscus as the most likely site of injury and source of hemorrhage (Orwig and Federle 1989).

28.3 Cause

28.3.1 Blunt Abdominal Trauma
The sentinel clot sign is an important clue that the bleeding source is an injured adjacent organ (Hamilton et al. 2008). It is a frequent and accurate sign that may help to focus attention on the traumatic lesion (Shinn et al. 2007). By facilitating diagnosis of trauma to a specific organ, it influences the management decision of surgical versus conservative therapy (Orwig and Federle 1989).

28.3.2 Gastrointestinal Bleeding
Nonbleeding protuberances in ulcer bases can be separated into vessels, which have a high risk of rebleeding, and sentinel clots, which have a low risk of rebleeding (Freeman et al. 1993).

28.3.3 Spontaneous Spleen Rupture
The formation of a clot close to the bleeding source may be a valuable sign in spontaneous spleen rupture (Gayer et al. 2003). During the subsequent course, clot lysis will progressively occur and the attenuation values of the fluid will decrease.

29 Small Bowel Feces Sign

29.1 Features

The small bowel feces sign was first described in 1995 by Mayo-Smith et al. (1995). It is defined by the presence of particulate (colonlike) feculent matter mingled with gas bubbles in the lumen of dilated loops of the small bowel (Fuchsjäger 2002) (Fig. 28).

29.2 Significance

The heterogeneous mottled particulate matter mixed with small gas bubbles observed in the small bowel feces sign resembles the appearance of stool in the large bowel on CT. It is the result of an abnormally low intestinal transit time, either mechanical or functional in origin, and is believed to be caused by incompletely digested food, bacterial overgrowth, or increased water absorption of the distal small bowel contents due to obstruction (Mayo-Smith et al. 1995; Catalano 1997).

29.3 Cause

29.3.1 Small Bowel Obstruction
The small bowel feces sign has been reported as a finding indicative of small bowel obstruction by many authors (Mayo-Smith et al. 1995; Catalano 1997; Delabrousse et al. 2005). Since the sign is usually seen immediately proximal to the level of obstruction, it may be helpful in recognition of the exact site and cause (Lazarus et al. 2004). The main source of the small bowel feces sign is small bowel obstruction due to adhesions. On the basis of the fact that this sign was initially described with subacute small bowel obstruction, Lazarus et al. (2004) stated that the small bowel feces sign may relate more to the chronic nature than to the degree of obstruction. Moreover, the small bowel feces sign has been reported to be secondary to incomplete obstruction with progressive

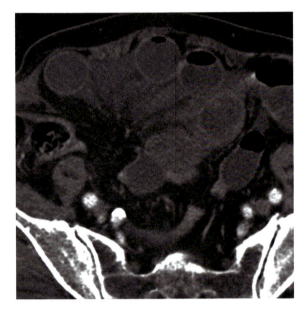

Fig. 29 The spoke wheel sign

slowing of small bowel transit as opposed to complete obstruction. Therefore, the notion that the small bowel feces sign could be a predictor of successful conservative management may be entertained (Delabrousse et al. 2005).

30 Spoke Wheel Sign

30.1 Features

The spoke wheel sign is defined as fluid-filled, dilated bowel loops that are radially arranged around converging thickened and stretched mesenteric vessels (Jaramillo and Raval 1986) (Fig. 29).

30.2 Significance

In small bowel volvulus, torsion at the root of the mesentery results in a shortened, tight mesentery with a funnel shape along the axis of rotation. The shortening and tightening of the mesentery causes the fluid-filled, dilated bowel loops that are attached to the twisted mesentery to lie in a concentric, more peripheral location, with engorged and thickened vascular structures occupying the center. Stretched and engorged mesenteric vessels that reach the concentrically arranged bowel loops and that converge toward the center of mesenteric torsion create folds of soft-tissue attenuation that ressemble spokes connected to the hub of a wheel. The resultant spoke wheel sign is best appreciated on cross sections when imaging is performed to the long axis of the bowel rotation (Rudloff 2005). Most often, a whirl sign may be demonstrated in association with the spoke wheel sign.

30.3 Cause

30.3.1 Small Bowel Volvulus

The spoke wheel sign is highly suggestive of small bowel volvulus. It incorporates diagnostics of both the mesentery and the small bowel, thereby aiding in the detection of closed loop obstruction (Balthazar et al. 1997). The association of this sign with bowel ischemia and infarction should lead to a search for other signs of bowel necrosis and raise suspicion of bowel strangulation.

31 String of Pearls Sign

31.1 Features

The string of pearls sign, which may be demonstrated on CT scans, was originally defined on abdominal radiographs (Maglinte et al. 1996). Also commonly referred to as the string of beads sign, this sign consists of a row of several small air bubbles trapped between the valvulae conniventes along the superior wall of dilated small bowel loops (Nevitt 2000) (Fig. 30).

31.2 Significance

The string of pearls sign corresponds to small amounts of air trapped between the valvulae conniventes. Dilatation of the small bowel stimulates the mucosa to secrete fluid. Thus, the distended bowel contains varying amounts of air and fluid. As the small bowel dilates, the valvulae conniventes widen, and this causes the small bowel air to be trapped (Nevitt 2000). The meniscal effect of the surrounding fluid gives the

Key CT Findings

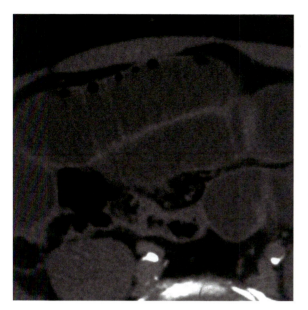

Fig. 30 The string of pearls sign

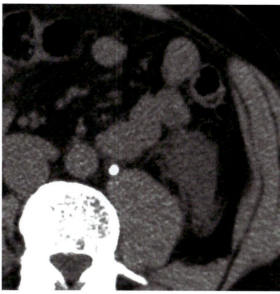

Fig. 31 The tissue rim sign

trapped air an ovoid or rounded shape, leading to the string of pearls appearance.

31.3 Cause

31.3.1 Mechanical Small Bowel Obstruction

Although the string of pearls sign is rarely seen in adynamic ileus, acute gastroenteritis, and saline catharsis, when present in the right clinical setting, it is considered to be diagnostic of mechanical small bowel obstruction (Levin 1973; Maglinte et al. 1996). The importance of recognizing the string of pearls sign is often related to the clinical and other CT findings of small bowel obstruction.

32 Tissue Rim Sign

32.1 Features

The tissue rim sign is a CT finding defined by the presence of a rim (or halo) of soft-tissue attenuation seen around the circumference of an intraureteral stone on unenhanced axial CT scans (Heneghan et al. 1997; Kawashima et al. 1997) (Fig. 31).

32.2 Significance

The tissue rim sign is believed to represent thickening of the ureteral wall secondary to edema from a stone lodged in the ureteral lumen (Smith et al. 1995). It has been reported to be useful in differentiating ureteral calculi from extraurinary calcifications (Smith et al. 1995; Smith et al. 1996) Stones without a rim sign are commonly larger than stones with a rim sign, likely because of stretching of the ureteral wall by the larger stones (Heneghan et al. 1997). For a time, the duration of obstruction was proposed as another explanation for the presence or absence of the rim sign. However, Heneghan et al. (1997) found no statistically significant difference in the duration of symptoms between patients with stones who exhibited a rim sign and those who did not.

32.3 Cause

32.3.1 Ureterolithiasis

A positive tissue rim sign is specific to the diagnosis of ureterolithiasis. However, a negative sign does not preclude such a diagnosis. The presence of the tissue rim sign should lead to careful inspection for other CT

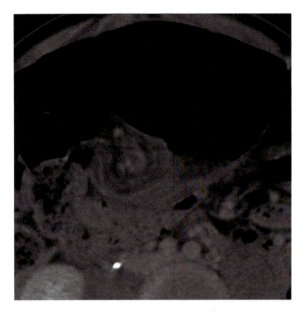

Fig. 32 The whirl sign

findings, such as ipsilateral dilatation, perinephretic edema, dilatation of intrarenal collecting system and renal swelling (Kawashima et al. 1997)

33 Whirl Sign

33.1 Features

The appearance of the whirl sign is that of soft-tissue mass with an internal architecture of swirling strands of soft-tissue and fat attenuation (Khurana 2003) (Fig. 32).

33.2 Significance

The whirl sign is highly suggestive of intestinal volvulus that occurs when afferent and efferent bowel loops rotate around a fixed point of obstruction, which results in tightly twisted mesentery along the axis of rotation. These twisted loops of bowel and mesenteric vessels create swirling strands of soft-tissue attenuation within a background of mesenteric fat attenuation, giving the appearance of a hurricane on a weather map (Moore et al. 2001). The whirl sign is best appreciated when CT scanning is performed perpendicular to the axis of bowel rotation (Khurana 2003).

33.3 Causes

33.3.1 Midgut Volvulus

The whirl sign was first described by Fisher (1981) as a CT finding of midgut volvulus, where the center of the whirl was the superior mesenteric artery, and the whirled appearance was created by the encircling loops of bowel .

33.3.2 Sigmoid Volvulus

Four years later, the definition of the whirl sign was extended to include the CT appearance of sigmoid volvulus where a whirl was formed by the afferent and efferent sigmoid loops with the central portion composed of tightly twisted bowel and mesentery. For some authors, the tightness of the whirl is proportional to the degree of rotation.

33.3.3 Cecal Volvulus

The whirl sign has also been reported in cecal volvulus. In cecal volvulus, the whirl sign comprises the twisted mesentery and the collapsed cecal loop (Frank et al. 1993). Pathophysiologically, three types of cecal volvulus are differentiated. In the loop type, the distal ileal loops may also participate in the creation of the whirl sign.

33.3.4 Small Bowel Volvulus

The main causes of small bowel volvulus are postoperative adhesions in which the bowel is fixed to a point that acts as a pivot, leading to closed loop obstruction, and hernia (Balthazar et al. 1997). In small bowel obstruction, the presence of a whirl sign is the very key feature that indicates a bowel volvulus.

References

Afagh A, Pancu D (2004) Radiologic findings in recurrent pyogenic cholangitis. J Emerg Med 26:343–346
Ahualli J (2007) The fat halo sign. Radiology 242:945–946
Aoyagi S, Kosuga T, Ogata T, Yasunaga M (2009) Spontaneous rupture of the spleen caused by bacillus infection: report of a case. Surg Today 39:733–737
Arita T, Matsunaga N, Takano K et al (1997) Abdominal aortic aneurysm: rupture associated with the high-attenuated crescent sign. Radiology 204:765–768

Baker SR (1996) Invited commentary: imaging of pneumoperitoneum. Abdom Imaging 21:413–414

Ballantyne GH (1982) Review of sigmoid volvulus: history and results of treatment. Dis Colon Rectum 25:494–501

Balthazar EJ, Megibow AJ, Fazzini E, Opulencia JF, Engel I (1985) Cytomegalovirus colitis in AIDS: radiographic findings in 11 patients. Radiology 155:585–589

Balthazar EJ, Birnbaum BA, Megibow AJ, Gordon RB, Whelan CA, Hulnick DH (1992) Closed-loop and strangulating intestinal obstruction: CT signs. Radiology 185:769–775

Balthazar EJ, Birnhaum BA, Megibow AJ, Gordon RB, Whelan CA, Hulnick DH (1997) Closed-loop and strangulating obstruction: CT signs. Radiology 185:769–775

Becker CD, Spring P, Glättli A, Schweizer W (1994) Blunt splenic trauma in adults: can CT findings be used to determine the need for surgery? AJR Am J Roentgenol 162:342–347

Benjaminov O, Atri M, Hamilton P, Rappaport D (2002) Frequency of visualization and thickness of normal appendix on nonenhanced helical CT. Radiology 225:400–406

Bergin D, Ennis ER, Keogh C, Fenlon HM, Murray JG (2001) The "dependant viscera" sign in CT diagnosis of blunt traumatic diaphragmatic rupture. AJR Am J Roentgenol 177:1137–1140

Bernard C, Lubrano J, Moulin V, Mantion E, Kastler B, Delabrousse E (2010) Value of Multidetector-row CT in the management of signoid Volvulus. J Radiol 91(2): 213–220

Breen DJ, Janzen DL, Zwirewich CV, Nagy AG (1997) Blunt bowel and mesenteric injury: diagnostic performance of CT signs. J Comput Assist Tomogr 21:706–712

Brennan GB, Rosenberg RD, Arora S (2004) Bouveret syndrome. RadioGraphics 24:1171–1175

Browse NL, Wilson NM, Russo F, al-Hassan H, Allen DR (1992) An etiology and treatment of chylous ascites. Br J Surg 9:1145–1150

Brunet WG, Greenberg HM (1991) CT demonstration of a ruptured splenic artery aneurysm. J Comput Assist Tomogr 15:177–178

Burrel HC, Baker DM, Wardrop P et al (1994) Signifiant plain film findings in sigmoid volvulus. Clin Radiol 49:317–319

Byun JY, Ha HK, Yu SY et al (1999) CT features of systemic lupus erythematosus in patients with acute abdominal pain: emphasis on ischemic bowel disease. Radiology 211:203–209

Cantwell CP (2006) The dependant viscera sign. Radiology 238:752–753

Catalano O (1997) The faeces sign: a CT finding in small-bowel obstruction. Radiologe 37:417–419

Chao TC, Wang CS, Wen MF (1999) Gastroduodenal perforation in cancer patients. Hepatogastroenterology 46:2878–2881

Checkoff JL, Weschler RJ, Nazarian LN (2002) Chronic inflammatory appendiceal conditions that mimic acute appendicitis on helical CT. AJR Am J Roentgenol 179:731–734

Chen S, Harisinghani MG, Wittenberg J (2003) Small bowel Ct fat density target sign in chronic radiation enteritis. Australas Radiol 47:450–452

Cho HS, Yoon SE, Park SH, Kim H, Lee YH, Yoon KH (2009) Distinction between upper and lower gastrointestinal perforation: usefulness of the periportal free air sign on computed tomography. Eur J Radiol 69:108–113

Choi BG (2001) The findings of ruptured hepatocellular carcinoma on helical CT. Br J Radiol 74:142–146

Chong WK, Tanner A, Wilkins RA (1987) Pneumoperitoneum, omental emphysema and intramural barium perforation following double contrast barium enema. Clin Radiol 38:319–320

Coulier B, Malbecq S, Brinon PE, Ramboux A (2008) MDCT diagnosis of ruptured tubal pregnancy with massive hemoperitoneum. Emerg Radiol 15:179–182

Daly KP, Ho CP, Persson DL, Gay SB (2008) Traumatic retroperitoneal injuries: review of multidetector CT findings. RadioGraphics 28:1571–1590

De Las Heras D, Pages M (2001) Abnormal hepatic enhancement on CT in congestive heart failure. J Hepatol 35:431

Delabrousse E, Bartholomot B, Sohm O, Wallerand H, Kastler B (2000) Gallstone ileus: CT findings. Eur Radiol 10:938–940

Delabrousse E, Baulard R, Sarliève P, Michalakis D, Rodière E, Kastler BA (2005) Value of the small bowel feces sign at CT in adhesive small bowel obstruction. J Radiol 86:393–397

Delabrousse E, Sarliève P, Sailley N, Aubry S, Kastler BA (2007) Cecal volvulus: CT findings and correlation with pathophysiology. Emerg Radiol 14:411–415

Delabrousse E, Lubrano J, Jehl J et al (2009) Small bowel obstruction from adhesive bands and matted adhesions: CT differentiation. AJR Am J Roentgenol 192:693–697

Demos TC, Solomon C, Posniak HV, Flisak MJ (1989) Computed tomography in traumatic defects of the diaphragm. Clin Imaging 13:62–67

Eisenbach C, Bläker H, Stremmel W, Sauer P, Schaible A (2008) Pneumoperitoneum following endoscopic mucosal resection without perforation of the colon. Endoscopy 40(Suppl 2):E64–E65

Eisenstat RS, Whitford AC, Lane MJ, Katz DS (2002) The flat cava sign revisited: what is it significance in patients without trauma? AJR Am J Roentgenol 178:21–25

Feldman D (2000) The coffee bean sign. Radiology 216:178–179

Fisher JK (1981) Computed tomographic diagnosis of volvulus in intestinal malrotation. Radiology 140:145–146

Fishman EK, Kavuru M, Jones B et al (1991) Pseudomembranous colitis: CT evaluation of 26 cases. Radiology 180:57–60

Frager DH, Goldman M, Beneventano TC (1983) Computed tomography in Crohn disease. J Comput Assist Tomogr 7:819–824

Frank AJ, Goffner LB, Fruauff AA, Losada RA (1993) Cecal volvulus: the CT whirl sign. Abdom Imaging 18:288–289

Freeman ML, Cass OW, Peine CJ, Onstad GR (1993) The non-bleeding visible vessel versus the sentinel clot: natural history and risk of rebleeding. Gastrointest Endosc 39:359–366

Fuchsjäger MH (2002) The small-bowel feces sign. Radiology 225:378–379

Furlan A, Fakhran S, Federle MP (2009) Spontaneous abdominal hemorrhage: causes, CT findings, and clinical complications. AJR Am J Roentgenol 193:1077–1087

Furuya Y, Yasuhara H, Ariki K et al (2002) Hepatic portal venous gas caused by blunt abdominal trauma: is it true ominous sign of bowel necrosis? Report of a case. Surg Today 32:655–658

Gale ME, Johnson WC, Gerzof SG, Robbins AH (1986) Problems in the CT diagnosis of ruptured abdominal aortic aneurysms. J Comput Assist Tomogr 10:637–641

Gayer G, Zandman-Goddard G, Kosych E, Apter S (2003) Spontaneous rupture of the spleen detected on CT as the initial manifestation of infectious mononucleosis. Emerg Radiol 10:51–52

Ghekiere O, Lesmik A, Millet I, Hoa D, Guillon F, Taourel P (2007) Direct visualization of perforation sites in patients with non-traumatic free pneumoperitoneum: added value of thin transverse slices and coronal and sagittal reformations for multidetector CT. Eur Radiol 17:2302–2309

Gore RM, Mathieu DG, White EM, Ghahremani GG, Panella JS, Rochester D (1994) Passive hepatic congestion: cross-sectional imaging features. AJR Am J Roentgenol 162:71–75

Gore RM, Balthazar EJ, Gharemani GG, Miller FH (1996) CT features of ulcerative colitis and Crohn's disease. AJR Am J Roentgenol 167:3–15

Ha HK, Park CH, Kim SK et al (1993) CT analysis of intestinal obstruction due to adhesions: early detection of strangulation. J Comput Assist Tomogr 17:386–389

Ha HK, Lee HJ, Yang SK et al (1998) Intestinal Behçet syndrome: CT features of patients with and patients without complications. Radiology 209:449–454

Haak HR, Kooymans-Coutinhao MF, von Teefelen ME, Adhin S, Falke TH (1990) Portal venous gas in a patient with diverticulitis. Hepatogastroenterology 37:528–529

Halliday KE, Al-Kutoubi A (1996) Draped aorta: CT sign of contained leak of aortic aneurysms. Radiology 199:41–43

Hamilton JD, Kumaravel M, Censullo ML, Cohen AM, Kievlan DS, West OC (2008) Multidetector CT evaluation of active extravasation in blunt abdominal and pelvic trauma patients. RadioGraphics 28:1603–1616

Harisingjhani MG, Wittenberg J, Lee W, Chen S, Guttierez AL, Mueller PR (2003) Bowel wall fat halo sign in patients without intestinal disease. AJR Am J Roentgenol 181:781–784

Harris AC, Swirewich CV, Lyburn ID, Torreggiani WC, Marchinkow LO (2001) CT findings in blunt renal trauma. RadioGraphics 21:201–214

Heneghan JP, Dalrymple NC, Verga M, Rosenfield AT, Smith RC (1997) Soft tissue rim sign in the diagnosis of ureteral calculi with use of unenhanced helical CT. Radiology 202:709–711

Heye S, Ghijselings L, van Campehoudt M (2002) Hepatic portal gas as a complication of diverticulitis with a colovenous fistula: a case report. Emerg Radiol 9:234–236

Holley HC, Koslin DB, Berland LL, Stanley RJ (1989) Inhomogeneous enhancement of liver parenchyma secondary to passive congestion: contrast-enhanced CT. Radiology 170:795–800

Hopper KD, Sherman JL, Ghaed N (1985) Aortic rupture into retroperitoneum. AJR Am J Roentgenol 145:435–437

Horton KM, Corl FM, Fishman EK (2000) CT evaluation of the colon: inflammatory disease. RadioGraphics 20:399–418

Horton KM, Lawler LP, Fishman EK (2003) CT findings in sclerosing mesenteritis (panniculitis): spectrum of disease. RadioGraphics 23:1561–1567

Iochum S, Ludig T, Walter F, Sebbag H, Grosdidier G, Blum AG (2002) Imaging of diaphragmatic injury: a diagnostic challenge? RadioGraphics 22:S103–S118

Jaramillo D, Raval B (1986) CT diagnosis of primary small bowel volvulus. AJR Am J Roentgenol 147:941–942

Javors BR, Baker SR, Miller JA (1999) The northern exposure sign: a newly described finding in sigmoid volvulus. AJR Am J Roentegenol 173:571–574

Jeffrey RB, Federle MP (1988) The collapsed inferior vena cava: CT evidence of hypovolemia. AJR Am J Roentgenol 150:431–432

Jeong YK, Ha HK, Yoon CH et al (1997) Gastrointestinal involvement in Henoch–Schönlein syndrome: CT findings. AJR Am J Roentgenol 168:965–968

Johnson KT, Julsrud PR, Johnson CD (2008) Constrictive pericarditis at abdominal CT: a commonly overlooked diagnosis. Abdom Imaging 33:349–352

Jones IT, Fazio VW (1989) Colonic volvulus: etiology and management. Dig Dis 7:203–209

Jones B, Fishman EK, Hamilton SR et al (1986) Submucosal accumulation of fat in inflammatory bowel disease: CT pathologic correlation. J Comput Assist Tomogr 10:759–763

Kane NM, Francis IR, Burney RE, Wheatley MJ, Ellis JH, Korobkin M (1991) Traumatic pneumoperitoneum. Implications of computed tomography diagnosis. Invest Radiol 26:574–578

Karaosmanoglu D, Karcaaltincaba M, Oguz B, Akata D, Ozmen M, Akhan O (2009) CT findings of lymphoma with peritoneal, omental and mesenteric involvement: peritoneal lymphomatosis. Eur J Radiol 71:313–317

Karcaaltincaba M, Haliloglu M, Akpinar E et al (2007) Multidetector CT and MRI findings in periportal space pathologies. Eur J Radiol 61:3–10

Kawamoto S, Horton KM, Fishman EK (1999) Pseudomembranous colitis: spectrum of imaging findings with clinical and pathologic correlation. RadioGraphics 19:887–897

Kawashima A, Sandler CM, Boridy IC, Takahashi N, Benson GS, Goldman SM (1997) Unenhanced helical CT of ureterolithiasis: value of the tissue rim sign. AJR Am J Roentgenol 168:997–1000

Kerry RL, Lee F, Ransom HK (1971) Roentgenologic examination in the diagnosis and treatment of colon volvulus. AJR Am J Roentgenol 113:343–348

Keyting WS, McCarver RR, Kovanik JL, Daywitt AL (1961) Pneumatosis intestinalis: a new concept. Radiology 76:733–741

Khurana B (2003) The whirl sign. Radiology 226:69–70

Killen KL, Mirvis SE, Shanmuganathan K (1999) Helical CT of diaphragmatic rupture caused by blunt trauma. AJR Am J Roentgenol 173:1611–1616

Kim JK, Ha HK, Byun JY et al (2001) CT differentiation of mesenteric ischemia due to vasculitis and thromboembolic disease. J Comput Assist Tomogr 25:604–611

Kleinman PK, Brill PW, Winchester P (1980) Pneumatosis intestinalis. Am J Dis Child 134:1149–1151

Knechtle SJ, Davidoff AM, Rice RP (1990) Pneumatosis Intestinalis: surgical management and clinical outcome. Ann Surg 212:160–165

Ko SF, Lee TY, Cheng TT, Ng SH, Lai HM, Cheng YF et al (1997) CT findings at lupus mesenteric vasculitis. Acta Radiol 38:115–120

Koslin BD, Stanley RJ, Campbell WL, Zakjo AB, Demetris AJ (1988) Hepatic perivascular lymphedema. AJR Am J Roentgenol 150:111–113

Laffargue P, Taourel P, Saguintaah L, Lesnik A (2002) CT diagnosis of abdominal compartment syndrome. AJR Am J Roentgenol 178:771–772

Larici AR, Gotway MB, Litt HI et al (2002) Helical CT with sagittal and coronal reconstructions: accuracy for detection of diaphragmatic injury. AJR Am J Roentgenol 179:451–457

Lawson TL, Thorsen MK, Erickson SJ, Perret RS, Quiroz FA, Foley WD (1993) Periportal halo: a CT sign of liver disease. Abdom Imaging 18:42–46

Lazarus DE, Slywotsky C, Bennett GL, Megibow AJ, Macari M (2004) Frequency and relevance of the small-bowel feces sign on CT in patients with small bowel obstruction. AJR Am J Roentgenol 183:1361–1366

Lee SS, Ha HK, Yang SK et al (2002) CT of prominent pericolic or perienteric vasculature in patients with Crohn's disease: correlation with clinical disease activity and findings on barium studies. AJR Am J Roentgenol 179:1029–1036

Lenchick L, Dovgan DJ, Kier R (1994) CT of the iliopsoas compartment: value in differentiating tumor, abscess and hematomas. AJR Am J Roentgenol 162:83–86

Levin B (1973) Mechanical small bowel obstruction. Semin Roentgenol 8:281–297

Levsky JM, Den EI, Dubrow RA, Wolf EL, Rozenblit AM (2010) CT findings of sigmoid volvulus. AJR Am J Roentgenol 194:136–143

Liebman PR, Patten MT, Manny J, Benfield JR, Hechtman HB (1978) Hepatic-portal venous gas in adults: etiology, pathology and clinical significance. Ann Surg 187:281–287

Lubner M, Menias C, Rucker C, Bhalla S, Peterson CM, Wang L, Gratz B (2007) Blood in the belly: CT findings of hemoperitoneum. RadioGraphics 27:109–125

Macari M, Balthazar EJ (2001) CT of bowel wall thickening: significance and pitfalls of interpretation. AJR Am J Roentgenol 176:1105–1116

Macari M, Balthazar EJ, Megibow AJ (1999) The accordion sign at CT: a non-specific finding in patients with colonic edema. Radiology 211:743–746

Macrander SJ, Lawson TL, Foley DW, Dodds WJ, Erickson SJ, Quiroz FA (1989) Periportal tracking in hepatic trauma: CT features. J Comput Assist Tomogr 13:952–957

Madura MJ, Craig RM, Shields TW (1982) Unusual causes of spontaneous pneumoperitoneum. Surg Gynecol Obstet 154:417–420

Madureira AJ (2004) The comb sign. Radiology 230:783–784

Maglinte DDT, Reyes BL, Harmon BH et al (1996) Reliability and role of plain film radiography and CT in the diagnosis of small-bowel obstruction. AJR Am J Roentgenol 167:1451–1455

Maniatis V, Chryssikopoulos H, Roussakis A et al (2000) Perforation of the alimentary tract: evaluation with computed tomography. Abdom Imaging 25:373–379

Marineck B, Barbier PA, Becker CD, Mettler D, Ruchti C (1986) CT appearances of impaired lymphatic drainage in liver transplant. AJR Am J Roentgenol 147:519–523

Marshak RH, Linder AE, Maklansky D (1977) Pneumatosis cystoides coli. Gastrointest Radiol 2:85–89

Mayo-Smith WW, Wittenberg J, Bennett GL, Gervais DA, Gazelle GS, Mueller PR (1995) The CT small bowel faeces sign: description and clinical relevance. Clin Radiol 50:765–767

Mehard WB, Heiken JP, Sicard GA (1994) High-attenuating crescent in abdominal aortic aneurysm wall at CT: a sign of acute or impending rupture. Radiology 192:359–362

Mellins HZ, Riger LG (1954) The roentgen finding in strangulating obstructions of the small intestine. AJR Am J Roentgenol 74:409–415

Merlin A, Soyer P, Boudiaf M, Hamzi L, Rymer R (2008) Chronic intestinal pseudo-obstruction in adult patients: multidetector row helical CT features. Eur Radiol 18:1587–1595

Messmer JM (1994) Gas and soft tissue abnormalities. In: Gore RM, Levine MS, Laufer I (eds) Textbook of gastrointestinal radiology. Saunders, Philadelphia, pp 175–176

Meyers MA (1994) Dynamic radiology of the abdomen: normal and pathologic anatomy, 4th edn. Springer-Verlag, Berlin, pp 55–57

Meyers MA, McGuire PV (1995) Spiral CT demonstration of hypervascularity in Crohn disease: "vascular jejunization of the ileum" or "the comb sign". Abdom Imaging 20:327–332

Meyers MA, Ghahremani GG, Clement JL Jr, Goodman K (1977) Pneumatosis intestinalis. Gastrointest Radiol 2:91–105

Mindelzun RE, Jeffrey RB Jr, Lane MJ, Silverman PM (1996) The misty mesentery on CT: differential diagnosis. AJR Am J Roentgenol 167:61–65

Mirvis SE, Shanmuganathan K, Erb R (1994) Diffuse small bowel ischemia in hypotensive adults after blunt trauma (shock bowel): CT findings and clinical significance. AJR Am J Roentgenol 163:1375–1379

Miyatani H, Yashida Y (2007) Retroperitoneal perforation caused by endoscopic biopsy in patients with ulcerative colitis and cytomegalovirus infection. Endoscopy 39(1):E246

Moore CJ, Corl FM, Fishman EK (2001) CT of the cecal volvulus. AJR Am J Roentgenol 177:95–98

Morehouse HT, Hochstein JG, Louie W, States L (1992) Pitfalls in the CT diagnosis of ruptured abdominal aortic aneurysms (abstract). Radiology 185:181

Muldowney SM, Balfe DM, Hammerman A, Wick MR (1995) Acute fat deposition in bowel wall submucosa: CT appearance. J Comput Assist Tomogr 19:390–393

Murray JG, Caoili E, Grunden JF, Evans SJJ, Halvorsen RA Jr, Mackersie RC (1996) Acute rupture of the diaphragm due to blunt trauma: diagnostic sensitivity and specificity. AJR Am J Roentgenol 166:1035–1039

Nakagawa Y, Masuda M, Shiihara H et al (1990) A chronic contained rupture of an abdominal aortic aneurysm complicated with severe back pain. Ann Vasc Surg 4:189–192

Nevitt PC (2000) The string of pearls sign. Radiology 214:157–158

Nghiem HV, Jeffrey RB Jr, Mindelzun RE (1993) CT of blunt trauma to the bowel and mesentery. AJR Am J Roentgenol 160:53–58

O'Sullivan SG (1998) The accordion sign. Radiology 206:177–178

Ormsby EL, Duffield C, Ostovar-Sirjani F, McGahan JP, Troppmann C (2007) Colonoscopy findings in end-stage liver disease patients with incidental CT colonic wall thickening. AJR Am J Roentgenol 189:1112–1117

Orwig D, Federle MP (1989) Localized clotted blood as evidence of visceral trauma on CT: the sentinel clot sign. AJR Am J Roentgenol 153:747–749

Patel A, Lall CG, Jennings SG, Sandrasegaran K (2007) Abdominal compartment syndrome. AJR Am J Roentgenol 189:1037–1043

Pereira JM, Sirlin CB, Pinto PS, Jeffrey RB, Stella DL, Casola G (2004) Disproportionate fat stranding: a helpful CT sign in patients with acute abdominal pain. RadioGraphics 24:703–715

Perrone L, Piacentini F, Minordi LM, Vecchioloi A (2005) Pneumomediastinum and abdominal pain: which correlation? Rays 30:63–69

Petrovic B, Nikalaidis P, Hammond NA, Grant TH, Miller FH (2006) Identification of adhesions on CT in small bowel obstruction. Emerg Radiol 12:88–93

Philpotts LE, Heiken JP, Westcott MA, Gore RM (1994) Colitis: use of CT findings in differential diagnosis. Radiology 190:445–449

Pickhardt PJ, Shimony JS, Heiken JP, Buchman TG, Fisher AJ (1999) The abdominal compartment syndrome: CT findings. AJR Am J Roentgenol 173:575–579

Power N, Atri M, Ryan S, Haddad R, Smith A (2007) CT assessment of anastomotic bowel leak. Clin Radiol 62:37–42

Pun E, Firkin A (2004) Computed tomography and complicated peptic ulcer disease. Australas Radiol 48:516–519

Puylaert JB (1992) Right-sided segmental infarction of the omentum: clinical, US and CT findings. Radiology 185:169–172

Rao PM, Wittenberg J, Lawrason JN (1997) Primary epiploic appendagitis: evolutionary changes in CT appearance. Radiology 204:713–717

Rha SF, Ha HK, Lee SH et al (2000) CT and MR findings of bowel ischemia from various primary causes. RadioGraphics 20:29–42

Riger LG (1944) Roentgen diagnosis of acute abdominal conditions. Bull Univ Minn Hosp 116:120–137

Ros PR, Bluetow PC, Pantograg-Brown L, Forsmark CE, Sobin LH (1996) Pseudmembranous colitis. Radiology 198:1–9

Rosenthal D, Clark MD, Stanton PE, Lamis PA (1986) Chronic contained ruptured abdominal aortic aneurysm: is it real? J Cardiovasc Surg 27:723–725

Rudloff U (2005) The spoke wheel sign: bowel. Radiology 237:1046–1047

Saku M, Yoshimitsu K, Murakami I et al (2006) Small bowel perforation resulting from blunt abdominal trauma: interval change of radiological characteristics. Radiat Med 24:358–364

Schulze CG, Blum U, Haag K (1995) Hepatic portal venous gas: imaging modalities and clinical significance. Acta Radiol 36:377–380

Schwartz SA, Taljanovic MS, Smyth S, O'Brien MJ, Rogers LF (2007) CT findings of rupture, impending rupture and contained rupture of abdominal aortic aneurysms. AJR Am J Roentgenol 188:57–62

Sebastia C, Quiroga S, Espin E, Boye R, Alvarez-Castells A, Armengol M (2000) Portomesenteric vein gas: pathologic mechanism. RadioGraphics 20:1213–1226

Seo BK, Ha HK, Kim AY et al (2003) Segmental misty mesentery: analysis of CT features and primary causes. Radiology 226:86–94

Shanmuganathan K, Mirvis SE (1998) CT evaluation of blunt hepatic trauma. Radiol Clin North Am 36:399–411

Shanmuganathan K, Mirvis SE, Amoroso M (1993) Periportal low density on CT in patients with blunt trauma: association with elevated venous pressure. AJR Am J Roentgenol 160:279–283

Shariatzadeh AN, Bolivar JC (1973) Transient incompetence of the sphincter of Oddi with pneumobilia: a case report. Am Surg 39:406–409

Sherman SC, Tran H (2006) Pneumobilia: benign or life-threatening. J Emerg Med 30:147–153

Shimono T, Nishimura K, Hayakawa K (1998) CT imaging of biliary enteric fistula. Abdom Imaging 23:172–176

Shinn SS, Jeong YY, Chung TW et al (2007) The sentinel clot sign: a useful CT finding for the evaluation of intraperitoneal bladder rupture following blunt trauma. Korean J Radiol 8:492–497

Siegel CL, Cohan RH (1994) CT of abdominal aortic aneurysms. AJR Am J Roentgenol 163:17–29

Silverman PM, Baker ME, Cooper C, Kelvin FM (1987) Computed tomography of mesenteric disease. Radio-Graphics 7:309–320

Smith RC, Rosenfield AT, Choe KA et al (1995) Acute flank pain: comparison of non-contrast-enhanced CT and intravenous urography. Radiology 194:789–794

Smith RC, Verga M, McCarthy S, Rosenfield AT (1996) Diagnosis of acute flank pain: value of unenhanced CT. AJR Am J Roentgenol 166:97–101

Sorbello MP, Utiyama EM, Parreira JG, Birolini D, Rasslan S (2007) Spontaneous intramural small bowel hematoma induced by anticoagulant therapy: review and case report. Clinics 62:785–790

Soyer P, Martin-Grivaud S, Boudiaf M et al (2008) Linear or bubbly: a pictorial review of CT features of intestinal pneumatosis in adults. J Radiol 89:1907–1920

Stallard DJ, Tu RK, Gould MJ, Pozniak MA, Pettersen JC (1994) Minor vascular anatomy of the abdomen and the pelvis: a CT atlas. RadioGraphics 14:493–513

Stein MG, Crues JV 3rd, Hamlin JA (1983) Portal venous air with barium enema. AJR Am J Roentgenol 140: 1171–1172

Stevens SD, Heiken JP, Brunt E, Hanto DW, Flye MW (1991) Low-attenuation periportal collar in transplanted liver is not reliable CT evidence of acute allograft rejection. AJR Am J Roentgenol 157:1195–1198

Stroud WH, Cullom JW, Anderson MC (1981) Hemorrhagic complications of severe pancreatitis. Surgery 90: 657–665

Taourel PG, Deneuvielle M, Pradel JA, Regent D, Bruel JM (1996) Acute mesenteric ischemia: diagnosis with contrast-enhanced CT. Radiology 199:623–626

Taylor GA, Fallat ME, Eichelberger MR (1987) Hypovolemic shock in children: abdominal CT manifestations. Radiology 164:479–481

Torres GM, Abbitt PL, Weeks M (1994) CT manifestations of infarcted epiploic appendages of the colon. Abdom Imaging 19:449–450

Torricelli P, Coriani C, Marchetti M, Rossi A, Manenti A (2001) Spontaneous rupture of the spleen: report of two cases. Abdom Imaging 26:290–293

Tsai JA, Calissendorff B, Hanczewski R, Permert J (2000) Hepatic portal venous gas and small bowel obstruction with no signs of intestinal gangrene after appendicectomy. Eur J Surg 166:826–827

Van Bresla Vriesman AC, Lohle PN, Coerkamp EG, Puylaert JB (1999) Infarction of omentum and epiploic appendage: diagnosis, epidemiology and natural history. Eur Radiol 9:1886–1892

Van Dyck P, Vanhoenacker P, D'Haenens P (2001) Acute emphysematous cholecystitis. JBR-BTR 84:77

Venkatesh SK, Wan JM (2008) CT of blunt pancreatic trauma: a pictorial essay. Eur J Radiol 67:311

Waraich NG, Hudson JS, Iftikhar SY (2007) Vibrator-induced fatal rectal perforation. N Z Med J 120:U2685

Wechsler RJ, Munoz SJ, Needeleman L et al (1987) The periportal collar sign: a CT sign of liver transplant rejection. Radiology 165:57–60

White EM, Ankenbrandt WJ, Gore RM, Gharemani GG, Golan JF (1992) CT manifestations of ruptured abdominal aortic aneurysms (abstract). Radiology 185:359

Wiesner W, Mortele KJ, Glickman JN, Hoon J, Ros P (2001) Pneumatosis intestinalis and portomesenteric venous gas in intestinal ischemia: correlation of CT findings with severity of ischemia and clinical course. AJR Am J Roentgenol 177:1319–1323

Wittenberg J, Harisinghani MG, Jhaveri K, Varghese J, Mueller PR (2002) Algorithmic approach to CT diagnosis of the abnormal bowel wall. RadioGraphics 22:1093–1109

Wu JM, Wang MY (2009) Hepatic portal venous gas in necrotizing pancreatitis. Dig Surg 26:119–120

Yagan N, Auh YH, Fisher A (2009) Extension of air into the right perirenal space after duodenal perforation: CT findings. Radiology 250:740–748

Yao DC, Jeffrey RB, Mirvis SE et al (2002) Using contrast-enhanced helical CT to visualize arterial extravasation after blunt abdominal trauma: incidence and organ distribution. AJR Am J Roentgenol 178:17–20

Yen C, Chen J, Tui C, Chou Y, Lee C, Chang C, Yu C (2005) Internal hernia: computed tomography diagnosis and differentiation from adhesive small bowel obstruction. J Chin Med Assoc 68(1):21–28

Yoon W, Jeong YY, Kim JK (2006) Acute gastrointestinal bleeding: contrast-enhanced MDCT. Abdom Imaging 31:1–8

Young WS, Engelbrecht HE, Stroker A (1978) A plain film analysis in sigmoid volvulus. Clin Radiol 29:553–560

Zissin R (2000) The significance of a positive round belly sign on CT. AJR Am J Roentgenol 175:267–268

Part III

CT Techniques

Volume CT of Acute Abdomen: Acquisition and Reconstruction Techniques

Samuel Mérigeaud, Ingrid Millet, Fernanda Curros-Doyon, and Patrice Taourel

Contents

1	**Introduction**	65
2	**CT Acquisition Protocols**	66
2.1	Patient Setting	66
2.2	Acquisition Parameters	66
2.3	Non-enhanced CT (NECT)	66
2.4	Intravenous Opacification	67
2.5	Intestinal Lumen Opacification	67
2.6	Focused CT	68
3	**Thin Slice Review**	68
4	**Multiplanar Reformatting**	69
5	**Average Intensity Projection and Ray Sum**	70
6	**Maximum Intensity Projection**	71
7	**Minimum Intensity Projection**	72
8	**3D Reconstructions**	73
8.1	Shaded Surface Display	73
8.2	Volume Rendering	73
8.3	Virtual Endoscopy	74
8.4	Segmentation	74
8.5	Utility of 3D in CT of Acute Abdomen	76
9	**Conclusion**	78
References		78

S. Mérigeaud (✉)
Hôpital Lapeyronie,
371 Avenue du Docteur Gaston Giraud,
34000 Montpellier, France
e-mail: s-merigeaud@chu-montpellier.fr

I. Millet · F. Curros-Doyon · P. Taourel
Department of Imaging,
CHU Montpellier, Hospital Lapeyronie,
371 Avenue du Doyen Gaston-Giraud,
34295 Montpellier Cedex 5, France

Abstract

Along with the development of MDCT, the rapidity of volumic acquisition over the entire abdomen and pelvis has allowed to tailor acquisition protocols to diagnosis indications and etiologic hypotheses of acute abdomen. Furthermore, advances in computer technology (hardware and software) have allowed fast post processing of large volume of data over extended areas using reconstruction algorithms. This chapter is thus aimed at detailing each steps from CT data acquisition to volumetric reconstruction techniques and their practical applications in CT studies of the acute abdomen.

1 Introduction

The development of multidetector computed tomography (MDCT) has revolutionized radiologic explorations, including acute abdomen studies, by introducing real three-dimensional (3D) imaging. For many years, scanner interpretation has been limited to axial examination, of up to 1-cm thick sections. The former MDCTs have allowed to start refining axial sections and developing multiplanar reformation and 3D of variable quality (one may remember 'stairs' impairing coronal or sagittal sections in the early 90s). Currently, the acquisition of large volumes in shorter duration, a good spatial resolution in all 3D and the obtention of isotropic voxels constitute a precise databank for different volumetric rendering techniques. Computed hardware and software have progressed over the last few years, allowing faster and

P. Taourel (ed.), *CT of the Acute Abdomen*, Medical Radiology. Diagnostic Imaging,
DOI: 10.1007/174_2011_162, © Springer-Verlag Berlin Heidelberg 2011

more ergonomic processing of large volume of data generated by MDCT. Most manufacturers offer consoles that try in integrating these different image processing for routine utilization. However, many radiologists still consider that 3D reconstructions may increase the complexity and interpretation time of a scan examination, which may account for the slow spreading of some of these reconstruction techniques. This chapter is thus aimed at detailing each CT volumetric reconstruction techniques and their practical applications in CT studies of the acute abdomen.

2 CT Acquisition Protocols

2.1 Patient Setting

The patient admission must be reassuring. His level of consciousness permitting, the different steps in CT examination must be clearly explained to him to improve the quality of acquisition, such as avoiding artifacts from kinetic fuzziness related to inopportune movement frequent in algesic patients.

A short and accurate interview must investigate the main contraindications to the use of X-rays (pregnancy) and intravenous iodinated contrast material (allergy, kidney failure, myeloma...). Indeed, in the emergency setting, management may be precipitated and a complete interview may not always be done before admission to the imaging department. If a contraindication arises then, the utility and type of imaging protocol must be discussed with the referring physician, without delaying management of the patient. In some cases, the benefit to risk ratio will lead to perform a scan with injection, despite a theoretical formal contraindication. Knowing whether the patient is treated with certain drugs that require some caution, such as biguanides or beta-blockers may be useful. Biguanide intake must be discontinued the same day and resumed after 48 h, eventually after checking for renal function. Beta-blockers intake should not be discontinued, but it must be known, as it requires increased doses of adrenaline in case of cardiac arrest resuscitation. Fasting may be difficult to observe in emergency conditions and should not delay CT scanning in any cases.

Following the interview, the patient is laid down in dorsal decubitus, with the arms up above the head when possible, to avoid artifacts from beam hardening impairing the reading of hepatic and splenic parenchyma (Delabrousse 2009).

2.2 Acquisition Parameters

A preliminary topogram (scout view) is performed in the anterior and often lateral views. It allows in plotting the anatomic landmarks to set the acquisition boxes at the area to explore. The field of view (FOV) is thus tailored to the patient's outline to allow optimal image reconstruction using a 512×512 scan matrix.

The constants (kV, mAs), preset in the manufacturer acquisition protocols must be sometimes modulated, such as with obese subjects requiring higher energy rays than young and lean subjects.

The collimation may be millimetric, more rarely sub-millimetric, with reconstructions in millimetric axial sections directly available for postprocessing on interpretation console.

2.3 Non-enhanced CT (NECT)

Non-enhanced CT is a fast and simple examination to perform. In non-traumatic acute abdomen, it can be performed in the setting of urolithiasis exploration or when a formal contraindication to iodinated contrast material exists. It can also be performed as the first step of a CT examination with intravenous iodinated contrast material (for example to investigate spontaneous bowel hematomas that are often seen in the setting of underlying coagulopathy (Lane et al. 1997)).

Most of the time, NECT must be performed using a low-dose technique allowing to reduce radiation exposure to the patient. However, the challenge is not to deteriorate the image, with the risk of misdiagnosis due to a decreased signal-to-noise ratio, especially in obese patients. New acquisition algorithms, such as ASIR (Adaptive Statistical Iterative Reconstruction, General Electric Healthcare, Milwaukee, WI, USA) allow in further reduce the doses to 20–80%, while eliminating the noise with no loss of image quality (Kambadakone et al. 2010).

In elderly patients, in whom biliary lithiasis is frequent, the low-dose technique must not be used to help detect low density lithiases within the bile duct.

Volume CT of Acute Abdomen

Table 1 CT acquisition protocols based on the diagnostic hypotheses in non-traumatic acute abdomen

CT techniques	Indications
Low-dose NECT	Acute renal colic
NECT + portal phase	Acute pancreatic and biliary system pathologies
NECT + arterial + portal phases	Acute abdominal pain with coagulopathy (spontaneous bowel hematomas)
Arterial + portal phases (±delayed phase at 3 min)	Abdominal aortic aneurysm rupture
	Acute abdominal hemorrhage
	Mesenteric ischemia
	Renal infarction
Portal Phase alone	Most of the indications:
	Non-specific abdominal pain
	Acute appendicitis
	Diverticulitis
	Bowel obstruction
	Peptic ulcer disease
	…
Portal + delayed phases	Urinary tract diseases (acute pyelonephritis)
	Characterization of a tumor found by chance on portal phase

One recent advance is dual energy technique, notably applied to characterization of urolithiasis: when a calculus is localized on a standard low-dose NECT, a targeted acquisition with dual energy (80/140 kV) is performed over the anatomical area containing the calculus. Post-processing softwares further permit in differentiating calculi based on their composition (uric acid, cystine and calcified stones) more accurately than with simple measurement of their density, which allow the therapy to be adapted (Hidas et al. 2010).

2.4 Intravenous Opacification

In the absence of contraindication to iodinated contrast material and besides renal colic evaluation, the majority of scanners indicated for non-traumatic abdominal pain are performed with intravenous opacification (Table 1). Indeed, opacification allows better evaluation of the vascular lumen, intestinal walls and parenchyma of intraabdominal organ (Urban and Fishman 2000a).

Most often, for example, in case of non-specific abdominal pain, or suspected acute appendicitis or diverticulitis, only one acquisition on portal phase is required to establish a diagnosis or to seek complications (acquisition starting 70 s after injection at a 1.5 mL/kg to 2.5 mL/s rate).

In some cases, especially in case of suspected mesenteric ischemia or intraabdominal hemorrhage (Ernst et al. 2003), an acquisition on arterial phase must be planned. It must be performed using fast intravenous injection (at least 3 mL/s), through a good quality venous line, eventually using contrast media with high iodine concentration (400 mg/mL) (Jaeckle et al. 2008a). The acquisition phase is started 20–30 s after the injection or using a bolus tracking technique.

A delayed acquisition may be performed, either after 10 min in studies of the urinary cavity lumen, or earlier after 3–4 min in studies aiming at
- characterizing a tumor-like lesion found by chance.
- confirm active leaking of intraabdominal bleeding only seen on portal phase (extravasation of contrast material, whose extent varies between acquisition phases).

2.5 Intestinal Lumen Opacification

Numerous protocols, including oral or intravenous intestinal opacification have been described in patients presenting with non-traumatic acute abdomen, in particular for evaluation of suspected acute appendicitis (Johnson et al. 2006; Kaewlai and Nazinitsky 2007; Thoeni and Cello 2006). Some authors even recommend enteroclysis opacification (Gollub 2005). However, recent studies have suggested that oral opacification might not be necessary in acute abdomen (Anderson et al. 2009; Lee et al. 2006b; Mun et al. 2006), as it presents certain risk and disadvantages. Indeed, the patient has to ingest the recommended 800–1,000 mL of contrast material (Pinto Leite et al. 2005). This can be an issue in a patient presenting with abdominal symptoms associated with nausea and vomiting, or in the elderly (with a risk of inhalation). Does performing the opacification justify the need for a nasogastric probe to be placed? The cost of examination and the side effects related to contrast material are increased. Last, the duration of examination is increased, as a 1–2 h time interval is required for the contrast material to reach the cecum, which could seem long in an emergency setting (Huynh et al. 2004).

Colorectal opacification and distension can be obtained by rectal administration of 800–1,000 mL of water or diluted contrast material (Macari and Balthazar 2003; Rao et al. 1997; Urban and Fishman 2000b) for evaluation of suspected acute appendicitis or diverticulitis. This technique is faster than oral opacification (around 15 min). However, it requires a logistic organization and involves non-negligible discomfort to the patient. Furthermore, cecal opacification is inconstant and contraindication exists in patients presenting with neutropenia or with peritoneal or perforation signs (Pinto Leite et al. 2005). It has been shown that one can do without this technique, with no loss of diagnostic efficacy in acute appendicitis (Dearing et al. 2008) and can be reserved for the occasional patient with equivocal findings in acute diverticulitis (Urban and Fishman 2000a).

2.6 Focused CT

In acute abdomen, the interest of only focussing CT acquisition on a part of the abdomen has been investigated in acute appendicitis and is discussed in the corresponding chapter of this book.

3 Thin Slice Review

The first step in scan interpretation is reading axial slices. The advent of multidetector row CT scanners has allowed routine acquisitions of large volume with millimetric and sub-millimetric collimations. However, axial reconstructions of thickness similar to the 5-mm collimation recommended few years ago for single detector row CT scanners are still in use (Johnson et al. 2006; Weltman et al. 2000). Nevertheless, small structures, such as the normal appendix may not be greater than 3 mm in diameter, which requires the use of reconstructed slices of <5 mm thickness for accurate detection (Fig. 1). The value of thin slices has been demonstrated by Johnson et al. (2009b). According to their analysis of 212 scanners with thinner and thinner axial reconstructed slices (5, 3 and 2 mm thick), thinner reconstruction would significantly improve the visualization rate of the appendix (79, 86 and 89%, respectively) and the confidence regarding the presence or absence of signs of acute appendicitis (mean sensitivities were 79.4, 82.4, and 82.4% for 5, 3, and 2 mm, respectively; specificities were 99.2, 98.7, and 98.2%). According to Ketelslegers et al. thin slices improve the detection and characterization of urinary calculi (Ketelslegers and Van Beers 2006). Similarly, it can help in distinguishing small distal ureteral calculi from pelvic phleboliths (Arac et al. 2005). In our department, we have shown the diagnostic value of thin slices in direct visualization of perforation sites in patients with a non-traumatic free pneumoperitoneum (Ghekiere et al. 2007).

Better findings in the use of thinner transversal slices are due to the partial volume effect resulting from the use of thick slices over small structures, in particular when they show not much contrast: the voxels are averaged, which render such structures more challenging to detect.

The two major drawbacks in the use of thinner reconstruction sections are, on one hand, a higher number of images to visualize and on the other hand an increased image noise. To counter the noise without increasing the radiation doses, some advocate reading thin slices with sliding slab ray—sum technique, which is available on many CT workstations (Seo et al. 2009).

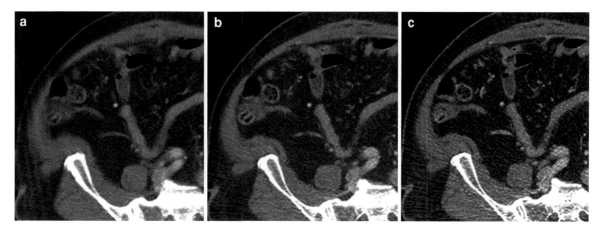

Fig. 1 Value of thin axial sections. Reconstructions in axial sections of decreasing thickness: a 10 mm, b 3 mm and c 1.25 mm, centered on the appendix. Details of the appendiceal wall and vessels are hardly visible in a while clearly better seen in b and c. In contrast, the noise increases from a to c, while the image is less and less smooth

4 Multiplanar Reformatting

Volume data generated by MDCT scanner can be represented by a cube constituted from sub-elements called voxels (by similarity with 2D image pixels). Isotropy means that voxels are of equal dimensions in all three spatial axes (x, y, z). The 16 and 64 MDCT currently available achieve sub-millimetric isotropic voxels in only one acquisition over the entire abdomen and pelvis. These data may then be analyzed in multi-planar reconstruction (MPR), with a spatial resolution close to that of axial reconstructions. Current consoles enable fast treatment of MPR data, with no waste of time for the physician. Coronal, sagittal or oblique sections can be easily generated (Fig. 2). Of all planes, coronal reconstructions appear as the most useful in evaluation of non-traumatic acute abdominal pain, such as for the diagnosis of a normal appendix (Jan et al. 2005), acute appendicitis, as well as for pitfalls and differential diagnoses of acute appendicitis (Kim et al. 2008; Lee et al. 2006a; Neville and Paulson 2009; Paulson et al. 2005), including in pediatric patients (Kim et al. 2009). Jaffe et al. (2006) have reported similar diagnostic value for coronal reformatted images in small-bowel obstruction. We have shown the added diagnostic value of coronal and sagittal reformations in direct visualization of perforation sites in patients with a non-traumatic-free pneumoperitoneum (Ghekiere et al. 2007).

Curved plane reconstructions (or curved MPR) are a variation of MPR. Instead of using a plane in a standard direction (axial, coronal, sagittal, oblique or double-oblique), the user draws a curve along the course of a structure, such as a vessel. All voxels localized within the plane of the curve are displayed on only one 2D image (the entire vessel is thereby displayed, even if its course is complicated). By changing the viewpoint around the curve initially drawn, one can rotate the curve plane on 360° (and see for example the vessel walls in all directions).

The main applications of curved MPR concern tubular structures, arteries in particular, as well as ureters or bowel (Sun 2006). Some stations include specific applications (such as Advantage Vessel Analysis (AVA), Advantage Workstation Volume Share 4, General Electric Healthcare, Milwaukee, WI, USA) allowing extraction of the lumen of a blood vessel in two clicks and obtention of a curvilinear and 3D image. It is then easy to detect, characterize and even quantify any abnormality of the vascular wall on curved plane reconstructions: beginning and end of a stenosis, percentage of maximal stenosis (in diameter and surface).

In another setting, Nino-Murcia et al. have shown that curved MPR allowed better characterization of dilations of the bile duct and pancreas system, for example by demonstrating the presence of a pancreas divisum responsible of an acute pancreatitis (Nino-Murcia et al. 2001). Other authors also propose to use curved MPR for improved detection of acute appendicitis (Stabile Ianora et al. 2010) or characterization of the site and cause of small-bowel obstruction (Aufort et al. 2005).

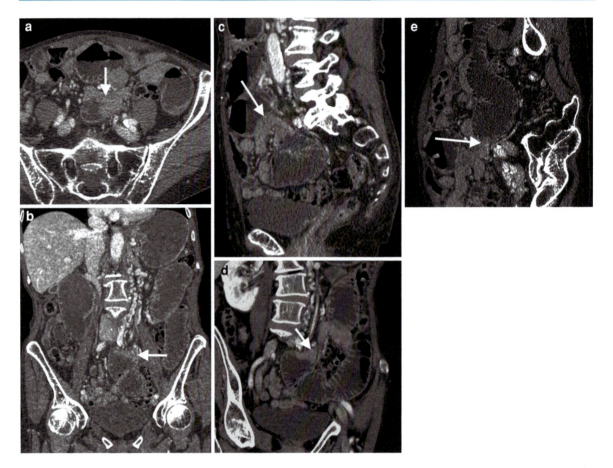

Fig. 2 Value of MPR reconstructions in CT of acute abdomen. Images seen in axial section (**a**), coronal (**b**), sagittal (**c**), oblique (**d**) and curved MPR (**e**) showing the transition area (*white arrow*) of an acute bowel obstruction by a band. Although axial and coronal sections are generally considered as more valuable, sagittal and oblique sections may prove useful, as in this case, whereby the transition level is best seen. Curved MPR images, more time consuming, mostly have iconographic value

Whichever the plane used for MPR, it is also possible to increase the slice thickness by using several types of projection algorithms (Fig. 3) such as average intensity projection (AIP), ray sum, maximum intensity projection (MIP), minimum intensity projection (MinIP) and volume rendering (VR).

5 Average Intensity Projection and Ray Sum

The average intensity projection is a reconstruction algorithm allowing in displaying the average attenuation value of voxels on a given thickness, for any MPR slice in a given plane. This results in a thick slice whose aspect is close to that of the thick axial slices often first reconstructed in most examinations. The usefulness, when compared with thin slices is to reduce the noise and enhance the contrast, while increasing artifacts from partial volume.

Another algorithm, Ray sum, consists in summing up the attenuation value of each voxel projecting on a given plane.

When thin slices are used, the appearance remains close to that of AIP, and would be useful in detecting anomalies of the appendix, for example (Seo et al. 2009). In contrast, the use of Ray sum on larger volumes lead to images close to conventional radiography (Dalrymple et al. 2005), which is expected as radiography produces images by summing up X-rays more or less attenuated through the targeted object. This may be valuable if one wanted to confirm the

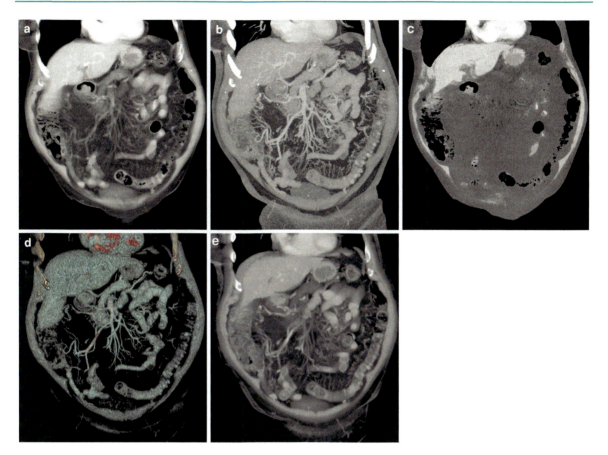

Fig. 3 Thick coronal sections using different reconstruction algorithms: **a** average intensity projection (AIP), **b** MIP, **c** MinIP and volume rendering using two different settings (**d, e**). MIP enables better view of dense structures, such as vessels, including smaller ones, such as in the meso (**b**). Structures filled with air better stand out in MinIP (**c**). Anatomical relationships between vessels and adjacent organs are best displayed in VR (**d, e**) than in MIP (**c**). In contrast, small vessels are best seen in MIP, with variable results in VR depending on the settings (**d, e**)

possibility to locate a calculus on a plain abdominal radiography without the need to actually perform the radiography, before proposing an extracorporeal lithotripsy, in the treatment of a renal colic first diagnosed on MDCT.

6 Maximum Intensity Projection

The MIP algorithm plots a ray perpendicular to the plane studied that crosses continuous slices in this plane. Of all voxels passed through, only the one with the highest density will be displayed. All denser structures in a given volume would be thus displayed on only one 2D image, irrespective of their location within the thickness of this volume (Parrish 2007; Perandini et al. 2010).

MIP is thus by definition tailored to representation of dense objects that strongly differentiate from adjacent tissues of lower density, whether these objects are spontaneously dense, such as lithiasis, calcifications, surgical clips or stercolith, or opacified structures, such as for CT angiography or urography. This algorithm is fast and simple to use. In studies of the urinary tract, coronal MIP allows in fast description of the morphology of the urinary tree, as well as of the location and shape of an eventual calculus before percutaneous treatment (Patel et al. 2009). However, it is in vascular studies that MIP is the most valuable for acute abdominal pathology (Fig. 4), by allowing straightforward and fast mapping of blood vessels (Duran et al. 2009; Wildermuth et al. 2005), both at the artery level in the setting of bleeding or ischemia, and at the vein level in the setting of portal hypertension.

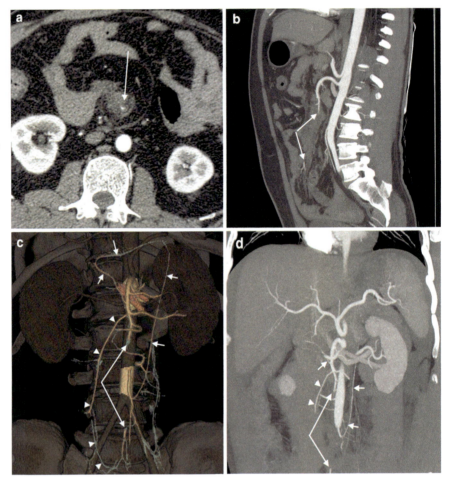

Fig. 4 Traumatic dissection with occlusion of superior mesenteric artery (SMA) (*big arrows*) in axial (**a**) and sagittal oblique thin MIP (**b**) reconstructions. The anastomosis between the SMA proximal and distal segments (*arrowheads*) as well as the Riolan arcade (*little arrows*) are much better depicted on a segmented VR image (**c**) than on a coronal MIP reconstruction (**d**)

Understanding MIP limitations is crucial for proper image interpreting. First of all, the presence of attenuating structures next to blood vessels can impair blood vessel analysis. Attenuating structures, such as bones may be deleted from the volume for better visualization of arteries (with the risk to loose some artery volume if the artery is in contact to the bone), using certain softwares. In case of atheromatous calcifications, studies of the arterial lumen become challenging and an eventual stenosis can prove difficult to depict. To minimize this disadvantages, sliding thin-slab MIP reconstructions may be used which might be more efficient than thicker slices in analysis of vascular lumen (Ertl-Wagner et al. 2006; Kim et al. 2004) and characterization of acute gastrointestinal bleedings (Jaeckle et al. 2008a). Finally, anatomical relationships between displayed structures are not easy to assess due to the absence of shades or 3D landmarks on images (Calhoun et al. 1999; Fishman et al. 2006). This can be partially overcome by generating a series of MIP images, each obtained from a viewpoint different from one to another around the object, thereby creating the illusion of volume rotation, useful in studies of complex vascular structures (Perandini et al. 2010).

MIP is a fast and straightforward technique to use provided that its limitations and how to overcome them are known. MIP is recommended at first intention, especially in studies of the arteries, before to eventually switch to VR as a complementary visualization method.

7 Minimum Intensity Projection

In contrast to MIP, the MinIP algorithm that projects voxels with the lowest density on a 2D image. This allows to preferentially represent hypodense

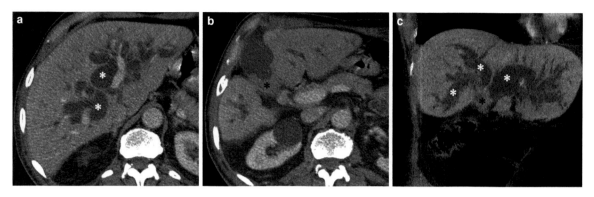

Fig. 5 Value of MinIP in obstructive pathologies of the bile duct. Axial sections (**a**, **b**) and oblique coronal MinIP (**c**) show a dilation of the intra hepatic biliary ducts (*white asterisk*) upper from an obstruction by a vesicular adenocarcinoma (*black asterisk*)

structures of a given acquisition volume. MinIP is not used commonly, except for representation of the central airways or areas of air trapping within the lungs (emphysema).

In acute abdomen, MinIP may be used to analyze the bile tree and pancreatic duct. Rao et al. (2005) described how they used computed tomography cholangiography in gallbladder carcinoma patients with obstructive jaundice. On thick coronal slabs of the portal vein phase (without the administration of biliary contrast media), they segmented manually the liver and all the visible bile ducts, trying to remove unwanted structures of low attenuation (fat and air) before to apply MinIP algorithm. This method is time consuming (from 15 to 40 min) and does not seem to give more information than 2D images, but it is useful in depicting the 3D anatomy of the biliary system. Therefore, another method, rapid and simple, is to use thin sliding slabs in a coronal or oblique plane, centered on the biliary system, with MinIP algorithm (Kamel et al. 2005) that can depict the site and cause of biliary obstruction (Johnson et al. 2003) (Fig. 5).

8 3D Reconstructions

Several methods allow 3D reconstructions of data generated by a scanner. The former, called shaded surface display (SSD), is progressively replaced by the volume rendering (VR) technique, which offers numerous advantages over SSD, as well as over other techniques including MIP. VR allows to perform quality virtual endoscopy (VE). By segmenting an object or anatomical structure, it is possible to calculate its volume or represent it in its anatomical relationships with the whole acquired volume using the various settings available on most consoles.

8.1 Shaded Surface Display

Shaded Surface Display, also called surface rendering, is a reconstruction algorithm allowing to only represent the surface of an object in 3D. In a first step, the object is segmented: voxels that correspond to the object of interest are selected (see Sect. 8.4. Segmentation). Most often, SSD segmentation is done using a threshold density value: only those values above the threshold are selected, while voxels of inferior value are not. The surface of the object thus defined is then represented in perspective by simulating shadows and light reflection effects using a virtual light source that intensifies the illusion of image relief and depth.

8.2 Volume Rendering

The VR technique is the 3D reconstruction technique that develops the most currently, as it offers wider possibilities over SSD or MIP. This development is possible due to the recent advances in computing power in recent computer hardware. Unlike other techniques that select voxels represented by their densities, all voxels of a same volume will contribute to the VRT image, independently from their densities: the

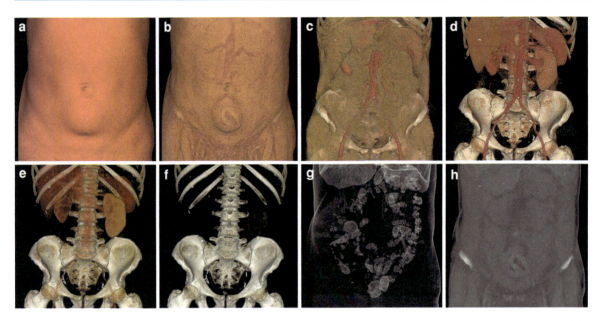

Fig. 6 Volume rendering. Using only one acquisition and by changing the settings thresholds of the voxels shown on the histogram, several images can be obtained showing the different anatomical structures from the skin to the bones (**a–f**). Other settings enable better view of the structures filled with air (**g**), of the muscular wall of the abdomen (a subumbilical parietal hernia is shown here) (**h**)

entire Hounsfield scale can be represented. This technique assigns a value of opacity ranging from 0% (total transparency) to 100% (total opacity) to each voxel along a virtual line directed in the observer viewpoint. The opacity value as well as the color are selected according to the density of each voxel and using an algorithm set for the type of tissue to be represented. This enables the display of a large variety of tissue structures of variable density in only one volume, from skin to bones (Fig. 6) and this avoids MIP overlays (Fig. 7). Gray scale shading is also used to enhance the 3D effect by adding surface reflections and projected shadows from a computed virtual light source.

8.3 Virtual Endoscopy

Virtual Endoscopy also called perspective volume rendering (pVR), is a special type of volume rendering (VRT), mainly used to make endoscopic views of hollow organs filled with air (paranasal sinuses, pharynx, larynx, bronchial tree, colon) or opacified fluids (arteries, veins, ureters, small-bowel lumen…). The course of a virtual endoscope through the cavity can be simulated ("fly through") and displayed either as successive images visible on a PACS system, or as a video animation (format:".avi"). The most developed indication to date is virtual colonoscopy.

8.4 Segmentation

Segmentation is the operation allowing to select a desired object within a volume, to better visualize it on 3D or to measure its volume (Fig. 8). Tools to help including or excluding the desired object voxels that are more or less accurate, either automated, semi-automated or not, are offered by certain manufacturers.

The simplest and fastest method is to only select within a given volume those voxels whose density ranges between two threshold values. This is easy for high density voxels (bones, calcifications or opacified structures including vessels, urinary or digestive tract) and low density voxels (airways, cutaneous surface). This operation can be automated in certain applications. In contrast, it is more difficult to segment structures of close densities, including internal organs, such as the liver, spleen, nodes, or muscles, using this method.

Fig. 7 Value of MIP and VR in acute vascular pathology of the abdomen. Right kidney ischemia over occlusive dissection of the right renal artery (*white arrow*) in axial (**a**) and sagittal (**b**) sections. Oblique coronal section in MIP (**c**) enables fast display of anatomical relationships between the proximal pre-occlusive part of this artery and a superior polar artery (*arrowhead*). VR (**d**) further improves studies of these relationships by avoiding MIP overlays and by visualizing on the same image the superior polar parenchyma, still vascularized (*asterisk*)

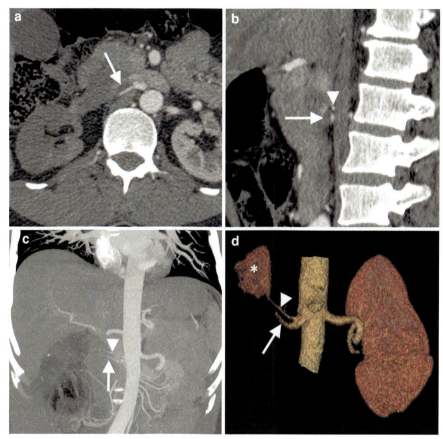

Another simple method is to define a region-of-interest (ROI) by plotting a rectangle, ellipse or any other shape centered on the studied object with a virtual scalpel that can be used on 2D MPR images or on 3D images.

The "paintbrush" tool allows in highlighting the object to isolate on 2D images for subsequent 3D reconstruction. The issue is to plot on every slice, which may require extensive work considering the hundreds of images obtained in current examinations. Growing region tools, like the "magic wand", can be also very useful. By setting the wand over a pixel of one of the 2D MPR images and maintaining the left click down, all neighboring pixels of density close to that of the targeted central pixel (within the range of preset thresholds) will be progressively selected, from one to another as an oil stain. Depending on the softwares, the selection of adjacent pixels can be performed on the only 2D image used, on all three planes systematically or even directly on the 3D image. This tool is very useful for fast segmentation of objects of similar densities, such as vascular structures. It can also be used to isolate a plain or intestinal organ or a foreign body. Indeed selected pixels can be easily checked (subtraction tools are also available). The issue is that this technique can become time consuming when the studied object is of complex shape, with different density voxels or when it is in direct contact to other structures of same density (the tool then cannot differentiate voxels of the studied object from voxels of the neighboring organ). Recently developed algorithms associate shape recognition, which renders this technique easier and faster. Segmenting a tumor within an organ, even with close densities is easy.

A very important notion to consider in segmentation is that whatever the technique used, it is imperative to check that the selected volume on 2D MPR images matches to the reality of the studied object. One can indeed miss an important structure, such as a polar artery when segmenting kidney vascularization, or add up voxels that do not belong to the studied object, but to

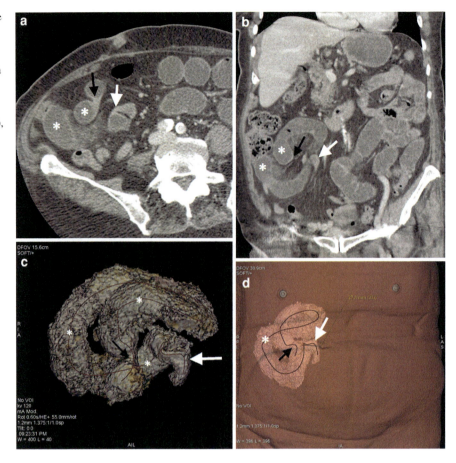

Fig. 8 Value of VR in acute bowel obstruction over band with a volvulated loop. The two beaks (*white* and *black arrows*) of the transition area are seen on axial (**a**) and coronal (**b**) sections as well as on segmentation (**c**) of the volvulated loop (*asterisk*), even without oral contrast administration. The center of digestive lumen is delineated by the *red line*. Entire view of the abdomen with the volvulated loop in transparency allows in mapping the band relative to the umbilicus (**d**)

a neighboring object thereby virtually misrepresenting the targeted object. In any cases, saving the 3D object data in a specific file that can be recorded into a PACS system is necessary. It can eventually allow in further completing the segmentation later on, without losing all the work previously done.

8.5 Utility of 3D in CT of Acute Abdomen

Some of the 3D reconstruction techniques will be useful in CT of acute abdomen (Fig. 9).

SSD is a simple technique that used to have the advantage, few years ago, to reduce the volume of 3D data to compute, as only the surface was represented. Recent advances in calculation power have pushed such limitations. Nevertheless, SSD has numerous disadvantages over VR. The segmentation of a given object using a threshold value is easy when one needs to select structures surrounded by soft tissues of completely different densities, such as bones. It becomes less convenient when the object to depict is surrounded of structures of close density. As an example, it is challenging and even hazardous to study arterial stenosis within a calcified plaque as densities of the calcified plaque and lumen may overlap, and the stenosis may therefore be under- or over-estimated with SSD.

Of note, this technique leads to a loss of information on the density of the represented voxels. When several structures over the segmentation threshold value are lined up in a given direction, only the closer structure to the observer is represented, even if the farther structure has a much more higher CT number. When considering all these limitations, SSD is only scarcely used in abdominal pathology, studies of surface being mostly valuable in osteoarticular trauma. More generally, volume rendering must be preferred to SSD in most if not all applications (Dalrymple et al. 2005).

Numerous publications address the utility of MIP and VR, especially in studies of acute vascular

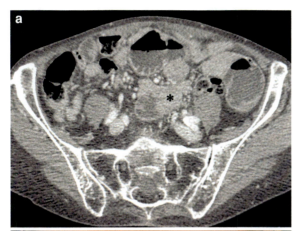

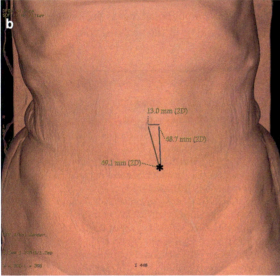

Fig. 9 Mapping of the transition level (*black asterisk*) in bowel acute mechanic obstruction over bands thanks to a cursor set on axial section (**a**) or any other MPR reconstruction. The cursor is then visible in VR (**b**) and allows to locate the band relative to cutaneous landmarks, such as the umbilicus, before surgical management

pathologies of the abdomen (Fig. 6). MIP is of simple use and fast in thick slices in a given plane (axial, coronal, sagittal, and oblique) or in the whole volume. The drawback is that the relationships between arteries and adjacent anatomical structures are much less visualized, with regard to the position of veins, organs, muscles or bones (Fishman et al. 2006). VR enables ranges of color and shadow display helpful in depicting complex 3D structures. Nevertheless, those two techniques are often used concomitantly, and one can switch from one to the other to describe vascular anomalies eventually responsible for mesenteric ischemia (Wildermuth et al. 2005), an acute gastrointestinal bleeding (Jaeckle et al. 2008a, b) or an abdominal aortic aneurysm before and after treatment (Sun 2006).

MIP and VR may also be useful although not necessary, in description of acute abdominal pathologies of intestinal origin, whether they are inflammatory (Crohn's disease), infectious (see Chapter Acute appendicitis) or obstructive pathology (Hong et al. 2006; Johnson et al. 2009a). In intestinal obstruction, 3D techniques actually allow better understanding of anatomical relationships, especially for the course of vessels within some internal herniation (Rezazadeh Azar et al. 2010), or to better localize an area of transition of a mechanic obstruction (Fig. 8). In the last case, density of unopacified loops is similar to that of adjacent organs, which renders proper visualization in VR challenging. Small-bowel opacification by enteroclysis has lead to esthetic results (Candocia and Goldman 2005; Gollub 2005). However, this technique complicates management of abdominal emergencies, especially during shifts, with risks of complications (perforation, enhanced ischemic stress of the intestinal loops, pain...) and impact on diagnosis yet to be evaluated. VR may be used on unenhanced CT examination, allowing better understanding of the organization of a volvulus of the sigmoid or cecum (Aufort et al. 2005) while in the same setting, 3D surfacic VR can be used to depict the distance between an adhesive band and umbilicus before an eventual celioscopic surgery (Fig. 9).

Both VR and MIP are also very much used in urology for better localization and characterization of the location and shape of stones as well as description of the anatomy of the patient's urinary tract before surgical intervention (Patel et al. 2009). VR may also assist in the planning of an intervention: using virtual endoscopy, the surgeon may be prepared to the eventual technical challenges he may actually face.

Lastly, the segmentation of objects within 3D volume, especially in VR, is currently developing. One of the leading applications is measurement of the tumor volume in oncology. In acute abdominal pathology, segmentation enables to, for example, accurately measure the volume of an abscess (Fig. 10), an hematoma or hemoperitoneum. A pathologic organ can also be segmented for better depiction of its

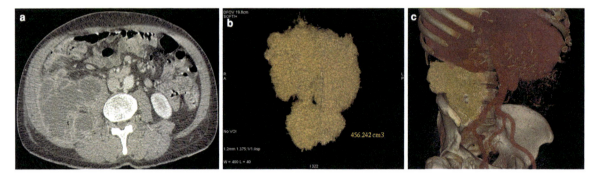

Fig. 10 Large appendicular abscess diffusing within the retroperitoneum on axial section (**a**). Segmentation in VR (*yellow*) allows to measure the volume (**b**) and to depict it relative to adjacent structures (**c**)

position and anatomical relationships with the adjacent structures (Fig. 3). All post-processing consoles may not offer all the tools required for fast 3D segmentation and manufacturers must put some efforts in further improving the ease of use and speed of such a promising technique, although some already have a non-negligible advance over the others.

9 Conclusion

Along with the development of MDCT, the rapidity of volumic acquisition over the entire abdomen and pelvis allow to tailor protocols to diagnosis indications and etiologic hypotheses of non-traumatic acute abdomen. As examinations performed using multiple acquisition phases are facilitated, the use of the lowest effective radiation dose for adequate diagnostic result must be highly considered.

The large volume of data generated by the making of thin sections with isotropic sub-millimetric voxels over extended areas have benefited from advances in computer technology (hardware and software) over the last few years. It is currently simple and fast to use thin sections or MPR in any different plane of interest, with the coronal plane often reported as the most valuable in studies of acute abdomen. Although certain reconstruction algorithms, such as MinIP have limited value, other 3D algorithms, such as MIP or volume rendering have proved useful in vascular pathology. Only recently have MIP and VR started to develop in the studies of intraabdominal organs, notably due to segmentation allowing volume calculations and spatial localization of a particular object. Post-processing techniques will certainly further benefit from computing advances, making them faster and more intuitive in the years to come.

References

Anderson SW, Soto JA, Lucey BC, Ozonoff A, Jordan JD, Ratevosian J, Ulrich AS, Rathlev NK, Mitchell PM, Rebholz C, Feldman JA, Rhea JT (2009) Abdominal 64-MDCT for suspected appendicitis: the use of oral and IV contrast material versus IV contrast material only. AJR Am J Roentgenol 193(5):1282–1288

Arac M, Celik H, Oner AY, Gultekin S, Gumus T, Kosar S (2005) Distinguishing pelvic phleboliths from distal ureteral calculi: thin-slice CT findings. Eur Radiol 15(1):65–70

Aufort S, Charra L, Lesnik A, Bruel J, Taourel P (2005) Multidetector CT of bowel obstruction: value of post-processing. Eur Radiol 15(11):2323–2329

Calhoun PS, Kuszyk BS, Heath DG, Carley JC, Fishman EK (1999) Three-dimensional volume rendering of spiral CT data: theory and method. Radiographics 19(3):745–764

Candocia FJ, Goldman I (2005) Three-dimensional computed tomography illustration of small bowel obstruction transition points in patients receiving oral contrast: report of 3 cases. J Comput Assist Tomogr 29(2):202–204

Dalrymple NC, Prasad SR, Freckleton MW, Chintapalli KN (2005) Informatics in radiology (infoRAD): introduction to the language of three-dimensional imaging with multidetector CT. Radiographics 25(5):1409–1428

Dearing DD, Recabaren JA, Alexander M (2008) Can computed tomography scan be performed effectively in the diagnosis of acute appendicitis without the added morbidity of rectal contrast? Am Surg 74(10):917–920

Delabrousse E (2009) TDM des urgences abdominales. Masson, Paris

Duran C, Uraz S, Kantarci M, Ozturk E, Doganay S, Dayangac M, Bozkurt M, Yuzer Y, Tokat Y (2009) Hepatic arterial mapping by multidetector computed tomographic angiography in living donor liver transplantation. J Comput Assist Tomogr 33(4):618–625

Ernst O, Bulois P, Saint-Drenant S, Leroy C, Paris JC, Sergent G (2003) Helical CT in acute lower gastrointestinal bleeding. Eur Radiol 13(1):114–117

Ertl-Wagner BB, Bruening R, Blume J, Hoffmann RT, Mueller-Schunk S, Snyder B, Reiser MF (2006) Relative value of sliding-thin-slab multiplanar reformations and sliding-thin-slab maximum intensity projections as reformatting techniques in multisection CT angiography of the cervicocranial vessels. AJNR Am J Neuroradiol 27(1):107–113

Fishman EK, Ney DR, Heath DG, Corl FM, Horton KM, Johnson PT (2006) Volume rendering versus maximum intensity projection in CT angiography: what works best, when, and why. Radiographics 26(3):905–922

Ghekiere O, Lesnik A, Millet I, Hoa D, Guillon F, Taourel P (2007) Direct visualization of perforation sites in patients with a non-traumatic free pneumoperitoneum: added diagnostic value of thin transverse slices and coronal and sagittal reformations for multi-detector CT. Eur Radiol 17(9):2302–2309

Gollub MJ (2005) Multidetector computed tomography enteroclysis of patients with small bowel obstruction: a volume-rendered "surgical perspective". J Comput Assist Tomogr 29(3):401–407

Hidas G, Eliahou R, Duvdevani M, Coulon P, Lemaitre L, Gofrit ON, Pode D, Sosna J (2010) Determination of renal stone composition with dual-energy CT: in vivo analysis and comparison with X-ray diffraction. Radiology 257(2):394–401

Hong SS, Kim AY, Byun JH, Won HJ, Kim PN, Lee MG, Ha HK (2006) MDCT of small-bowel disease: value of 3D imaging. AJR Am J Roentgenol 187(5):1212–1221

Huynh LN, Coughlin BF, Wolfe J, Blank F, Lee SY, Smithline HA (2004) Patient encounter time intervals in the evaluation of emergency department patients requiring abdominopelvic CT: oral contrast versus no contrast. Emerg Radiol 10(6):310–313

Jaeckle T, Stuber G, Hoffmann MH, Freund W, Schmitz BL, Aschoff AJ (2008a) Acute gastrointestinal bleeding: value of MDCT. Abdom Imaging 33(3):285–293

Jaeckle T, Stuber G, Hoffmann MH, Jeltsch M, Schmitz BL, Aschoff AJ (2008b) Detection and localization of acute upper and lower gastrointestinal (GI) bleeding with arterial phase multi-detector row helical CT. Eur Radiol 18(7):1406–1413

Jaffe TA, Martin LC, Thomas J, Adamson AR, DeLong DM, Paulson EK (2006) Small-bowel obstruction: coronal reformations from isotropic voxels at 16-section multi-detector row CT. Radiology 238(1):135–142

Jan YT, Yang FS, Huang JK (2005) Visualization rate and pattern of normal appendix on multidetector computed tomography by using multiplanar reformation display. J Comput Assist Tomogr 29(4):446–451

Johnson PT, Heath DG, Hofmann LV, Horton KM, Fishman EK (2003) Multidetector-row computed tomography with three-dimensional volume rendering of pancreatic cancer: a complete preoperative staging tool using computed tomography angiography and volume-rendered cholangiopancreatography. J Comput Assist Tomogr 27(3):347–353

Johnson PT, Horton KM, Mahesh M, Fishman EK (2006) Multidetector computed tomography for suspected appendicitis: multi-institutional survey of 16-MDCT data acquisition protocols and review of pertinent literature. J Comput Assist Tomogr 30(5):758–764

Johnson PT, Horton KM, Fishman EK (2009a) Nonvascular mesenteric disease: utility of multidetector CT with 3D volume rendering. Radiographics 29(3):721–740

Johnson PT, Horton KM, Kawamoto S, Eng J, Bean MJ, Shan SJ, Fishman EK (2009b) MDCT for suspected appendicitis: effect of reconstruction section thickness on diagnostic accuracy, rate of appendiceal visualization, and reader confidence using axial images. AJR Am J Roentgenol 192(4):893–901

Kaewlai R, Nazinitsky KJ (2007) Acute colonic diverticulitis in a community-based hospital: CT evaluation in 138 patients. Emerg Radiol 13(4):171–179

Kambadakone AR, Eisner BH, Catalano OA, Sahani DV (2010) New and evolving concepts in the imaging and management of urolithiasis: urologists' perspective. Radiographics 30(3):603–623

Kamel IR, Liapi E, Fishman EK (2005) Liver and biliary system: evaluation by multidetector CT. Radiol Clin North Am 43(6):977–997

Ketelslegers E, Van Beers BE (2006) Urinary calculi: improved detection and characterization with thin-slice multidetector CT. Eur Radiol 16(1):161–165

Kim JK, Kim JH, Bae SJ, Cho KS (2004) CT angiography for evaluation of living renal donors: comparison of four reconstruction methods. AJR Am J Roentgenol 183(2):471–477

Kim HC, Yang DM, Jin W, Park SJ (2008) Added diagnostic value of multiplanar reformation of multidetector CT data in patients with suspected appendicitis. Radiographics 28(2):393–405 discussion 405-396

Kim YJ, Kim JE, Kim HS, Hwang HY (2009) MDCT with coronal reconstruction: clinical benefit in evaluation of suspected acute appendicitis in pediatric patients. AJR Am J Roentgenol 192(1):150–152

Lane MJ, Katz DS, Mindelzun RE, Jeffrey RB Jr (1997) Spontaneous intramural small bowel haemorrhage: importance of non-contrast CT. Clin Radiol 52(5):378–380

Lee KH, Kim YH, Hahn S, Lee KW, Lee HJ, Kim TJ, Kang SB, Shin JH, Park BJ (2006a) Added value of coronal reformations for duty radiologists and for referring physicians or surgeons in the CT diagnosis of acute appendicitis. Korean J Radiol 7(2):87–96

Lee SY, Coughlin B, Wolfe JM, Polino J, Blank FS, Smithline HA (2006b) Prospective comparison of helical CT of the abdomen and pelvis without and with oral contrast in assessing acute abdominal pain in adult emergency department patients. Emerg Radiol 12(4):150–157

Macari M, Balthazar EJ (2003) The acute right lower quadrant: CT evaluation. Radiol Clin North Am 41(6):1117–1136

Mun S, Ernst RD, Chen K, Oto A, Shah S, Mileski WJ (2006) Rapid CT diagnosis of acute appendicitis with IV contrast material. Emerg Radiol 12(3):99–102

Neville AM, Paulson EK (2009) MDCT of acute appendicitis: value of coronal reformations. Abdom Imaging 34(1):42–48

Nino-Murcia M, Jeffrey RB Jr, Beaulieu CF, Li KC, Rubin GD (2001) Multidetector CT of the pancreas and bile duct system: value of curved planar reformations. AJR Am J Roentgenol 176(3):689–693

Parrish FJ (2007) Volume CT: state-of-the-art reporting. AJR Am J Roentgenol 189(3):528–534

Patel U, Walkden RM, Ghani KR, Anson K (2009) Three-dimensional CT pyelography for planning of percutaneous nephrostolithotomy: accuracy of stone measurement, stone depiction and pelvicalyceal reconstruction. Eur Radiol 19(5):1280–1288

Paulson EK, Harris JP, Jaffe TA, Haugan PA, Nelson RC (2005) Acute appendicitis: added diagnostic value of coronal reformations from isotropic voxels at multi-detector row CT. Radiology 235(3):879–885

Perandini S, Faccioli N, Zaccarella A, Re T, Mucelli RP (2010) The diagnostic contribution of CT volumetric rendering techniques in routine practice. Indian J Radiol Imaging 20(2):92–97

Pinto Leite N, Pereira JM, Cunha R, Pinto P, Sirlin C (2005) CT evaluation of appendicitis and its complications: imaging techniques and key diagnostic findings. AJR Am J Roentgenol 185(2):406–417

Rao PM, Rhea JT, Novelline RA, Mostafavi AA, Lawrason JN, McCabe CJ (1997) Helical CT combined with contrast material administered only through the colon for imaging of suspected appendicitis. AJR Am J Roentgenol 169(5):1275–1280

Rao ND, Gulati MS, Paul SB, Pande GK, Sahni P, Chattopadhyay TK (2005) Three-dimensional helical computed tomography cholangiography with minimum intensity projection in gallbladder carcinoma patients with obstructive jaundice: comparison with magnetic resonance cholangiography and percutaneous transhepatic cholangiography. J Gastroenterol Hepatol 20(2):304–308

Rezazadeh Azar A, Abraham C, Coulier B, Broze B (2010) Ileocecal herniation through the foramen of Winslow: MDCT diagnosis. Abdom Imaging 35(5):574–577

Seo H, Lee KH, Kim HJ, Kim K, Kang SB, Kim SY, Kim YH (2009) Diagnosis of acute appendicitis with sliding slab ray-sum interpretation of low-dose unenhanced CT and standard-dose i.v. contrast-enhanced CT scans. AJR Am J Roentgenol 193(1):96–105

Stabile Ianora AA, Moschetta M, Lorusso V, Scardapane A (2010) Atypical appendicitis: diagnostic value of volume-rendered reconstructions obtained with 16-slice multidetector-row CT. Radiol Med 115(1):93–104

Sun Z (2006) 3D multislice CT angiography in post-aortic stent grafting: a pictorial essay. Korean J Radiol 7(3):205–211

Thoeni RF, Cello JP (2006) CT imaging of colitis. Radiology 240(3):623–638

Urban BA, Fishman EK (2000a) Tailored helical CT evaluation of acute abdomen. Radiographics 20(3):725–749

Urban BA, Fishman EK (2000b) Targeted helical CT of the acute abdomen: appendicitis, diverticulitis, and small bowel obstruction. Semin Ultrasound CT MR 21(1):20–39

Weltman DI, Yu J, Krumenacker J Jr, Huang S, Moh P (2000) Diagnosis of acute appendicitis: comparison of 5- and 10-mm CT sections in the same patient. Radiology 216(1):172–177

Wildermuth S, Leschka S, Alkadhi H, Marincek B (2005) Multislice CT in the pre- and postinterventional evaluation of mesenteric perfusion. Eur Radiol 15(6):1203–1210

Part IV

CT Diagnosis in Non Traumatic Abdomen

Acute Liver Disease

Valérie Vilgrain and François Durand

Contents

1 Introduction 83

2 Hemorrhagic Hepatic Lesions 83
2.1 Hepatocellular Carcinoma 84
2.2 Hepatocellular Adenoma 85
2.3 Liver Metastases 85
2.4 Other Lesions 86

3 Acute Vascular Diseases of the Liver 86
3.1 Budd–Chiari Syndrome 86
3.2 Portal Vein Thrombosis 87
3.3 Hepatic Infarction 87

4 Hypoxic Hepatitis 88

5 Acute Hepatitis 88
5.1 Paracetamol (acetaminophen) Overdose 89
5.2 Hepatitis Viruses 89
5.3 Toxic Hepatitis 89

6 Wilson Disease 89

7 Reye Syndrome 89

8 Malignant Infiltration of the Liver 90

9 Acute Liver Disease in Pregnancy 90
9.1 HELLP Syndrome 90
9.2 Acute Fatty Liver 91

References 91

V. Vilgrain (✉)
Department of Radiology, Hôpital Beaujon,
Paris, France
e-mail: valerie.vilgrain@bjn.aphp.fr

F. Durand
Department of Hepatology, Hôpital Beaujon,
Paris, France

Abstract

Acute liver disease may be due to various causes and different mechanisms. Although the contribution of imaging to diagnosis is low in paracetamol (acetaminophen) overdose (the most common cause of acute liver failure in Western countries) and viral hepatitis, imaging, and especially CT, plays an important role in diagnosis of hemorrhagic hepatic lesions or acute vascular disorders.

1 Introduction

In this chapter, we discuss the contribution of CT in acute liver disease. The most common causes will be covered: hemorrhagic hepatic lesions, acute vascular disorders, hypoxic hepatitis, acute hepatitis, acute presentation of chronic diseases, and acute liver disease in pregnancy.

2 Hemorrhagic Hepatic Lesions

Spontaneous hepatic bleeding is a rare condition. In the absence of trauma or anticoagulant therapy, hepatic hemorrhage is usually due to underlying liver disease. The most common causes of nontraumatic hepatic hemorrhage are hepatocellular carcinoma and hepatocellular adenoma. Less commonly, other liver tumors may be responsible for hemorrhage, such as liver metastases. Other conditions associated with this entity include HELLP syndrome (see Sect. 9.2), amyloidosis, and miscellaneous causes.

P. Taourel (ed.), *CT of the Acute Abdomen,* Medical Radiology. Diagnostic Imaging,
DOI: 10.1007/174_2010_93, © Springer-Verlag Berlin Heidelberg 2011

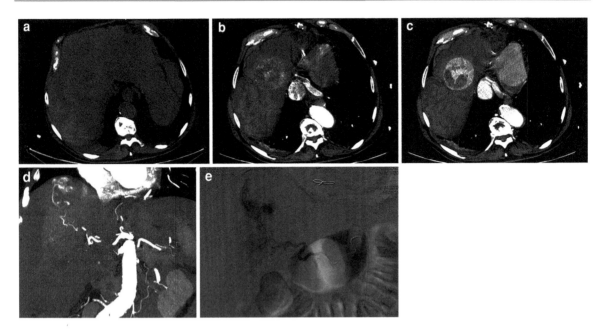

Fig. 1 Hemorrhagic hepatocellular carcinoma. Unenhanced (**a**) and multiphasic contrast-enhanced (**b**, **c**) CT scans show hemorrhagic tumor in the liver dome with clotting around the liver and intra-abdominal fluid effusion. Active bleeding is seen at the upper part of the tumor on the coronal CT image (**d**) and during preembolization angiography (**e**)

2.1 Hepatocellular Carcinoma

Hepatocellular carcinoma (HCC) is the most common primary malignant tumor of the liver and has the highest prevalence of rupture (6.9–14% of cases) (Miyamoto et al. 1991). It also represents the most common cause of nontraumatic acute hemoperitoneum in male patients (Casillas et al. 2000). Clinical symptoms differ according to the degree of rupture: epigastric or right upper quadrant pain in patients with subcapsular hematoma of the liver to hypotension, shock, and signs of peritonitis or abdominal distention in patients with rupture of the liver capsule. Predictive factors have been identified: a large tumor located at the periphery of the liver which protrudes into the abdominal cavity and without normal hepatic parenchyma between the tumor and the liver capsule are key findings (Kanematsu et al. 1992). The prognosis of patients with ruptured HCC is variable and is mainly depends on the severity of the underlying liver disease. Bilirubin level seems a good indicator of patient prognosis, a high bilirubin level being associated with higher mortality rates.

Diagnosis of ruptured HCC is suspected when a hemorrhagic tumor is seen in patients with chronic liver diseases. When the diagnosis of chronic liver disease has not been established, imaging findings suggestive of cirrhosis are helpful, such as morphologic changes of the liver, liver surface nodularity, and portal hypertension. Figure 1 shows CT findings of tumor hemorrhage in the presence of hyperattenuation within the tumor on unenhanced CT. HCCs are hypervascular in most cases in the arterial-dominant phase; however, tumor hypervascularization is often lacking in hemorrhagic HCCs. Subcapsular hematoma appearing as a hyperattenuated crescent is often seen as is hemoperitoneum which exhibits high-attenuation peritoneal fluid around the liver and spleen. When layering of the clot is detected, it is located next to the hemorrhagic site and it indicates the origin of bleeding. Tumor hyperattenuation decreases over time and is no longer seen several weeks after the bleeding.

The goal of the treatment is to stop bleeding. Transcatheter arterial embolization is the recommended treatment. During acute bleeding, transarterial chemoembolization could worsen the prognosis and should not be performed. If arterial embolization is ineffective, surgical hemostasis is indicated, often associated with arterial ligation.

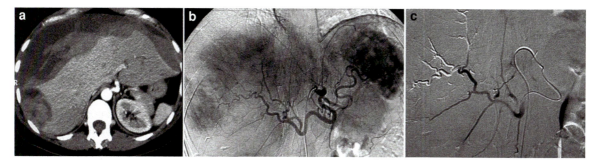

Fig. 2 Hemorrhagic hepatocellular adenoma. Contrast-enhanced CT (**a**) shows hemorrhagic tumor in the right side of the liver with clotting around the liver and intra-abdominal fluid effusion. Preembolization (**b**) and postembolization (**c**) angiography demonstrate bleeding control

2.2 Hepatocellular Adenoma

Hepatocellular adenomas (HCA) are benign hepatocellular lesions mostly observed in women. They are composed of cords of well-differentiated hepatocytes but lack bile ducts and venous tracts. Recently, HCAs have been considered as heterogeneous lesions on the basis of genotypic and phenotypic features leading to different morphologic presentations (Bioulac-Sage et al. 2009; Zucman-Rossi et al. 2006). At least three subtypes of HCA were initially recognized: steatotic liver fatty acid binding protein negative HCA associated with HNF1α mutation, telangiectatic/inflammatory serum amyloid A positive HCA, and HCA with atypical cells that are frequently β-catenin mutated. A small group of HCAs with no specific morphologic and immunophenotypic features is still observed, named as unclassified HCA.

Hemorrhage is a classic complication of HCAs and appears mostly in large tumors. It also represents a common cause of nontraumatic acute hemoperitoneum in female patients. Bleeding may occur at the end of pregnancy. In a large single-center surgical series of HCAs, microscopic hemorrhage was seen in 19 and 68% of HCAs of 2–5 cm and more than 5 cm, respectively, whereas macroscopic hemorrhage was detected in 5 and 24% of HCAs of 2–5 cm and more than 5 cm, respectively (Dokmak et al. 2009). Thus, a cutoff at 5 cm seems reasonable for predicting the risk of hemorrhage in HCAs. Moreover, with comparable size, the risk of hemorrhage is lower in markedly steatotic HCAs than in the other subgroups. Similarly to HCCs, clinical symptoms differ according to the severity of the hemorrhage and the presence of subcapsular hematoma or hemoperitoneum.

Diagnosis of hemorrhagic HCA is suspected when a hemorrhagic tumor is seen in a female patient (Fig. 2). The presence of fatty (with marked hypoattenuation on unenhanced CT) or telangiectatic (hypervascularization in the arterial-dominant phase followed by sustained enhancement in the delayed phase) components strengthen the diagnosis of HCAs.

In patients with active bleeding, transarterial embolization is the treatment of choice and allows delayed surgical resection to be performed in better conditions. Interestingly, in some patients pathologic examination of the resected HCA does not show any residual tumor. In patients with features of intratumoral hemorrhage but no clinical symptoms, transarterial embolization is not mandatory.

2.3 Liver Metastases

Liver metastases from lung carcinoma, renal carcinoma, and melanoma are the most frequent types that cause hepatic bleeding (Casillas et al. 2000). Clinical findings range from unexplained blood loss and shock to signs consistent with acute abdomen. The diagnosis is very difficult when liver metastases are not known. Multiple liver lesions in oncologic patients should raise the possibility of hemorrhagic metastases. A differential diagnosis to HCA is a hemorrhagic liver metastasis from a choriocarcinoma, which should be suspected in women who have delivered recently and in whom serum human chorionic gonadotropin beta level is increased (Fig. 3).

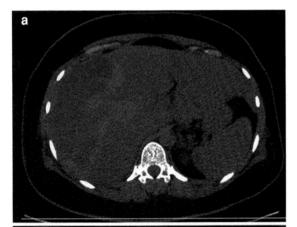

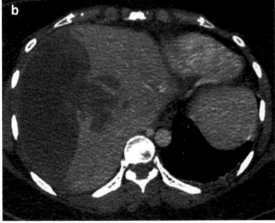

Fig. 3 Young woman who presented with evidence of recent hemorrhage and a tumor of the liver due to hemorrhagic choriocarcinoma. This patient had a markedly elevated serum human chorionic gonadotropin level. Unenhanced (a) and contrast-enhanced (b) CT shows hemorrhagic tumor in the liver dome with clotting around the liver and intra-abdominal fluid effusion

2.4 Other Lesions

Very rarely, other liver lesions may bleed. This has been reported in focal nodular hyperplasia and hemangioma (Becker et al. 1995; Soyer and Levesque 1995).

3 Acute Vascular Diseases of the Liver

3.1 Budd–Chiari Syndrome

Budd–Chiari syndrome (BCS) is characterized by an obstruction of the hepatic venous outflow tract located at the level of the small or large hepatic veins, or on the suprahepatic portion of inferior vena cava. When the blockage is caused by invasion or compression by a tumor, BCS is considered as secondary.

BCS is favored by underlying prothrombotic conditions either acquired (such as myeloproliferative diseases) or inherited (such as antithrombin deficiency, protein C deficiency, protein S deficiency, heterozygous factor V Leiden). BCS can occur at any age, and is more common in women.

The disease is usually characterized by a progressive involvement of the hepatic veins, explaining why most patients have subacute or chronic clinical presentations (Valla 2009). However, in a minority of patients, BCS first results in acute liver failure with abdominal pain, high serum transaminase levels, and a rapid decrease in the levels of coagulation factors. Even though the manifestations are similar to those of acute liver failure, almost all patients have underlying liver lesions corresponding to a previously asymptomatic liver disease. These patients have developed partial or complete thrombosis of the main hepatic veins. Acute decompensation, mimicking acute liver failure, results from additional thrombosis of patent segments of the hepatic veins and/or collaterals. Ascites, liver and spleen enlargement, and portal hypertension are often observed. Jaundice may also be seen.

In acute BCS, the morphologic features of the liver are usually normal, but enlargement may also be seen because the liver is engorged with blood (Buckley et al. 2007). Occlusion of the hepatic veins with severe ascites is the typical finding. The liver exhibits patchy, decreased peripheral enhancement caused by portal and sinusoidal stasis and stronger enhancement of the central portion of the liver parenchyma (Cura et al. 2009). The thrombosed hepatic veins are hypoattenuating on contrast-enhanced CT, and the inferior vena cava is compressed by the enlarged caudate lobe (Brancatelli et al. 2007). Yet, hyperattenuation within thrombosed hepatic veins on unenhanced CT is a feature of recent thrombosis (Fig. 4). In the acute phase, varices are usually absent and splenic enlargement is unusual. Concomitant portal vein thrombosis (PVT) may be present in 9–20% of patients (Buckley et al. 2007).

Again, most patients have an acute presentation in chronic BCS. In these cases, morphologic changes in the liver are common and are the result of the type of

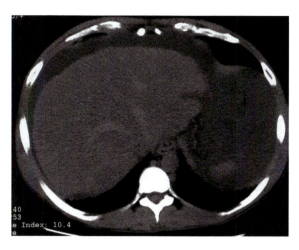

Fig. 4 Acute Budd–Chiari syndrome. Unenhanced CT (**a**) shows massive ascites and hyperattenuation within the main hepatic veins. The latter is related to recent clotting

venous involvement. Portosystemic and intrahepatic collateral vessels are often found as is splenic enlargement. Hypervascular liver nodules may be seen in patients with an acute presentation in chronic BCS but never in acute disease.

Early diagnosis of acute BCS is important for establishing appropriate treatment. Imaging plays an important role because biopsy findings might be normal at this stage, whereas CT nicely shows liver congestion. Doppler ultrasonography is more accurate for the assessment of hepatic veins. Treatment should be started promptly and is based on anticoagulation. Conversely to PVT, BCS patients often need additional treatment, which ranges from hepatic venous angioplasty or stenting, to transjugular intrahepatic portosystemic stent shunt or liver transplantation (Plessier et al. 2006).

3.2 Portal Vein Thrombosis

PVT is defined by the formation of a thrombus within the portal vein, the mesenteric veins, and/or the splenic vein. Occlusion can be complete or partial, acute or chronic. Local risk factors (mainly abdominal inflammatory diseases) are seen in 30% of patients with acute PVT, whereas the remnant patients have a general risk factor for PVT, most commonly myeloproliferative disease (Condat and Valla 2006). Patients with acute PVT usually present with abdominal or lumbar pain of sudden onset and moderate abdominal distension. A systemic inflammatory response syndrome is often detected.

Because of the nonspecific symptoms, imaging plays a crucial role in diagnosis of PVT, especially ultrasonography and CT. CT findings of PVT are the lack of endoluminal enhancement after administration of intravenous contrast medium and the increased hepatic enhancement of the obstructed segments in the arterial-dominant phase (Fig. 5). These transient hepatic attenuation differences have straight borders corresponding to anatomic landmarks when the PVT is limited to intrahepatic branches. On the other hand, they are localized in the peripheral liver segments when the portal vein itself is completely obstructed because portal venous supply is maintained in the central portion of the liver. Some additional findings strongly support the acute obstruction, such as vessel enlargement, high-attenuation thrombus on unenhanced CT, and absence or minimal cavernomatous transformation of the portal vein (Mori et al. 1987). The role of CT is also to assess PVT extension and severity. Features of intestinal congestion or ischemia should be searched for.

Early initiation of anticoagulation therapy for acute PVT is associated with complete and partial success in 50 and 40% of patients, respectively (Condat and Valla 2006). Unrecognized or untreated patients usually develop chronic PVT leading to complications such as portal hypertension and development of portosystemic collaterals, and portal cholangiopathy.

3.3 Hepatic Infarction

Hepatic infarction is a very rare disease characterized by parenchymal necrosis involving at least two entire lobules, in relation to a local circulatory insufficiency requiring impairment of both arterial and portal venous flow (Francque et al. 2004). In most cases, hepatic infarction is caused by portal venous thrombosis associated with severe systemic hemodynamic problems. Very rarely, it is due to combined portal venous and arterial thrombosis.

CT shows portal venous thrombosis and lack of enhancement of the corresponding segments on multiphasic examination. A lack of visualization of the hepatic artery may also be found. These findings

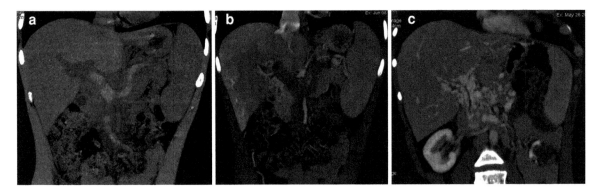

Fig. 5 Acute portal vein thrombosis. Unenhanced (a) and portal venous-phase contrast-enhanced (b) CT shows acute obstruction of the portal vein with spontaneous hyperattenuation and lack of enhancement of the portal vein after administration of intravenous contrast medium. Despite anticoagulation, the portal vein was not recanalized. Portal venous-phase contrast-enhanced CT (c) performed 2 years later demonstrates cavernous transformation of the portal vein

differ from those for biliary necrosis due to arterial thrombosis only. In the latter, liver hypoattenuation is mostly depicted around intrahepatic bile ducts and bilomas or bile ducts dilatation is often seen.

4 Hypoxic Hepatitis

Hypoxic hepatitis, also known as ischemic liver or shock liver, is due to inadequate oxygen uptake by the centrilobular hepatocytes resulting in necrosis (Ebert 2006). In a 10-year period, Henrion et al. (2003) analyzed 142 episodes of hypoxic liver injury. They were due to decompensated congestive heart failure (58%), acute cardiac failure (14%), exacerbated chronic respiratory failure (14%), and toxic/septic shock (14%). The mechanisms are varied:
- Ischemia with hypoxia of the liver resulting from decreased hepatic blood flow in heart failure
- Hypoxemia in chronic respiratory failure
- Increased oxygen needs in toxic/septic shock

Hypoxic hepatitis is defined by three factors: a typical clinical setting of hemodynamic failure; a massive but rapidly reversible increase in serum transaminase levels; and the exclusion of other causes of hepatocyte necrosis such as viral hepatitis and drug-induced hepatitis (Henrion 2007). Cirrhotic patients are at particular risk of developing hypoxic hepatitis (Ebert 2006). Generally, hypoxic hepatitis occurs in elderly patients (older than 60 years) and in poor general condition (more than 80% have primary heart disease) (Ebert 2006; Henrion 2007) but a shock state is observed in only about 50% of cases (Henrion 2007). Indeed, there is a weak correlation between manifestations related to systematic circulatory changes and the consequences in terms of liver cell necrosis. Clinical symptoms are weakness, shortness of breath, and right upper abdominal pain.

Imaging has been rarely reported. Imaging findings include hepatomegaly and dilation of hepatic veins due to passive congestion of the liver. On CT, hypoattenuating lesions have been described, which could correspond to large areas of necrosis (Kahn et al. 2000).

In the setting of cardiac or respiratory failure, the diagnosis of hypoxic hepatitis may be assumed without liver biopsy. There is no specific liver therapy and the prognosis is poor, depending on the severity of the underlying condition.

5 Acute Hepatitis

In only a minority of patients with acute hepatitis does it lead to acute liver failure. The main causes of acute liver failure are currently represented by paracetamol (acetaminophen) overdose, viral hepatitis, and idiosyncratic drug reactions. Jaundice may also be seen. Moderate ascites can be present, especially in patients with subacute diseases. Serum transaminase levels (alanine transaminase and aspartate transaminase) are constantly and markedly increased, whereas the levels of coagulation factors are constantly decreased. Imaging and CT in particular are not very helpful. CT may show nonspecific features such as hepatomegaly, thickening of gallbladder wall, and ascites. Signs of portal hypertension are absent. Some patients with subfulminant liver failure and a prolonged interval between jaundice and encephalopathy may present with large, tumorlike, regenerative nodules, and irregular margins (Durand and Bernuau 2007). These nodules may be hypervascular, thus mimicking malignant tumors. On the other hand, CT is accurate for diagnosing brain edema which might complicate acute liver failure by showing diffuse hypoattenuation of the brain, a loss of distinction between gray and white matter, swollen gyri, and compressed or absent cisterns.

5.1 Paracetamol (acetaminophen) Overdose

Paracetamol overdose has become the predominant cause of acute liver failure in most Western countries. However, only a minority (less than 10%) of patients with paracetamol overdose eventually develop acute liver failure (Durand and Bernuau 2007). The hepatotoxicity of paracetamol is dose-dependent. Acute liver failure is almost always observed in patients who ingested single doses exceeding 15 g in an attempt at suicide. However, lower doses may produce significant liver damage when predisposing factors are present, such as starvation, poor nutritional status, alcoholism, concomitant ingestion of enzyme inducers, and concomitant ingestion of isoniazid.

5.2 Hepatitis Viruses

Acute liver failure only develops in 0.05–0.01% of patients with symptomatic hepatitis A. The diagnosis is based on the presence of anti-hepatitis A virus IgM in the serum.

Hepatitis B virus (HBV) can be responsible for acute liver failure in two distinct ways: (1) recent HBV infection and (2) acute exacerbation (or reactivation) in chronic HBV carriers. The risk of developing acute liver failure during the course of symptomatic acute hepatitis B is about 1% (Durand and Bernuau 2007). The diagnosis is based on the presence of anti-HBV IgM in the serum.

It seems that hepatitis C virus infection alone never results in acute liver failure.

Other viruses may induce acute liver failure, such as hepatitis D (delta) virus, hepatitis E virus, and herpes simplex viruses.

5.3 Toxic Hepatitis

Amanita phalloides is a highly toxic white mushroom occurring in many places in Europe and the USA, and contains toxins that cause liver cell necrosis. Industrial solvents, herbal medicines, drugs, and illicit drugs such as cocaine and ecstasy can also cause severe liver damage.

6 Wilson Disease

Wilson disease (WD) is an inherited, autosomal recessive disorder which leads to copper accumulation mainly in the liver, but also in the brain, cornea, and kidney. The most frequent clinical presentation of WD is liver involvement (Cope-Yokoyama et al. 2010). Hepatic manifestations may range from hepatomegaly and fatty liver, to acute hepatitis (especially in children and young adults) with high serum transaminase levels, liver failure, jaundice, and cirrhosis. In the absence of specific treatment, the outcome is almost always fatal unless emergency liver transplantation is performed. Early administration of D-penicillamine, before the onset of encephalopathy, may rapidly reverse liver insufficiency.

Almost all patients with acute-like presentation have underlying chronic liver disease, cirrhosis in most cases. WD patients with acute hepatitis may show nonspecific CT findings such as liver, enlargement and ascites. However, changes in liver attenuation could suggest the underlying disease. The metallic deposition may result in diffuse increased attenuation on CT owing to the high atomic number of copper. On the other hand, steatosis related to WD causes decreased attenuation (Akpinar and Akhan 2007). CT of patients with acute WD may also show findings of cirrhosis and portal hypertension.

7 Reye Syndrome

Reye syndrome is a rare disorder affecting children and occasionally young adults. Patients may present with acute liver disease. It is characterized by the occurrence of diffuse microvesicular steatosis following a benign viral infection and/or the ingestion of salicylates.

8 Malignant Infiltration of the Liver

Massive infiltration of the liver is an uncommon cause of acute liver failure. Hodgkin and non-Hodgkin lymphoma, other types of leukemia, breast cancer, and melanoma are among the most frequently implicated malignancies. Early recognition of this condition is of particular importance since it obviously represents a contraindication for transplantation. On CT, the liver usually appears diffusely heterogeneous and enlarged. Liver biopsy is indicated and may show lymphoma or leukemia that requires rapid treatment.

9 Acute Liver Disease in Pregnancy

Abnormal findings from liver tests occur in 3–5% of pregnancies but liver dysfunction is quite rare. Most liver dysfunction in pregnancy is due to one of the following diseases: hyperemesis gravidarum, intrahepatic cholestasis of pregnancy, preeclampsia, the HELLP syndrome, and acute fatty liver (AFL) of pregnancy (Hay 2008). Only the latter two, which are acute and severe diseases, will be covered in this chapter.

9.1 HELLP Syndrome

Severe preeclampsia is complicated in 2–12% of cases by the HELLP syndrome, defined by hemolysis (elevated indirect serum bilirubin levels and LDH levels above 600 U/l), elevated levels of liver enzymes (asparate transaminase level above 70 U/l), and low platelet count (below 150,000). Most patients present between 27 and 36 weeks' gestation, but 25–30% present in the postpartum period (Hay 2008; Mihu et al. 2007). The HELLP syndrome is a microangiopathic hemolytic anemia associated with vascular endothelial injury, fibrin deposition in blood vessels, and platelet activation with platelet consumption, resulting in areas of hemorrhage and necrosis leading to severe complications such as hematomas, liver rupture, and intraperitoneal bleeding (Hay 2008). The pathogenesis of HELLP syndrome is not completely understood. Most patients present with right upper quadrant abdominal pain, nausea, vomiting, malaise, and edema with significant weight gain (Lee and Brady 2009). Occasionally jaundice, hepatomegaly, hepatic encephalopathy, and hypertension may be present.

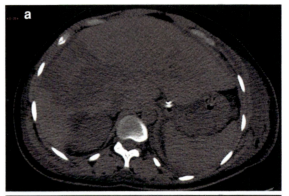

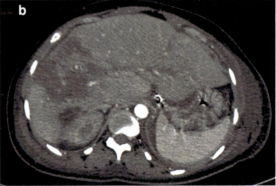

Fig. 6 HELLP syndrome. Unenhanced (**a**) and portal venous-phase contrast-enhanced (**b**) CT shows hypoattenuating lesions in the right side of the liver that are not enhanced after administration of contrast medium. There was neither abdominal fluid effusion nor rupture of the liver capsule

On CT, the most common imaging findings are subcapsular and intraparenchymal hematomas (Nunes et al. 2005) (Fig. 6). These hematomas are predominantly seen in the right side of the liver (Rooholamini et al. 1993). Hepatic rupture, which occurs less often, may be suspected when the interface between the intraparenchyma and the perihepatic hemorrhage is irregular. Hemoperitoneum is usually seen in those patients (Nunes et al. 2005). Hepatic infarction may also be observed and appears as nonenhanced low-attenuation areas ranging in configuration from peripheral, well-defined, wedge-shaped lesions to large abnormalities (Kronthal et al. 1990).

Imaging also enables one to detect severe extrahepatic complications such as cerebral hemorrhage and pulmonary edema.

The diagnosis of HELLP syndrome must be quickly established because of maternal and fetal risk and the necessity for immediate delivery. Hepatic hemorrhage without rupture is managed conservatively. There is no consensus regarding treatment of liver rupture, which is a rare, life-threatening complication of HELLP syndrome. Although hepatic artery ligation or partial hepatectomy can be performed, hepatic artery embolization is indicated in hemodynamically stable women.

9.2 Acute Fatty Liver

AFL of pregnancy is a sudden disease defined by microvesicular fatty infiltration of the liver. AFL occurs almost exclusively in the third trimester, from 28 to 40 weeks, rarely in the late second trimester (Hay 2008). Rarely, it may be diagnosed in the postpartum period. The pathophysiologic processes in AFL involve defects in mitochondrial fatty acid β-oxidation. The presentation can range from asymptomatic to fulminant liver failure with encephalopathy. Typically women present with 1–2 weeks' history of nausea, vomiting, abdominal pain, and fatigue. Jaundice occurs frequently. About 50% of patients with AFL have preeclampsia, and this disease can overlap with HELLP syndrome.

Although CT can demonstrate hepatomegaly and diffusely diminished attenuation of the liver parenchyma in some patients, this technique is less reliable for detecting microvesicular fatty infiltration than for detecting macrovesicular fatty infiltration (Lee and Brady 2009; Rooholamini et al. 1993). Therefore, the definitive diagnosis is based on liver biopsy that shows swollen, pale hepatocytes in the central zones with microvesicular fatty infiltration.

Similarly to HELLP syndrome, AFL requires prompt delivery.

References

Akpinar E, Akhan O (2007) Liver imaging findings of Wilson's disease. Eur J Radiol 61:25–32

Becker YT, Raiford DS, Webb L, Wright JK, Chapman WC, Pinson CW (1995) Rupture and hemorrhage of hepatic focal nodular hyperplasia. Am Surg 61:210–214

Bioulac-Sage P, Laumonier H, Couchy G et al (2009) Hepatocellular adenoma management and phenotypic classification: the Bordeaux experience. Hepatology 50:481–489

Brancatelli G, Vilgrain V, Federle MP et al (2007) Budd-Chiari syndrome: spectrum of imaging findings. AJR Am J Roentgenol 188:W168–W176

Buckley O, O'Brien J, Snow A et al (2007) Imaging of Budd-Chiari syndrome. Eur Radiol 17:2071–2078

Casillas VJ, Amendola MA, Gascue A, Pinnar N, Levi JU, Perez JM (2000) Imaging of nontraumatic hemorrhagic hepatic lesions. Radiographics 20:367–378

Condat B, Valla D (2006) Nonmalignant portal vein thrombosis in adults. Nat Clin Pract Gastroenterol Hepatol 3:505–515

Cope-Yokoyama S, Finegold MJ, Sturniolo GC et al (2010) Wilson disease: histopathological correlations with treatment on follow-up liver biopsies. World J Gastroenterol 16:1487–1494

Cura M, Haskal Z, Lopera J (2009) Diagnostic and interventional radiology for Budd-Chiari syndrome. Radiographics 29:669–681

Durand F, Bernuau J (2007) In: Rodes J, Rizzetto M, Benhamou JP, Blei A, Reichen J (eds) The textbook of hepatology: from basic sciences to clinical practice, 3rd edn. Wiley, Hoboken, pp 1523–1535

Dokmak S, Paradis V, Vilgrain V et al (2009) A single-center surgical experience of 122 patients with single and multiple hepatocellular adenomas. Gastroenterology 137:1698–1705

Ebert EC (2006) Hypoxic liver injury. Mayo Clin Proc 81:1232–1236

Francque S, Condat B, Asselah T et al (2004) Multifactorial aetiology of hepatic infarction: a case report with literature review. Eur J Gastroenterol Hepatol 16:411–415

Hay JE (2008) Liver disease in pregnancy. Hepatology 47:1067–1076

Henrion J (2007) Hypoxic hepatitis: the point of view of the clinician. Acta Gastroenterol Belg 70:214–216

Henrion J, Schapira M, Luwaert R, Colin L, Delannoy A, Heller FR (2003) Hypoxic hepatitis: clinical and hemodynamic study in 142 consecutive cases. Medicine (Baltimore) 82:392–406

Kahn JA, Haker KM, Petrovic LM, Arnaout WS, Koobatian G, Fong TL (2000) Radiographic findings of ischemic hepatitis in a cirrhotic patient. J Comput Assist Tomogr 24:887–889

Kanematsu M, Imaeda T, Yamawaki Y et al (1992) Rupture of hepatocellular carcinoma: predictive value of CT findings. AJR Am J Roentgenol 158:1247–1250

Kronthal AJ, Fishman EK, Kuhlman JE, Bohlman ME (1990) Hepatic infarction in preeclampsia. Radiology 177:726–728

Lee NM, Brady CW (2009) Liver disease in pregnancy. World J Gastroenterol 15:897–906

Mihu D, Costin N, Mihu CM, Seicean A, Ciortea R (2007) HELLP syndrome—a multisystemic disorder. J Gastrointestin Liver Dis 16:419–424

Miyamoto M, Sudo T, Kuyama T (1991) Spontaneous rupture of hepatocellular carcinoma: a review of 172 Japanese cases. Am J Gastroenterol 86:67–71

Mori H, Hayashi K, Uetani M, Matsuoka Y, Iwao M, Maeda H (1987) High-attenuation recent thrombus of the portal vein: CT demonstration and clinical significance. Radiology 163:353–356

Nunes JO, Turner MA, Fulcher AS (2005) Abdominal imaging features of HELLP syndrome: a 10-year retrospective review. AJR Am J Roentgenol 185:1205–1210

Plessier A, Sibert A, Consigny Y et al (2006) Aiming at minimal invasiveness as a therapeutic strategy for Budd-Chiari syndrome. Hepatology 44:1308–1316

Rooholamini SA, Au AH, Hansen GC et al (1993) Imaging of pregnancy-related complications. Radiographics 13:753–770

Soyer P, Levesque M (1995) Haemoperitoneum due to spontaneous rupture of hepatic haemangiomatosis: treatment by superselective arterial embolization and partial hepatectomy. Australas Radiol 39:90–92

Valla DC (2009) Primary Budd-Chiari syndrome. J Hepatol 50:195–203

Zucman-Rossi J, Jeannot E, Nhieu JT et al (2006) Genotype-phenotype correlation in hepatocellular adenoma: new classification and relationship with HCC. Hepatology 43:515–524

Biliary Emergencies

Yves Menu, Julien Cazejust, Ana Ruiz,
Louisa Azizi, and Lionel Arrivé

Contents

1	**Introduction**	93
2	**CT Technique**	94
2.1	How Many Rows?	94
2.2	Plain Images	95
2.3	Contrast Enhancement	95
2.4	Acquisition Parameters	95
2.5	Main Protocols	96
3	**Gallbladder Disease**	96
3.1	Acute Cholecystitis	96
3.2	Mirizzi Syndrome	105
3.3	Phlegmonous Cholecystitis	107
3.4	Gallbladder Haemorrhage	109
4	**Intrahepatic and Extrahepatic Bile Duct Diseases**	109
4.1	Cholangitis	109
4.2	Significance of Pneumobilia	110
4.3	Common Bile Duct Stones	110
4.4	Liver Biliary Abscesses	112
4.5	Ischemic Cholangitis	113
5	**Conclusion**	113
References		113

Abstract

Computed tomography (CT) is an important tool in the workup of patients with biliary emergencies. Optimal settings are mandatory to take full advantage of multidetector CT and to obtain the best multiplanar images with the lowest achievable radiation dose. CT is also part of an imaging strategy together with ultrasonography and magnetic resonance imaging. CT is a problem solver in the case of cholecystitis, most often complementary to ultrasonography, especially in the case of complications such as abscesses. CT is also an important tool to assess unusual diseases such as Mirizzi syndrome and ischemic cholangitis. Because CT is a tool that is available 24/7, the radiologist should be familiarize himself or herself with appropriate protocols and with interpretation of common and/or severe diseases, because most of clinical situations will require urgent medical decisions, mainly based on imaging.

1 Introduction

Although computed tomography (CT) is the workhorse of imaging in the case of abdominal emergencies, examination of the biliary tract is one field where ultrasonography (US) and magnetic resonance imaging (MRI) challenge CT. US has been the initial procedure for years and is still recommended when acute cholecystitis is suspected or when bile duct dilatation is anticipated in a patient with a potential obstructive jaundice. It has also been proposed as an adjunct to the clinical examination. This bedside US

Y. Menu (✉) · J. Cazejust · A. Ruiz · L. Azizi · L. Arrivé
Hôpital Saint Antoine,
182 rue du Faubourg Saint Antoine,
75012 Paris, France
e-mail: yves.menu@sat.aphp.fr

P. Taourel (ed.), *CT of the Acute Abdomen*, Medical Radiology. Diagnostic Imaging,
DOI: 10.1007/174_2011_158, © Springer-Verlag Berlin Heidelberg 2011

would help in the triage of patients (Endo 2010). Although the role of MRI in emergency patients has been very low until now, some authors are now exploring the capability of MRI in these conditions. MRI has some advantages, such as high tissue contrast, sensitivity to fluid and inflammation, allowing cholangiopancreatography, and improved spatial resolution and examination duration (Tkacz et al. 2009). Conversely, with CT it might be difficult to identify bile duct stones when they are poorly mineralized, and the radiation dose is a drawback (Brenner 2010). Also, although US and MRI have native 3D capabilities, CT was primarily a 2D method. The third dimension really appeared as a competitive adjunct with the development of multidetector CT (MDCT), especially with machines that include at least 16 detector rows, opening the possibility of nearly isotropic imaging (Choi et al. 2007). For bile ducts, volumetric examination through multiplanar navigation is clearly a necessity (Choi et al. 2007).

The availability of CT machines is also an important feature in emergency conditions. CT has definitely taken a leading role in the management of abdominal emergencies at large, and is now widely available 24/7 in most institutions that are in a position to take care of these patients (Mills et al. 2010). Therefore, availability is less a problem for CT than for other modalities such as MRI. For some institutions that do not host a specialized radiologist, sending images through a teleradiology system for remote reporting is also a possibility.

Because patients with acute abdomen should be examined with short notice, there are three competing major modalities, and the radiologist who is in charge of these patients should know how to manage all three modalities and make the best use of each as far as necessary, dealing with complementarities and substitution. Therefore, the clinician will appreciate this integrated management of imaging modalities.

Finally, in some situations, interventional radiology can be helpful, because it can solve the problem itself, become a temporary substitute for surgery in fragile patients, or even be a complement to surgery. Therefore, every radiologist should know the potential role of interventional radiology in these conditions, and appreciate the anatomical possibilities, as well as the optimal method for guidance, which is very commonly either CT or a combination of US and fluoroscopy.

In this chapter, the role of CT will be stressed, but in every situation the reader will be reminded of the role of US and MRI and the possibility of interventional radiology to help the radiologist become a complete global imaging expert.

2 CT Technique

2.1 How Many Rows?

Although CT examination of the bile ducts can be performed with virtually all CT machines, MDCT is a clear advance owing to the possibility to perform isotropic or nearly isotropic imaging. Given the complex anatomic orientation of the bile ducts and gallbladder, appreciation of all structures requires at least axial, coronal, and sagittal views with a similar spatial resolution (Choi et al. 2007).

It is also obvious that examination should never be focussed on the usual area of the bile ducts, for several reasons. First, although there are many anatomical variants, a distended gallbladder may be found as low as the right iliac fossa. Second, the bile ducts accompany the liver when it is displaced or enlarged. Again, finding the gallbladder in the right iliac fossa is possible in the case of liver enlargement. Third, some diseases of the bile ducts may lead to bile leakage, and therefore may be associated with peritoneal or even sometimes retroperitoneal fluid, which could be found down in the pelvis. Finally, the examination is usually motivated by symptoms that may correspond to disease of bile ducts as well as to many other emergency conditions. Therefore, the minimum examination should include the abdomen and the pelvis. Relying on clinical background, and also age characteristics, one should discuss if the inclusion of chest CT during the same examination is desirable or not. In a patient with severe infection, examination of the chest is recommended. Conversely, if the symptoms are clearly located to the bile ducts and if the patient is young, one can question if the additional radiation dose given for additional chest CT acquisition is justified or not. However, in this case, US would have been a better option from the beginning.

To compromise between the acquisition volume, duration of apnea, and the necessity to provide isotropic images, MDCT machines with 16 rows and above are most appropriate. If machines with fewer than 16 rows are used, the compromise would probably be to increase the pitch and decrease the volume to maintain spatial resolution. Obviously, 64-row machines are best adapted to the examination of the bile ducts, given the necessity to examine the whole abdomen, as well as the chest in many cases.

2.2 Plain Images

Another question is the necessity to perform plain imaging and/or postcontrast imaging. The main advantage of plain images is that they allow the detection of calcifications. This might be critical because, unlike urinary stones, the vast majority of biliary stones, at least those found in the common bile duct, are only faintly calcified or not calcified at all. Therefore, postcontrast images carry the risk of overlooking common bile duct stones (Neitlich et al. 1997). Conversely, adding another acquisition will increase the overall radiation dose (Brenner 2010).

Therefore, there is no unique answer to this question. The decision to perform plain imaging should be taken by the radiologist, in the context of clinical symptoms and previous US examination. Schematically, if there is suspicion of a common bile duct stone, if US findings are inconclusive, and if MRI is unavailable, CT should probably be performed using both plain and enhanced imaging.

In rare cases, iodine cannot be injected into the patient, owing to the presence of a contraindication. Although the amount of information will be much less, plain CT might, however, provide some useful information, such as the presence of calcifications, blood, or gas or the identification of a large tissue mass.

2.3 Contrast Enhancement

In most cases, intravenous contrast medium injection is mandatory, in order to better delineate normal tissue, tumor, and inflammation.

There are no specific requirements for contrast medium injection related to bile duct examination, and the injection rate and the iodine concentration are similar to those in most routine abdominal protocols.

A total dose of 2 ml/kg and an injection rate of 1–2 ml/s are common and suitable settings.

The best single acquisition is performed in the portal phase, starting 70–90 s after injection has started. These slices are optimal to evaluate normal and abnormal bile duct wall and surrounding tissues and vessels.

In very rare instances, additional acquisition could be useful. In the case of bleeding of unknown origin, or suspicion of ischemic disease of the bile ducts, it might be useful to include an acquisition in the arterial phase as well. These situations are uncommon.

Delayed images are usually unnecessary.

2.4 Acquisition Parameters

Slice thickness is a confusing issue with MDCT. Slice collimation, primary reconstruction, and secondary reconstruction are usually completely different. Slice collimation is dependent on the detector characteristics. Most modern devices can acquire images with a collimation of approximately 0.6–1 mm. However, these slices are raw data and are seldom reconstructed as images, because the signal-to-noise ratio is not optimal, at least for an acceptable radiation dose (Gallix et al. 2006).

Most commonly, thicker slices are reconstructed. There are several options depending on the machine and the workstation. Because the biliary tree is a somewhat complex anatomic structure, multiplanar reconstructions are very useful, and sometimes not just in the common three planes (axial, coronal, sagittal). Oblique reconstructions are interesting, and specific planes should be adapted to the patient's specific anatomy, and to the findings for a disease.

Therefore, it is desirable to reconstruct a set of thin slices (approximately 1–1.25 mm) with an overlapping reconstruction to improve the quality of images reconstructed in alternative planes. Some workstations provide on-the-fly fast reconstruction in all directions, using the set of thin slices, and making easier the navigation in the volume. However, there are drawbacks: the signal-to-noise ratio is still not optimal and the number of slices is very high, which is a problem for storage and image transmission.

As a compromise, most centers now produce systematic and automatic reconstruction of 2–3-mm-thick slices in axial, coronal, and sagittal planes. Thinner slices are available on workstations in order to perform additional postprocessing, but may or may not be recorded on storage systems (picture archiving and communication system) and are usually not recorded on mobile media such as a CD-ROM.

The voltage is a very important issue for the optimization of the radiation dose to which the patient is exposed. Except in severely overweight patients, the voltage should not be set over 120 kV. In very thin patients, it is sufficient to use 100 kV. Most machines come with different software aiming to decrease an unnecessarily high radiation dose. A radiation dose report is provided for each examination. It is the radiologist's responsibility to check that the CT dose index and LDP are within acceptable limits.

2.5   Main Protocols

As a summary, there are four different protocols for CT of the bile ducts:

1. The most common protocol consists in a single acquisition, in the portal phase (70–90 s) after injection of iodine.
2. If there is suspicion of a common bile duct stone, a noncontrast acquisition should be added.
3. If the patient's general condition is poor, for instance, with intense fever, and if the symptoms are unclear, it is wise to include a chest CT acquisition as well.
4. In the case of bleeding, an arterial phase acquisition is mandatory.

However, these are general orientations and the radiologist should fine-tune the protocol according to the clinical questions. He or she should keep in mind that the expected quality of the examination and the radiation dose should be appropriately adapted to the patient's characteristics and symptoms.

Because CT is only one tool among others for these patients, the radiologist should be familiar with the indications, possibilities, and limits of alternative methods such as US and MRI. Ideally, the radiologist could be able to decide which examination is best suited to the patient or which sequence of examinations is appropriate. In that case, it is likely that US will be the first examination performed in the vast majority of cases.

3   Gallbladder Disease

3.1   Acute Cholecystitis

Acute cholecystitis is a very common disease. It accounts for 3–10% of all patients with abdominal pain (Brewer et al. 1976). Most of the patients are over 50 years old. In 90–95% of patients, it is attributable to gallbladder stones. It is likely that the stones in the gallbladder are deleterious for several reasons. First, there could be a direct mechanical inflammation related to contact of the stone with the mucosa. Second, this inflammation may cause a small hemorrhage that might increase inflammation again and favor infection. However, the third process might be the most important one. The stone may block the outflow, increasing the pressure within the gallbladder and favoring the development of infection. The degree of obstruction and its duration are important factors. If the obstruction is incomplete and short, the patient has biliary colic. If the obstruction is total and durable, acute cholecystitis can develop (Kimura et al. 2007).

In less than 10% of cases, cholecystitis may develop in a gallbladder with no preexisting stones. This "acalculous" cholecystitis is mainly observed in patients with a severe general condition, such as in patients in an intensive care unit for any reason, in the postoperative period in patients who have undergone heavy surgery, and more commonly in patients with a recent polytrauma or blunt trauma of the abdomen. For this reason, it should be remembered that the absence of a gallbladder stone does not preclude the possibility of a cholecystitis. The pathogenesis is somewhat similar to that of calculous cholecystitis. Even if there is no stone, stasis and functional obstruction of the bile outflow is probably the main reason for infection and inflammation. There is a lack of stimulation for gallbladder emptying, which is also enhanced by medications such as opioid analgesics. Gallbladder ischemia and the presence of mediators of inflammation due to the associated disease are also cofactors.

A specific situation is the patient with recent chemoembolization, who is exposed to ischemic cholecystitis (Wagnetz et al. 2010). In this case, the diagnosis is easy, given the clinical background. Cholecystitis related to radioembolization is a similar issue (Atassi et al. 2008).

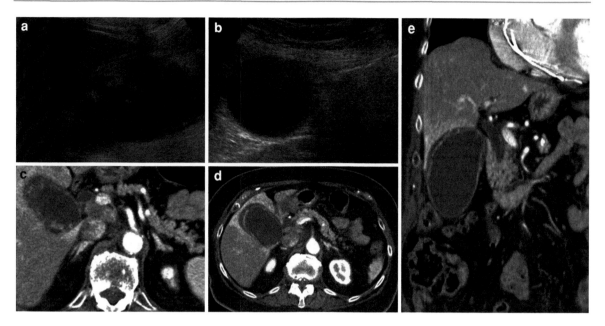

Fig. 1 A 88-year-old woman with abdominal pain and a Murphy sign on clinical examination. **a** Ultraonography (US) findings were misleading because there was some material within the gallbladder but it was "floating". Shadowing was mild. **b** No definite wall thickening in the gallbladder fundus. Although the diagnosis of acute cholecystitis was likely, computed tomography (CT) was performed because of some ambiguous features. **c–e** Postcontrast CT in the axial (**c, d**) and in the coronal (**e**) planes. Obvious thickening of the gallbladder wall was seen. On the upper slice (**c**), the gallbladder wall seemed highly inflammatory, with some mucosal disruption. On the lower slice (**d**) the wall appeared as homogeneously thickened. On the coronal image (**e**), the difference between the obviously thickened wall in the upper part of the gallbladder contrasts with the rather normal appearance of the fundus, as noticed on US. See also in **c** slightly hyperdense material appearing within the gallbladder as well as hyperemia of the surrounding liver, related to gallbladder inflammation

There are several stages of acute cholecystitis (Kimura et al. 2007). Initially, the cholecystitis is only edematous. There is no damage to the gallbladder wall except reversible edema. Necrotizing cholecystitis is the second stage. There is damage to the mucosa, but lesions are not transmural. Suppurative cholecystitis is the third stage. Active necrosis is present and there is a risk of perforation and pericholecystic abscesses. Finally, chronic cholecystitis is the result of repeated occurrences of attenuated episodes. Mucosal atrophy is observed as well as fibrosis.

Acute cholecystitis presents as a progressively increasing pain of the right upper quadrant or of the epigastric area. Pain may be continuous or acuminated. One major characteristic is that the palpation of the gallbladder area reinforces the pain, which should be same as the spontaneous pain, and should prevent the patient from breathing in deeply. If the palpation is done in the same condition, but in a slightly different area, the same characteristics do not appear. This is known as the Murphy sign. Hyperthermia is present, but moderate. In the case of very severe hyperthermia, one should suspect a complication such as perforation.

In most circumstances, US should be the first examination performed for the detection of cholecystitis, at least if it is clinically suspected. US has the potential to identify the gallbladder stone, thickening of the gallbladder wall, and hypervascularization of the inflamed wall, as depicted with color Doppler US (Ralls et al. 1985, Jeffrey et al. 1995). Also, US has the potential to reproduce the clinical Murphy maneuver, and to check that the target area for palpation is really related to the gallbladder (Ralls et al. 1982).

There have not been so many studies comparing the results of US and CT for the detection of acute cholecystitis. Only Mirvis et al. (1986) found that the final results were very similar, and their study was limited to a very short series of 15 cases, in which sensitivity and specificity were both 100%. Because technology has improved so much, MDCT should

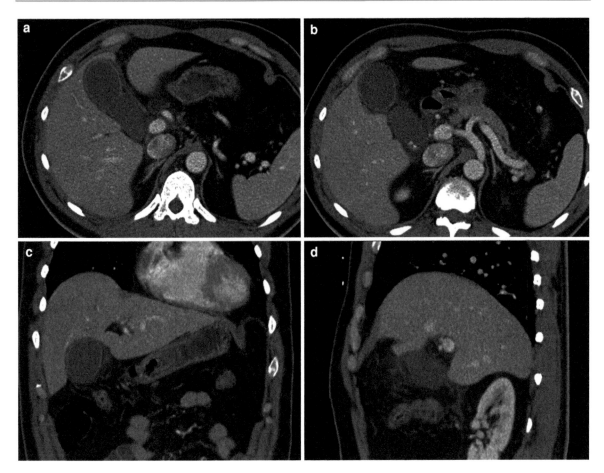

Fig. 2 Typical cholecystitis associated with gallstones. A 44-year-old man with right upper quadrant pain, fever, and a Murphy sign. CT in the axial (**a**, **b**) coronal (**c**), and sagittal (**d**) planes confirms gallbladder wall thickening, hyperattenuation of the perivesicular fat, and stranding, associated with calcified gallstones in the neck of the gallbladder

also be an excellent tool for this purpose. Compared with US, the only drawback of CT was that gallstones were not always identified. However, this did not prevent the correct diagnosis being made using the other signs for inflammation.

When US findings are positive and typical, there is no need for additional CT. However, US has limitations. Access to the gallbladder area may be difficult owing to gas interposition and a small stone in the gallbladder neck might be challenging to identify. Finally, in not all cases of cholecystitis is there a thickened wall and even wall thickening can be heterogeneous (Fig. 1). Gangrenous cholecystitis may have with a very thin wall, and carry a high risk of perforation.

Because CT is typically performed in challenging cases, and because the identification of a stone in the gallbladder neck might be difficult, it is advisable to start the examination with plain images acquired through the upper abdomen only. Arterial phase images are not mandatory. Portal phase images are the best adapted sequence. Thin slices are desirable because the anatomy of the gallbladder is rather complex. In addition to conventional axial, coronal, and sagittal planes, oblique reconstructions through the long axis and the short axis of the gallbladder allow optimal analysis of the gallbladder wall. This is critical because one of the goals of CT examination is to detect fistulization through the gallbladder wall, mainly to the liver parenchyma.

The most common feature of cholecystitis is thickening of the gallbladder wall (Figs. 1, 2, 3, 4). Usually the threshold is 3 mm. Measurement of the gallbladder wall is not so easy because there are several layers, with enhanced mucosa, and edematous submucosa (Fig. 3) One should measure the whole gallbladder wall, and not only the enhanced layer, which is often limited to the mucosa. After contrast medium injection, there is a marked enhancement of the gallbladder wall, either homogeneous or layered owing to preferential enhancement of the mucosa (Fig. 2). Edema of the periphery of the gallbladder wall may be seen as a hypodense ring, which is often interpreted as a perivesicular localized peritoneal fluid collection (Fig. 3). Actually, this cannot be the case because there is no peritoneal recess between the superior part of the fundus and the liver. Fluid can be present as well. A very small quantity is only the result of local inflammation and is not necessarily pejorative.

Gallbladder wall thickening is not specific to cholecystitis, as it can be found in other circumstances, such as portal hypertension, adenomyomatosis, and acute hepatitis. Portal hypertension is not a problem because there are no clinical symptoms for a cholecystitis. Adenomyomatosis can be associated with colic pain, in the case of a commonly associated gallbladder stone. However, there is no fever or inflammation of the gallbladder wall, and the appearance of very small cystic lesions within the wall is rather characteristic. Conversely, acute hepatitis can occur with a very similar pain. Evaluation of liver test results is useful because cholecystitis is rarely associated with a very high level of transaminases, whereas hepatitis is usually associated with marked cytolysis.

Mucosal sloughing is another sign for cholecystitis (Fig. 5). However, it is difficult to identify owing to mild changes of attenuation between the mucosa and the bile, which can be hyperattenuating itself.

Hyperemia of the surrounding liver is often associated with cholecystitis and can be a helpful ancillary sign. Of course, it is likely that localized liver hyperemia is related to inflammation of the gallbladder wall, and this may help one differentiate inflammation from other causes of wall thickening (Fig. 1).

Stranding and hyperattenuation of the perivesicular fat is a second sign frequently observed. Although this appearance is consistent with regional inflammation, its specificity is rather low.

Difficulty to see gallstones on CT sometimes makes it difficult to differentiate between calculous

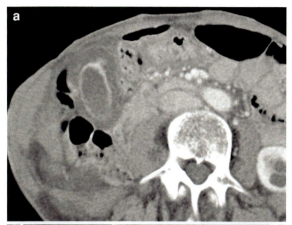
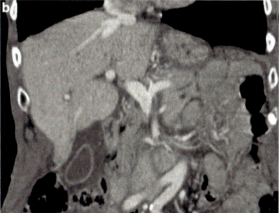
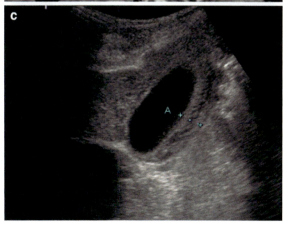

Fig. 3 Edematous thickening of the gallbladder wall in a patient with acute cholecystitis. A 91-year-old man without any medical record with abdominal pain and fever. Because the clinical features were unclear, CT was performed initially. Postcontrast CT in the axial (**a**) and coronal (**b**) planes shows a hypoattenuating rim surrounding the gallbladder. The initial report concluded there was peritoneal perivesicular accumulation of fluid. US performed immediately thereafter (**c**) showed that this was part of a markedly enlarged gallbladder wall

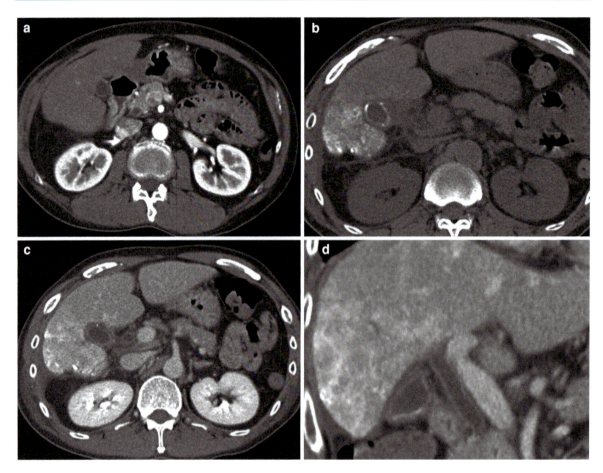

Fig. 4 Ischemic cholecystitis after chemoembolization. A 55-year-old man underwent chemoembolization for palliative treatment of hepatocellular carcinoma. Three days after chemoembolization, the patient complained of severe pain in the right upper quadrant. **a** On CT performed 1 month before, the gallbladder was unremarkable. **b** CT on the third day after chemoembolization. Plain image showing the presence of Lipiodol within the gallbladder wall. **c–d** After injection, the gallbladder wall is thickened and appears layered on the axial (**c**), and coronal (**d**) images

and acalculous cholecystitis. Stones can be completely overlooked because their attenuation can be similar to that of bile. In some cases, narrowing the window allows visualization of slightly hyperattenuating stones within the gallbladder (Fig. 1). Finally, the clinical background helps in differentiating calculous and acalculous cholecystitis when the context is, for instance, that of an ischemic cholecystitis related to chemoembolization (Fig. 4), severe associated disease or trauma, or the complication of bile duct stenting.

Some CT criteria have been gathered to facilitate the diagnosis and are reported in Table 1.

Complications of cholecystitis are as follows:
- Emphysematous cholecystitis is an exceptional occurrence characterized by the presence of gas within the gallbladder wall or even within the cavity (Wu et al. 2010b). The presence of air is related to necrosis and/or development of anaerobic bacteria. Obviously, if the air is within the lumen, it should not be confused with a common aerobilia, following surgery, endoscopic sphincterotomy, or sometimes spontaneous fistulization within the bowel. The presence of some air within the gallbladder wall is one of the signs for acute cholecystitis, although it is rarely encountered.
- Perforation of the gallbladder within the peritoneum is a rare but life-threatening event. A very small amount of peritoneal fluid is usually associated with inflammation and is not pejorative. If the quantity of fluid increases, and moreover if the clinical presentation is more a peritonitis than a

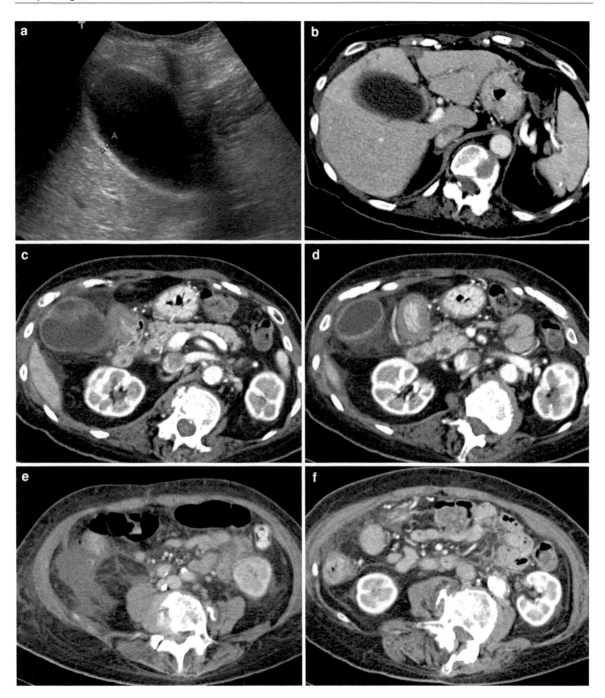

Fig. 5 Acalculous acute cholecystitis. An 82-year-old man with pulmonary embolism in an intensive care unit. On the basis of abdominal pain and an elevated white cell blood count, acalculous cholecystitis was suspected. The diagnosis was made by CT after inconclusive US findings. Antibiotics were given, but there was deterioration on the second day. CT showed increased peritoneal effusion, and the patient was successfully treated with percutaneous cholecystostomy a US findings were inconclusive, showing a moderate thickening of the wall as well as gallbladder distension. It was unclear if there was a Murphy sign. b–d CT performed the same day shows perfusion abnormalities in the liver next to the gallbladder bed (b), thickened gallbladder wall as well as sloughing (c), and hyperattenuation of the surrounding fat. e CT on the second day shows peritoneal effusion. f A percutaneous cholecystostomy was performed under bedside US guidance. The recovery was uneventful

Table 1 Criteria for the diagnosis of acute cholecystitis on computed tomography. Either two major criteria or one major criterion and two minor criteria satisfy the CT diagnosis of acute cholecystitis. (Adapted from Barie and Eachempati 2010)

Major criteria	Minor criteria
Gallbladder wall thickening more than 3 mm	Gallbladder distention (more than 5 cm in transverse diameter)
Subserosal halo sign (intramural lucency caused by edema)	
Pericholecystic infiltration of fat	High-attenuation bile (sludge)
Pericholecystic fluid (without either ascites or hypoalbuminemia)	
Mucosal sloughing	
Intramural gas	

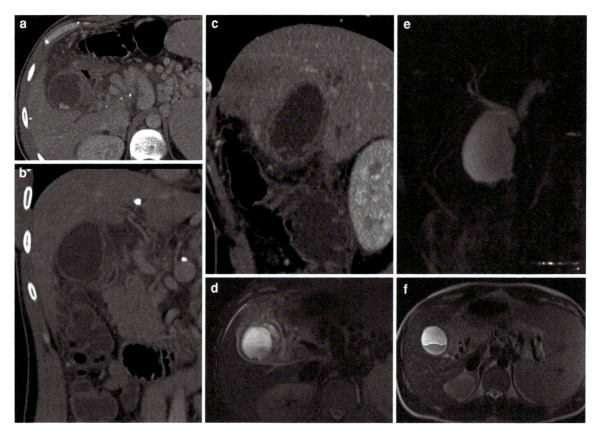

Fig. 6 Perforated cholecystitis in a patient with portal cavernoma. A 30-year-old patient with a history of portal cavernoma. US findings were inconclusive owing to the presence of portal collaterals. Postcontrast CT in the axial (**a**), coronal (**b**), and sagittal (**c**) planes shows abnormalities of the gallbladder wall, and a localized defect in the gallbladder wall. Magnetic resonance imaging (MRI) confirms the irregularities of the gallbladder wall in the fundus on T2-weighted axial images (**d**) and on magnetic resonance cholangiopancreatography (**e**) and fluid–fluid level on a T2-weighted half-Fourier acquisition single shot turbo spin echo sequence (**f**)

localized pain, perforation of the gallbladder and peritoneal bile leakage should be suspected. Subtle perforation of the gallbladder wall can sometimes be suspected before leakage (Fig. 6).

- Gangrenous cholecystitis is related to necrosis of the wall. Consequently, the gallbladder wall thickening might be absent, and, by virtue of necrosis, there is no enhancement after injection of contrast medium

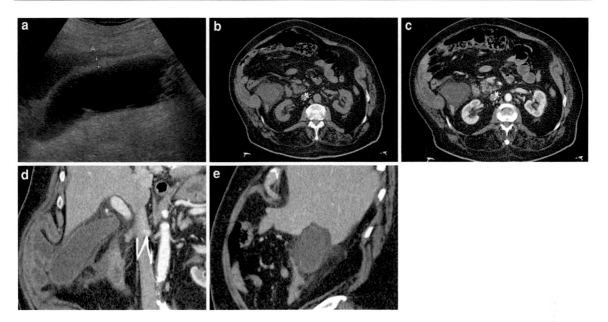

Fig. 7 Acute gangrenous cholecystitis. Am 85-year-old patient with fever and pain in the right flank. On surgery, gangrenous cholecystitis with minimal localized perforations was seen. **a** US shows a distended gallbladder with stones and thickening of the gallbladder wall. Gallstones are not identified, **b** Plain CT shows the gallbladder with hyperattenuation surrounding fat. **c–e** Post contrast CT in the axial (**c**), coronal (**d**), and sagittal (**e**) planes show that there is virtually no enhancement of the gallbladder wall

(Fig. 7). However, the wall is usually irregular, some places showing thickening and enhancements, others being thin and without enhancement. Gangrenous cholecystitis is usually associated with severe clinical symptoms, prompting rapid surgery. It occurs in up to 7.1% of cases of cholecystitis (Tokunaga et al. 1997). There are some discriminating CT signs for gangrenous cholecystitis. One is the presence of perfusion defects in the gallbladder wall, either localized or generalized. The appearance could be that of a poorly enhanced gallbladder wall (Wu et al. 2010a). In a series of 25 patients, the presence of a perfusion defect was 100% predictive of gangrenous cholecystitis, whereas conversely, 30% of gangrenous cholecystitis did not come with such defects.

- The most common complication of cholecystitis is liver abscess formation (Fig. 8). Abscesses usually develop in segments IV or V of the liver and are related to direct fistulization through a perforation of the superior aspects of the gallbladder wall. The role of CT in the depiction of liver abscesses is extremely important because US may fail to detect these complications, at least when they are small. However, this is a critical issue for treatment planning. It precludes the possibility for simple laparoscopic surgery and alternatively may require initial percutaneous drainage or even open surgery. The detection of liver abscesses requires careful multiplanar examination. The abscess is best depicted on portal phase imaging. Enhanced wall of the abscess is very common. It is sometimes associated with nonspecific regional liver enhancement; however, this hyperemia can be seen even in the absence of any liver abscess (Fig. 1). Conversely, gallbladder cancer can mimic cholecystitis with liver abscess (Fig. 9). The appearance can be extremely confusing because a gallbladder stone can be associated and there could be hypervascularization of the adjacent liver parenchyma as well (Fig. 10).

- Generally speaking, CT is slightly superior to US for the exact depiction of the disease, not only the presence or absence of abscesses, and also to appreciate the amount of inflammation. As some of these patients are fragile because of age or comorbidities, there are alternatives to classic surgery, such as percutaneous drainage of the gallbladder, which can often facilitate delayed surgery,

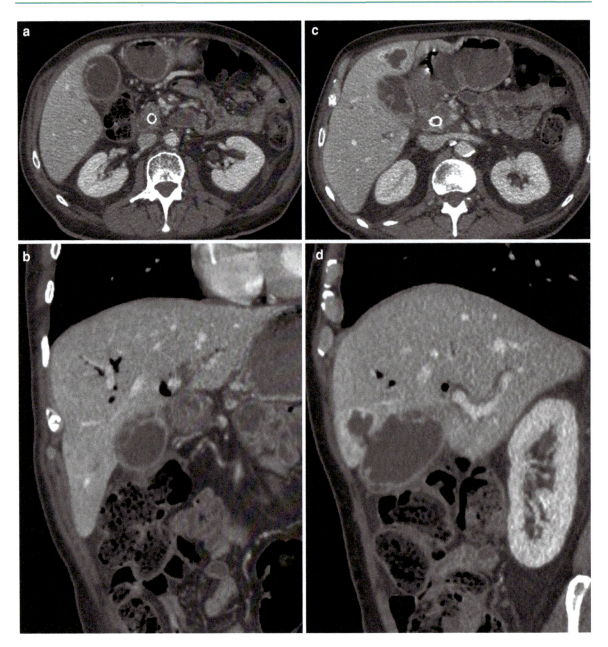

Fig. 8 A 72-year-old man with cancer of the pancreas treated with chemotherapy and metallic stenting of the common bile duct, experiencing fever and tenderness of the right upper quadrant. Postcontrast CT shows the pancreatic tumor and the stent, and a gallbladder with thickened wall and mucosal sloughing in the axial (**a**) and coronal (**b**) planes. In the adjacent liver, there is a hypoattenuating mass with enhanced contours (**c**). Communication between this liver abscess and the inflamed gallbladder is better visualized in the sagittal plane (**d**)

or even partial resection of the gallbladder, trying to avoid difficult dissections near the cystic duct and the common bile duct, in order to avoid severe complications such as intraoperative injury of the common bile duct or of the right hepatic duct. Even if US findings are positive, in these fragile patients it might be wise to perform CT to provide a more precise topographical evaluation of the disease. CT

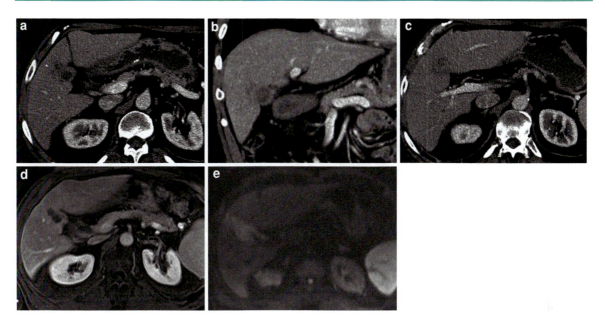

Fig. 9 Gallbladder cancer mimicking cholecystitis. A 64-year-old patient is treated for lymphoma of the neck. He presented with mild fever and increasing pain of the right upper quadrant. US shows enlargement of the gallbladder wall without the Murphy sign. CT and MRI could not differentiate between chronic cholecystitis and cancer. Fine-needle aspiration was performed and confirmed malignancy. The tumor was surgically removed. CT shows enlargement of the gallbladder wall on axial (**a**) and coronal (**b**) planes. **c** In the segments IV and V of the liver, there is a hypoattenuating area. MRI was performed. Gd-enhanced T1-weighted images in the portal phase (**d**) confirmed gallbladder wall thickening and a hypointense area in adjacent liver, whereas the diffusion-weighted image (**e**) showed diffuse restriction of the area

can also be a useful tool for close follow-up of fragile patients when the risk of surgery seems high and there is discussion whether an interventional or a surgical is best (Fig. 7).

3.2 Mirizzi Syndrome

Mirizzi syndrome is a rare and challenging situation. A stone is impacted in the cystic duct. This stone mechanically erodes the duct wall, and produces an inflammatory mass. Because the cystic duct is in very close relationship with the hepatic duct, this mass at least compresses the common bile duct, at the level of the hepatic duct, or even creates a complex fistula. Depending on the severity, Mirizzi syndrome can be classified as stage I if there is only a compression of the common bile duct and stages II–V according to the presence of fistulas of the common bile duct and the duodenum, with or without stone ileus (Solis-Caxaj 2009). This classification may not be universally accepted, but it translates the fact that surgical procedures can widely differ from one stage to another. The role of imaging is to delineate the existence or at least the risk of fistulas.

Usually, the main clinical finding is jaundice, owing to the obstruction of the hepatic duct. Surgery can be very difficult because there is at least inflammation of the hepatic duct, if not fistulas and some destruction of the common bile duct wall. Resection of the stone and the gallbladder is not easy.

Mirizzi syndrome should be suspected when a patient presents with bile duct dilatation at the level of the common hepatic duct and above, with a stone located in the area of the obstruction (Fig. 11). Because the stone is surrounded by inflammation, the appearance might be challenging. Sometimes irregular enhancement is seen, mimicking a tumor. The gallbladder stone is sometimes only faintly calcified, only at the periphery, and the calcified ring might be incomplete. For this reason, Mirizzi syndrome is frequently overlooked as a tumor, unless the specific location is identified, leading to consideration of this possibility.

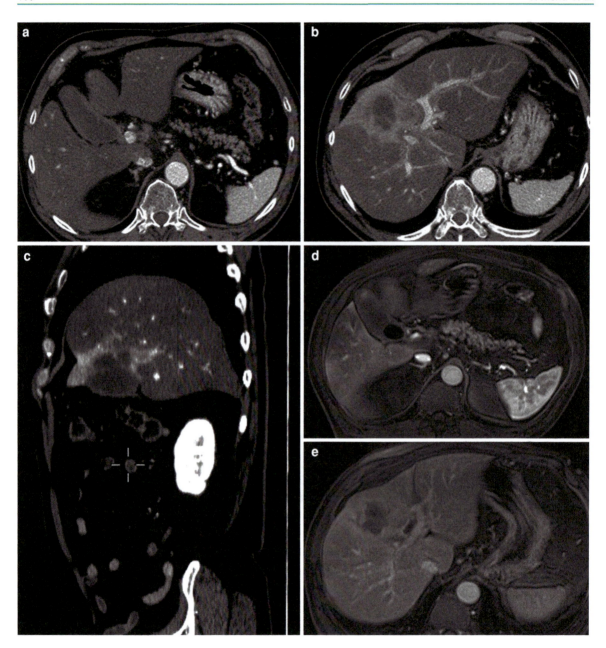

Fig. 10 Gallbladder cancer mimicking perforated cholecystitis. A 66-year-old patient with abdominal pain and fever. CT and MRI favor the hypothesis of a calculous cholecystitis with intrahepatic abscess formation related to gallbladder wall perforation. Surgery demonstrated that it was in fact a large bulky gallbladder carcinoma, associated with inflammatory changes. Contrast-enhanced CT shows a gallbladder with an irregular wall (a) and a hypoattenuating mass within segments IV and V of the liver (b) associated with liver perfusion changes of inflammatory type. There is an obvious communication with the gallbladder on the sagittal plane (c) MRI (T1-weighted Gd-enhanced) confirms the presence of a large gallstone, not apparent on CT (d), and the adjacent mass within the liver (e)

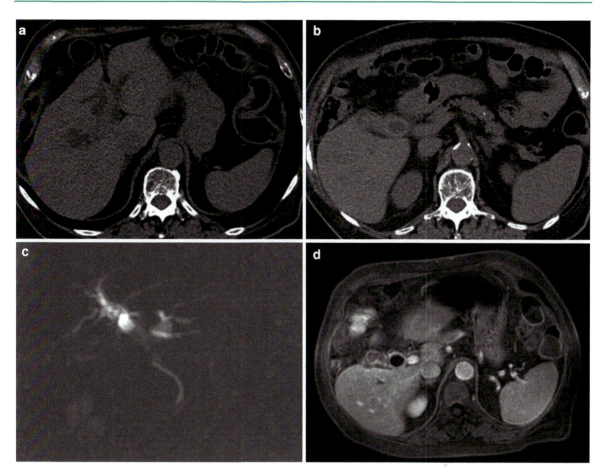

Fig. 11 Mirizzi syndrome. A 72-year-old man with progressive jaundice. US shows dilatation of intrahepatic bile ducts, but not of the lower common bile duct. The gallbladder area is difficult to analyze. Plain CT (**a**, **b**) and MRI (**c**, **d**) were performed. On plain CT, intrahepatic dilation of the bile duct is seen (**a**). On a lower slice (**b**), a stone is detected, appearing as hypoattenuating in the center and slightly hyerattenuating at the periphery. In the gallbladder fossa, the stone is seen in the gallbladder neck area, and the gallbladder seems to be collapsed. On the magnetic resonance cholangiogram (**c**), intrahepatic dilatation is confirmed and the lower common bile duct is normal. On contrast-enhanced images in the axial plane (**d**), the stone is clearly visible and the gallbladder seems atrophic. On surgery, Mirizzi syndrome was confirmed. The hepatic duct was inflammatory and there were two small fistulas between the cystic duct and the hepatic duct. Cholecystectomy and drainage of the common bile duct were performed and the postoperative period was uneventful

The diagnosis benefits greatly from the complementary of CT and magnetic resonance cholangiopancreatography (MRCP). In a study of 52 patients, the overall sensitivity, specificity, positive predictive value, negative predictive value, and accuracy of the combination of MRCP and CT were 96.0, 93.5, 83.5, 98.5, and 94.0%, respectively. Corresponding values for CT were 42.0, 98.5, 93.0, 83.5, and 85.0%, respectively (Yun et al. 2009).

From a treatment point of view, surgery is mandatory. The stone and the gallbladder should be removed, but the inflammatory mass is usually not resected. Cautious intubation of the hepatic duct and postoperative drainage, sometimes prolonged, allows progressive healing and hopefully a satisfactory recovery of the bile duct continuity (Hubert et al. 2010).

3.3 Phlegmonous Cholecystitis

"Phlegmonous cholecystitis" means that inflammatory processes related to acute cholecystitis resolve in part,

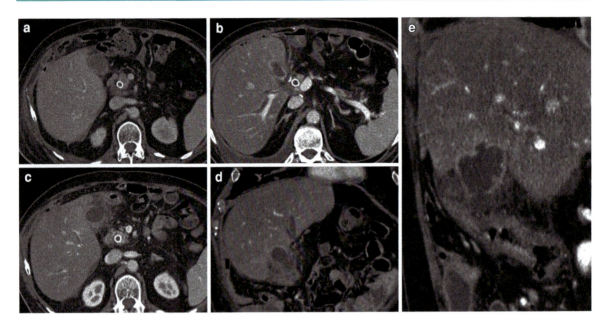

Fig. 12 Phlegmonous cholecystitis in a patient with a biliary stent. A 58-year-old patient had biliary stenting as a palliative treatment of unresectable pancreatic adenocarcinoma. He presented with mild fever, and permanent pain of the right upper quadrant. **a** CT 2 months before showed no abnormalities of the gallbladder. **b** CT upon admission showed enhanced wall of the gallbladder after contrast medium injection. **c** On a lower level, CT shows a heterogeneous mass surrounding the gallbladder and extending to the transverse colon. There is a discontinuity of the gallbladder wall. **d** The coronal plane image shows that the perforation of the gallbladder extends toward the transverse colon, which is included within the inflammatory mass. **e** The sagittal plane image confirms the extension of this mass and shows also small perforation of the upper aspect of the gallbladder

most commonly because cholecystitis has initially been overlooked, and because a treatment had been administered, including antibiotics. From an acute disease, it evolves into a subacute disease. The inflammatory process tends to self-limit, and produces an inflammatory mass near the gallbladder fossa. This mass is a combination of the inflammatory gallbladder itself, inflamed perivesicular fat, and also adhesion of small bowel caused by regional inflammation (Fig. 12).

From a clinical point of view, the patient has subacute pain, fatigue, tenderness of the right upper quadrant without a Murphy sign. The patient may have moderate hyperthermia. Weight loss can be observed. Biologically, inflammation is constant, but the white cell counts are not always increased. From this clinical and biological description, one can imagine that a gallbladder tumor is suspected as the first hypothesis.

On US, it is a challenging situation because the palpated mass is poorly limited and the gallbladder may not be recognizable. CT has a clear advantage in this case, but one might nevertheless hesitate in deciding between the two hypotheses of subacute inflammation and gallbladder cancer.

There are several features that help one differentiate the two diseases. In the case of cancer, the gallbladder wall thickening is usually irregular and poorly limited. In subacute cholecystitis, enhanced images commonly show a layered pattern of the gallbladder wall, mainly due to the presence of perivesicular fat which is inflamed, but remains nevertheless hypodense and may in that case produce a halo. This halo is clearly absent in the case of a tumor.

In the case of subacute cholecystitis, it is exceptional to observe discrete collected abscesses. In that case, seeing round hypoattenuating lesions within segments IV or V of the liver would clearly be more indicative of a tumor. Finally, gallbladder tumors have a tendency to invade the infundibulum and the common bile duct, whereas subacute cholecystitis does not produce common bile duct obstruction, with the exception of Mirizzi syndrome, which is a clinically different situation.

However, none of these features are absolutely specific. There are some difficult cases in which a percutaneous biopsy might be recommended.

Although the positive findings are helpful in most cases, there are still situations in which it is appropriate to combine the advantages and complementarities of US and CT. However, one last advantage of CT is its very high specificity. If the CT findings are normal, the hypothesis of a cholecystitis might reasonably not be considered.

3.4 Gallbladder Haemorrhage

This is a very exceptional situation. Haemorrhage in the gallbladder is a rare cause of abdominal pain encountered in the setting of trauma, malignancy, and bleeding diathesis, such as renal failure, cirrhosis, and anticoagulation (Parekh and Corvera 2010). It happens also when chronic or acute lesions of the gallbladder erode a branch of the cystic artery. In most cases, the hemorrhage is only seen as melena. Only when it is extremely abundant does it develop into hematemesis. However, the hemorrhage does not always communicate with the gallbladder lumen. In this case, the consequence is either a hemoperitoneum or a localized hematoma. When such a complication is suspected, it is better to plan an acquisition in the arterial phase; however, this situation is extremely rare and not necessarily suspected clinically if there is no exteriorized digestive bleeding. Nevertheless, in most cases, extravasation of contrast medium is still visible in the portal phase and even sometimes more clearly. Identification of the bleeding is important because it can be life-threatening, and might be treated with transarterial embolization rather than surgery, which is difficult in such a situation.

4 Intrahepatic and Extrahepatic Bile Duct Diseases

Emergencies related to intrahepatic and extrahepatic bile duct lesions are mainly related to cholangitis and its consequences. This is a life-threatening condition,

because infection in the bile ducts may lead to liver abscesses and moreover septicemia.

4.1 Cholangitis

Cholangitis is a condition with acute inflammation and infection in the bile duct. Acute obstructive cholangitis is defined by the association of lethargy, mental confusion and shock, fever jaundice, and abdominal pain (Reynolds and Dargan 1959). This so-called Reynolds pentad is indicative of a very severe condition requiring emergency biliary decompression, which is the only way to treat the disease. The prognosis is rather poor because the mortality ranges from 10 to 30% (Kimura et al. 2007). There are no direct signs of cholangitis on imaging. Cholangitis is a clinical diagnosis and imaging helps to define the cause of the biliary disease and to evaluate the consequences. Cholangitis is potentially a life-threatening condition and is a true emergency (Lee 2009). The two commonest causes are obstructive and iatrogenic.

Obstruction of the bile duct induces stasis and favors the development of infection. However, this very seldom happens in the case of progressive obstruction, mainly represented by tumors, whether biliary or pancreatic. Usually, cholangitis is associated with bile duct stones. The reason is not completely clear. However, one can imagine that stones are foreign bodies that produce inflammation of the mucosa and that this may favor the development of infection. Another possibility is that common bile duct stones are commonly multiple. Some small stones are able to go through the papilla and are eliminated. However, during this process, the papilla might experience a transient dysfunction, allowing retrograde communication of duodenal lumen and bile ducts, and consequently bacterial contamination of the bile. Iatrogeny is probably the commonest cause of cholangitis. Previous biliary surgery such as choledocoduodenal or hepaticojejunal anastomosis, endoscopic sphincterotomy, and percutaneous or endoscopic biliary stenting and drainage are the commonest situations. Rarely, contamination is related to direct cholangiography, especially after endoscopic retrograde

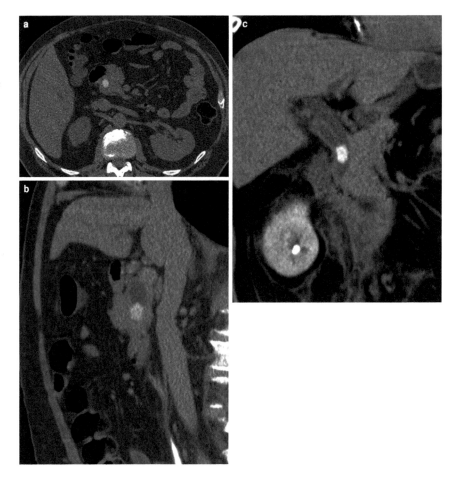

Fig. 13 Choledocolithiasis. A 66-year-old man with Reynolds pentad. US was initially performed and detected mild bile duct dilatation but the lower part of the common bile duct could not be examined. CT was performed and identified a common bile duct stone. As this stone is rather large and calcified, it is seen on plain images, in the axial (**a**) and sagittal (**b**) planes. The coronal image (**c**) is from the image set acquired after injection of contrast medium. In this case, because of stone characteristics, injection did not impair stone visualization

cholangiopancreatography (ERCP). However, this method is likely to induce cholangitis only if there is an associated biliary disease such as tumor obstruction or sclerosing cholangitis. For this reason, and because of the development of noninvasive imaging with CT and moreover MRCP, ERCP is only seldom performed for diagnostic purposes. There are exceptional circumstances of cholangitis not related to stones or to previous intervention. Single cases of direct perforation by a duodenal ulcer have been reported.

4.2 Significance of Pneumobilia

CT is able to identify the signs of previous surgery, either because of the findings related to the presence of an anastomotic jejunal loop or because of aerobilia. However, the presence of air in the bile ducts greatly differs according to the type of previous surgery and between individuals. The presence of air is not a complete guarantee that the anastomosis is patent, and absence of air in the bile ducts does not mean that the anastomosis is abnormal. Air is only an ancillary sign drawing the attention to potential previous intervention on the bile ducts.

4.3 Common Bile Duct Stones

Detection of common bile duct stones is a common problem with imaging. US is widely used for detection. However, the reported sensitivity is disappointing because of technical difficulties to access the lower bile duct area in some patients, and also related to the small size of the stone, which might be undetectable. Although the sensitivity has been improved recently, with a highest reported score of 86% (Ripolles et al. 2009), it should be kept in mind that the stone is easier to identify by US if the bile

Biliary Emergencies

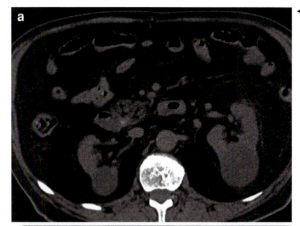
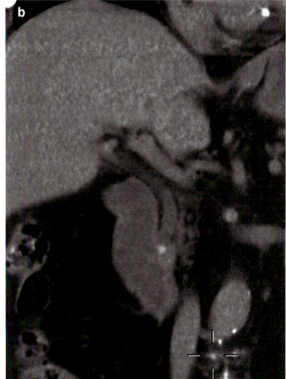
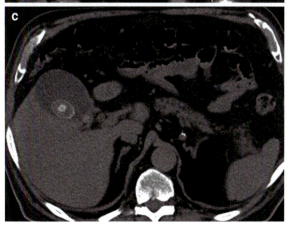

◀ **Fig. 14** Small stone of the common bile duct. An 82-year-old man with recent episodes of right upper quadrant pain and mild fever. US shows a gallstone but no sign of cholecystitis. The common bile duct was not dilated. Plain CT shows a small stone in the lower common bile duct, seen because of its mild hyperattenuation on the axial plane image (**a**). Coronal multiplanar reconstruction shows the stone and the common bile duct, which is not enlarged (**b**). CT shows a gallbladder stone as well (**c**)

ducts are dilated and if the stone is larger than 4 mm. Conversely, MRCP and endoscopic US (EUS) have the highest scores for sensitivity and specificity. Consequently, US can be an easy initial examination because it is best suited to detect bile duct dilatation and to localize the level of obstruction. EUS has a sensitivity of nearly 100%, but conversely a specificity of 95%, owing to some ambiguous findings that may be confused with very small stones (Lee et al. 2010). In the study of Lee et al. (2010), comparing US, CT, and EUS, the sensitivity of US and CT was only 26%, whereas the specificity was 93% and the negative predictive value was 70%. CT sensitivity has been reported at very different levels. Since the initial enthusiasm (Neitlich et al. 1997) and a score as high as 88%, based on the identification, on plain CT, of hyperdense stone, other reports have shown that the sensitivity is likely to be much lower, especially when comparing CT and MRCP (Soto et al. 2000). Soto et al. (2000) reported a sensitivity was 65% for unenhanced helical CT and 96% for magnetic resonance cholangiography. The specificity was 84% for unenhanced helical CT and 100% for magnetic resonance cholangiography. Differences in sensitivity were significant, but they were not significant for specificity.

In summary, it appears that CT might clearly overlook common bile duct stones, especially when contrast-enhanced studies are performed only, because the hyperattenuation is lacking or is minimal (Figs. 12, 13, 14). Therefore, it is highly recommended to perform plain imaging when one of the goals of the examination is to detect potential common bile duct stones. If stone detection is the only question for the examination, it is advisable to propose a substitution by MRI if this is available because of its much higher sensitivity.

Recently, the performance of CT for the identification of biliary stones as the cause of acute pancreatitis

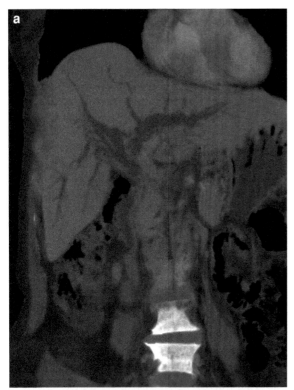

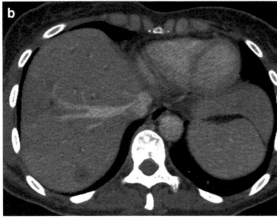

Fig. 15 A 43-years-old woman who underwent laparoscopic cholecystectomy. A few weeks later, she presented with mild jaundice, complicated with fever and right upper quadrant pain. The patient had a surgical injury of the common bile duct during cholecystectomy. CT with minimum-intensity projection reconstruction in the coronal plane (**a**) showed dilatation of intrahepatic ducts and the hepatic duct, whereas the lower common bile duct was normal. Axial enhanced CT (**b**) shows a heterogeneous mass in the posterior sector of the right lobe of the liver, consistent with abscess formation. After antibiotic therapy, the patient had surgery for biliary-enteric anastomosis

was reported and the role of CT was enhanced, but rather as a provider of several signs, including pericholecystic increased attenuation of the liver parenchyma, gallbladder wall enhancement and thickening, pericholecystic fat stranding, and stones in the gallbladder and common bile duct (Yie et al. 2010). In this series, the stone in the common bile duct was identified in 50% of cases.

4.4 Liver Biliary Abscesses

Biliary infection is one of the major causes of liver abscesses. Identification of abscesses is usually easy, as they are usually multiple and associated with an obvious biliary disease (Cerwenka 2010) such as surgical injuries related to cholecystectomy (Fig. 15). However, there might be some difficulties in the identification of the abscesses.

- In the case of small abscesses, it might be difficult to differentiate peripheral dilated bile ducts and small abscesses. Usually, this is solved using multiplanar reconstruction, showing that the abscesses are not tubular in shape in any direction.
- When a malignant tumor is the cause of bile duct obstruction and infection, it is very challenging, though extremely important, to differentiate abscesses and metastases. CT is usually limited for this purpose as it displays only a focal hypoattenuating image with some peripheral vascularization, which is in accordance with either possibility. Moreover, central necrosis of a metastatic tumor and liquefaction of the abscess are exactly the same. In this case, MRI might be very helpful given the clinical importance of such a diagnosis. Nevertheless it should be kept in mind that patients with malignant obstruction of the bile duct seldom have cholangitis, unless previous direct access to the bile ducts has been performed.

CT in an easy tool for guidance when drainage is planned. However, the initial step is usually to treat the biliary obstruction, because resolution of bile outflow interruption might be sufficient to improve the situation, in combination with antibiotics. Drainage of biliary abscesses is necessary only when they are large or when they persist after correct biliary drainage.

4.5 Ischemic Cholangitis

Ischemic-type biliary lesions are of increasing importance. Virtually all cases are related to previous intervention. This disease accounts for a major part of patients' morbidity and mortality after orthotopic liver transplantation. The exact origin of this type of biliary complication remains unknown (Heidenhain et al. 2010). These lesions can also be secondary to pancreatic surgery when there is an impairment of the liver arteries. Ischemic cholangitis can also be secondary to endoscopic retrograde maneuvers, to chemoembolization, or to arterial infusion chemotherapy (Shrikhande et al. 2002).

In some cases, ischemia is localized and its consequence is the development of a bile duct stenosis. In other cases, ischemia is dramatic and a diffuse destruction of the bile ducts is observed. There is no specific direct sign for ischemic cholangitis. However, the diagnosis is rather clear given the clinical background. In severe cases, extensive destruction of the bile ducts is observed, with the formation of intrahepatic irregular bile lakes. These bilomas are commonly contaminated and this may lead to dramatic infections and risk of liver failure, septicemia, and death.

5 Conclusion

Biliary emergencies are common, mainly represented by cholecystitis and cholangitis. CT is one of the available tools. However, in many cases, US should be performed first. CT has the advantages, in clinically equivocal cases, of being able to perform a more exhaustive survey of potential diseases in several areas. The technique should be appropriate, with the permanent necessity to an produce examination with the quality adapted to the clinical questions and with a radiation dose which is as low as possible. The role of MRI is also increasing. The radiologist should therefore be regarded as the person who will decide which is the best examination or the most logical combination in order to achieve emergency diagnosis and optimal preparation and staging for the treatment.

References

Atassi B, Bangash AK, Lewandowski RJ et al (2008) Biliary sequelae following radioembolization with yttrium-90 microspheres. J Vasc Interv Radiol 19:691–697

Barie PS, Eachempati SR (2010) Acute acalculous cholecystitis. Gastroenterol Clin North Am 39:343–357

Brenner DJ (2010) Should we be concerned about the rapid increase in CT usage? Rev Environ Health 25:63–68

Brewer BJ, Golden GT, Hitch DC, Rudolf LE, Wangensteen SL (1976) Abdominal pain. An analysis of 1,000 consecutive cases in a university hospital emergency room. Am J Surg 131:219–223

Cerwenka H (2010) Pyogenic liver abscess: differences in etiology and treatment in Southeast Asia and Central Europe. World J Gastroenterol 16:2458–2462

Choi JY, Lee JM, Lee JY et al (2007) Assessment of hilar and extrahepatic bile duct cancer using multidetector CT: value of adding multiplanar reformations to standard axial images. Eur Radiol 17:3130–3138

Endo Y (2010) A prospective evaluation of emergency department bedside ultrasonography for the detection of acute cholecystitis. Ultrasound Q 26:228

Gallix BP, Aufort S, Pierredon MA, Garibaldi F, Bruel JM (2006) Une angiocholite: comment la reconnaître? Quelles conduites à tenir? J Radiol 87:430–440

Heidenhain C, Pratschke J, Puhl G et al (2010) Incidence of and risk factors for ischemic-type biliary lesions following orthotopic liver transplantation. Transpl Int 23:14–22

Hubert C, Annet L, van Beers BE, Gigot JF (2010) The "inside approach of the gallbladder" is an alternative to the classic Calot's triangle dissection for a safe operation in severe cholecystitis. Surg Endosc 24:2626–2632

Jeffrey RB Jr, Nino-Murcia M, Ralls PW, Jain KA, Davidson HC (1995) Color Doppler sonography of the cystic artery: comparison of normal controls and patients with acute cholecystitis. J Ultrasound Med 14:33–36

Kimura Y, Takada T, Kawarada Y et al (2007) Definitions, pathophysiology, and epidemiology of acute cholangitis and cholecystitis: Tokyo guidelines. J Hepatobiliary Pancreat Surg 14:15–26

Lee JG (2009) Diagnosis and management of acute cholangitis. Nat Rev Gastroenterol Hepatol 6:533–541

Lee JH, Lee SR, Lee SY et al (2010) The usefulness of endoscopic ultrasonography in the diagnosis of choledocholithiasis without common bile duct dilatation. Korean J Gastroenterol 56:97–102

Mills AM, Baumann BM, Chen EH et al (2010) The impact of crowding on time until abdominal CT interpretation in emergency department patients with acute abdominal pain. Postgrad Med 122:75–81

Mirvis SE, Vainright JR, Nelson AW et al (1986) The diagnosis of acute acalculous cholecystitis: a comparison of sonography, scintigraphy, and CT. AJR Am J Roentgenol 147: 1171–1175

Neitlich JD, Topazian M, Smith RC, Gupta A, Burrell MI, Rosenfield AT (1997) Detection of choledocholithiasis: comparison of unenhanced helical CT and endoscopic retrograde cholangiopancreatography. Radiology 203:753–757

Parekh J, Corvera CU (2010) Hemorrhagic cholecystitis. Arch Surg 145:202–204

Ralls PW, Halls J, Lapin SA, Quinn MF, Morris UL, Boswell W (1982) Prospective evaluation of the sonographic Murphy sign in suspected acute cholecystitis. J Clin Ultrasound 10:113–115

Ralls PW, Colletti PM, Lapin SA et al (1985) Real-time sonography in suspected acute cholecystitis. Prospective evaluation of primary and secondary signs. Radiology 155:767–771

Reynolds BM, Dargan EL (1959) Acute obstructive cholangitis; a distinct clinical syndrome. Ann Surg 150:299–303

Ripolles T, Ramirez-Fuentes C, Martinez-Perez MJ, Delgado F, Blanc E, Lopez A (2009) Tissue harmonic sonography in the diagnosis of common bile duct stones: a comparison with endoscopic retrograde cholangiography. J Clin Ultrasound 37:501–506

Shrikhande S, Friess H, Kleeff J et al (2002) Bile duct infarction following intraarterial hepatic chemotherapy mimicking multiple liver metastasis: report of a case and review of the literature. Dig Dis Sci 47:338–344

Solis-Caxaj CA (2009) Mirizzi syndrome: diagnosis, treatment and a plea for a simplified classification. World J Surg 33:1783–1784 (author reply 1786–1787)

Soto JA, Alvarez O, Munera F, Velez SM, Valencia J, Ramirez N (2000) Diagnosing bile duct stones: comparison of unenhanced helical CT, oral contrast-enhanced CT cholangiography, and MR cholangiography. AJR Am J Roentgenol 175:1127–1134

Tkacz JN, Anderson SA, Soto J (2009) MR imaging in gastrointestinal emergencies. Radiographics 29:1767–1780

Tokunaga Y, Nakayama N, Ishikawa Y et al (1997) Surgical risks of acute cholecystitis in elderly. Hepatogastroenterology 44:671–676

Wagnetz U, Jaskolka J, Yang P, Jhaveri KS (2010) Acute ischemic cholecystitis after transarterial chemoembolization of hepatocellular carcinoma: incidence and clinical outcome. J Comput Assist Tomogr 34:348–353

Wu CH, Chen CC, Wang CJ, Wong YC, Wang LJ, Huang CC, Lo WC, Chen HW et al (2010a) Discrimination of gangrenous from uncomplicated acute cholecystitis: accuracy of CT findings. Abdom Imaging. doi:10.1007/s00261-010-9612-x

Wu JM, Lee CY, Wu YM (2010b) Emphysematous cholecystitis. Am J Surg 200:e53–e54

Yie M et al (2010) Diagnostic value of CT features of the gallbladder in the prediction of gallstone pancreatitis. Eur J Radiol. doi:10.1016/j.ejrad.2010.05.022

Yun EJ, Choi CS, Yoon DY et al (2009) Combination of magnetic resonance cholangiopancreatography and computed tomography for preoperative diagnosis of the Mirizzi syndrome. J Comput Assist Tomogr 33:636–640

Acute Splenic Disease

Eric Delabrousse

Contents

1 Introduction 116

2 Pyogenic Splenic Abscess 116
2.1 Introduction 116
2.2 Clinical Presentation 116
2.3 Laboratory Findings 116
2.4 Radiographic and Ultrasonographic Findings 116
2.5 CT Findings 117
2.6 Differential Diagnosis 117

3 Fungal Splenic Abscess 117
3.1 Introduction 117
3.2 Clinical Presentation 117
3.3 Laboratory Findings 117
3.4 Radiographic and Ultrasonographic Findings 118
3.5 CT Findings 118
3.6 Differential Diagnosis 118

4 Splenic Infarction 118
4.1 Introduction 118
4.2 Clinical Presentation 119
4.3 Laboratory Findings 119
4.4 Radiographic and Ultrasonographic Findings 119
4.5 CT Findings 119
4.6 Differential Diagnosis 119

5 Acute Torsion of a Wandering Spleen 120
5.1 Introduction 120
5.2 Clinical Presentation 120
5.3 Laboratory Findings 120
5.4 Radiographic and Ultrasonographic Findings 120
5.5 CT Findings 120
5.6 Differential Diagnosis 121

6 Acute Splenic Sequestration Crisis 121
6.1 Introduction 121
6.2 Clinical Presentation 121
6.3 Laboratory Findings 121
6.4 Radiographic and Ultrasonographic Findings 121
6.5 CT Findings 122
6.6 Differential Diagnosis 122

7 Spontaneous Splenic Rupture 122
7.1 Introduction 122
7.2 Clinical Presentation 122
7.3 Laboratory Findings 122
7.4 Radiographic and Ultrasonographic Findings 123
7.5 CT Findings 123
7.6 Differential Diagnosis 123

References 123

E. Delabrousse (✉)
Service de Imagerie Digestive et Génito-urinaire,
CHU Besançon, Hôpital Jean Minjoz 3 bd Fleming,
25030 Besançon, France
e-mail: edelabrousse@chu-besancon.fr

Abstract

The spleen is a lymphopoietic organ, which is part of the immunoprotective system of the body, in the same way as the lymph nodes. Its situation, under the left hemidiaphragm, in the immediate neighborhood of the abdominal wall and ribs, as well as its very important natural fragility, can explain the importance of its blunt trauma pathology. Because of the lymphoid nature of the spleen, infectious lesions are rare, and are seen almost exclusively in immunocompromised patients. Conversely, splenic infarction is frequent, and of various causes. Spontaneous splenic rupture is a rare, but life-threatening condition.

P. Taourel (ed.), *CT of the Acute Abdomen*, Medical Radiology. Diagnostic Imaging,
DOI: 10.1007/174_2010_94, © Springer-Verlag Berlin Heidelberg 2011

1 Introduction

The spleen is a lymphopoietic organ, which is part of the immunoprotective system of the body, in the same way as the lymph nodes. Its situation, under the left hemidiaphragm, in the immediate neighborhood of the abdominal wall and ribs, as well as its very important natural fragility, can explain the importance of its blunt trauma pathology. Because of the lymphoid nature of the spleen, infectious lesions are rare, and are seen almost exclusively in immunocompromised patients. Conversely, splenic infarction is frequent, and of various causes. Spontaneous splenic rupture is a rare, but life-threatening condition.

2 Pyogenic Splenic Abscess

2.1 Introduction

Pyogenic splenic abscess is defined by focal collection of liquefied pus within splenic parenchyma. It has been reported to occur in less than 1% of large autopsy series (Chun et al. 1980). In the preantibiotic era, splenic abscess had a high mortality rate (Rice et al. 1977). If not treated, a splenic abscess is invariably fatal (Green 2001). Splenic abscess usually follows hematogenous dissemination, but may occur with infection of a splenic infarct or spread of infection from adjacent organs (Joazlina et al. 2006). Although regarded as a rare condition, splenic abscess is now being seen with increasing frequency because of the use of immunosuppressive agents, treatment with chemotherapy, especially for leukemia, patients with HIV, and intravenous drug abusers who often have concomitant endocarditis (Ng et al. 2002). Several factors have been incriminated as leading causes in the development of splenic abscesses. Among them are diabetes mellitus (Joazlina et al. 2006), endocarditis (Nores et al. 1998), typhoid fever, malaria (Bae and Jeon 2006), trauma, sickle cell disease (Roshkow and Sanders 1990), and a variety of pyogenic infections. In many instances, the development of a splenic abscess is related not only to the presence of bacteremia, but also to intrinsic splenic disease that damages the splenic architecture (Balthazar et al. 1985). High exposure to infectious agents and susceptibility to splenic infarction are important causative factors that often explain the occurrence of splenic abscesses. In occidental countries, the most encountered infecting organisms are *Staphylococcus aureus*, *Escherischia coli*, and *Salmonella*.

Pyogenic abscesses in the spleen are commonly multiple, variable in location, and typically 3–5 cm in diameter. CT is the most accurate modality for imaging the spleen, and CT of the abdomen is used to investigate patients with unexplained fever (Drevelengas 2000). Thus, CT is the best imaging modality for the diagnosis of pyogenic splenic abscess. However, it is often not possible to predict the infecting agent on the basis of the CT features.

The surgical literature has stressed splenectomy as the treatment for splenic abscess. The serious complication of splenic abscess is spleen rupture, in which case surgery is mandatory. However, with the awareness of the value of conserving the spleen, treatment eith antibiotics and, if the abscess is unruptured and is large enough, percutaneous drainage under ultrasonography or CT guidance can be undertaken, with a reported success rate of 75–100% (van der Laan et al. 1989; Thanos et al. 2002).

2.2 Clinical Presentation

Pyogenic splenic abscess classically presents with fever and abdominal left upper quadrant pain. However, pain may be absent (50%), making the diagnosis difficult.

2.3 Laboratory Findings

Leukocytosis is often present. A raised erythrocyte sedimentation rate occurs inconsistently. Most often, blood culture findings are positive. Nevertheless, microbiological examination of the spleen by aspiration or after surgery remains the gold standard for the diagnosis of splenic abscess.

2.4 Radiographic and Ultrasonographic Findings

Abdominal plain films may show rare gas bubbles in projection of the spleen and left-sided pleural effusion. Ultrasonography may reveal within the spleen one or

Acute Splenic Disease

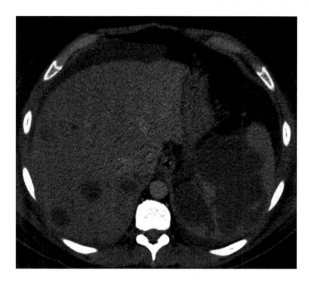

Fig. 1 Pyogenic splenic abscesses. Axial contrast-enhanced CT scan showing multiple hypoattenuating lesions within the liver and the spleen consistent with abscesses caused by *Escherischia coli*

several hypoechoic collections with septations and internal echoes representing pus. No internal flow is present on color Doppler ultrasonography.

2.5 CT Findings

Pyogenic splenic abscess is characterized on CT scans by the following (Fig. 1):
- One or several rounded hypoattenuation complex fluid collections in the spleen (3–5 cm), with enhanced rims when intravenous contrast material is administrated
- Gas or air–fluid level within the lesions (rare)
- Mass effect on the splenic capsule and the vascular structures
- Frequent splenomegaly
- Left-sided pleural effusion

2.6 Differential Diagnosis

Fungal splenic abscesses are often small and multiple and occur in immunocompromised patients or in patients undergoing chemotherapy, particularly for leukemia (Chew et al. 1991). Splenic infarct is typically in a peripheral location and is wedge-shaped. However, in endocarditis, splenic infarct is due to seeding with infected emboli, and is prone to become a splenic abscess (Ng et al. 2002). Splenic tumors are solid or cystic. Splenic trauma is associated with perisplenic hematoma and/or hemoperitoneum. A history of blunt injury is always present. There may be a sentinel clot sign.

3 Fungal Splenic Abscess

3.1 Introduction

Fungal splenic abscesses represent 25% of infectious splenic disorders. Hematogenous dissemination of infection to the spleen is the main cause. Fungal splenic abscesses develop most often in immunocompromised patients or patients undergoing chemotherapy, particularly for leukemia (Joazlina et al. 2006). Fungal infections are more common in this population. The most frequent infecting agents are *Candida*, *Aspergillus*, and *Cryptococcus* (Chew et al. 1991). Patients with AIDS only infrequently develop the fungal microabscesses encountered in other immunocompromised patients. More often, the presence of splenic microlesions is the result of granulomas or microabscesses caused by *Mycobacterium avium-intracellulare* or *Pneumocystis carinii*. Disseminated *Pneumocystis carinii* infection in AIDS patients commonly involves both the liver and the spleen (Freeman et al. 1993). Mostly, it is difficult to isolate the fungi. Multiple lesions in patients with leukemia or immunocompromised status are presumed to be fungal abscesses, even if culture findings are negative (Lim et al. 2003).

3.2 Clinical Presentation

The clinical presentation is often nonspecific. In immunocompromised patients, the diagnosis of fungal splenic abscesses should be evoked when fever, splenomegaly, and weight loss are present.

3.3 Laboratory Findings

Neutropenia due to leukemia or secondary to an immunocompromised status is often present. A raised erythrocyte sedimentation rate occurs inconsistently.

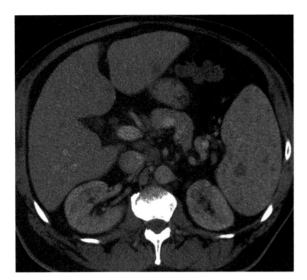

Fig. 2 Fungal splenic abscesses. Axial contrast-enhanced CT scan of an immunocompromised patient showing multiple round areas of decreased attenuation scattered throughout the liver and the spleen. Candidiasis was confirmed on biopsy

A positive blood culture finding is rare. Moreover, microbiological examination of the spleen by aspiration is not a reliable method because of the substantial number of false-negative results (Pastakia et al. 1988).

3.4 Radiographic and Ultrasonographic Findings

Abdominal plain films typically show normal findings. Fungal abscesses in neutropenic patients are often very small, multiple, and may not be detectable on ultrasonography, even with disseminated infection.

3.5 CT Findings

Fungal splenic abscesses are characterized on CT scans by the following (Fig. 2):
- Multiple scattered rounded areas of low attenuation (less than 10 mm) within the spleen, with no enhancement after intravenous contrast material injection
- Typical (but rare) bull's eye lesions (also called wheels-in-wheels lesions) corresponding to hypoattenuating areas with central cores of increased attenuation
- Innumerable punctate calcifications scattered throughout the spleen, particularly in AIDS patients
- Frequent splenomegaly
- Similar lesions within the liver

3.6 Differential Diagnosis

Pyogenic abscesses are often larger. Metastases, lymphoma, and granulomatous involvement with sarcoidosis can mimic splenic infection, but the clinical presentation is different.

4 Splenic Infarction

4.1 Introduction

Splenic arterial branches are end arteries that do not intercommunicate; therefore, occlusion leads to infarction (Freeman et al. 1993). Splenic infarction is defined by global or partial parenchymal splenic ischemia and necrosis. Splenic infarcts are relatively common and usually result from embolic occlusion of the splenic arterial system. Although they are generally not clinically significant, early diagnosis is crucial to exclude more serious intra-abdominal diseases that may also cause left upper quadrant pain. In most cases, occlusion of the splenic artery is precipitated by emboli originating from the heart (Nores et al. 1998). Relative ischemia produced by splenomegaly (Taylor et al. 1991), especially when associated with sickle cell disease (Roshkow and Sanders 1990), myeloproliferative syndromes, and other hemoglobinopathies, predisposes a patient to splenic infarction secondary to thrombosis or functional ischemia (Shadle et al. 1982; Balcar et al. 1984). Local thromboses, as may occur in atherosclerosis (Frippiat et al. 1996), arteritis, coagulopathy, and splenic artery aneurysm, account for the minority of infarcts (Freeman and Tonkin 1976). Pancreatitis (Fishman et al. 1995; Rypens 1997), pancreatic adenocarcinoma, and acute torsion of a wandering spleen (Nemcek et al. 1991; Ben Ely et al. 2006) have also been associated with this condition. Infarcts range in size, but rarely involve the entire organ. In their global form (particularly in pancreatitis and torsion of a wandering spleen), they may enlarge the spleen. Splenic infarcts are generally bland and anemic, with the infectious variety almost always caused by endocarditis (Nores et al. 1998). Many authors reported CT to be the best imaging tool for the diagnosis of splenic infarction (Pierkarski et al. 1980; Maier 1982). Loss of splenic parenchyma is generally not clinically significant, and is treated with sedation and bed rest. However, splenectomy remains mandatory for increasing pain or splenic rupture.

4.2 Clinical Presentation

Splenic infarcts can be asymptomatic or cause left upper quadrant pain (often radiating to the left shoulder), chills, and abdominal guarding.

4.3 Laboratory Findings

Laboratory findings are not specific. Anemia is seen in 50% of patients and leukocytosis is seen in 40% of patients.

4.4 Radiographic and Ultrasonographic Findings

Abdominal plain films are able to demonstrate very little in splenic infarction. Occasionally, a left-sided pleural effusion, elevation of the left hemidiaphragm, or splenomegaly is seen.

The ultrasonographic appearance is variable, depending on whether the splenic infarct is acute or chronic. Acute hemorrhagic splenic infarcts are usually triangular and hypoechoic, whereas healed infarcts appear hyperechoic, due to deposition of fibrous tissue (Goerg et al. 1990). Flow is absent in areas of infarction on color Doppler ultrasonography (Nemcek et al. 1991).

4.5 CT Findings

Splenic infarct is characterized on CT scans by the following (Fig. 3):
- Peripheral wedge-shaped, nonenhanced, low-density lesion with its base at the splenic capsule and apex toward the hilum (in partial ischemia)

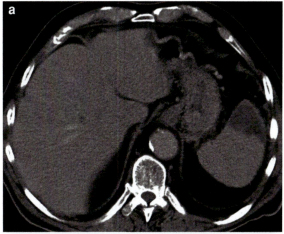

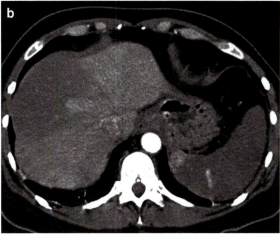

Fig. 3 Splenic infarction in two different patients. **a** Axial contrast-enhanced CT scan showing peripheral wedge-shaped hypoattenuating lesions secondary to emboli. Note the peripheral hyperdense rim. **b** Axial contrast-enhanced CT scan showing subtotal nonenhancement of the spleen due to thrombosis of the splenic artery

- Complete nonenhancement and possible enlargement of the spleen (in global ischemia)
- A peripheral hyperdense rim corresponding to the splenic capsule

4.6 Differential Diagnosis

Splenic abscess, splenic laceration, neoplasm, benign tumor, hematoma, and even complicated cyst may have a similar CT appearance (Balcar et al. 1984). In general, the clinical setting will help differentiate them. In difficult cases, percutaneous needle aspiration biopsy can be useful in establishing a specific diagnosis.

5 Acute Torsion of a Wandering Spleen

5.1 Introduction

The wandering spleen is defined by an abnormally mobile spleen. This anomaly is rare, with a reported incidence of less than 0.5% in several large series of splenectomies (Gayer 2002). It is found mainly in children (Raaissaki et al. 1998) and in women aged 20–40 years (Sty and Conway 1985). The increased mobility of the spleen results from absence, underdevelopment, or laxity of the supporting gastrosplenic and splenorenal ligaments that normally anchor the spleen in the left upper quadrant (Gayer et al. 2001). Splenic hypermobility may be congenital or acquired. Acquired wandering spleen is caused by underlying conditions that weaken the supporting splenic ligaments, such as hormonal effects of pregnancy (Gilman and Thomas 2003), abdominal surgery, and abdominal wall laxity (Heydenrych and Du Toit 1978; Nemcek et al. 1991). A wandering spleen may be incidentally detected as an abdominal or pelvic mass on physical examination or on imaging examinations of the abdomen. Acute, chronic, or intermittent torsion of the spleen is a major complication of wandering spleen, caused by its increased mobility. Acute splenic torsion is a potentially fatal surgical emergency. Involvement of the pancreatic tail in the torsion has been reported to occur (Parker et al. 1984; Sheffin et al. 1984). Accurate clinical diagnosis of torsion of a wandering spleen is difficult because of the rarity of the condition and the nonspecific presenting symptoms (Ben Ely et al. 2006). With the widespread use of CT in the evaluation of abdominal pain, positive diagnosis and information on the viability of the splenic parenchyma may be provided preoperatively. This information is valuable for the surgeon in deciding whether splenopexy rather than splenectomy is an option, particularly in young patients, even if splenectomy remains mandatory in the case of acute torsion with complete infarction of the spleen (Cavazos et al. 2004).

5.2 Clinical Presentation

Acute torsion of a wandering spleen presents with severe abdominal pain due to marked congestion and capsule stretching (Gayer 2002). Physical examination may reveal a tender abdominal or pelvic mass (Raaissaki et al. 1998). Previous intermittent abdominal pain, presumably due to spontaneous splenic torsion and detorsion, and a palpable abdominal mass are often reported by patients on questioning (Gayer 2002).

5.3 Laboratory Findings

Laboratory values are not specific, and include a normal hemoglobin level, a very increased white blood cell count, and a normal platelet count.

5.4 Radiographic and Ultrasonographic Findings

Abdominal plain films may demonstrate absence of the splenic shadow under the left hemidiaphragm and a comma-shaped opacity in the left flank of the mid-abdomen or the left side of the pelvis.

Ultrasonography may show an abdominal or pelvic soft-tissue mass and absence of spleen in its typical location in the left upper quadrant (Kinori and Rifkin 1988; Nemcek et al. 1991). The normal homogenous, medium-level echogenicity of the spleen may be replaced by a heterogeneous appearance (Sheffin et al. 1984). Color flow and duplex Doppler ultrasonography reveal no detectable flow in the intrasplenic arteries and high resistive index in the main splenic artery just distal to the celiac trunk. These findings are considered diagnostic of splenic infarction due to torsion.

5.5 CT Findings

Acute torsion of a wandering spleen is characterized on CT scans by the following (Fig. 4):
- The spleen in an ectopic position in the left flank of the mid-abdomen or the left side of pelvis
- Enlargement and rotation of the spleen
- Low attenuation of the spleen with high density of the splenic capsule relative to parenchyma before intravenous contrast material administration
- Partial or complete nonenhancement of the spleen (as an indication of infarction) after intravenous contrast material administration
- Possible but rare involvement of the pancreatic tail

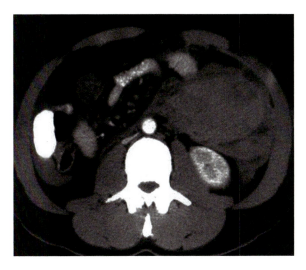

Fig. 4 Acute torsion of a wandering spleen. Axial contrast-enhanced CT scan showing the spleen in the left flank of the mid-abdomen. Note the heterogeneity of the splenic parenchyma and important perisplenic fat stranding due to spleen infarction

- A whirl sign usually at the splenic hilum, corresponding to the twisted splenic vascular pedicle
- Hyperdense fresh thrombus within the splenic vein or/and within the splenic artery on precontrast CT scans and no contrast enhancement of the vessels on postcontrast CT scans
- Frequent marked stranding of perisplenic fat and ascites

5.6 Differential Diagnosis

In clinical practice, the diagnosis of acute torsion of a wandering spleen shows no differential diagnosis because the CT features of torsion of an ectopic spleen are virtually pathognomonic.

6 Acute Splenic Sequestration Crisis

6.1 Introduction

Acute splenic sequestration crisis is a rare complication in adults with sickle cell disease (Geola et al. 1978). It occurs predominantly in young children with homozygous sickle cell disease but can also occur in adults with heterozygous sickle cell disease, particularly those with sickle cell–thalassemia and sickle cell–hemoglobin C disease (Roshkow and Sanders 1990). A major episode is defined as one in which the hemoglobin level is less than 6 g/dL and has fallen more than 3 g/dL, whereas a minor episode is one in which the hemoglobin level remains above 6 g/dL (Roshkow and Sanders 1990). The rarity of acute splenic sequestration crisis in adults may be due to a relatively low susceptibility to this complication or to underdiagnosis, particularly in minor episodes (Solanki et al. 1986). The pathogenesis of acute splenic sequestration crisis is not clear. The triggering event may be acute obstruction to venous outflow from the spleen leading to sequestration of red cells and often platelets as well (Solanki et al. 1986). Experimental ligation of the splenic vein in animals produces a similar syndrome (Altman et al. 1951).

The initial treatment of acute splenic sequestration crisis is transfusion. Splenectomy is reserved for adults with recurrent episodes or red cell alloantibodies that may hamper transfusion (Solanki et al. 1986). Splenic rupture has been reported as a rare complication of acute splenic sequestration crisis.

6.2 Clinical Presentation

Acute splenic sequestration crisis presents with left upper quadrant pain and massive sudden splenic enlargement.

6.3 Laboratory Findings

The hemoglobin level is often less than 6 g/dL. A rapid fall in hematocrit is a very valuable finding for the diagnosis. Often thrombocytopenia is seen as well. A reticulocyte count greater than or equal to steady-state values is evidence of bone marrow activity and serves to distinguish acute splenic sequestration crisis from aplasia (Topley et al. 1981).

6.4 Radiographic and Ultrasonographic Findings

Abdominal plain films are able to demonstrate very little in acute splenic sequestration crisis. Occasionally, splenomegaly or left-sided pleural effusion is seen.

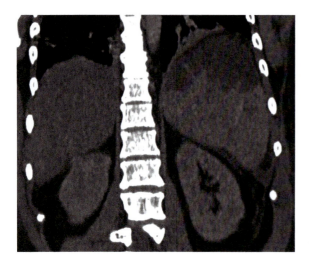

Fig. 5 Acute splenic sequestration crisis. Coronal contrast-enhanced CT scan in a patient with sickle cell disease showing splenomegaly and nonenhanced areas consistent with partial splenic infarction

Ultrasonography may show massive splenomegaly with multiple hypoechoic areas in a peripheral distribution consistent with hemorrhage or infarction. Doppler ultrasonography examination often shows a patent splenic vein, as well as patency of large intrasplenic veins.

6.5 CT Findings

Acute splenic sequestration crisis is characterized on CT scans by the following (Fig. 5):
- Massive splenomegaly
- Areas of low attenuation interspersed with areas of high attenuation due to recent hemorrhage on unenhanced CT scans
- Multiple nonenhanced areas, most commonly in a peripheral location, better seen after intravenous contrast material administration
- Rarely, splenic rupture

6.6 Differential Diagnosis

Splenic infarcts secondary to other causes may have a similar CT appearance. In general, the clinical and laboratory settings will help distinguish them.

7 Spontaneous Splenic Rupture

7.1 Introduction

Spontaneous splenic rupture is a rare condition. Splenic abscesses (Joazlina et al. 2006), splenic angiosarcoma (Levy et al. 1986), leukemic spleen (Freeman et al. 1993), amyloidosis (Kozicky et al. 1987), large or multiple hemangiomas (Rolfes and Ros 1990), peliosis, malarial spleen (Yagmur et al. 2000), mononucleosis, acute splenic sequestration crisis (Bowcock et al. 1988; Roshkow and Sanders 1990), and mainly acute pancreatitis (Warshaw et al. 1972; Hastings et al. 1978; Fishman et al. 1995) have been reported as etiologic causes of spontaneous splenic rupture. In all these diseases, acute enlargement of the spleen causes intrasplenic hemorrhage. If the hemorrhage is important enough, laceration, capsular disruption, or actual rupture of the spleen may occur (Vujic 1989). If the diagnosis is delayed, the patient may rapidly go into hypovolemic shock. Although subcapsular hematoma and limited splenic parenchymal lesions resolve conservatively, splenic rupture requires urgent surgery (Donckier et al. 1992). Percutaneous drainage is contraindicated in spontaneous splenic rupture because of the risk of causing massive intraperitoneal hemorrhage (Fishman et al. 1995).

7.2 Clinical Presentation

Spontaneous splenic rupture often presents with left upper quadrant pain, associated with guarding and sudden hypotension, and the patient may go rapidly into hypovolemic shock.

7.3 Laboratory Findings

Laboratory values are variable and depend mainly on the cause of the splenic rupture. The hemoglobin level often drops.

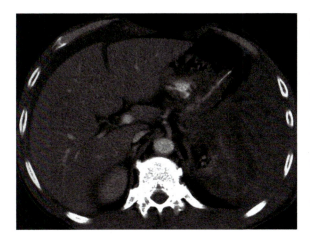

Fig. 6 Spontaneous splenic rupture. Axial contrast-enhanced CT scan showing a very heterogeneous appearance of the spleen associated with hemoperitoneum

7.4 Radiographic and Ultrasonographic Findings

The findings from abdominal plain films are not specific. Ultrasonography demonstrates a heterogeneous splenic parenchyma, and peritoneal fluid.

7.5 CT Findings

Spontaneous splenic rupture is characterized on CT scans by the following (Fig. 6):
- A very heterogeneous appearance of the spleen
- Areas of high attenuation (60 HU) within the splenic parenchyma due to recent hemorrhage before intravenous contrast material administration
- Areas of nonenhancement in the spleen after intravenous contrast material administration
- A possible sentinel clot sign
- Splenic capsule tear and an associated hemoperitoneum
- Signs from the causal disease

7.6 Differential Diagnosis

The differential diagnosis mainly depends on the search for signs of the causal disease.

References

Altman KI, Wattman RN, Solomon K (1951) Surgically induced splenogenic anemia in the rabbit. Nature 168:827

Bae K, Jeon KN (2006) CT findings in malarial spleen. Br J Radiol 79:145–147

Balcar I, Seltzer SE, Davis S, Geller S (1984) CT patterns of splenic infarction: a clinical and experimental study. Radiology 151:723–729

Balthazar EJ, Hilton S, Naidich D, Megibow A, Levine R (1985) CT of splenic and perisplenic abnormalities in septic patients. AJR 114:53–56

Ben Ely A, Zissin R, Copel L et al. (2006) The wandering spleen: CT findings and possible pitfalls in diagnosis. Clin Radiol 61:954–958

Bowcock SJ, Nwabueze ED, Cook AE, Aboud HH, Hugues RG (1988) Fatal splenic sequestration in adult sickle cell disease. Clin Lab Haematol 10:95–99

Cavazos S, Ratzer ER, Fenoglio ME (2004) Laparoscopic management of the wandering spleen. J Laparoendosc Adv Surg Tech A 14:227–229

Chew FS, Smith PL, Barboriak D (1991) Candidal splenic abscesses. AJR Am J Roentgenol 156:474

Chun CH, Raff MJ, Contreras L et al. (1980) Splenic abscess. Medicine 59:550–565

Donckier V, Rypens F, van de stadt J (1992) Unusual splenic complication of acute pancreatitis. J Clin Gastroenterol 15:245–247

Drevelengas A (2000) The spleen in infectious disorders. JBR-BTR 83:208–210

Fishman EK, Soyer P, Bliss DF, Bluemke DA, Devine N (1995) Splenic involvement in pancreatitis: spectrum of CT findings. AJR Am J Roentgenol 164:631–635

Freeman MH, Tonkin AK (1976) Focal splenic defects. Radiology 121:689–692

Freeman JL, Zafar H, Jafri S, Roberts JL, Mezwa DG, Shirkhoda A (1993) CT of congenital and acquired abnormalities of the spleen. Radiographics 13:597–610

Frippiat F et al. (1996) Splenic infarction: report of three cases of atherosclerotic embolization originating in the aorta and retrospective study of 64 cases. Acta Clin Belg 51:395–402

Gayer G (2002) Torsion of a wandering spleen. IMAJ 4:658–659

Gayer G, Zissin R, Apter S et al. (2001) CT findings in congenital anomalies of the spleen. Br J Radiol 74:767–772

Geola F, Kukreja SC, Schade SG (1978) Splenic sequestration with sickle cell-C disease. Arch Intern Med 138:307–308

Gilman RS, Thomas RL (2003) Wandering spleen presenting as acute pancreatitis in pregnancy. Obstet Gynecol 101:1100–1102

Goerg C et al. (1990) Splenic infarction: sonographic patterns, diagnosis, follow-up, and complications. Radiology 174:803–807

Green BT (2001) Splenic abscess: report of six cases and review of the literature. Am Surg 67:80–85

Hastings OM, Jain KM, Khademi M, Lazaro EJ (1978) Intrasplenic pancreatic pseudocyst complicating severe acute pancreatitis. Am J Gastroenterol 69:182–186

Heydenrych JJ, Du Toit DF (1978) Torsion of the spleen and associated 'prune belly syndrome'. A case report and review of the literature. S Afr Med J 53:637–639

Joazlina ZY, Wastie ML, Ariffin N (2006) Computed tomography of focal splenic lesions in patients presenting with fever. Singapore Med 4:37–41

Kinori I, Rifkin MD (1988) A truly wandering spleen. J Ultrasound Med 7:101–105

Kozicky OJ, Brandt LJ, Lederman M, Milcu M (1987) Splenic amyloidosis: a case report of spontaneous splenic rupture with a review of the pertinent literature. Am J Gastroenterol 82:582–587

Levy DW, Rindsberg S, Friedman AC et al. (1986) Thoratrast-induced hepatosplenic neoplasia: CT identification. AJR Am J Roentgenol 146:997–1004

Lim PC, Chang TT, Jang RC et al. (2003) Hepatosplenic abscesses in pediatric leukemia. Kaohsiung J Med Sci 19:368–374

Maier W (1982) Computed tomography in the diagnosis of splenic infarction. Eur J Radiol 2:202–204

Nemcek AA Jr, Miller FH, Fitzgerald SW (1991) Acute torsion of a wandering spleen: diagnosis by CT and duplex Doppler and color flow sonography. AJR Am J Roentgenol 157:307–309

Ng KK, Lee TY, Wan YL et al. (2002) Splenic abscess: diagnosis and management. Hepatogastroenterology 49:567–571

Nores M, Phillips EH, Morgenstern L et al. (1998) The clinical spectrum of splenic infarction. Am Surg 64:182–188

Parker LA, Mittelstaedt CA, Mauro MA, Mandell VS, Jacques PF (1984) Torsion of a wandering spleen: CT appearance. J Comput Assist Tomogr 8:1201–1204

Pastakia B, Shawker TH, Thaler M, O'Leary T, Pizzo PA (1988) Hepatosplenic candidiasis: wheels within wheels. Radiology 166:417–421

Pierkarski J, Federle MP, Moss AA, London SS (1980) Computed tomography of the spleen. Radiology 135:683–689

Raaissaki M, Prassopoulos P, Daskalogiannaki M, Magkanas E, Gourtsoyianis N (1998) Acute abdomen due to torsion of wandering spleen. Eur Radiol 8:1409–1412

Rice LJ, Rosenstein R, Swikert NC, Williams HC (1977) Splenic abscess: review of the literature and report of cases. J Ky Med Assoc 75:375–378

Rolfes RJ, Ros PR (1990) The spleen: an integrated imaging approach. Crit Rev Diagn Imaging 30:41–83

Roshkow JE, Sanders LM (1990) Acute splenic sequestration crisis in two adults with sickle cell disease: US, CT, and MR imaging findings. Radiology 177:723–725

Rypens F (1997) Splenic parenchymal complications of pancreatitis: CT findings and natural history. J Comput Assist Tomogr 21:89–93

Shadle CA, Scott ME, Ritchie DJ, Seliger G (1982) Spontaneous splenic infarction in polysplenia syndrome. J Comput Assist Tomogr 6:177–179

Sheffin JR, Lee CM, Kretchmar KA (1984) Torsion of wandering spleen and distal pancreas. AJR Am J Roentgenol 142:100–101

Solanki DL, Kletter GG, Castro O (1986) Acute splenic sequestration crises in adults with sickle cell disease. Am J Med 80:985–990

Sty JR, Conway JJ (1985) The spleen: development and functional evaluation. Semin Nucl Med 15:276–298

Taylor AJ, Dodds WJ, Erickson SJ, Stewart ET (1991) CT of acquired abnormalities of the spleen. AJR Am J Roentgenol 157:1213–1219

Thanos L, Dailana T, Papaioannou G et al. (2002) Percutaneous CT-guided drainage of splenic abscess. AJR Am J Roentgenol 179:629–632

Topley JM, Rogers DW, Stevens MCG, Serjeant GR (1981) Acute splenic sequestration and hypersplenism in the first five years in homozygous sickle cell disease. Arch Dis Child 56:765–769

van der Laan RT, Verbeeten B Jr, Smits NJ, Lubbers MJ (1989) Computed tomography in the diagnosis and treatment of solitary splenic abscesses. J Comput Assist Tomogr 13:71–74

Vujic I (1989) Vascular complications of pancreatitis. Radiol Clin North Am 27:81–91

Warshaw AL, Chesney TM, Evans GW et al. (1972) Intra-splenic dissection of pancreatic pseudocysts. N Engl J Med 287:72–75

Yagmur Y, Kara IH, Aldemir M, Buyukbayram H, Tacyildiz IH, Keles C (2000) Spontaneous rupture of malarial spleen: two case reports and review of the literature. Crit Care 4:309–313

Acute Pancreatitis

Catherine Ridereau-Zins and Christophe Aubé

Contents

1	**Introduction**	125
2	**Epidemiology**	126
3	**Physiopathology**	126
4	**Clinical Findings**	127
5	**CT Findings**	127
5.1	MDCT Technique	128
5.2	Initial Lesions	128
5.3	CT Score	131
5.4	Etiological Orientations	133
5.5	Complications	135
6	**CT Pitfalls**	138
7	**Impact of CT on the Management**	138
7.1	Positive Diagnosis	138
7.2	CT Scoring	138
7.3	Looking for Acute Complications	139
7.4	First Etiological Orientations	139
7.5	Following Acute Pancreatitis by CT	140
7.6	Radiological Treatments	140
8	**Diagnostic Strategy**	140
References		141

Abstract

Acute pancreatitis is an inflammatory disease that is mild and resolves without serious morbidity in 80% of patients. In the remaining 20%, it is complicated by substantial morbidity and mortality. The early distinction of these two groups of patients is desirable, as it is essential for their proper management. Even though positive diagnosis of acute pancreatitis is based on clinical and biological data, imaging, especially abdominal multidetector computed tomography (MDCT), has a key role in the initial phases of the disease. It allows the establishment of radiologic scoring systems with the aim of predicting which patients will have a severe debilitating hospital course and which patients will recover without major physiologic insult. The time of realization and the technique of MDCT are presently well defined. In the initial phase of the disease, MDCT allows firstly assessment of extension of initial lesions (pancreatic necrosis and fluid collections) and secondly depiction of early complications. Later, MDCT in association with MRI contributes to the etiological diagnosis and to the detection of late complications. Moreover, MDCT is helpful to plan and perform the treatment of the complications.

1 Introduction

Acute pancreatitis is an inflammatory disease that is mild and resolves without serious morbidity in 80% of patients. In the remaining 20%, it is complicated by substantial morbidity and mortality (Frossard et al. 2008).

C. Ridereau-Zins (✉) · C. Aubé
Radiologie A, Centre Hospitalier, 4 rue Larrey,
49000 Angers, France
e-mail: caridereauzins@chu-angers.fr

P. Taourel (ed.), *CT of the Acute Abdomen,* Medical Radiology. Diagnostic Imaging,
DOI: 10.1007/174_2010_138, © Springer-Verlag Berlin Heidelberg 2011

The early distinction of these two groups of patients is desirable, as it is essential for their proper management. Even though positive diagnosis of acute pancreatitis is based on clinical and biological data, imaging, especially abdominal multidetector computed tomography (MDCT), has a key role in the initial phases of the disease. It allows the establishment of radiologic scoring systems with the aim of predicting which patients will have a severe debilitating hospital course and which patients will recover without major physiologic insult. The time of realization and the technique of MDCT are presently well defined. In the initial phase of the disease, MDCT allows firstly assessment of extension of initial lesions (pancreatic necrosis and fluid collections) and secondly depiction of early complications. Later, MDCT in association with MRI contributes to the etiological diagnosis and to the detection of late complications (Maher et al. 2004). Moreover, MDCT is helpful to plan and perform the treatment of the complications (Cannon et al. 2009; Kirby et al. 2008).

2 Epidemiology

The incidence of acute pancreatitis has been rising in the western world during the last 20 years (Whitcomb 2006), (5–80 per 1,000,000 inhabitants). But the incidence, varying widely depending on the country, is partly explained by the difference in alcohol consumption in the various countries (Yadav and Lowenfels 2006).

Complications are clearly related to severe pancreatitis (in opposition to mild pancreatitis), where in up to 20% of cases acute pancreatitis is complicated by substantial morbidity and mortality. However, the frequency of severe pancreatitis remains stable and the overall population mortality rate has remained unchanged in the 20 last years (Yadav and Lowenfels 2006).

The main causes of acute pancreatitis are chronic alcohol consumption, cholelithiasis, pancreatic tumors, and iatrogenic causes including following endoscopic retrograde cholangiopancreatography (ERCP), following gastric, pancreatic, or splenic surgery, and following blunt or penetrating trauma (Maher et al. 2004). Other causes are secondary to use of drugs, infection, hyperlipidemia, hypercalcemia, inflammatory bowel disease (Pitchumoni et al. 2010), and

Table 1 Causes of acute pancreatitis

Common causes
Choledocholithiasis
Chronic alcohol consumption
Traumatic (blunt, endoscopic retrograde cholangiopancreatography, abdominal surgery)
Less common causes
Pancreatic or ampullary tumors
Pancreas divisum
Choledochocele
Oddi sphincter dysfunction
Autoimmune
Congenital anomalies
Drug-induced hypertriglyceridemia
Hypercalcemia, hyperparathyroidism
Hypothermia
Infections
Vascular
Idiopathic

anatomic variations. In about 15–20% of cases, no cause of acute pancreatitis was found (Table 1) (Carroll et al. 2007)

The main cause, gallstones or alcohol consumption, depends on the country (Whitcomb 2006). Gallstone pancreatitis is more common in women, and alcoholic pancreatitis is more common in men. However, in the last 20 years, the incidence of gallstone pancreatitis has increased in all counties (Yadav and Lowenfels 2006; Nøjgaard et al. 2010). Alcohol-induced acute pancreatitis is associated with a greater incidence of severe acute pancreatitis (Lankisch et al. 1999).

3 Physiopathology

According to most authors, acute pancreatitis is caused by the unregulated activation of trypsinogen to trypsin within pancreatic acinar cells that leads to the autodigestion of the gland and local inflammation. The triggers of the activation are mainly gallstones, probably caused by an increase in intraductal pressure, and alcohol abuse.

The severity of pancreatic damage is not related to the cause that triggers the disease, but to the injury of acinar cells and to the activation of inflammatory and endothelial cells. Local complications (acinar cell necrosis, peripancreatic fat necrosis, acute fluid collection, then pseudocyst formation) might develop. Release of several mediators from the pancreas or from extrapancreatic organs such as the liver could lead to injury in remote organs (e.g., lungs, kidney) and could contribute to visceral failure (Pastor et al. 2003).

Classically, acute pancreatitis is classified as mild pancreatitis (called interstitial or edematous pancreatitis) and severe acute pancreatitis (called necrotizing pancreatitis). In mild pancreatitis, the inflammation is limited; there is no organ failure and there is spontaneous regression without complications. In 20% of cases, the acute pancreatitis is severe. This form will lead to high morbidity, and high mortality (death rates 30–50%) (McKay and Buter 2003; Papachristou et al. 2007).

In the literature, the terms "necrotizing pancreatitis" and "severe acute pancreatitis" are often used interchangeably. In many cases the clinical diagnosis of severe acute pancreatitis corresponds to the radiological diagnosis of necrotizing pancreatitis, but this is not necessarily true. Thus, patients with pancreatic necrosis may have minimal discomfort and no organ dysfunction in up to 50% of cases (Delrue et al. 2010).

Severe acute pancreatitis evolves in two phases. In the first 2 weeks there is an expansion of the inflammation, and the pancreatic and peripancreatic ischemia. Organ failure is the main determinant of the disease outcome. The second phase is marked by infection that occurs in 40–70% of cases (Takahashi et al. 2008).

4 Clinical Findings

There is constant acute abdominal pain. It begins in the epigastric area or in the right upper quadrant and becomes diffuse with irradiations to the back. Nausea and vomiting can be associated.

Physical findings depend on the severity of the disease. In mild disease, there is tenderness in the upper abdomen contrasting with the intensity of the abdominal pain. For 20% of patients, the disease is severe with some extrapancreatic complications which appear quickly. Physical examination can reveal ascites, ileus, hypovolemic shock, and hypoxemia.

Increased capillary permeability, which conveys fluid accumulation within the interstitium, contributes to the decreased intravascular volume. Renal dysfunction is a severe complication that results from inadequate fluid resuscitation and septic complications. The incidence of pulmonary complications is high in severe pancreatitis (15–55% of cases), with a first peak upon admission (15% of patients); later, pulmonary injury might result from septic shock and complicate infection of the necrotic pancreas. Hepatic injury is usually mild during acute pancreatitis (Whitcomb 2006).

Biochemical findings supported the diagnosis of acute pancreatitis: a high serum lipase concentration of 3 times the normal upper limit indicates acute pancreatitis but it has no role in the assessment of disease severity. The serum trypsinogen level is not commonly available (Ueda et al. 2007).

Others markers are valuable to score the severity of the disease: serum creatinine level, white blood cell count, glucose level, lactate dehydrogenase (LDH) level, aspartate transaminase level, calcium serum level, and hematocrit.

Several clinical scoring systems are helpful for clinicians to assess the severity of the disease and to identify patients at risk of having adverse outcomes; they are based on physical and biochemical data. Many scores have been established: the SOFA scoring system, the Marshall scoring system, the Acute Physiology and Chronic Health Evaluation II (APACHE II), and the Ranson scoring system (Table 2). It is important to note that the Ranson score cannot be obtained before 48 h after admission and APACHE II can be calculated after 24 h.

The Atlanta classification, introduced in 1992, was a step toward a global consensus and is widely accepted. It divides acute pancreatitis into mild and severe. Severe acute pancreatitis is defined if a patient suffers at least one of the criteria detailed in Table 3. Moreover, the Atlanta classification includes the important role of computed tomography (CT) in describing disease severity.

5 CT Findings

CT has several goals:
- To confirm the diagnosis of acute pancreatitis by excluding other diagnoses of acute abdominal pain

Table 2 Apache II and Ranson criteria

Apache II	Ranson
Age >55 years	Age >55 years
White blood cell count <3,000 or >14,900/mL	White blood cell count >16,000/mL
Rectal temperature <36°C or >38.4°C	Glucose >200 mg/dL
Mean arterial pressure <70 or >109 mmHg	LDH >350 IU/mL
Heart rate <70 or >109 bpm	AST >250 IU/L
Respiratory rate <12 or >24 cpm	Hematocrit decrease >10
pH <7.33 or >7.49	Blood urea nitrogen increase >5 mg/dL
Na^+ <130 or >149 mmol/L	Calcium <8 mg/dL
K^+ <3.5 or <5.4 mmol/L	PO_2 <60 mmHg
PO_2 <70 or >200 mmHg	Base deficit >4 mEq/L
Creatinine <0.6 mg or >1.4 mg/100 mL	Fluid sequestration >6 L
Hematocrit <30% or >45.9%	
15 Glasgow Coma Scale chronic health points	

LDH lactate dehydrogenase, *AST* aspartate transaminase

Table 3 Atlanta definition of severe acute pancreatitis

Criteria	Signs or biological values
Organ failure	Pulmonary insufficiency (paO_2 <60 mmHg) or renal failure (creatinine >177 mol/L after rehydration)
Shock	Systolic arterial pressure <90 mmHg
Gastrointestinal bleeding	Evidence of digestive hemorrhage at a rate >500 mL/day
Local complications	Necrosis, infection, presence of an abscess
Diseminated intravascular coagulation	Platelets <100 g/L, fibrinogen <1 g/L, fibrin split products >80 µg/mL
Metabolic disturbance	Calcium ≤1.87 mmol/L
Ranson criteria	≥3
Apache II criteria	≥8

- To assess the severity of the disease
- To diagnose early an obstructive biliary cause
- To assess complications and to manage their treatment

5.1 MDCT Technique

The best time for staging acute fluid collection is at 72 h and the appreciation of parenchymal necrosis is optimal at 96 h after the first symptoms (abdominal pain). Usually, CT is performed within 48–72 h following the clinical diagnosis of pancreatitis. The CT protocol must include two acquisitions:

- The first acquisition without injection of iodine contrast medium is helpful to show biliary or pancreatic stones and to asses hemorrhage.
- The second acquisition after injection of 2 mL of iodine contrast medium per kilogram (concentration 350 g/L) at 3 mL/s, performed in the portal phase (delay of 70 s). Neither gastric nor bowel opacification is necessary.

5.2 Initial Lesions

Initial lesions contribute to scoring the acute pancreatitis; they can be isolated or associated with each other.

Acute Pancreatitis

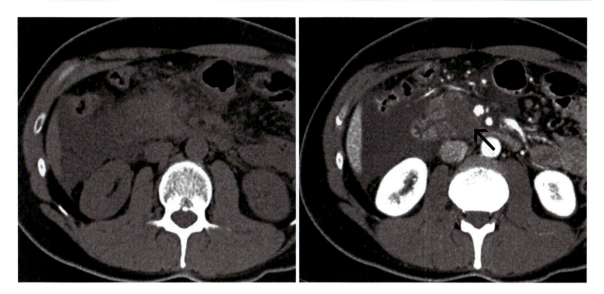

Fig. 1 Severe pancreatitis with necrosis of the head of the pancreas. Nonenhanced and contrast-enhanced computed tomography (CT) examination shows the necrosis in the head of the pancreatic parenchyma that fails to be enhanced (*arrow*)

5.2.1 Pancreatic Necrosis

Pancreatic necrosis is defined as an area of nonviable pancreatic parenchyma; it consists of focal or a diffuse lack of parenchymal enhancement demonstrated after intravenous contrast medium administration (Fig. 1). This necrosis can involve a part or the entire pancreas, and can go over the pancreas in peripancreatic fat (Fig. 2). It is present in 5–20% of patients with acute pancreatitis. It can be hemorrhagic (Fig. 3), with hyperattenuation on the series before contrast medium injection. Its evolution to walled-off pancreatitis necrosis (WOPN) leads to an irregular fluid collection that develop within the area of pancreatic necrosis and can extend into the peripancreatic space. These WOPN have solid luminal content that develops as a late consequence of necrotizing pancreatitis (Fig. 4). They must be well differentiated from pseudocyst because the therapeutic options are different (Takahashi et al. 2008).

5.2.2 Acute Fluid Collections

Fluid collections contain enzymatic fluid secretions. They can be homogeneous or hetrogeneous. The presence of gas inside is a sign of gravity. A well-defined wall encloses fluid collections. They are more often located near the pancreatic gland and on the left and right anterior pararenal spaces (Fig. 5). This collection can have visceral atypical locations, such

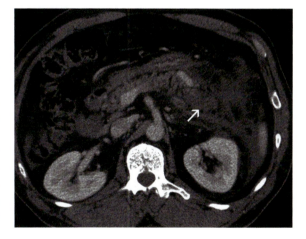

Fig. 2 Severe pancreatitis with necrosis of the pancreatic tail. Contrast-enhanced CT examination shows the nonenhanced tail of the pancreas (*arrow*), associated with significant stranding of the peripancreatic fat

as hepatic, splenic, and even pleural. Present in 40% of patients with acute pancreatitis, they have a spontaneous resolution in 50% of patients. In the case of nonresolution, they evolve as pseudocyst (in a minimal time of 4 weeks) (Table 4).

5.2.3 Size and Morphology of the Pancreatic Gland

The size of the pancreas can be normal or increased owing to edema. This increase is diffuse or localized.

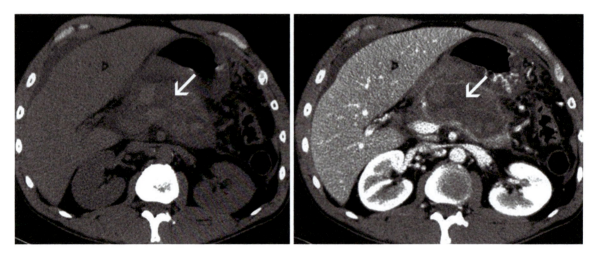

Fig. 3 Severe pancreatitis with hemorrhagic necrosis. In the nonenhanced CT examination, necrosis appears heterogeneous (*arrow*), with spontaneous increased attenuation, without enhancement after injection of contrast medium

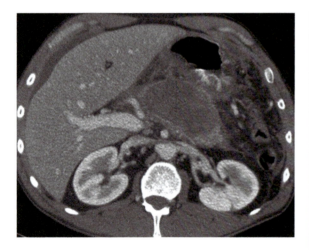

Fig. 4 Severe pancreatitis with walled-off necrosis. In the enhanced CT examination, a large heterogeneous low-attenuated collection replaces almost the entire body of the pancreas. Pancreatic parenchyma necrosis is associated with an important stranding of the peripancreatic fat

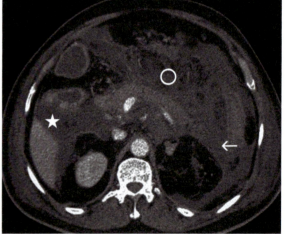

Fig. 5 Severe pancreatitis without pancreatic necrosis classified as Balthazar E or CT severity index (CTSI) 4. The pancreas has a smooth-contour appearance. The prepancreatic collection (*circle*) is heterogeneous and could correspond to fat necrosis or acute fluid collection. Perihepatic (*star*) and prerenal (*arrow*) collections are classified as acute fluid collections

Normal lobular contours can disappear with a smooth-contour appearance in a diffuse or focal way (Fig. 6).

5.2.4 Peripancreatic Fat Infiltration

A reticulation of the peripancreatic fat reveals fat stranding (Fig. 7). This infiltration is evident when it is associated with parenchyma necrosis, but even if there is no parenchyma necrosis on the CT scan, peripancreatic fat infiltration can be present.

5.2.5 Ascites

Ascites as a peritoneal reaction can be observed especially around the liver and the spleen, and in the pelvis. It is often associated with pleural effusion. It is important, but not easy, to differentiate ascites and acute fluid collection, to avoid an overestimation of the different CT scores that take into account this last sign but not the ascites.

Table 4 Summary of Atlanta classification terminology of the computed tomography (CT) finding in acute pancreatitis (from Cannon et al. 2009)

Pathological finding	Characteristics
Acute fluid collections	Occur in the first hours (less than 72 h) in the course of the disease. Located in or near the pancreas. Do not have a wall of granulation
Pancreatic necrosis	Diffuse or focal area of nonviable pancreatic parenchyma. Typically associated with peripancreatic fat necrosis
Acute pseudocyst	Collection of pancreatic juice enclosed by a wall of fibrous or granulation tissue. Arises as a consequence of acute pancreatitis. Have a well-defined wall. Require 4 weeks or more from the onset of acute pancreatitis
Pancreatic abscess	Circumscribed intra-abdominal collection of pus. Occurs later in the course of severe acute pancreatitis, often 4 weeks or more after onset. The presence of pus and a positive culture for bacteria or fungi, but little or no pancreatic necrosis, differentiate a pancreatic or peripancreatic abscess from infected necrosis

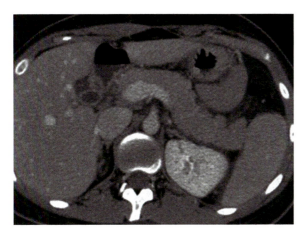

Fig. 6 Mild pancreatitis without pancreatic necrosis, classified as Balthazar B or CTSI 1. The initial enhanced CT examination demonstrates an enlarged edematous pancreas and effacement of the lobular contours

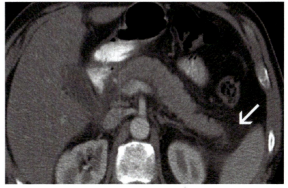

Fig. 7 Mild pancreatitis without pancreatic necrosis, classified as Balthazar C or CTSI 2. In addition to the enlargement of the pancreas and smooth contours, CT examination shows peripancreatic inflammatory change with fat stranding around the pancreatic tail (*arrow*)

5.3 CT Score

The establishment of a prognostic of the severity of the disease allows the best orientation and the best management of the patient. The CT scores mostly used are the Balthazar score and the CT severity index (CTSI). But new scores have been described, such as the extrapancreatic inflammation on CT (EPIC) score and the simple prognostic score, that try to take into account the visceral dysfunction, which remains the main factor determining outcome in the first period of severe acute pancreatitis. Other scores such as the pancreatic severity index (London et al. 1989) and the mesenteric edema and peritoneal score (King et al. 2003) have been proposed but are not often used in clinical practice.

5.3.1 Balthazar Score

The Balthazar score is based on a five-grade scale (Table 5). The parameters recorded are a reflection of the pancreatic and peripancreatic inflammation and the presence of fluid collection. The main advantages of this score are its simplicity and that contrast medium injection is not required. The main disadvantages are the lack of precision regarding the fluid collection (acute fluid collection, organized necrosis, walled-off pancreatic necrosis, postnecrotic fluid collection) and, above all, not taking into account the pancreatic necrosis. Morbidity and mortality are, respectively, 4 and 0% in patients with CT grade A, B, or C and 54 and 14% in patients with CT grade D or E. To obtain the best results, the CT must not be performed too early. One must wait at least 48–72 h

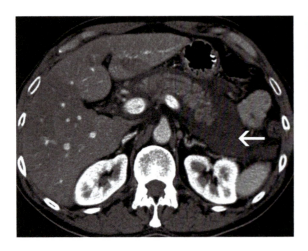
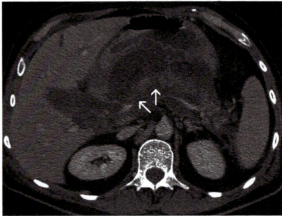

Fig. 8 Mild pancreatitis without pancreatic necrosis, classified as Balthazar D or CTSI 3. There is only one acute fluid collection on the initial CT examination. Notice the heterogeneous hypoattenuation of the liver that could correspond to steatosis

Fig. 9 Severe pancreatitis with pancreatic necrosis, classified as Balthazar E or CTSI 8. CT examination shows multiple acute fluid collections. The enhancement of the pancreatic parenchyma is poor and heterogeneous (*arrows*). Almost all of the gland seems to be involved in the necrosis but not in a homogeneous way

Table 5 Balthazar CT score

Balthazar CT score	Finding
A	Normal pancreas
B	Enlarged edematous pancreas; effacement of the lobular contours
C	Peripancreatic stranding
D	In addition, one single fluid collection
E	In addition, multiple or extensive fluid collection

Table 6 CT severity index

CT signs	Points
Pancreatic inflammation signs	
Normal pancreas	0
Enlarged edematous pancreas; effacement of the lobular contours	1
Peripancreatic stranding	2
In addition, one single fluid collection	3
In addition, multiple or extensive fluid collection	4
Pancreatic necrosis	
None	0
≤30%	2
>30% to ≤50%	4
>50%	6

after the beginning of the symptoms (Delrue et al. 2010; Casas et al. 2004; Balthazar et al. 1985) (Figs. 5, 6, 7, 8).

5.3.2 CT Severity Index

The CTSI is probably the most used CT score. It is based on the Balthazar score, but, in addition, it takes into account the percentage of pancreatic necrosis (Table 6). This score has a better correlation than the Balthazar score with the morbidity and the mortality, which are, respectively, 3 and 8% when the CTSI is 3 or less and 92 and 17% when it is 7 or more (Delrue et al. 2010; Balthazar et al. 1990; Vriens et al. 2005). The main advantage of this CTSI is the introduction of pancreatic necrosis, and thus the difference between edematous and necrotic pancreatitis (Fig. 9). As reported in "Pancreatic necrosis," this is closely related to a high morbidity and mortality, in contrast to interstitial and edematous pancreatitis. The disadvantages of the CTSI are, firstly, the requirement of contrast medium injection, which has been reported by some authors to aggravate the course of the disease (Schmidt et al. 1995), and, secondly, the need for a delay of 72 h or better 96 h to define well the pancreatic necrosis. It is important to note that the potential aggravation by iodine contrast medium has been invalidated by more recent studies (Arvanitakis et al. 2004; Balthazar et al. 1990).

Table 7 Extrapancreatic inflammation on CT (EPIC) score

	CT signs	Points
Pleural effusion	None	0
	Unilateral	1
	Bilateral	2
Ascites in any of these locations: perisplenic, perihepatic, interloop, or pelvis	None	0
	One location	1
	More than one location	2
Retroperitoneal inflammation	None	0
	Unilateral	1
	Bilateral	2
Mesenteric inflammation	Absent	0
	Present	1

A modified CTSI has been proposed (Mortelé et al. 2004) that associates with the signs of inflammation and necrosis of the classical CTSI the signs of extrapancreatic complications. This score seems to be more strongly correlated to the outcome of the disease than the traditional CTSI, but it has been poorly evaluated and the delay before CT is very long (within 1 week).

5.3.3 EPIC Score

The EPIC score is based not on pancreatic or peripancreatic lesions but only on extrapancreatic manifestations of the disease (Table 7). An EPIC score of 4 or more is predictive of a severe acute pancreatitis with a sensitivity of 100% and a specificity of 70.8%. The main advantages of the EPIC score are that injection of contrast medium is not required and that it can be performed in the first 24 h following the start of the symptoms (De Waele et al. 2007).

5.3.4 Simple Prognosis Score

The simple prognosis score is a composite score based on the presence (1 point) or the absence (0 points) of the following biological and CT data: (1) serum LDH level (900 IU/L or higher), (2) blood urea nitrogen level (25 mg/dL or higher), and (3) the presence of pancreatic necrosis on the CT performed within the first 2 days of admission. A score higher than 2 or 3 is considered to reflect severe pancreatitis. The mortality rate, percentage of infection, and rate of organ failure are, respectively, 10, 7, and 37% when the score is 0 or 1 and 58, 51, and 91% when the score is 2 or 3.

The main advantages of this score are that it reflects through the biological data the visceral dysfunction and its simplicity. The main disadvantage is its poor evaluation in the literature (Delrue et al. 2010).

5.3.5 Classification in Three Groups

A new classification in three categories has recently been proposed taking into account the CT score and multiple or persistent organ failure. Severe acute pancreatitis was defined as death, persistent organ failure (over 48 h), or multiple organ failure. Moderate acute pancreatitis was defined as the presence of acute collections and/or pancreatic necrosis. Mild acute pancreatitis was defined by exclusion. This classification seems to distinguish three homogeneous groups of severity but needs validation (De Madaria et al. 2010).

5.4 Etiological Orientations

5.4.1 In the Early Stage Some Cause Could Be Suspected

A common bile duct stone migration is the most important cause to diagnose initially because of its clinical impact (therapeutic ERCP). It could be suggested in the case of gallstones or a common bile duct dilatation visible on CT. Common bile duct stones are rarely obvious on CT. Ultrasonography has good sensibility performance for the diagnosis of gallstones (more than 90%) but poor sensibility for the diagnosis of common duct stones (40–60%). Nevertheless, ultrasonography in the first 24 h is mandatory to depict bile duct dilatation, small lithiasis in the gallbladder (large lithiasis do not migrate), or biliary duct lithiasis (Fig. 10).

An alcoholic cause can be suggested in the case of liver abnormalities: steatosis (hepatic size increased with attenuation of the parenchyma) or cirrhosis (dysmorphism of the liver and portal hypertension signs) (Fig. 11).

Iatrogenic and traumatic causes are obvious causes because of the clinical context: ERCP, pancreatic surgery, car crash, for example.

5.4.2 Different Pancreatic Diseases

Different pancreatic diseases are to blame for acute pancreatitis. They are difficult to diagnose in the early stage of the disease because of the pancreatic

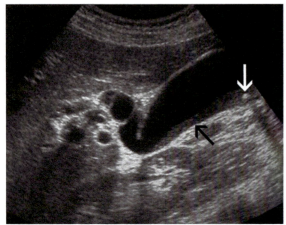

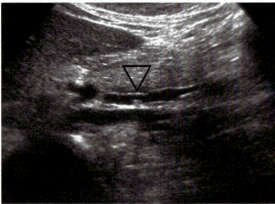

Fig. 10 Ultrasonography performed 24 h after the beginning of the symptoms of pancreatitis shows sludge (*black arrow*) and a small stone (*white arrow*) in the gallbladder. The extrahepatic bile duct is visible and ultrasonography demonstrates a small stone (*head of arrow*). These findings enable one to make the diagnosis of biliary pancreatitis and lead to the performance of an endoscopic retrograde cholangiography associated with a sphincterectomy

parenchyma change. An exploration by CT or MRI is mandatory later.

Pancreatic Duct Abnormalities

- Stenosis or intraductal stones in the case of chronic pancreatitis: CT features include pancreatic lithiasis, irregular ductal dilatation, and parenchyma atrophy.
- Intraductal papillary mucinous tumors of the pancreas: the enlargement of the main pancreatic duct and/or branch ducts is well identified on MRI (Fig. 12) (Vullierme et al. 2005).

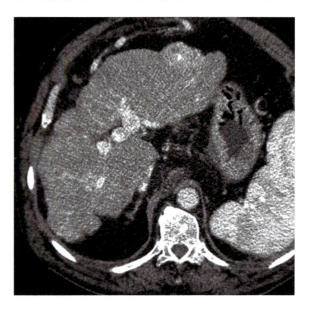

Fig. 11 Patient with mild pancreatitis. The morphological change of the liver, typical of cirrhosis, could lead to suspicion of an alcoholic cause of the pancreatitis

- Congenital anomalies of the pancreatic duct (annular pancreas or pancreas divisum) explored by magnetic resonance cholangiopancreatography.

Tumors

- Adenocarcinoma induces an enlargement of the main pancreatic duct but it is difficult to differentiate a hyperattenuating mass in the early phase due owing inflammation and necrosis from a pancreatic tumor. Although the diagnosis of adenocarcinoma is usually easy to perform by CT, it is important not to perform the examination too early after the acute episode (Fig. 13).
- Lymphoma. Pancreas localization is more often secondary to a general disease; it can appear as a nodular or diffuse infiltrative lesion.

Autoimmune Pancreatitis

This disease is characterized by an autoimmune inflammatory process and can initially be revealed by an acute pancreatitis. It mimics a tumoral lesion with enlargement of the pancreas associated with a minimal peripancreatic stranding and a nondilated or diffusely narrowed pancreatic duct. The diagnosis is

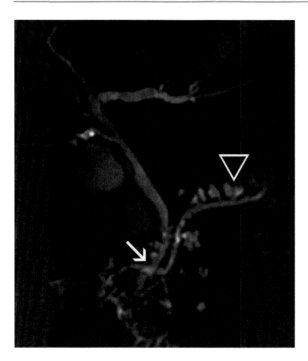

Fig. 12 Magnetic resonance cholangiopancreatography. Intraductal papillary tumor of branch duct. Magnetic resonance cholangiopancreatography shows multiple cysts branched on the main duct (*head of arrow*). Notice the association with a pancreas divisum (*arrow*)

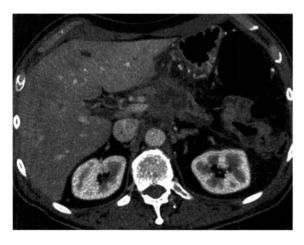

Fig. 13 Patient with mild pancreatitis from adenocarcinoma. CT examination shows a heterogeneous hypoattenuation of the pancreas, with a local enlargement and peripancreatic fat spreading. In this situation of pancreatitis, this aspect should not be mistaken for a pancreatic necrosis

based on the association with extrapancreatic manifestations of autoimmune diseases, serologic markers (autoantibodies), and the response to corticosteroid treatment (Fig. 14) (Sahani et al. 2004).

General metabolic diseases

General metabolic diseases (hypercalcemia, hypertriglyceridemia) can be incriminated for acute pancreatitis, but they have no particular CT features.

5.5 Complications

CT allows the diagnosis of complications which can appear during the clinical course of the disease.

5.5.1 In the Acute Phase

In the acute phase complications are dominated by organ failures, but some local complications can occur.

Thrombosis usually concerns veins more than arteries, such as splenic, mesenteric, or portal vein (Fig. 15).

Pseudoaneurysms are rare during the initial phase of acute pancreatitis and are more often discovered on CT in the follow-up of the disease. They are due to direct erosion of the artery wall by the pancreatic enzymes of the fluid collection. They appear as an image of addition, enhanced with the same timing as the arterial vessels. CT should be considered as the first investigation in diagnosis and for planning intervention. Multiplanar reformation and maximum intensity projection reconstructions allow one to identify the artery from which the pseudoaneurysm rises and the pseudoaneurysm morphology. Their treatment must be endovascular first (Fig. 16) (Kirby et al. 2008).

Acute fluid collection can injure abdominal organs such as liver, spleen, gallbladder, and gut and may be responsible for necrosis (Fig. 17), infarction, hematoma, and even spleen rupture (Habib et al. 2000).

Intestinal perforation is rare but can occur owing to spread of pancreatic enzymes to the intestinal wall (Van Minnen et al. 2004). According to the literature, this complication seems to involve almost exclusively the colon and not the small bowel. Diagnosis is often difficult because the signs of colon perforation (pericolitis, bubble of gas) are frequent in acute pancreatitis.

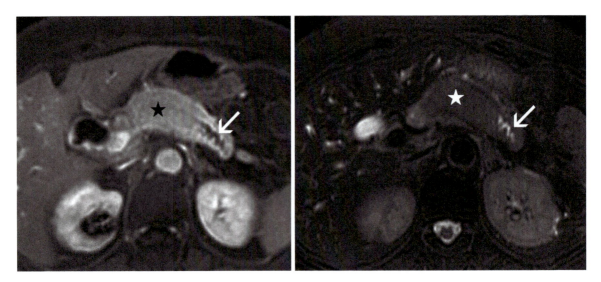

Fig. 14 Autoimmune pancreatitis. MRI T1-weighted sequence after gadolinium injection and T2-weighted sequence. Focal enlargement of the body of the pancreas, homogeneously enhanced (*star*), responsible for a dilated pancreatic duct of the tail

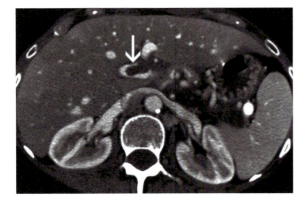

Fig. 15 Mild pancreatitis without pancreatic necrosis. The partial portal vein thrombosis (*arrow*) is well displayed in the enhanced CT examination surrounded by the normal enhancement of the vessel

Infection of necrosis is a frequent and severe complication (Whitcomb 2006). The diffuse or local area of nonviable parenchyma is initially sterile and can become infected by bacteria of gut origin. Mortality in sterile and infected necrosis is, respectively, 10 and 25%. This complication develops during the second or third week in 40–70% of patients with severe pancreatitis. Suspicion of infection of the necrosis is made on the basis of clinical and biological criteria. The only CT sign is the presence of a bubble of gas within the necrosis area. But this sign is not very sensitive (Fig. 18). Thus, to discriminate between sterile and infected pancreatic necrosis, CT-guided needle aspirations of pancreatic or peripancreatic tissues are done repeatedly.

A positive diagnosis of infection can lead to surgical debridement. Endoscopic or percutaneous drainage is limited in the case of infected necrosis because these lesions are mainly made up of solid residues with a poor liquid component (Freeny et al. 1998). But percutaneous drainage can be performed when surgery is contraindicated or for residual collections after surgical debridement (Fig. 19).

Disconnection of the pancreatic duct (Sandrasegaran et al. 2007) is underestimated. However, patients with a disconnected pancreatic duct are at a increased risk of persistent pancreatic fistula. Therefore, surgical treatment should be discussed in this situation.

Diagnosis of disconnected pancreatic duct could be advocated if all of the following signs are present: necrosis of at least 2 cm of pancreas; viable pancreatic tissue upstream of the site of necrosis, and extravasation of contrast medium injected into the main pancreatic duct on pancreatography or on MRI with secretin injection.

5.5.2 In a Later Phase (After 4 Weeks)

Local complications are mainly due to a pseudocyst. Pseudocysts are the evolution of the acute fluid collection that has not been resolved. On CT,

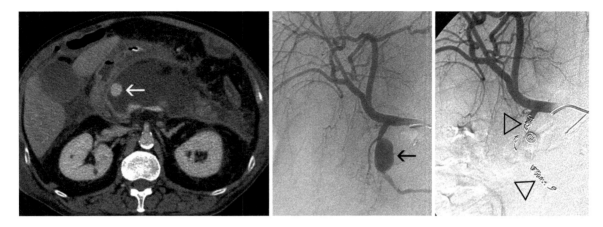

Fig. 16 Severe pancreatitis with pancreatic necrosis, complicated by a pseudoaneurysm. The enhanced CT examination performed 16 days after the beginning of the disease shows a pseudoaneurysm (*arrow*) of the gastroduodenal artery close to a voluminous collected necrosis. Embolization by the sandwich technique (*heads of arrow*) allows complete exclusion of the pseudoaneurysm

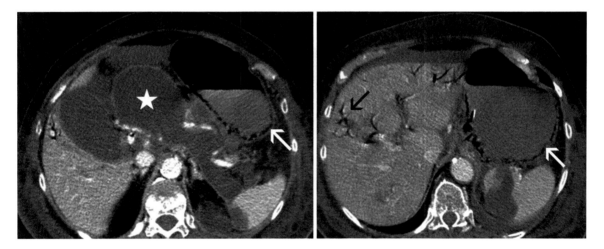

Fig. 17 Severe pancreatitis with digestive necrosis and spleen infarction. Enhanced CT examination shows a voluminous acute fluid collection in the omental bursa (*star*). Presence of gas in the gastric wall (*white arrow*) and in the intrahepatic portal vessel (*black arrow*) demonstrates the digestive necrosis. Well-delineated segmental hypoattenuation of the spleen corresponds to an infarction

pseudocysts appear at least after 4 weeks of evolution of the acute pancreatitis (Fig. 20). Pancreatic pseudocysts are defined as localized amylase-rich fluid collections located within the pancreatic tissue or adjacent to the pancreas (Yeo et al. 1990). They are more frequently unilocular than multilocular and are surrounded by a fibrous wall without epithelial lining. The CT findings of a pseudocyst include a round or oval fluid collection, well delineated, with an homogeneous content and a thin or thick, but regular wall enhanced after contrast medium injection (Kim et al. 2005). They occur in 5–40% of patients with acute pancreatitis.

Classic complications of pseudocyst are compression on digestive, biliary, or vascular structures, rupture, infection, and hemorrhage. In the literature, an etiological or morphological factor is predictive of the evolution (regression or complication of the pseudocyst) (Maringhini et al. 1999).

Infection of the pseudocyst does not dramatically change the feature of the pseudocyst on CT, but a light heterogeneity of the content could appear.

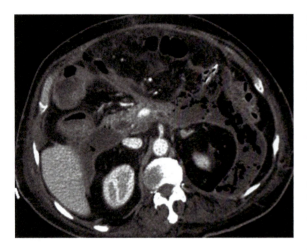

Fig. 18 CT examination performed 3 weeks after the beginning of a severe pancreatitis with necrosis. A large area of necrosis containing numerous bubbles of gas enables the diagnosis of infection. Infection was confirmed by CT-guided aspiration

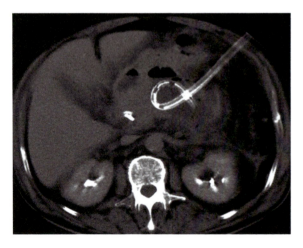

Fig. 19 Percutaneous drainage of a pancreatic necrosis. Notice the large diameter of the catheter (28G), which is essential to drain the thick collection with debris

Treatment consists in drainage that could be endoscopic or per cutaneous (Loveday et al. 2008).

Compression can involve the gut, the biliary system, or vessels (Fig. 21). CT is used to determine the relation between the pseudocyst and its adjacent structures, and thus to guide the choice of the therapeutic management, which can be endoscopic or surgical.

Intracystic hemorrhage is due to the erosion of an artery by the pancreatic enzymes of the pseudocyst fluid. Diagnosis could follow a hypovolemic shock, but it is more often made following a systematic CT examination in the follow-up of the acute pancreatitis. The density of the pseudocyst is spontaneously high and after contrast medium injection leakage of contrast medium within the pseudocyst is observed (Fig. 22). The first treatment should be endovascular.

6 CT Pitfalls

Considering that the diagnosis of acute pancreatitis is based on clinical and biological data, any pancreatic or peripancreatic abnormality noticed on CT is used to classify the severity of the disease. Thus, the only pitfalls are the etiological diagnosis that could be hidden by the signs of pancreatitis.

7 Impact of CT on the Management

7.1 Positive Diagnosis

The only rule of CT on positive diagnosis is to exclude other causes of acute abdominal pain such as bowel perforation, mesenteric ischemia, or aortic aneurysm rupture.

7.2 CT Scoring

The main rule of CT is to establish the severity of the disease (mild or severe) to determine the gravity of the disease, leading to a specific management.

The choice of the score to use is not so easy because, on one hand, it is important to have an early risk stratification of patients with acute pancreatitis. On the other hand, scoring systems based on necrosis are limited because they need an evolution of the disease of at least 48 h or better 72 h to be efficient. In this situation, more recent radiologic scoring systems based on signs of organ dysfunction could be useful in the prediction of severity.

Thus, we suggest two options. For a patient without any clinical sign of severity, i.e., with no problems other than low to moderate abdominal pain, we can wait 72 h to perform the CT and use the CTSI. (Of course, if the patient is referred to the clinician more than 72 h after the beginning of the symptoms, the situation is the same.) For a patient with serious

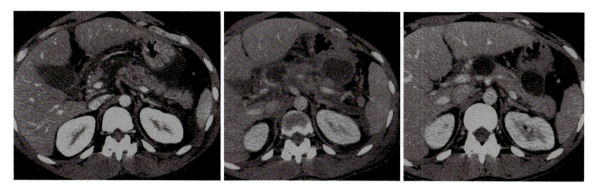

Fig. 20 Evolution of the acute fluid collections to a pseudocyst, in a mild pancreatitis. CT examinations were performed at 48 h, 3 weeks, and 6 weeks in the course of the pancreatitis

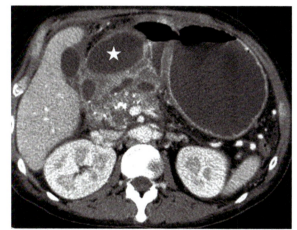

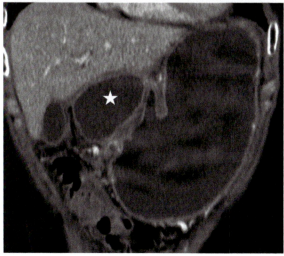

Fig. 21 Pseudocyst (*stars*) 2 months after the beginning of a severe pancreatitis. The compression of the pseudocyst on the antrum is responsible for an important gastric dilatation and will be treated by endoscopic drainage

symptoms, i.e., serious pain, abdominal tenderness, hypovolemic or respiratory symptoms, CT is performed without contrast medium in the first 24 h and the EPIC score is used; the scoring is then completed after 72 h with a CT scan with injection of contrast medium.

7.3 Looking for Acute Complications

Complications of acute pancreatitis generally do not appear in the first few days of the evolution of the disease but appear in the first few weeks, or later in the case of pseudocyst complications. But even then uncommon early complications can occur. Thus, first CT, even it is mainly performed to establish a predictive score, should be used to look carefully for vascular, digestive, or visceral associated lesions.

7.4 First Etiological Orientations

During the first scoring CT scan, it is essential to look for signs that could be oriented to specific causes: hepatic abnormality (steatosis, cirrhosis); biliary or pancreatic lithiasis.

Other causes are, in most of cases, impossible to affirm in the early stage of the disease, especially when acute pancreatitis is severe, owing to the pancreatic parenchymal change. Therefore, when the etiological investigations (including clinical, biological, and first CT examinations) are not successful, new morphological examinations, which could be CT

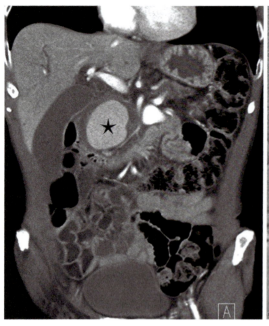 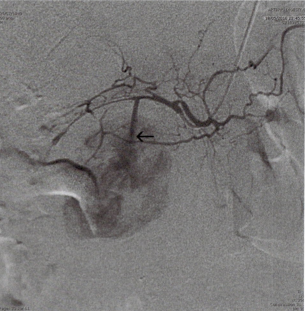

Fig. 22 Pseudocyst close to the head of the pancreas, responsible for an erosion of the gastroduodenal artery with intracystic hemorrhage. On enhanced CT examination, the pseudocyst is filled by contrast medium (*star*). On angiography, the gastroduodenal artery is pushed into a horizontal position by the pseudocyst. Leakage of contrast medium in the pseudocyst is clearly demonstrated (*arrow*)

or MRI depending on the clinical suspicions, must be carried out after the clinical resolution of the acute pancreatitis. In this situation, it is important not to perform the examination too early after the acute episode, to prevent an inconclusive examination.

7.5 Following Acute Pancreatitis by CT

- There is no well-established rhythm for following acute pancreatitis by CT. It is not so easy to determine a good delay between the beginning of the symptoms and the first CT examination regarding the opposing needs of an early risk stratification and establishment of an accurate score (48–72 h).
- After this first CT examination has been performed to stage and score the disease, there is no need for a new CT examination until at least 4 weeks later, except in the case of a clinical or biological change. In this specific situation, a new CT examination could lead to the discovering of complications, worsening of score graduation or a change from edematous to necrotic pancreatitis (in 13 and 8%, respectively) (Lankisch et al. 2001).
- At 4 weeks CT could be performed in the following cases: (1) when there have been no etiological findings; (2) in the case of resolute pancreatitis if it was necrotic or with a Balthazar grade of D or higher, with the goal of detecting complications; (3) and when the disease is not yet resolved. In this latest case, a CT scan is performed during the course of the disease in accordance with the clinical evolution.

7.6 Radiological Treatments

CT has a major role in the therapeutic management, to guide bacteriologic necrosis or fluid collection samples, to diagnose and plan treatment of abscess or vascular complications.

8 Diagnostic Strategy

1. Positive diagnosis of acute pancreatitis is based on clinical symptoms and blood pancreatic enzyme level.

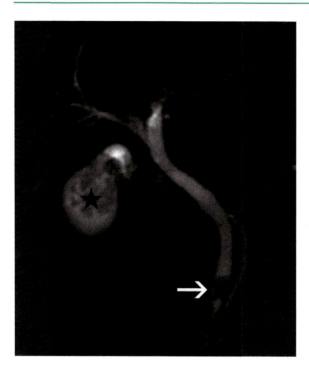

Fig. 23 Magnetic resonance cholangiopancreatography. Gallstones (*star*) and choledocholithiasis (*arrow*) are well demonstrated

2. CT is the unique morphological examination to perform at the initial stage of the disease. The ideal delay between the beginning of the symptom and this CT is 48–72 h. This CT allows the first staging of the lesions and predicts the evolution risk of the pancreatitis through the use of CT scores.
3. In the first 24 h it could be useful to perform biliary ultrasonography. The goal of this examination is definitively not to detect any pancreatic signs but to look after signs of lithiasis. If a biliary pancreatitis is diagnosed or suspected, an early ERCP with endoscopic sphincterotomy is recommended (Wada et al. 2010; Johnson and Lévy 2010).
4. The place of MRI in acute pancreatitis has not been established. Regarding detection of necrosis and acute fluid collection, as well as predicting scoring, the performance of MRI is reported to be equivalent to that of CT (Arvanitakis et al. 2007; Xiao et al. 2010). Potential advantages of MRI are the lack of radiation, which might be suitable for patients with multiple follow-up reviews, and providing in the same examination information regarding the pancreatic parenchyma and biliary tree (Fig. 23), as well as the visualization of the pancreatic duct to evaluate integrity or rupture (Lau et al. 2001). The main disadvantages are the lower availability of MRI, the difficulty to achieve breathhold in patients with great pain, which could alter image quality, and the difficulty to manage the intensive care devices, in the case of severe patient conditions, in a magnetic environment.

In practice, MRI is rarely used in the initial staging of acute pancreatitis, but it could have an important place in the etiological assessment.

References

Arvanitakis M, Delhaye M, De Maertelaere V, Bali M, Winant C, Coppens E, Jeanmart J, Zalcman M, Van Gansbeke D, Devière J, Matos C (2004) Computed tomography and magnetic resonance imaging in the assessment of acute pancreatitis. Gastroenterology 126:715–723

Arvanitakis M, Koustiani G, Gantzarou A, Grollios G, Tsitouridis I, Haritandi-Kouridou A, Dimitriadis A, Arvanitakis C (2007) Staging of severity and prognosis of acute pancreatitis by computed tomography and magnetic resonance imaging—a comparative study. Dig Liver Dis 39:473–482

Balthazar EJ, Ranson JHC, Naidich DP et al (1985) Acute-pancreatitis—prognostic value of CT. Radiology 3:767–772

Balthazar EJ, Robinson DL, Megibow AJ, Ranson JH (1990) Acute pancreatitis: value of CT in establishing prognosis. Radiology 2:331–336

Cannon JW, Callery MP, Vollmer CM Jr (2009) Diagnosis and management of pancreatic pseudocysts: what is the evidence? J Am Coll Surg 209(3):385–393

Carroll JK, Herrick B, Gipson T, Lee SP (2007) Acute pancreatitis: diagnosis, prognosis, and treatment. Am Fam Physician 10:1513–1520

Casas JD, Diaz R, Valderas G, Mariscal A, Cuadras P (2004) Prognostic value of CT in the early assessment of patients with acute pancreatitis. AJR Am J Roentgenol 3:569–574

De Madaria E, Soler-Sala G, Lopez-Font I, Zapater P, Martínez J, Gómez-Escolar L, Sánchez-Fortún C, Sempere L, Pérez-López J, Lluís F, Pérez-Mateo M (2010) Update of the Atlanta classification of severity of acute pancreatitis: should a moderate category be included. Pancreatology 10(5):613–619

De Waele JJ, Delrue L, Hoste EA et al (2007) Extrapancreatic inflammation on abdominal computed tomography as an early predictor of disease severity in acute pancreatitis—evaluation of a new scoring system. Pancreas 2:185–190

Delrue LJ, De Waele JJ, Duyck PO (2010) Acute pancreatitis: radiologic scores in predicting severity and outcome. Abdom Imaging 35(3):349–361

Freeny PC, Hauptmann E, Althaus SJ, Traverso LW, Sinanan M (1998) Percutaneous CT-guided catheter drainage of infected acute necrotizing pancreatitis: techniques and results. AJR Am J Roentgenol 170(4):969–975

Frossard JL, Steer ML, Pastor CM (2008) Acute pancreatitis. Lancet 371(9607):143–152

Habib E, Elhadad A, Slama JL (2000) Diagnosis and treatment of spleen rupture during pancreatitis. Gastroenterol Clin Biol 24(12):1229–1232

Johnson C, Lévy P (2010) Detection of gallstones in acute pancreatitis: when and how? Pancreatology 10(1):27–32

Kim YH, Saini S, Sahani D, Hahn PF, Mueller PR, Auh YH (2005) Imaging diagnosis of cystic pancreatic lesions: pseudocyst versus nonpseudocyst. Radiographics 25(3):671–685

King NK, Powell JJ, Redhead D, Siriwardena AK (2003) A simplified method for computed tomographic estimation of prognosis in acute pancreatitis. Scand J Gastroenterol 4:433–436

Kirby JM, Vora P, Midia M, Rawlinson J (2008) Vascular complications of pancreatitis: imaging and intervention. Cardiovasc Intervent Radiol 31(5):957–970

Lankisch PG, Assmus C, Pflichthofer D, Struckman K, Lehnick D (1999) Which etiology causes the most severe pancreatitis? Int J Pancreat 26:55–57

Lankisch PG, Struckmann K, Assmus C, Lehnick D, Maisonneuve P, Lowenfels AB (2001) Do we need a computed tomography examination in all patients with acute pancreatitis within 72 h after admission to hospital for the detection of pancreatic necrosis? Scand J Gastroenterol 36(4):432–436

Lau ST, Simcuck EJ, Kozarek RA, Traverso W (2001) A pancreatic ductal leak should be sought to direct treatment in patients with acute pancreatitis. Am J Surg 181:411–417

London NJ, Neoptolemos JP, Lavelle J, Bailey I, James D (1989) Contrast-enhanced abdominal computed tomography scanning and prediction of severity of acute pancreatitis: a prospective study. Br J Surg 3:268–272

Loveday BP, Mittal A, Phillips A, Windsor JA (2008) Minimally invasive management of pancreatic abscess, pseudocyst, and necrosis: a systematic review of current guidelines. World J Surg 32(11):2383–2394

Maher MM, Lucey BC, Gervais DA, Mueller PR (2004) Acute pancreatitis: the role of imaging and interventional radiology. Cardiovasc Intervent Radiol 27(3):208–225

Maringhini A, Uomo G, Patti R et al (1999) Pseudocysts in acute nonalcoholic pancreatitis: incidence and natural history. Dig Dis Sci 44:1669–1673

McKay CJ, Buter A (2003) Natural history of organ failure in acute pancreatitis. Pancreatology 2:111–114

Mortelé KJ, Wiesner W, Intriere L et al (2004) A modified CT severity index for evaluating acute pancreatitis: improved correlation with patient outcome. AJR Am J Roentgenol 5:1261–1265

Nøjgaard C, Bendtsen F, Matzen P, Becker U (2010) The aetiology of acute and chronic pancreatitis over time in a hospital in Copenhagen. Dan Med Bull 57(1):A4103

Papachristou GI, Clermont G, Sharma A, Yadav D, Whitcomb DC (2007) Risk and markers of severe acute pancreatitis. Gastroenterol Clin N Am 2:277–296

Pastor CM, Matthay M, Frossard JL (2003) Pancreatitis-associated lung injury: new insights. Chest 124:2341–2351

Pitchumoni CS, Rubin A, Das K (2010) Pancreatitis in inflammatory bowel diseases. J Clin Gastroenterol 44(4):246–253

Sahani DV, Kalva SP, Farrell J, Maher MM, Saini S, Mueller PR, Lauwers GY, Fernandez CD, Warshaw AL, Simeone JF (2004) Autoimmune pancreatitis: imaging features. Radiology 233(2):345–352

Sandrasegaran K, Tann M, Jennings SG, Maglinte DD, Peter SD, Sherman S, Howard TJ (2007) Disconnection of the pancreatic duct: an important but overlooked complication of severe acute pancreatitis. Radiographics 27(5):1389–1400

Schmidt J, Hotz HG, Foitzik T et al (1995) Intravenous contrastmedium aggravates the impairment of pancreatic microcirculation in necrotizing pancreatitis in the rat. Ann Surg 3:257–264

Takahashi N, Papachristou GI, Schmit GD, Chahal P, LeRoy AJ, Sarr MG, Vege SS, Mandrekar JN, Baron TH (2008) CT findings of walled-off pancreatic necrosis (WOPN): differentiation from pseudocyst and prediction of outcome after endoscopic therapy. Eur Radiol 18(11):2522–2529

Ueda T, Takeyama Y, Yasuda T et al (2007) Simple scoring system for the prediction of the prognosis of severe acute pancreatitis. Surgery 1:51–58

Van Minnen LP, Besselink MG, Bosscha K, Van Leeuwen MS, Schipper ME, Gooszen HG (2004) Colonic involvement in acute pancreatitis. A retrospective study of 16 patients. Dig Surg 21(1):33–38

Vriens PW, van de Linde P, Slotema ET, Warmerdam PE, Breslau PJ (2005) Computed tomography severity index is an early prognostic tool for acute pancreatitis. J Am Coll Surg 4:497–502

Vullierme MP, Giraud M, Hammel P, Couvelard A, Sauvanet A, Belghiti J, Ruszniewski P, Vilgrain V (2005) Intraductal papillary mucinous tumours of the pancreas: imaging features. J Radiol 86(6 Pt 2):781–794

Wada K, Takada T, Hirata K, Mayumi T, Yoshida M, Yokoe M, Kiriyama S, Hirota M, Kimura Y, Takeda K, Arata S, Hirota M, Sekimoto M, Isaji S, Takeyama Y, Gabata T, Kitamura N, Amano H (2010) Treatment strategy for acute pancreatitis. J Hepatobiliary Pancreat Sci 17(1):79–86

Whitcomb DC (2006) Acute pancreatitis. N Engl J Med 20:2142–2150

Xiao B, Zhang XM, Tang W, Zeng NL, Zhai ZH (2010) Magnetic resonance imaging for local complications of acute pancreatitis: a pictorial review. World J Gastroenterol 16(22):2735–2742

Yadav D, Lowenfels AB (2006) Trends in the epidemiology of the first attack of acute pancreatitis: a systematic review. Pancreas 33:323–330

Yeo CJ, Bastidas JA, Lynch-Nyhan A et al (1990) The natural history of pancreatic pseudocysts documented by computed tomography. Surg Gynecol Obstet 170:411–417

Acute Appendicitis

Samuel Mérigeaud, Ingrid Millet, and Patrice Taourel

Contents

1	**Introduction**	144
2	**Anatomy and Embryology**	144
3	**Pathophysiology**	145
3.1	Role of the Vermiform Appendix	145
3.2	Mechanism of Appendiceal Lesions	145
4	**Clinical, Laboratory, and Ultrasonography Findings**	146
4.1	Clinical and Laboratory Findings	146
4.2	Ultrasound Semiology	147
5	**CT Protocols**	148
5.1	CT with or Without Intravenous Administration of Iodinated Contrast Material?	148
5.2	Focused or Nonfocused CT?	148
5.3	CT with or Without Digestive Opacification?	149
5.4	Low-Dose or Standard-Dose CT?	149
5.5	Which Image Processing?	150
5.6	Our Protocol	150
6	**CT Findings**	151
6.1	The Normal Appendix	151
6.2	Acute Appendicitis	153
6.3	Complications of Acute Appendicitis	156
7	**CT Pitfalls**	161
7.1	Normal and Variant Anatomy	161
7.2	Appendiceal Crohn Disease	162
7.3	Distal (or Tip) Appendicitis	162
7.4	Stump Appendicitis	162
7.5	Recurrent and Chronic Appendicitis	162
7.6	Abscessed Mass in the Right Iliac Fossa	164
7.7	Acute Appendicitis in Pregnant Women	164
7.8	Acute Appendicitis in the Elderly	165
8	**Differential Diagnosis**	167
8.1	Mesenteric Adenitis	167
8.2	Extra-appendiceal Digestive Conditions	167
8.3	Appendiceal Digestive Conditions	171
8.4	Gynecologic Disorders	173
8.5	Urologic Disorders	173
8.6	Nonspecific Abdominal Pain	173
9	**CT Accuracy and Diagnosis Strategy**	173
10	**Conclusion: Impact of CT on Management of Acute Appendicitis**	176
References		176

S. Mérigeaud (✉) · I. Millet · P. Taourel
Department of Imaging,
CHU Montpellier, Hospital Lapeyronie,
371 Avenue du Doyen Gaston-Giraud,
34295 Montpellier, Cedex 5, France
e-mail: s-merigeaud@chu-montpellier.fr

Abstract

Acute appendicitis is the most frequent cause of nontraumatic acute abdominal pain that requires emergency surgery. Its diagnosis remains challenging when relying only on clinical and laboratory findings, which explains the high rate of normal appendix after appendectomy. During the past 20 years, imaging techniques and particularly computed tomography (CT) have allowed preoperative diagnosis of appendicitis to be more reliable, related complications to be evaluated, the negative appendectomy rate and costs of caring to be lowered, and differential diagnosis to be sought. After an anatomical and pathophysiological review, we will highlight the use and impact of CT in the diagnosis and management of acute appendicitis.

P. Taourel (ed.), *CT of the Acute Abdomen*, Medical Radiology. Diagnostic Imaging,
DOI: 10.1007/174_2010_142, © Springer-Verlag Berlin Heidelberg 2011

1 Introduction

Acute appendicitis is currently the most frequent cause of nontraumatic acute abdominal pain that requires emergency surgery. It affects about 250,000 persons per year in the USA (Addiss et al. 1990), with a similar incidence in other industrialized countries. It is less frequent in developing countries (Walker and Segal 1990).

Described as early as 1886 by Fitz (1886), acute appendicitis is surgically treated by appendectomy. From the beginning, this procedure has been performed following the least equivocal physical examination, with the aim to operate as early as possible to prevent perforation-related complications (McBurney 1889). For years, only clinical evaluation by the surgeon's hand would allow a decision for or against surgery to be made. Currently, diagnosing acute appendicitis remains challenging when relying only on clinical and laboratory findings. Indeed, the rate of histologically normal appendix is 20%, with a rate as high as 42% in women of childbearing age (Raman et al. 2008; Poortman et al. 2009; Birnbaum and Wilson 2000). However, during the past 20 years, ultrasonography and computed tomography (CT) have progressively changed the practices. These new imaging technologies, in particular CT, allow preoperative diagnosis of appendicitis to be more reliable, related complications to be evaluated, the negative appendectomy rate and costs of caring to be lowered, and differential diagnosis to be sought.

2 Anatomy and Embryology

The vermiform appendix is a wormlike diverticulum of the cecum, only present in man and anthropoid apes, among primates. Its length varies from 8 to 10 cm on average, ranging from 1 to 25 cm (Schumpelick et al. 2000; Whitley et al. 2009). It arises from the posteromedial wall of the cecum, where the three tenia coli converge, 1.5–2.5 cm caudally to the ileocecal junction, which is a major landmark in imaging. The appendix is vascularized and innervated by its own meso, the mesoappendix, to which it is attached, to the lower end of the small bowel mesentery.

Both the cecum and the vermiform appendix arise from the cecal diverticulum. The vermiform appendix appears in the sixth week of embryonic development.

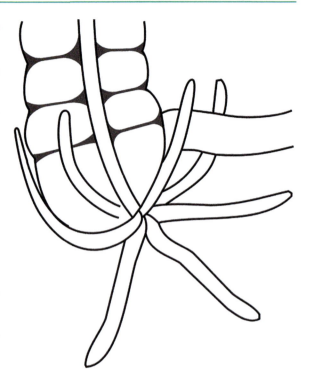

Fig. 1 Positions of the appendix relative to the cecum

The cecal diverticulum is the last to position itself, first below the liver. It then progressively descends into the right lower quadrant. The vermiform appendix begins to form during this descent, at the distal aspect of the cecum, which may explain the frequent retrocecal location of the appendix. The growth of the cecal walls is not uniform at the origin of the medial location of the appendix.

Peritoneal attachments will fix some parts of the gut. The meso of the right and the left colon attach to the posterior parietal peritoneum, forming the Toldt fascia. The cecum, appendix, and sigmoid do not attach and retain a meso. The appendix is thus free. It is simply related to the other adjacent organs through the mesoappendix. It may have variable location relative to the cecum (Fig. 1):

- Mediocecal, the most frequent, which corresponds to the McBurney point
- Laterocecal
- Retrocecal, anterior to the psoas-iliacus muscle, responsible for pso
- Subcecal, either anterior or posterior
- Prececal
- Ileocecal, either anterior or posterior

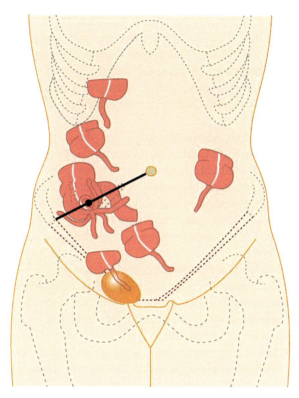

Fig. 2 Variable position of the vermiform appendix and cecum

Depending on the variable location of the cecum and the length of the appendix, the appendix may lie in different positions (Fig. 2):
- Subhepatic, either prececal or retrocecal.
- Pelvic.
- Mesoceliac, either because the appendix is long on an orthotopic cecum, or because the cecum is heterotopic (by lack of attachment of the right Toldt fascia).
- Hernial, inguinal, or crural, rarely in a Spiegel hernia (Mathias et al. 2008). The presence of the vermiform appendix in inguinal hernia, referred to as Amyand hernia, is rare (1% of inguinal hernias).

In rare cases of a common mesentery or situs inversus, the cecum and vermiform appendix may lie in the left lower quadrant.

3 Pathophysiology

3.1 Role of the Vermiform Appendix

The role of the vermiform appendix is still controversial. It has long been regarded as a vestigial organ with no function, only manifesting itself as acute appendicitis. However, in recent years, studies have shown that its mucosa is lined, as the entire gut, with a biofilm containing immunoglobulins as well as commensal bacteria essential to digestion. It also prevents pathogenic bacteria from invading the digestive lumen. During diarrhea episodes, a large amount of the colonic biofilm is purged, leaving the mucosa exposed to infections. The appendiceal biofilm, denser, is preserved, with the appendix shunting the cecum. Hence, the colonic biofilm can progressively replenish itself from the appendix. The vermiform appendix plays a role in facilitating faster recovery from diarrhea, with a more important role in developing countries where inhabitants are prone to this type of infection (Randal Bollinger et al. 2007). Inversely, inhabitants of industrialized countries are less exposed to pathogenic viruses and bacteria. Organisms are poorly prepared to fight against invading pathogens, leading to an impaired immune response. A virus can, for example, induce a severe lymphoid hyperplasia obstructing the appendiceal lumen, or mucosal lesions followed by bacterial infection (Barker 1989; Walker and Segal 1990, 1995). This would account for the higher incidence of acute appendicitis encountered in industrialized countries than in developing countries (Walker and Segal 1990).

3.2 Mechanism of Appendiceal Lesions

Luminal obstruction typically causes acute appendicitis. Causes of obstruction include:
- Thickening of the parietal wall, which could be related to lymphoid hyperplasia (induced by some viruses), and a cecal or appendiceal tumor (both primary and metastatic tumors) (Hermans et al. 1993; Kim et al. 2008a)
- The presence of an obstacle within the lumen: appendicoliths, parasites (ascaris, shistosomiasis) (Nandipati et al. 2008; Misra et al. 1999; York 2003), or a foreign body, either ingested, such as a tooth crown, or iatrogenic, such as a biliary stent (Klingler et al. 1998; Tzovaras et al. 2007; Basu et al. 2009)

Obstruction of the appendiceal lumen induces a stasis of the appendiceal content, associated with bacterial proliferation and followed by an infection worsening with the parietal involvement. Catarrhal appendicitis (or endoappendicitis) is characterized by mucosal ulcerations. In suppurative appendicitis, either multiple parietal microabscesses (pseudo phlegmonous appendicitis) or a purulent luminal collection (appendiceal empyema) can be found. Parietal necrosis of gangrenous appendicitis is related to a venous obstruction secondary to edema, with a high risk of perforation (D'Acremont et al. 1995).

Inflammation is typically more important at the tip of the appendix. The base may be prevented and look normal, which could be an ultrasonography pitfall, for example.

Gram-negative (*Escherichia coli*) and anaerobic bacteria are the most frequent germs involved. In the case of a delayed diagnosis, the most frequent evolution is ischemic perforation followed by necrosis of the appendiceal wall. It can occur within a free peritoneum and lead to generalized peritonitis. Most often, the adjacent organs, namely, the small-bowel loops, greater omentum, and bladder, attach to the appendiceal source in order to limit the spreading of infection: this is the appendiceal plastron or periappendiceal phlegmon. This localized form of peritonitis can spread in the entire peritoneal cavity, leading to two-step peritonitis. A periappendiceal abscess can form: its rupture can eventually induce a three-step generalized peritonitis.

4 Clinical, Laboratory, and Ultrasonography Findings

Physical examination, later associated with laboratory findings, has long allowed acute appendicitis to be diagnosed. Ultrasonography and CT scanning allowed this diagnosis to be refined, especially in the case of atypical presentation. Although this chapter focuses on CT scanning in acute appendicitis, a brief summary of the use of ultrasonography among other diagnostic tools appears essential.

4.1 Clinical and Laboratory Findings

4.1.1 Clinical Presentation
Clinical presentation classically begins with continuous epigastric or periumbilical pain, poorly localized, getting worse when walking, coughing, or stressing.

Pain progressively migrates within a few hours to the right iliac fossa. It is often associated with low-grade fever (38–38.5°C) and dyspeptic disorders manifesting themselves as anorexia, nausea, and vomiting. Digestive disorders, such as constipation (predisposing to stercolith) and more rarely diarrhea, may also occur.

Physical examination classically shows pain and tenderness localized to the McBurney point (situated a third externally between the anterosuperior right iliac spine and the umbilicus), with psoitis or not. Rebound tenderness (right iliac fossa pain felt upon release of the abdominal pressure at a distance) related to parietal peritoneum irritation can be observed.

As previously described, the location of the vermiform appendix may differ depending on its length and the position of the cecum to which it is attached. Clinical presentation will also differ depending on the position of the appendix:

- Retrocecal: lumbar pain, with no abdominal tenderness, diminished when flexing the thigh but worsened when extending it (psoitis)
- Pelvic: subpubic pain sometimes accompanied with pain when internally rotating the thigh (obturator indicator caused when flexing the obturator internus muscle near an inflamed appendix), rectum tender at examination, urinary signs
- Subhepatic: pain and guarding of the right hypochondrus with Murphy sign
- Mesoceliac: febrile occlusive syndrome
- Hernial, inguinal, or crural

4.1.2 Laboratory Findings
Hyperleukocytosis with predominating polynuclear neutrophils (more than 10^{10}/L) can be observed. An elevated C-reactive protein value (more than 10 mg/L) is another classic finding despite its average negative predictive value: normal laboratory findings do not rule out the diagnosis of acute appendicitis (Gronroos et al. 2009; Gronroos and Gronroos 2001; Kessler et al. 2004).

4.1.3 Alvarado Score
Owing to the frequency of acute appendicitis and a challenging clinical diagnosis, Alvarado (1986) proposed a scoring system including six clinical items and two laboratory measurements, with a maximum score of 10 (Table 1). The diagnosis of appendicitis is

Acute Appendicitis

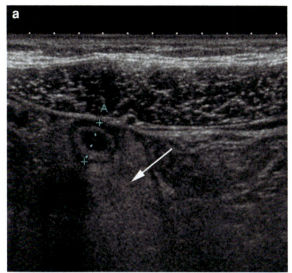

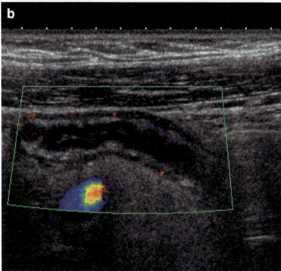

Fig. 3 Ultrasonography findings in acute appendicitis. **a** Mode B transverse cross section of a thick-walled appendix with 10-mm diameter and hyperechoic surrounding fat (*white arrow*). **b** Longitudinal cross section in color Doppler ultrasonography showing an incompressible, blind-ended, fluid-filled tubular structure with hyperemic walls

possible with a score of 5 or 6, probable with a score of 7 or 8, and highly probable with a score of 9 or 10.

A mnemonic aid is "MANTRELS":
Migration to the right iliac fossa
Anorexia, Nausea/vomiting
Tenderness in the right iliac fossa
Rebound pain
Elevated temperature (fever)

Table 1 Alvarado score for acute appendicitis

	Score
Symptoms	
Migratory right iliac fossa pain	1
Nausea/vomiting	1
Anorexia	1
Signs	
Tenderness in right iliac fossa	2
Rebound tenderness in right iliac fossa	1
Elevated temperature	1
Laboratory findings	
Leukocytosis	2
Shift to the left of neutrophils	1
Total	10

Leukocytosis
Shift of leukocytes to the left.

4.2 Ultrasound Semiology

Since the early 1990s, ultrasonography has allowed reliable analysis of the vermiform appendix, notably thanks to the graded-compression ultrasonography technique (Kessler et al. 2004; Lim et al. 1996; Rioux 1992). The examination is done using high-frequency linear probes (at least 7–8 MHz).

Acute appendicitis will show as a blind-ended tubular structure, larger than 6 mm in diameter, noncompressible, with a laminated wall (Fig. 3). The periappendiceal fat can be stranded, appearing hyperechoic. Color Doppler ultrasonography shows hypervascularization of the appendiceal wall (Fig. 3). Pressure on the appendix by the handheld ultrasonography transducer elicits elective pain, known as the McBurney sign. Intraperitoneal leaking from the Douglas pouch is frequently encountered. A drawback of ultrasonography is poor echogenicity or obesity of some patients, making the diagnosis of acute appendicitis challenging even for a skilled operator. Furthermore, the detection rate for normal appendix does not exceed 60–80%, depending on the series (Lee et al. 2005), which is a limitation to this technique, as the appendix must be visualized and diagnosed for acute appendicitis to be excluded. This may be one of the reasons why CT scanning has progressed so much in this indication.

5 CT Protocols

The optimal abdominal CT scanning technique when acute appendicitis is suspected has been controversial. The most used CT protocol incorporates helical acquisition in the entire abdomen and pelvis aided by oral and intravenous opacification (Birnbaum and Wilson 2000). Many publications, until recently (Paulson and Coursey 2009), have discussed the use of intravenous administration of iodinated contrast material or digestive opacification. Volume and acquisition parameters as well as image processing may also be adapted.

5.1 CT with or Without Intravenous Administration of Iodinated Contrast Material?

Intravenous administration of contrast material is associated with a higher evaluation cost or patient discomfort. A nonnegligible risk of allergic reaction, extravasation (possibly leading to tissue lesions at the puncture site), or renal failure exists. That is why some authors advocate nonenhanced CT (NECT), with good results (Ege et al. 2002; Funaki 2000; Lane et al. 1999).

A nonnegligible part of the symptoms in acute appendicitis has been described with contrast-enhanced CT. Homogeneous or heterogeneous enhancement or localized defect in enhancement of the appendiceal wall are important signs, which cannot be found with NECT.

Identification of the appendix, whether normal or not, is not always easy in the absence of contrast enhancement, especially in lean patients or patients with little abdominal fat (Macari and Balthazar 2003). Ganguli et al. (2006) have shown that a nonvisualized appendix on enhanced CT mostly corresponds to an absence of acute appendicitis, al though to our knowledge no NECT study has proved this.

Tamburrini et al. (2007) reported a reliable NECT evaluation in 75% of cases: a second evaluation with contrast material is thus required in 25% of cases, hence both wasting time and resulting in overexposure to X-rays. Letting alone our colleagues, who, in a routine clinical setting, would more likely hear "The appendix is normal", rather than "We cannot find the appendix, but we see no evidence of acute appendicites" (Paulson and Coursey 2009).

Some severe complications of acute appendicitis (perforation, abscess, pylephlebitis) are best characterized with intravenous contrast enhancement (Urban and Fishman 2000a). This is of note, as many surgeons are more likely to initially treat an abscess with antibiotics, eventually followed by percutaneous drainage (with appendectomy performed secondary), than with emergency surgery (Andersson and Petzold 2007).

Lastly, contrast-enhanced CT has been shown to allow improved differential diagnosis of those diseases which mimic acute appendicitis (including mesenteric ischemia, inflammatory bowel disease, and pyelonephritis) (Urban and Fishman 2000a; Seo et al. 2009; Urban and Fishman 2000b), as well as improved detection and characterization of accidental discovery disorders that can affect management.

We, as other teams, thus recommend that a localized right iliac fossa pain be evaluated by enhanced CT with intravenous administration of iodinated contrast material in the absence of contraindications (Holden and Einstein 2007; Macari and Balthazar 2003).

5.2 Focused or Nonfocused CT?

CT scanning of the submesocolic abdomen and pelvis, with different combinations of oral, rectal, and intravenous contrast opacification, has been advocated by some authors. This technique would allow accurate analysis of both direct and indirect signs of acute appendicitis at the cecal apex, while exposing the patient to a lower dose of ionizing radiation, which can be of particular importance, especially in pediatric patients (Fefferman et al. 2001; Rao et al. 1997e, f; Rhea et al. 1997).

However, two teams have clearly demonstrated that the lack of sus-mesocolic abdomen studies in a patient presenting with a right lower quadrant pain would significantly decrease CT scanning sensitivity for all acute abdominal disorders requiring surgical management (Jacobs et al. 2001; Kamel et al. 2000). That may be why this technique is merely recommended by teams proficient in abdominal emergency imaging and is no longer discussed by Paulson and Coursey (2009) and in a recent report dedicated to CT protocols for acute appendicitis (Holden and Einstein 2007; Macari and Balthazar 2003).

5.3 CT with or Without Digestive Opacification?

5.3.1 Oral Opacification

Opacification with iodinated oral contrast material for abdominal CT studies, including right lower quadrant pain examination, is still in use in North America (Holden and Einstein 2007; Macari and Balthazar 2003). Described many years ago, bowel loop opacification may help to distinguish the appendix from a bowel loop or any other digestive tubular structure, including abnormal fallopian tubes, ureteral vessels,or blood vessels (Rao et al. 1997d, f). The use of thin sections and cine-loop display of images has allowed digestive structures to be easily identified, despite the lack of opacification of their lumen. Hence, an opacified appendix is supposed to rule out acute appendicitis. However, in some cases the proximal aspect relative to the appendiceal obstruction could fill in and lead to a false negative (tip appendicitis) (Rao et al. 1997c). The lack of opacification does not allow one to reliably diagnose acute appendicitis, as normal appendix does not always opacify with oral contrast material (Funaki et al. 1998; Tamburrini et al. 2005).

Two recent studies have shown no difference in specificity, sensitivity, positive or negative predictive value in patients who underwent CT scanning with or without oral opacification (Anderson et al. 2009; Keyzer et al. 2009).

This technique raises several problems. The patient has to ingest the recommended 800–1,000 mL of contrast material (Pinto Leite et al. 2005). This can be an issue in a patient presenting with abdominal symptoms associated with nausea and vomiting, or in the elderly (with a risk of inhalation). Does performing the opacification justify the need for a nasogastric probe to be placed? The cost of examination and the side effects related to contrast material are increased. Last, the duration of examination is increased, as a 1–2-h time interval is required for the contrast material to reach the cecum, which be long in an emergency setting (Huynh et al. 2004; Lee et al. 2006c).

5.3.2 Rectal Opacification

Opacification and cecal distension can be obtained by rectal administration of 800–1,000 mL of water or diluted contrast material (Macari and Balthazar 2003; Rao et al. 1997f; Urban and Fishman 2000b). This would improve evaluation of the cecal wall thickness and opacification of a nonobstructed appendix. Some cecal signs, which we will describe later, such as the arrowhead sign, would be best detected. This technique is faster than oral opacification (around 15 min). However, it requires logistic organization and involves nonnegligible discomfort for the patient. Furthermore, cecal opacification is inconstant and contraindication exists in patients presenting with neutropenia or with peritoneal or perforation signs (Pinto Leite et al. 2005). It has been shown that one can do without this technique with no loss of diagnostic efficacy (Dearing et al. 2008).

5.4 Low-Dose or Standard-Dose CT?

Ever since the introduction of multidetector CT (MDCT), the increase in the volume studied and the increase in the overall number of CT examinations have led to the effects of medical irradiation being questioned (Brenner and Hall 2007). Reducing the patient radiation dose for each examination while retaining a signal over noise ratio allowing the necessary image quality for interpretation has been proposed. Of note, the term "low dose" is only valid in NECT examination, as using contrast material increases the noise over the image quality, thus usually requiring a higher number of milliamperes, noncompatible with the "low-dose" label.

No difference is observed in the visualization of the normal appendix at low or standard dose (Karabulut et al. 2007), and no significant difference is found between the different CT signs of acute appendicitis, except for signs related to appendiceal enhancement (Keyzer et al. 2004).

The low-dose technique is useful in seeking acute appendicitis on NECT scans. However, many teams, including ours, use intravenous injection of contrast material. In the study by Seo et al. (2009), including 207 patients, no significant differences in sensitivity and specificity in diagnosis of acute appendicitis between low-dose NECT and standard-dose contrast-enhanced CT were found. In contrast, diagnostic confidence, visualization of the appendix, and alternative diagnoses tended to be compromised with low-dose NECT, which still impairs routine management of emergency acute abdominal pain in the emergency setting.

5.5 Which Image Processing?

As for most CT scans, the first step in interpretation is the review of axial slices. MDCT has allowed routine acquisition of wide volumes, with millimeter and submillimeter collimations. However, axial reconstruction with 5-mm thickness, as recommended a few years ago for monodetector CT scanners, is still in use (Johnson et al. 2006; Weltman et al. 2000). As the normal appendix measures up to 3 mm in diameter (Tamburrini et al. 2005), the use of reconstructed sections of less than 5 mm is required to visualize it.

Johnson et al. (2009) first demonstrated the utility of thin sections. According to their analysis of 212 scans with thinner and thinner axial reconstruction (5, 3, and 2 mm thick), thinner reconstruction would significantly increase the visualization rate of the appendix (79, 86, and 89%, respectively) and the confidence in the presence or absence of acute appendicitis signs (the mean sensitivities were 79.4, 82.4, and 82.4% and the specificities were 99.2, 98.7, and 98.2% for 5, 3, and 2 mm, respectively).

'The two main drawbacks in using thinner reconstruction sections are the requirement for a larger number of images to be visualized and the increase in the noise background within the image. Reviewing thin sections with the sliding slab ray-sum technique, which is available on many CT workstations, appears useful to avoid the noise in detecting the appendix abnormalities (Lee et al. 2006a, 2008; Seo et al. 2009).

Sixteen and 64 MDCT scanners that are currently available allow submillimeter isotropic voxels to be obtained in one acquisition of the entire abdomen and pelvis. The data can then be analyzed with multiplanar reconstruction (MPR), with a spatial resolution similar to that of axial reconstructions. The consoles that are currently in use show fast processing of MPR data, with no waste of time for the clinician. This facilitates image visualization in the diagnosis of the normal appendix (Jan et al. 2005), acute appendicitis, as well as in that of pitfall types and alternative diagnoses (Kim et al. 2008b; Lee et al. 2006b; Neville and Paulson 2009; Paulson et al. 2005), including in children (Kim et al. 2009). The possible utility of curved reconstruction and volume rendering for improved detection of acute appendicitis has been advanced recently (Stabile Ianora et al. 2010). In our hands, these two techniques mainly have iconographic value in communicating with visceral surgeons for accurate depiction of acute appendicitis with atypical location: one can, for example, segment the appendix (i.e., only selecting the volume of this organ), and have it stand out relative to the rest of the abdominal volume by transparency (Fig. 4). The appendix is then easy to detect, using a surface anatomic element, such as the umbilicus, as reference, which allows the surgeon to adapt the incision approach (Figs. 4, 5). Coronal reconstructions as well as—with least impact—sagittal and oblique reconstructions are routinely helpful when facing any interpretation difficulty.

5.6 Our Protocol

Our protocol has been designed to be quick, and reliable in addressing most of the concerns that the emergency physicians with whom we are working might have. Indeed, before right iliac fossa abdominal pain, one has to make sure the appendix can be visualized, even if it is normal or very thin in a fat-free abdomen. Any possible semiologic argument supporting the diagnosis of acute appendicitis, or its related complications, has to be given. Last, in the case of a normal appendix, this examination has to allow differential diagnosis to be sought the for patien's management to be well oriented.

We perform a direct acquisition after intravenous administration of nonionic iodinated contrast material (iobitridol, Xenetix 350®, 350 mg I/mL, Guerbet), at 1.5 mL/kg and 2.5 mL/s, in the absence of contraindication. The volume is acquired in the portal phase using a 64-channel MDCT scanner (Lightspeed VCT, General Electric Healthcare, Milwaukee, WI, USA). It starts 70 s after the injection. This allows for proper detection of defects in enhancement of the appendiceal wall and characterization of all possible related complications, including pylephlebitis or hepatic abscess, that are difficult to identify without injection. Most other acute abdominal syndromes belonging to differential diagnosis of acute appendicitis can be characterized at this injection time (see Sect. 4.1).

The explored volume is not focused on the right iliac fossa. It extends across the entire abdomen and pelvis for the cecoappendiceal region to be properly visualized even in the case of anatomical variation (see Fig. 2), for sus-mesocolic (especially hepatic) complications to be diagnosed, and differential diagnosis to be made (see Sect. 4.2).

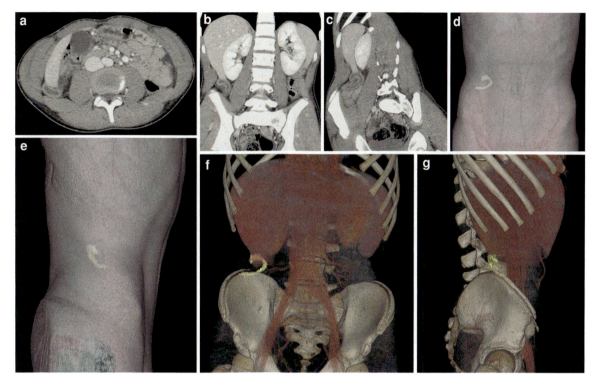

Fig. 4 Use of volume rendering (VR) in atypical anatomical forms of acute appendicitis. Transverse (**a**) and coronal (**b**) cross sections show a subhepatic acute appendicitis. A thick double-oblique cross section with VR can scroll through the entire appendix (**c**). After segmentation of the appendix (in *yellow*), VR helps one to localize the appendix from superficial skin benchmarks such as the umbilicus (**d**, **e**), or deeper ones such as the liver (**f**, **g**)

Finally, oral or rectal opacification is not used when looking for acute appendicitis signs as it delays the evaluation (15 min at least rectally and at least 1 h orally), with a relative efficacy and discomfort to the patient (see Sect. 4.3).

The collimation is either millimeter or submillimeter. Raw data are then reconstructed in axial slices of 1.25 mm, which are visualized in MPR using a workstation (Advantage Workstation Volume Share 4, General Electric Healthcare, Milwaukee, WI, USA).

Each examination is interpreted by two readers, including a resident and an experienced reader.

6 CT Findings

6.1 The Normal Appendix

In theory, the outer wall to outer wall diameter of the normal appendix is 6 mm or less, and the wall is 1–2 mm thick (Macari and Balthazar 2003). Nevertheless, in a nonnegligible number of cases (up to 45% depending on the series), this diameter may be more than 6 mm and less than 10 mm (Tamburrini et al. 2005; Benjaminov et al. 2002). This size criterion is thus not sufficient and characterization of the appendix content, the wall appearance (hence the utility of intravenous contrast material), and periappendiceal fat is required.

The content of the normal appendix is variable. The appendiceal lumen can be collapsed, not visible, or partially filled with air or fluid, provided that the liquid does not exceed 2.6 mm in depth (Moteki et al. 2009). Although the presence of an appendicolith increases the risk of acute appendicitis (Rabinowitz et al. 2007), appendiceal stercolith with no appendiceal disorder can be described on CT (Lowe et al. 2000), and does not constitute an indication for appendectomy in the absence of other associated signs. Periappendiceal surroundings have to be well studied. No stranding fat, intraperitoneal leaking, or periappendiceal collection is to be seen (Tamburrini et al. 2005).

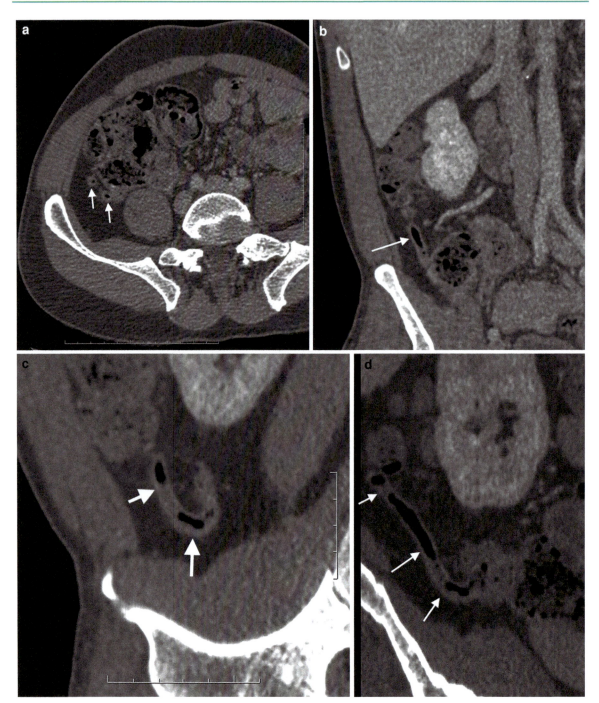

Fig. 5 Normal retrocecal appendix. Its tortuous course is difficult to follow on transverse (**a**) and coronal (**b**) computed tomography (CT) images but it can be seen entirely in oblique (**c**) and curved (**d**) images. Its diameter is 7 mm, but its wall is not thickened. It is filled with air with no surrounding fat stranding

Recent technical advances in MDCT and MPRs have allowed improved CT visualization of the normal appendix. Jan et al. (2005) described a visualization rate of 93% of normal appendix, with a small amount of intra-abdominal fat remaining a limiting factor. Nevertheless, the lack of a defect on

Acute Appendicitis

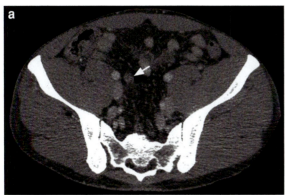

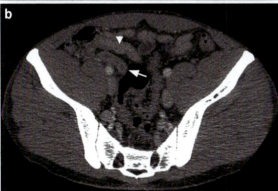

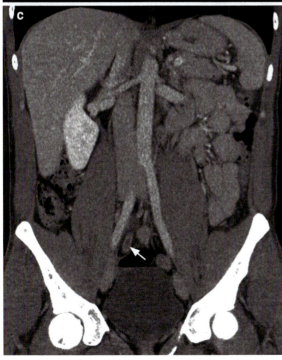

Fig. 6 Typical noncomplicated acute appendicitis: main findings. Enlarged appendix (*white arrow*) with wall thickening and hyperenhancement. The normal last ileal loop (*arrowhead*) is seen in the neighborhood (**a, b**). The appendix is blind-ended in the coronal plane (**c**)

abdominopelvic CT retains a high negative predictive value, even in the absence of a visible appendix, in adults as in children (Nikolaidis et al. 2004; Garcia et al. 2009; Ganguli et al. 2006).

6.2 Acute Appendicitis

6.2.1 Main Findings in Acute Appendicitis

Thickening of the appendix is one of the main signs of acute appendicitis. Classically, thickening is retained when the outer wall to outer wall transverse diameter is greater than 6 mm. However, this definition has been extrapolated from findings from ultrasonography, in which the appendix is analyzed by graduated compression of the right lower quadrant, which can eventually modify the appendiceal diameter.

CT images are obtained without compression, which may explain the possible CT visualization of appendix greater than 6 mm in diameter, in asymptomatic patients. That is why some authors have defined the upper limit of normal as 10 mm (Benjaminov et al. 2002; Tamburrini et al. 2005). Use of 6–10-mm appendiceal diameter for a definitive diagnosis of acute appendicitis is challenging. Searching for additional signs, including appendiceal wall thickening (3 mm or more), appendiceal wall hyperenhancement, mural stratification of the appendiceal wall, and intramural gas, is then useful (Fig. 6).

6.2.2 Ancillary Findings

The presence of gas within the appendiceal lumen can be found in up to 20% of acute appendicitis patients on CT (Rao et al. 1997a), and does not rule out this diagnosis, even if intraluminal gas is more often observed in normal than in inflammatory appendix (Rettenbacher et al. 2000) (Figs. 7, 8).

One to several appendicoliths can be described in acute appendicitis, although they are not specific as they can be frequently found in asymptomatic adults. Similarly, appendicoliths in acute appendicitis are more frequent in children (65% of cases) than in adults, but are not sufficient for diagnosing this disorder when no other associated findings are found on CT (Lowe et al. 2000). According to some authors, the use of bone window settings when reviewing CT scans is helpful in detecting appendicoliths (Alobaidi and Shirkhoda 2003; Giuliano et al. 2006).

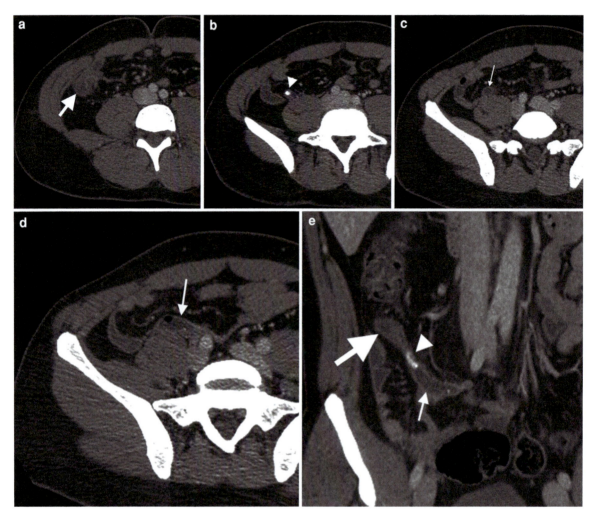

Fig. 7 Typical noncomplicated acute appendicitis: ancillary findings. As often, the coronal plane (**e**) is very valuable as the entire appendix is seen best as compared with the transverse plane (**a–d**). The appendix (*little arrow*) is thickened to more than 1 cm in diameter (**c**). Its wall is not very thick but is enhanced (without any focal defect). It is fluid-filled with just a small intraluminal gas bubble (**d**). Appendicoliths are located at the base (*arrowhead*) and at the end of the appendix, with thickening of the cecal wall (*big arrow*)

Asymetric thickening of the cecal wall relative to the appendiceal base reduces the cecal lumen to an arrowhead shape that points to the appendix: this arrowhead sign is even more visible with intraluminal contrast material (Rao et al. 1997g). A "cecal bar" refers to the thickening of the cecal wall where the inflammatory appendix separates from the contrast-filled cecal lumen.

Signs of inflammation of the right lower quadrant, periappendiceal in particular, are easily identified and are often determined in the positive diagnosis of acute appendicitis, despite their lack of specificity (Fig. 9) (Pinto Leite et al. 2005). They include:
- Periappendiceal fat stranding
- Right retroperitoneal fascia thickening (lateroconal in particular)
- Mesoappendix thickening
- Extraluminal fluid
- Ileocecal mild lymph node enlargement
- Inflammatory thickening of adjacent organs, including the terminal ileum ascending or sigmoid colon, and bladder

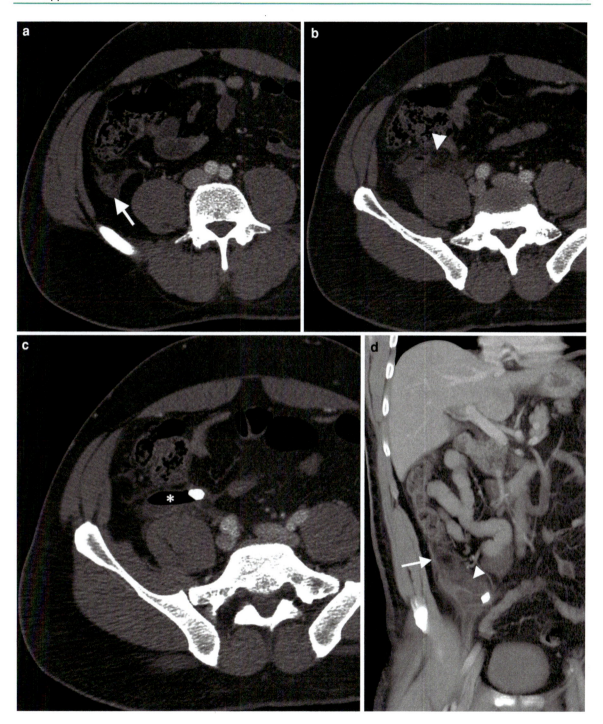

Fig. 8 Retrocecal acute appendicitis: ancillary findings. Transverse images (**a–c**) and a thick oblique VR image (**d**): thickening of the right retroperitoneal fascia (*white arrow*) and periappendicular fat stranding (*arrowhead*). The presence of intraluminal air (*asterisk*) does not rule out acute appendicitis

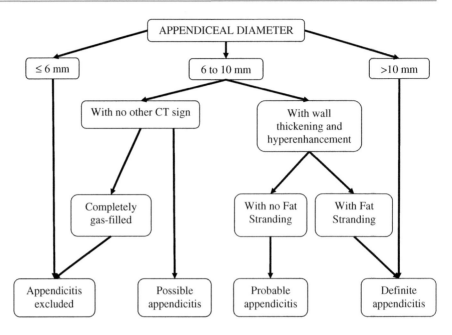

Fig. 9 Diagnostic strategy for suspected acute appendicitis according to CT findings

6.3 Complications of Acute Appendicitis

6.3.1 Gangrenous Appendicitis

Gangrenous (or emphysematous) appendicitis is a severe complication of acute appendicitis, rapidly evolving toward perforation. Edema and inflammatory mechanisms induce an obstruction of the periappendiceal wall vessels, with ensuing necrosis. CT findings show intramural air (pneumatosis) with a focal defect in enhanced appendiceal wall (Clarke 1987; Pinto Leite et al. 2005; Rao and Mueller 1998).

6.3.2 Appendiceal Perforation

As described in Sect. 2.2, untreated acute appendicitis often develops to ischemic perforation and necrosis of the appendiceal wall. Specific signs in the diagnosis of perforated appendicitis have been sought, in the aim of adapting the therapeutic approach. Either preoperative medical treatment or percutaneous drainage (either ultrasonography-guided or CT-guided) of a possible collection can be performed before surgery, or the surgical technique is modified (Singh et al. 2008; Simillis et al. 2010; Ein et al. 2005; Marin et al. 2010).

Horrow et al. (2003) showed that a dedicated search for five specific CT findings allowed an overall sensitivity of 94.9% for perforated appendicitis:

- Focal defect in enhanced appendiceal wall (Fig. 10)
- Extraluminal air
- Extraluminal appendicolith
- Abscess
- Phlegmon.

A focal defect in the enhanced appendiceal wall achieved the highest sensitivity (96–100%) for several authors (Horrow et al. 2003; Tsuboi et al. 2008). For others (Foley et al. 2005), extraluminal air and moderate or severe periappendiceal inflammatory stranding were statistically significant independent predictors for appendiceal perforation and were associated with increased hospital stay.

Of note, a free fecalith in the right lower quadrant associated with inflammatory signs is consistent with perforated acute appendicitis even in the absence of a visualized appendix (Sivit 1993; Pinto Leite et al. 2005).

6.3.3 Periappendiceal Inflammatory Masses: Phlegmon and Abscess

Periappendiceal phlegmon and abscess are both complications related to appendiceal perforation. They are both responsible for periappendiceal inflammatory masses that are difficult to differentiate on physical examination, but are easily diagnosed on CT (Jeffrey et al. 1988; Delabrousse 2009; Shapiro et al. 1989).

A periappendiceal phlegmon is a mass resulting from the agglutination of periappendiceal organs and tissues, including the cecum, ileal loops, and

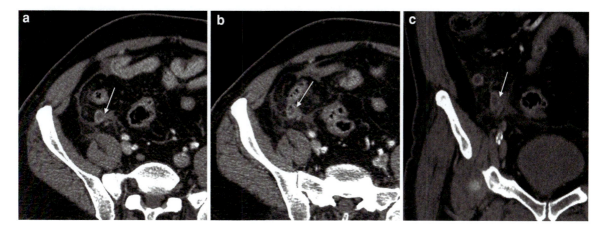

Fig. 10 Appendiceal perforation. Transverse (**a**, **b**) and coronal (**c**) CT images with a focal defect in the enhanced appendiceal wall (*white arrow*) associated with periappendiceal inflammatory stranding

particularly the greater omentum. The aim is to isolate the inflamed appendiceal focus, and to avoid a perforation in a free peritoneum occurring. CT scanning (Fig. 11) allows visualization of a heterogeneous tissue mass, poorly delineated, which corresponds to periappendiceal organ agglutination around the appendix. The appendix showing a nonenhanced area, more or less expanded, is not always visible within the mass. An appendicolith within the phlegmon is supportive of an appendiceal origin. Phlegmons may also complicate other disorders of the right lower quadrant, including right colon acute diverticulitis, Meckel diverticulitis, Crohn disease, and pyosalpinx, that will have to be evoked in the differential diagnosis of appendicitis.

Periappendiceal abscess (Fig. 12) is a frequent complication, and it can rupture and lead to generalized peritonitis in the absence of effective therapy. Peritoneal abscess may also form at a distance from the appendiceal focus, including the Douglas pouch, or the subhepatic region. CT shows a loculated, rim-enhanced fluid collection, which may contain air bubbles with an hydroaeric level. An appendicolith can be seen within this collection, which is a pathognomonic sign of an appendiceal origin.

Among the possible differential diagnoses are an abscess complicating Crohn disease, a cecal diverticulitis or typhlitis in a neutropenic patient, a right tubo-ovarian abscess, and an abscess of the iliopsoas muscle. Percutaneous drainage with antibiotherapy followed by delayed appendectomy is the treatment of periappendiceal abscess (Marin et al. 2010).

6.3.4 Bacterial Peritonitis

This is a severe complication that can develop either by macroscopic perforation of the appendix in the free peritoneal cavity or by rupture of a periappendiceal abscess.

Generalized peritonitis is more frequent in young children, in whom the greater omentum is incompletely formed and cannot reach the appendiceal region, and in whom the inflammation will more aggressively progress to perforation (which would not allow time for periappendiceal inflammatory adherences to clog the infectious foci) (Hopkins et al. 2001; Pinto Leite et al. 2005).

CT shows intraperitoneal fluid (interloop, paracolic gutters, hepatorenal, subhepatic and pelvic spaces) with peritoneal enhancement and thickening (Fig. 13), associated with more classic signs of acute appendicitis, with or without abscess.

6.3.5 Septic Pylephlebitis

Pylephlebitis or septic thrombophlebitis of the mesenteric and portal veins is an acute ascending infection often arising from a primary gastrointestinal inflammatory lesion, as acute appendicitis (other causes include colonic diverticulitis, inflammatory bowel disease, suppurative pancreatitis, acute cholangitis, bowel perforation, and pelvic infection). This is a severe complication with a mortality rate reaching up to 30–50%. CT scanning shows distended mesenteric or portal vein, with spontaneous internal hyperdensity corresponding to the intravascular

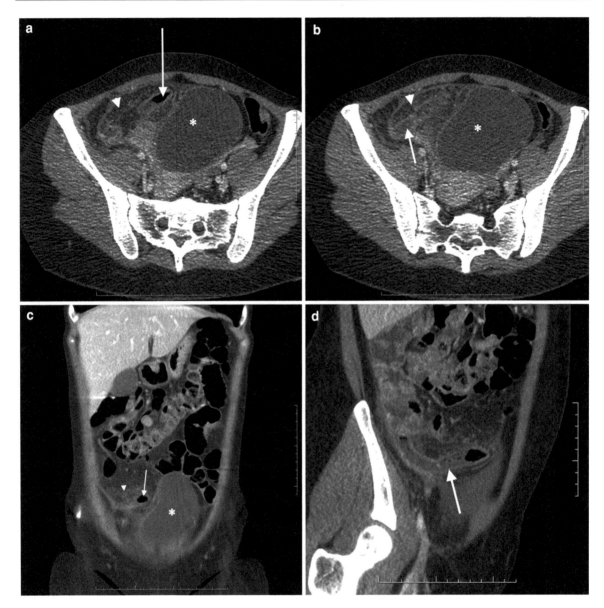

Fig. 11 Periappendiceal phlegmon. Transverse (a, b), coronal (c), and oblique (d) CT images showing an appendicitis (*arrow*) with important defects of enhancement in the appendiceal wall d. A large periappendiceal heterogeneous fatty mass (*arrowhead*) pushes the bladder (*asterisk*) to the left, without visible collection

thrombus. A complete defect in the enhanced vascular lumen or a simple focal enhancement defect (Fig. 14) can occur, due to thrombosis. Perivascular fat stranding is found. The presence of gas within the thrombus is a sign of the septic origin of the acute thrombosis. Signs of intestinal venous ischemia, including parietal thickening and intraperitoneal leaking, as well as hepatic microabscesses, resulting from septic spreading, can also be observed (Balthazar and Gollapudi 2000; Delabrousse 2009; Chang et al. 2008).

6.3.6 Dropped (or Retained) Appendicolith

Following appendectomy for acute appendicitis, one or several appendicoliths may remain in the abdomen, as also described for gallstones remaining after cholecystectomy. When acute appendicitis perforates, an appendicolith can be expulsed and not retrieved

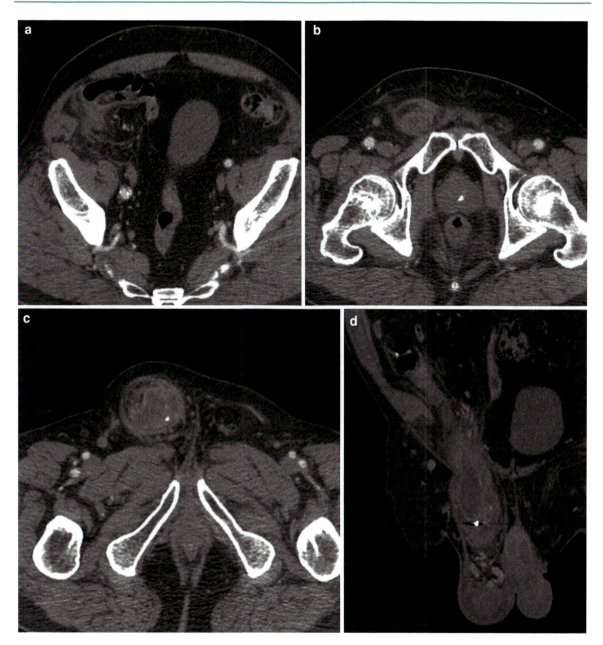

Fig. 12 Perforated appendix and periappendicular abscess within a right inguinal hernia. Transverse CT images showing thickened cecal (a) and appendiceal (b) walls. The appendix travels down through the right inguinal canal, then its tip is lost in the hernia sac (c, d). An inguinal abscess contains an appendicolith and an ingested metallic foreign body (*lead shot*). It is a rare complication of Amyand hernia

during surgery. In this rare complication, the appendicolith may remain asymptomatic or induce formation of an abdominal abscess, sometimes at a distance from the surgical focus, with a delay of a few days to a few years. Other causes of spontaneously hyperdense abdominal structure have to be evoked in the differential diagnosis, including dropped gallstones, calcified mesenteric lymph nodes, calcified epiploic appendagitis, and dropped surgical clips. Typical management of symptomatic appendicolith with abscess consists of open or laparoscopic surgery with abscess drainage and extraction of the

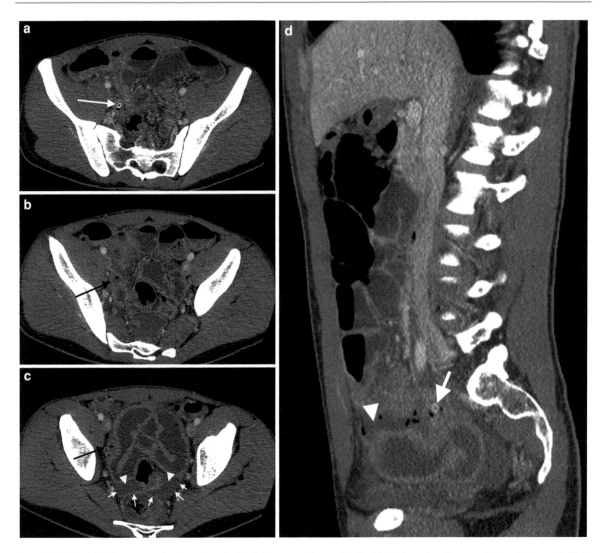

Fig. 13 Peritonitis. Transverse (**a–c**) and sagittal (**d**) images showing an enlarged appendix (*black arrow*) with an appendicolith (*big white arrow*) and focal defects in the enhanced appendiceal wall. Note an air-fluid intraperitoneal collection (*arrowhead*) with thickened peritoneum (*little white arrow*). Note also an ileus (overall distention of the intestine without transition zone)

appendicolith. Cases of percutaneous retrieval of an appendicolith using a stone basket passed through a 12-French sheath have been described (Singh et al. 2008; Kim et al. 2004; O'Shea and Martin 2003).

6.3.7 Other Complications of Acute Appendicitis

Other rarer complications are possible. Appendiceal perforation can occur in a neighboring organ such as the bladder, colon, ileum, etc., or at the skin, thus leading to appendicovesical, appendicocolic or appendicocutaneous fistula (Izawa et al. 1998; Athanassopoulos and Speakman 1995; Deorah et al. 2005).

Sometimes the infection proceeds to retroperitoneum and/or abdominal wall, leading to possible life-threatening necrotizing fasciitis (Wilharm et al. 2010; Chen et al. 2010).

Scrotal and/or inguinal abscesses following appendicitis have been described as rare events, occurring mostly when a processus vaginalis is present (Bingol-Kologlu et al. 2006) in Amyand's hernia (Fig. 12)

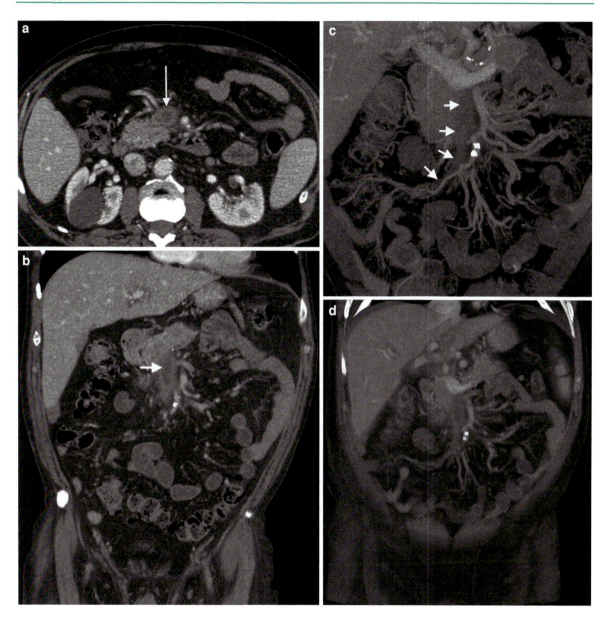

Fig. 14 Pylephlebitis. Thrombosis of the superior mesenteric vein (*white arrow*), with stranding of the perivascular fat in transverse (**a**) and coronal (**b**) images. The boundaries of the maximum intensity projection technique are represented here: the central low-attenuation lumen of the thrombosed veins is difficult to see on this coronal thick maximum intensity projection image (**c**), whereas the thrombotic expansion into the ileocolic vein is much better appreciated on thick sections in VR mode (**d**)

7 CT Pitfalls

7.1 Normal and Variant Anatomy

The position of the appendix is highly variable between individuals, depending both on the cecum location and on appendiceal length (see Sect. 1), which makes the detection of an appendix that is not located in the right lower quadrant challenging, with risks of false negatives. Similarly, in a pregnant woman, the appendix can be cranially and laterally moved by a developing gravid uterus, which can compromise a diagnosis of acute appendicitis.

Other anatomical abdominal structures, such as blood vessels or intestinal loops, can be confused with a pathologic appendix. To distinguish between them, a thin-slice dynamic analysis allows one to see that blood vessels are denser and more homogeneous than the appendix after injection, and are connected to other vessels. A bowel loop is followed along its length on both sides by other loops, whereas the appendix has a blind end on one side and is connected to the cecum on the other side. The use of intravenous contrast material helps in distinguishing between an inflammatory appendix and bowel loops with the highly enhanced appendiceal mucosa.

7.2   Appendiceal Crohn Disease

Crohn disease is a chronic inflammatory condition, more frequently involving the last ileal loop and cecum. Differentiating acute appendicitis leading to inflammation of the adjacent ileum from Crohn disease with appendiceal involvement can be challenging. Involvement of several digestive segments separated by normal area may orientate the diagnosis toward Crohn disease (Whitley et al. 2009; Pinto Leite et al. 2005; Rao and Mueller 1998).

Importantly, Crohn disease exclusively localized within the appendix is rare but possible. Differentiating it from a typical acute appendicitis on CT is thus very challenging. However, this appendiceal form isolated from Crohn disease would be less aggressive than when are involved other bowel segments, with a low rate of recurrence and postoperative fistula-type complications (Prieto-Nieto et al. 2001; Agha et al. 1987).

7.3   Distal (or Tip) Appendicitis

Acute appendicitis classically begins with a luminal obstruction occurring at a distance from its orifice in 8% of cases. This distal appendicitis manifests itself on CT with a normal proximal appendiceal portion. Its lumen can be either collapsed or filled with air (Fig. 15) or even with contrast material, when a digestive opacification has been performed. The distal aspect shows the typical presentations of acute appendicitis (see Sect. 5.2.1). A progressive thickening

of the appendiceal wall to the site of luminal obstruction can be observed between both distal and proximal portions.

As the inflammatory aspect is at a distance from the cecum, there is neither thickening of the cecal wall, nor arrowhead sign. Visualization of a normal portion of the appendix is not sufficient to rule out the diagnosis of acute appendicitis: following the appendix along its entire length, from its origin to its distal tip, is required for a false negative to be avoided (Levine et al. 2004; Rao et al. 1997c).

7.4   Stump Appendicitis

Stump appendicitis is a rare condition, related to inflammation of an appendiceal stump remaining after appendectomy. The clinical signs are similar to those of acute appendicitis, and the diagnosis is rarely evoked. Contrast-enhanced CT shows an enlarged tubular structure extending from the base of the cecum, the appendiceal stump, with enhanced wall and local inflammatory signs as stranding fat (Baek et al. 2008; Shin et al. 2005).

7.5   Recurrent and Chronic Appendicitis

When related to partial obstruction or mucus overproduction in the appendiceal lumen, poorly severe appendiceal inflammation may resolve spontaneously with no surgical treatment.

Recurrent appendicitis presents with repeated episodes of right lower quadrant pain, associated with a symptoms similar to those of typical acute appendicitis, including, anorexia, nausea or vomiting, tenderness, increased C-reactive protein levels, and hyperleukocytosis. Unlike acute appendicitis, the clinical signs regress spontaneously within 2 days, sometimes within a few hours, and a new episode may occur within a few weeks or a few years; 20–30% of patients with appendectomy would have experienced a previous similar episode, with spontaneous regression (Migraine et al. 1997). The CT signs are the same as those for typical acute appendicitis, except that the scan may appear normal, between painful episodes.

Chronic appendicitis is less frequent than recurrent appendicitis. It manifests itself as right iliac

Acute Appendicitis

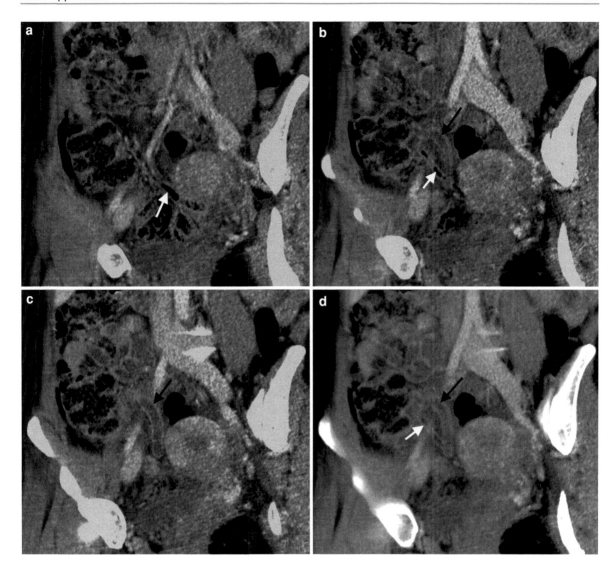

Fig. 15 Tip appendicitis. On oblique images (**a–c**), the proximal portion of the appendix, arising from a pelvic cecum, is normal and partially filled with air (*white arrow*). The appendix folds in the iliac vessel region and travels back down to the pelvis. Its distal portion is enlarged, fluid-filled, with a contrast-enhanced wall (*black arrow*). The set is best shown on an oblique thick image in VR mode (**d**)

fossa pain that lasts for at least 3 weeks and completely resolves after appendectomy (Pinto Leite et al. 2005). The clinical presentation (as shown by the Alvarado score) and laboratory findings such as hyperleukocytosis are milder than for acute appendicitis (Mussack et al. 2002). Chronic appendicitis is favored by coprostasis, according to some authors (Sgourakis et al. 2008). It could also result from undiagnosed acute appendicitis, with inefficient antibiotherapy, in children suspected of having urinary tract infection, or in adults suspected of having colic diverticulitis. Pathophysiological examination shows an inflammatory aspect with or without fibrosis of the appendiceal wall (Mussack et al. 2002), with no findings other than those typical of acute appendicitis, except for less periappendiceal fat stranding (Checkoff et al. 2002). Emergency appendectomy is not mandatory. Surgery can be delayed for a few weeks if antibiotherapy is started at time of diagnosis.

7.6 Abscessed Mass in the Right Iliac Fossa

An etiologic diagnosis of an abscessed mass in the right iliac fossa may sometimes be challenging. The anatomical relationships between the different structures of this area can be modified by the mass effect and inflammatory processes. The organ responsible may also be so altered that it is no longer distinguishable.

Phlegmon and periappendiceal abscesses are frequent complications, whose diagnosis is easy when the acute appendicitis is well visualized in close proximity. Their diagnosis becomes more challenging when acute appendicitis is not visualized, such as for necrosis or wide perforation. One of the quasi-pathognomonic signs of appendiceal origin is the presence of an appendicolith within the collection, including in the absence of a visualized appendix (Sivit 1993; Pinto Leite et al. 2005). Nevertheless, in the case of a perforated inflamed diverticulum, cecal cancer, or cecal ischemia, a stercolith can also be visualized within a right iliac fossa collection, which leads to one being cautious about this sign.

7.7 Acute Appendicitis in Pregnant Women

Acute appendicitis is the most common cause of nonobstetrical acute abdominal pain requiring surgical treatment in pregnant women. It is associated with a higher risk of premature labor, fetal and mother morbidity, and mortality. Its clinical presentation is even less suggestive than in the rest of the population, as anorexia, nausea, and vomiting are all frequently present, especially during the first trimester of pregnancy. The gravid uterus progressively pushes away the appendix; therefore, the abdominal pain may be localized at a distance from the right iliac fossa. This may lead to a delayed diagnosis, increasing the risk of appendiceal perforation in pregnant women (43 vs. 4–19% in the general population) (Tamir et al. 1990). That is why immediate surgery is often undertaken, with no delay, with a negative appendectomy rate often increased, reaching up to 25–50% depending on the series (Pedrosa et al. 2009). Unfortunately, surgical complications may occur, including preterm labor, fetal loss, and decreased birth weight, and makes the use of preoperative diagnosis techniques necessary.

Despite its variable sensitivity, partly due to the operator-dependency of this procedure, ultrasonography-graded compression is always indicated as a primary imaging modality, owing to its lower cost, availability, lack of ionizing radiation exposure, and efficacy in searching for differential diagnosis such as ovarian torsion, ovarian cyst, or salpingitis.

The detection of the appendix of a pregnant woman is easier in the first trimester and at beginning of the second, but it becomes more challenging in the third trimester because of the modifications in the anatomical relationships (examination in the left lateral decubitus may be useful) (Lim et al. 1992). If positive diagnosis of acute appendicitis is made by ultrasonography, no further confirmatory test other than surgery is required (Freeland et al. 2009). If a normal appendix is visualized on ultrasonography, with no sign of appendicitis, close clinical follow-up is required, especially in the absence of any differential diagnosis. In the case of a clinical change or any doubt, ultrasonography evaluation will have to be repeated or even confirmed by CT or MRI evaluation. If the appendix is not visualized, as frequently occurs in the third trimester, CT or MRI is required (Freeland et al. 2009; Patel et al. 2007).

In recent years, several studies have reported on the utility of MRI in excluding acute appendicitis in pregnant women when ultrasonography is not contributive. With a 100 % sensitivity, a 93.6% specificity, a 100% NPV, and an 94% accuracy, MRI, which does not require radiation, must be preferred to CT. The major difficulty of MRI is its availability in emergency conditions. A simple and fast protocol including T1, T2, and T2 fat-suppression breathhold sequences has been proposed. An oral negative contrast material (mix of ferumoxsil and barium sulfate) can be used to decrease susceptibility artifacts and to increase visualization of a normal appendix filled with liquid. Of course, the contraindication of intravenous administration of gadolinium chelates makes the enhanced periappendiceal wall impossible to study (Singh et al. 2007; Cobben et al. 2009; Pedrosa et al. 2009).

When ultrasonography is not contributive and MRI is not available or is contraindicated, CT can be useful in ruling out acute appendicitis in a pregnant woman, especially in the second and third trimesters (Fig. 16). Lazarus et al. (2007) have shown that a CT scan in this indication has a sensitivity of 92%, a specificity of 99%, and a negative predictive value close to 100%, which has been confirmed by another study

Acute Appendicitis

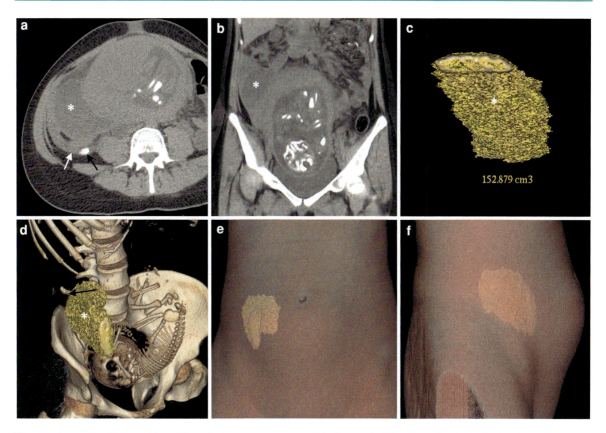

Fig. 16 Appendiceal abscess in a 27-week pregnant woman. The appendix was not seen on ultrasonography. A CT scan was performed (nonenhanced CT as the patient had a history of allergic reaction to iodinated radiological contrast media). The appendix (*white arrow*) is enlarged with an appendicolith (*black arrow*). The appendiceal tip is lost in an abscessed collection (*asterisk*) with air-fluid level, surrounding the right side of the gravid uterus (**a, b**). The segmentation of the abscess enables one to measure its volume (**c**) and to localize it from the pregnant uterus and skin benchmarks in VR mode (**d–f**)

(Shetty et al. 2010). The drawback is that CT scanning exposes the fetus to ionizing radiation, with possible teratogenic and carcinogenic effects. A CT scan for suspected acute appendicitis in a pregnant woman would expose the fetus to doses ranging up to 0.024 Gy in the first term and up to 0.046 Gy in the third term, which would be below teratogenic doses (from 0.05 to 0.15 Gy) (Lazarus et al. 2007). The risk of developing a tumor during childhood following a fetal exposure of 0.05 Gy would range from 1 in 2,000 to 2 in 2,000 (Lazarus et al. 2007). Adapting the acquisition protocol to minimize as much as possible the dose delivered is thus necessary. The kilovolt peak and milliampere-seconds can be decreased while retaining sufficient image quality, pitch can be increased, collimation can be thickened, and a z-axis modulation can be used. The only known risk related to fetal exposure to iodinated contrast material, crossing the placenta, would be neonatal hypothyroidism, requiring monitoring of thyroid function in the first week of life (Chen et al. 2008). The benefits over risk ratio must be discussed case by case between the radiologist, the surgeon, and the patient, depending on the imaging modalities available in an emergency in the different centers. Indeed, if ultrasonography is not contributive, CT remains an easy access compared with MRI, and its high NPV allows the negative appendectomy rate to be lowered while decreasing the risk of appendiceal perforation (Fig. 17).

7.8 Acute Appendicitis in the Elderly

Nontraumatic abdominal pain is a frequent cause of consultation for the elderly (older than 75 years for most authors) in the emergency department. Several reasons render the etiologic diagnosis often challenging. Firstly, an interview may be limited by cognitive

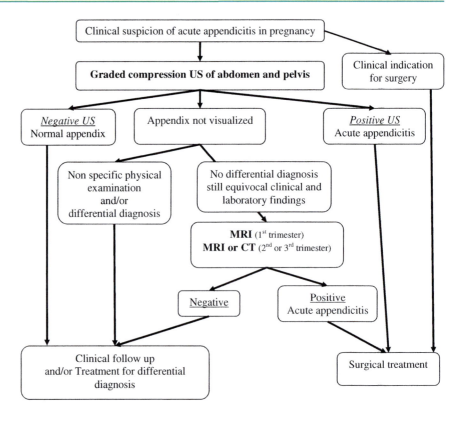

Fig. 17 Diagnostic strategy for suspected acute appendicitis in a pregnant woman

impairment, deafness, or memory loss. Secondly, the symptoms are less intense and less specific than in younger patients. Sometimes, abdominal pain is not the primary concern and the elderly may be addressed for symptoms with very poor specificity, such as fatigue, anorexia, fever, or confusion. Lastly, the physical examination may be altered by the preexisting status of the patient (bedridden) or by analgesic or steroid drug intake (Chang and Wang 2007). Although less frequent than in younger patients, with only 10% of acute appendicitis affecting the elderly, acute appendicitis in the elderly is often more severe, with a perforation rate up to 50%. The mortality rate is increased as well, with half of the deceases related to appendicitis affecting this group (Horattas et al. 1990; Lau et al. 1985; Rusnak et al. 1994). The differential diagnosis of acute appendicitis among acute abdominal pain diagnoses in the elderly is challenging owing to the lack of specificity of the clinical signs. The most frequently encountered include biliary tract diseases, bowel obstruction, malignancy, diverticulitis, and mesenteric ischemia.

The ability of CT to alter clinical decision-making in the evaluation of elderly emergency department patients with abdominal pain (Chang and Wang 2007; Esses et al. 2004; Lewis et al. 2007) has been shown in several studies. In a series including 104 patients aged 65 years and older, Esses et al. (2004) showed that CT scanning would modify the admission decision in 26% of cases, the need for surgery in 12% of cases, the need for antibiotics in 21% of cases, and the suspected diagnosis in 45% of cases. The degree of diagnosis certainty increased from 36% before CT to up to 77% after CT. CT therefore shows its efficacy, whereas ultrasonography is limited in this indication, except for biliary conditions, owing to difficulties in performing the examination, including digestive gas interposition and poor patient echogenicity.

The renal function is often altered with age, which questions the use of intravenous administration of contrast material. Oral or even percutaneous hydration is required in the case of poor or moderate renal failure. In the case of a too low creatinine clearance, or in the case of another contraindication, such as severe allergy to iodinated contrast materials, an NECT scan can be performed, with interesting results (Lane et al. 1999), despite a challenging evaluation of differential diagnoses, such as a vascular origin.

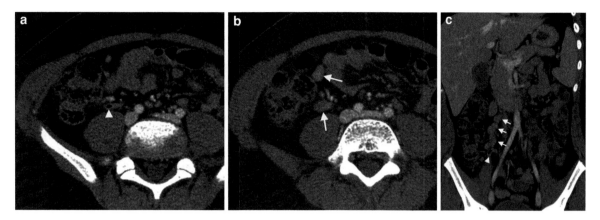

Fig. 18 Mesenteric adenitis. Axial (a, b) and coronal (c) CT scans obtained with intravenous contrast material show a cluster of lymph nodes (*white arrows*) in the right lower quadrant mesentery and abnormal appendix (*arrowhead*)

8 Differential Diagnosis

Nontraumatic acute abdominal pain is a frequent reason for admission to the emergency department. Many conditions present with nonspecific abdominal pain. In a series of 2,222 CT examinations for acute abdominal pain, Stromberg et al. (2007) reported the following distribution of evoked diagnosis, in descending order: nonspecific abdominal pain 44.3%, acute appendicitis 15.9%, bowel obstruction 9%, diverticulitis 8%, urological disease 5.9%, pancreatitis 3.2%, gynecological disease 2.4%, gastrointestinal perforation 2.3%, intra-abdominal malignancy 1.5%, vascular disease 1.5%. One can see that acute appendicitis is one of the most frequent causes, coming in second position. Nevertheless, it only represents 16% of all diagnoses. Physical examination is inadequate in definitely distinguishing acute appendicitis from another condition, even when pain is localized in the right lower quadrant. Knowing the differential diagnoses and exploring the conditions with noninvasive imaging tools is invaluable, as many need medical treatment only, with no surgery (Hoeffel et al. 2006; Pinto Leite et al. 2005).

8.1 Mesenteric Adenitis

Mesenteric adenitis is a common condition in children, rarely occurring in adults. Mesenteric adenitis manifests itself as inflammatory mesenteric lymph nodes, maximum of 10 mm in diameter, in the right lower quadrant small-bowel mesentery or ventral to the psoas muscle (Fig. 18).

Primary and secondary mesenteric adenitis can be distinguished. The former does not present with any evident inflammatory cause, except for a slight wall thickening of the last ileal loop (less than 5 mm), whereas the appendix is normal. In the secondary form, an intra-abdominal inflammatory process, such as acute appendicitis, is responsible for a lymph node reaction. It is therefore important to diagnose primary mesenteric adenitis, as it requires medical treatment only, with no surgery (Macari et al. 2002; Rao et al. 1997b).

8.2 Extra-appendiceal Digestive Conditions

8.2.1 Crohn Disease

Crohn disease is a chronic granulomatous inflammatory condition, involving any segment of the gastrointestinal tract. The most frequent localization involves the last ileal loop and right colon, thereby mimicking the appendiceal pattern. CT shows a circumferential thickening of the digestive wall, which can be stratified (target sign). A sclerolipomatous reaction with mesenteric fat hypertrophy, abscess, phlegmon, and even fistula, especially enteroenteric, can form. It may sometimes be difficult to differentiate an ileal inflammation reactional to acute appendicitis from Crohn disease with last ileal loop and appendix involvement (Figs. 19, 20). The presence of several affected intestinal segments separated by

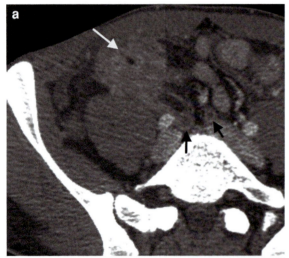

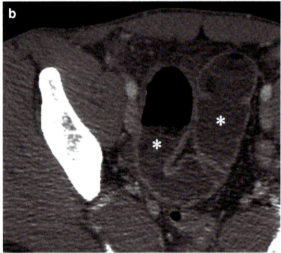

Fig. 19 Crohn disease. The transverse CT scan (**a**) shows an enlarged fluid-filled appendix (*black arrow*) with a hyperenhanced wall. These appendiceal inflammatory changes can be seen in Crohn disease, whose typical signs are concentric thickening of the cecum (*white arrow*), concentric mural thickening, and hyperenhancement of the last ileal loop (*asterisk*) (**b**)

normal areas, as well as the clinical history, can point the diagnosis toward Crohn disease (Whitley et al. 2009; Pinto Leite et al. 2005; Rao and Mueller 1998).

8.2.2 Epiploic Appendagitis

Related to an inflammation, torsion, or spontaneous thrombosis of the central vein of an epiploic appendage, epiploic appendagitis is most frequently left-sided, where it can be clinically mistaken for the onset of acute diverticulitis. However, epiploic appendagitis can involve an epiploic appendage of the right colon, and can therefore mimic acute appendicitis (Fig. 21). CT allows a noninvasive diagnosis, showing a fatty mass delineated by a hyperattenuating rim with infiltration of the pericolonic fat. Sometimes, the central thrombosed vein is seen as a spontaneous hyperdense focus in the center of the mass. Surgery is not necessary as epiploic appendagitis resolves within 5–7 days of analgesic medical treatment (Boudiaf et al. 2000; Almeida et al. 2009).

8.2.3 Omental Infarction

Idiopathic segmental infarction of the greater omentum is a rare disorder with the same pathophysiological characteristics as epiploic appendagitis (torsion or spontaneous thrombosis). When the greater omentum is located in the right lower quadrant, its infarction can mimic acute appendicitis. CT images show a heterogeneous fatty mass, well defined, with a hyperattenuating rim, between the anterior abdominal wall and the colon. Adjacent fat stranding and reactive thickening of the adjacent colonic wall can occur. CT allows the diagnosis to be made and surgical treatment to be avoided (Cianci et al. 2008; Pereira et al. 2005; Singh et al. 2006).

8.2.4 Acute Diverticulitis of the Right Colon

Acute diverticulitis of the right colon and cecum is uncommon in occidental countries (about 10% of colonic diverticulitis), and is more frequent in Asian populations. The CT signs are similar to those of typical sigmoid diverticulitis, and include the following: presence of one or several diverticula, parietal thickening of the colon, pericolonic fat stranding. The visualization of a normal appendix confirms the diagnosis, whereas differential diagnosis is difficult when the appendix is not seen. Indeed, an acute appendicitis adjacent to a colonic diverticulum can manifest itself with similar signs on CT (Balthazar et al. 1987).

8.2.5 Cecal Adenocarcinoma

Representing 25% of all colonic adenocarcinomas, cecal adenocarcinoma can evolve asymptomatically for long periods, until it occupies a large volume of the right iliac fossa. Typical complications include acute occlusion, invagination, and even perforation,

Acute Appendicitis

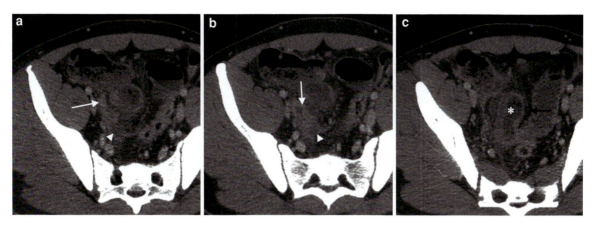

Fig. 20 Appendiceal perforation with abscess and secondary terminal ileitis. Transverse CT scan (**a**): enlarged appendix (*white arrow*) with focal defects in its thickened hyperenhanced wall (**b**). Perforation is confirmed by the presence of a periappendiceal abscess (*arrowhead*). **c** Nonconcentric wall thickening of a dilated terminal ileal loop (*asterisk*) near the abscess with diametrically opposed normal fat (*black arrow*) is in favor of a secondary ileitis, confirmed on surgery

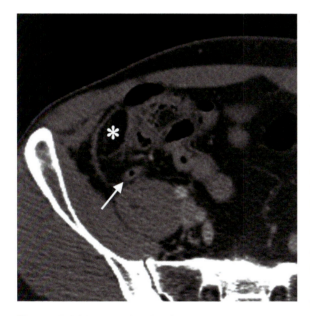

Fig. 21 Epiploic appendagitis of the right lower quadrant. Fatty mass delineated by a hyperattenuating rim (*asterisk*) with thickening of the lateral conal fascia and a normal appendix (*arrow*)

whose differential diagnosis with acute appendicitis is not always evident clinically, especially in the elderly.

8.2.6 Ischemic Necrosis of the Cecum

Isolated cecal infarction is a rare but severe cause of acute pain in the right lower quadrant (Fig. 22). This condition affects elderly patients with a low-flow state or small vessel disease (diabetes mellitus, vasculitis, etc.), or both. Most of the time, there is no evidence of major vessel occlusion. The cecum is more vulnerable to ischemia than other bowel segments because it is supplied by end arteries, whereas the ileum, appendix, and ascending colon are generally served by a dual blood supply. The CT findings are circumferential cecal wall thickening, mural stratification induced by submucosal edema, intramural spontaneous hyperdensity (hemorrhage), focal dilatation, engorged mesentery, pneumatosis intestinalis, portal or mesenteric venous gas, and pneumoperitoneum (Simon et al. 2000; Taourel et al. 2008).

8.2.7 Typhlitis

Neutropenic colitis, or typhlitis, is an inflammatory colitis affecting a neutropenic patient, classically a patient treated by chemotherapy for a hemopathy. The affected segments mainly include the cecum and ascending colon, but the appendix and the last ileal loop can also be involved. The differential diagnosis is not evident, neither clinically nor on CT, although some semiologic elements can aid the diagnosis. Parietal thickening of the cecum is more asymmetric in acute appendicitis than in typhlitis, in which the colonic involvement is more circumferential and extended (Fig. 23). Focalized cecal parietal hypodensities may correspond to ischemia or necrosis areas, which can complicate with perforation. Pericolonic effusion and fat stranding are frequent.

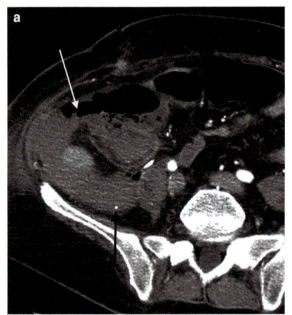

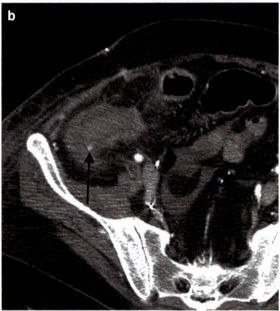

Fig. 22 Ischemic colitis with cecal perforation on two successive axial images (**a**, **b**). Large right lower quadrant collection with air-fluid level and stercoliths (*black arrows*). This abscess communicates with colic lumen through a wide breach in the thickened and nonenhanced cecal wall (*white arrow*). It should be differentiated from an abscess due to appendiceal perforati,on which is the first cause of a right lower quadrant collection containing a stercolith

Parietal pneumomatosis, pneumoperitoneum, and pericecal collection are complications requiring surgical management. This severe condition in fragile

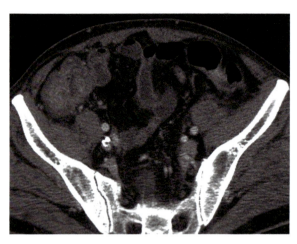

Fig. 23 Typhlitis. Circumferential thickening of the cecal wall with low attenuation secondary to the edema (accordion sign) and with no involvement of other intestinal segments in a neutropenic patient receiving chemotherapy for acute leukemia

patients requires early diagnosis for rapid treatment to be undertaken and perforation to be avoided (Hoeffel et al. 2006; Horton et al. 2000).

8.2.8 Ileal Diverticulitis

Ileal diverticulitis is another rare cause of right lower quadrant pain. The diagnosis can be evoked on CT when a diverticulum is visible on the mesenteric side of the ileum, with peripheral inflammatory signs such as fat stranding, enhancement, and thickening of the peridiverticular ileal walls (Bennett et al. 2004; Coulier et al. 2007).

8.2.9 Meckel Diverticulitis

Meckel diverticulitis is the most frequent of all congenital abnormalities of the intestine (2% of the population), with inflammation as one of the classic complications. Meckel diverticulitis has no specific clinical or laboratory findings, and can mimic acute appendicitis, especially when it lies in the right lower quadrant. CT displays a blind tubular digestive structure, thickened and enhanced, with variable content, whose aspect is similar to that of acute appendicitis (Fig. 24). The differential diagnosis may therefore be challenging in the absence of a visualized normal appendix or when an inflammation of the appendix adjacent to the diverticulitis is depicted. CT may sometimes show that the tip of the Meckel diverticulum is related to the umbilicus (Bennett et al. 2004).

Acute Appendicitis 171

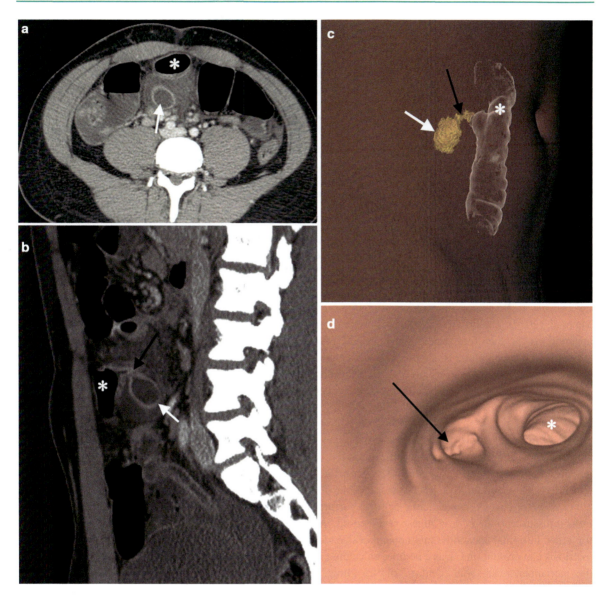

Fig. 24 Meckel diverticulitis. Transverse (**a**) and sagittal (**b**) CT scans show a blind-ended, fluid-filled tubular structure with hyperemic walls (*white arrow*). A neck (*black arrow*) communicates with the adjacent small bowel lumen (*asterisk*), easy to identify after segmentation in VR mode (**c**). A virtual endoscopy shows the diverticular neck connected to the ileum (**d**)

8.3 Appendiceal Digestive Conditions

8.3.1 Isolated Crohn Disease of the Appendix

As previously seen, Crohn disease isolated to the appendix is rare, but possible. Differentiating it from acute appendicitis on CT is very challenging. However, this isolated appendiceal form of Crohn disease is less aggressive than Crohn disease at other site of the digestive tract, with a low rate of recurrence and fistula-type postoperative complications (Prieto-Nieto et al. 2001; Agha et al. 1987).

8.3.2 Appendiceal Diverticulitis

An appendiceal diverticulum is rare, and most often asymptomatic. It may sometimes complicate with inflammation, with 2.7% of all appendectomies being due to appendiceal diverticulitis according to

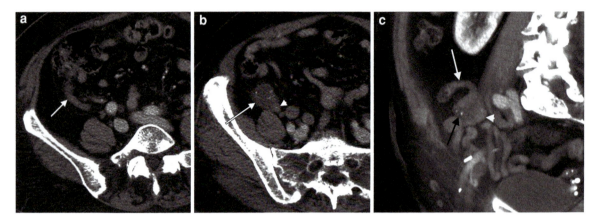

Fig. 25 Mucocele of the appendix on an axial CT scan (**a**, **b**) and with thick oblique cross section in VR mode (**c**). The appendix (*white arrow*) has an enlarged tip, 3 cm in diameter (*black arrow*) with low-attenuation and mural calcifications. There is no enhanced nodule. A small bowel loop is in close contact (*arrowhead*) with the lesion. Ruptured appendiceal mucocele, with no diffusion at a distance was found at surgery

Ma et al. (2010). The differential diagnosis with acute appendicitis is therefore challenging on CT. An appendiceal diverticulum is significantly associated with appendiceal neoplasia, which justifies a prophylactic appendectomy when such a diverticulum, even asymptomatic, is discovered (Abdullgaffar 2009).

8.3.3 Endometriosis of the Appendix

Appendiceal endometriosis refers to the presence of ectopic endometriosic tissue in the vermiform appendix. This condition may be responsible for either acute or chronic appendicitis, or for a perforation, intussusception, or low digestive bleeding. As for other intestinal locations, this appendiceal endometriosis can present on CT as a nodule, enhancing at the periappendiceal wall contact or invading it (Whitley et al. 2009; Akbulut et al. 2009; Biscaldi et al. 2007a, b; Hoeffel et al. 2006).

8.3.4 Appendiceal Tumors

Numerous appendiceal tumors are discovered in the course of appendectomy for acute appendicitis. When the clinical pattern is not typical with an isolated thickening of the appendix on CT and there is no other sign for acute appendicitis, an appendiceal tumor must be systematically evoked. Of course, most tumors can induce obstruction of the appendiceal lumen by their mass effect, and complicate with a true acute appendicitis.

- Appendiceal carcinoid tumor is the most frequent of all malignant tumors of the appendix. Often small in size, and located in the distal part of the appendix, it has a low complication rate. The size of the tumor permitting, CT can sometimes display a diffuse parietal appendiceal thickening, and even metastatic lesions at a distance (Pickhardt et al. 2003; Whitley et al. 2009).
- Appendiceal adenocarcinomas are much less frequent and can be divided into two types: nonmucinous and mucinous. In nonmucinous adenocarcinomas, the appendix is increased in size (greater than 15 mm in diameter) by a tissular mass without an associated mucocele. Clinical management is similar to that of cecum adenocarcinoma, including hemicolectomy and lymph node dissection. Mucinous adenocarcinomas represent the majority of all appendiceal epithelial tumors. Mucin-rich, they are often associated with a mucocele and have characteristics similar to those of mucinous epithelial lesions of the ovary. On CT, a tissular parietal thickening, a parietal irregularity of the mucocele, or peripheral fat stranding may suggest an underlying adenocarcinoma.
- Appendiceal mucocele refers to an appendix whose lumen is distended upon abnormal mucus collection (Fig. 25). Mural calcifications can suggest the diagnosis but are seen in less than 50% of cases (Bennett et al. 2009). Below 2 cm in diameter, the mucocele is most often secondary to a nontumoral obstruction of the appendiceal lumen (simple retention cyst), such as resulting from an inflammatory episode. When the diameter is 2 cm

and greater, the underlying presence of a mucinous cystadenoma or cystadenocarcinoma is suspected, in particular when a parietal nodular enhancement is depicted. Pseudomyxoma peritonei is a mucinous ascites, rarely complicating some mucoceles of neoplasic origin and requiring very specialized surgical management (Whitley et al. 2009; Pickhardt et al. 2003; Pinto Leite et al. 2005).

- Other appendiceal tumors

Appendiceal lymphoma is rare. The overall shape of the appendix is conserved on CT, but a diffuse wall thickening and a much greater diameter than in acute appendicitis (around 3 cm on average according to Pickhardt et al. 2002) are depicted. A lesion extending into the neighboring fat can be expected in the case of fat stranding. Intra-abdominal adenopathy is not necessarily visible.

Appendiceal metastases are most often of mammary origin and can manifest themselves as acute appendicitis (Whitley et al. 2009).

8.4 Gynecologic Disorders

The differential diagnosis between acute appendicitis and acute gynecologic disorder is often clinically challenging to make. This is why the negative appendectomy rate is more important in women of childbearing age, averaging 43.8 per 10,000 population per year (about 12 times more than in men of matching age, 35–44 years old; Addiss et al. 1990). Moreover, Bendeck et al. (2002) have shown that, in a given population, women would benefit much more from preoperative imaging examination. According to this study, there was a significantly lower negative appendectomy rate in women who underwent CT (7%), or ultrasonography (8%) examination than in women who did not undergo imaging (28%). Among all acute gynecologic disorders, the most classic ones can mimic acute appendicitis when they localize to the right lower quadrant. Imaging allows hemorrhagic ovarian cyst, ruptured ovarian cyst, toision of adnexa, salpingitis (Fig. 26), or a thrombosed right ovarian vein to be diagnosed. Importantly, the plasma HCG level must be known before any imaging exploration of right iliac fossa pain in a woman of childbearing age so as not to miss any extrauterine pregnancy.

8.5 Urologic Disorders

Right nephrolithiasis is a frequent differential diagnosis (Stromberg et al. 2007). When the clinical presentation is not typical, the presence of flank or right iliac fossa pain, with acute manifestation, may suggest right nephrolithiasis. Urine laboratory test findings may show hematuria. Ultrasonography or CT generally displays ureteral and pyelocaliceal dilatation, upstream a more or less radiopaque calculus, with a higher sensitivity and specificity for CT, including low-dose NECT. Acute right pyelonephritis occurring over urinary obstruction cannot be diagnosed using laboratory findings, with negative results with urinary strips and cytobacteriological examination of urine. Diagnosis then becomes easy on enhanced CT.

8.6 Nonspecific Abdominal Pain

Acute nonspecific abdominal pain is a common cause of emergency surgical admission for abdominal pain (13–40%; Sheridan et al. 1992; Irvin 1989). It refers to abdominal pain lasting more than 6 h and less than 8 days, without fever, leukocytosis, or obvious peritoneal signs and uncertain diagnosis after physical examination and baseline or more sophisticated investigations, including in some cases abdominal ultrasonography or CT (Morino et al. 2006). Simple follow-up with symptomatic treatment shows the lack of progression.

9 CT Accuracy and Diagnosis Strategy

Numerous studies have shown the excellent results obtained by CT in the diagnosis of appendiceal syndrome (Table 2). They have reported sensitivities of 88–100%, specificities of 91–98%, positive predictive values of 92–98%, negative predictive values of 95–100%, and accuracies of 94–98% (Lane et al. 1999; Balthazar et al. 1991, 1994; Rao et al. 1997e).

These results are better than those obtained by ultrasonography in this indication, with reported sensitivity of 76%, specificity of 91%, positive predictive value of 95%, negative predictive value of

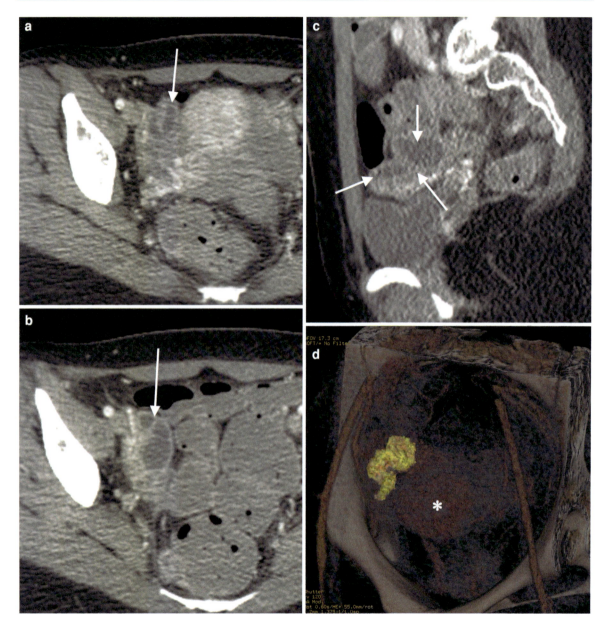

Fig. 26 Right acute salpingitis. Axial (**a**, **b**) and sagittal (**c**) CT scans showing a tubular, blind-ended, fluid-filled structure with contrast-enhanced wall (*white arrow*). The course of this inflammatory fallopian tube is clearly visible in VR mode after segmentation (in *yellow*), the thinnest extremity projecting to the right uterus horn (*asterisk*, **d**), thereby confirming its hollow organ origin. Its morphology is very different from that of an acute appendicitis after segmentation (Fig. 4)

76%, and accuracy of 83% (Balthazar et al. 1994). With regard to its lower cost, its availability, its performance in gynecologic disorders, and its lack of radiation exposure, ultrasonography still remains widely used as the primary imaging modality in the following situations: lean patients, children or young patients, and women of childbearing age. In all other situations, as well as when ultrasonography is not contributive, CT is the examination of choice to make a definite diagnosis or to exclude a diagnosis of acute appendicitis, owing to its high negative predictive value.

Table 2 Computed tomography (*CT*) in the diagnosis management of appendiceal syndrome

	Number of patients	Prevalence of acute appendicitis (%)	Sensitivity (%)	Specificity (%)	PPV (%)	NPV (%)	Appendix visualization (%)	CT technique	Alternative diagnoses (%)
Balthazar et al. (1991)	100	64	98	83	–	–	–	Oral and IV contrast material	17
Rao et al. (1998)	100	53	98	98	98	98	94	Focused CT with rectal opacification	–
Kamel et al. (2000)	100	24	96	100	100	99	100	Oral and IV contrast material	–
Bendeck et al. (2002)	462	91	96	–	96	–	97	Various with or without oral contrast material with or without IV contrast material	–
Tamburrini et al. (2007)	530	19.6	91	95	82	98	–	Nonenhanced CT with selective use of contrast material (IV, oral, or rectal)	35
Stromberg et al. (2007)	2,222	15.3	–	–	–	–	–	IV contrast material	–
Dearing et al. (2008)	238	93.7	90	98	98	91	–	Without rectal contrast material	–
Anderson et al. (2009)	303	8.9	100	97.1	77.8	100	–	IV contrast material with or without oral contrast material	–

PPV positive predictive value, *NPV* negative predictive value, *IV* intravenous

10 Conclusion: Impact of CT on Management of Acute Appendicitis

The performance of imaging, CT in particular, in the positive diagnosis of acute appendicitis and related complications, is now widely accepted. Nevertheless, several studies have shown controversies regarding the impact of CT on acute appendicitis management. Rao et al. (1998) demonstrated that systematic CT use in suspected appendicitis was cost effective, by decreasing the negative appendectomy rate as well as the number of patients hospitalized for observation. Flum et al. (2001) replied to Rao et al.'s enthusiastic conclusions by reporting a similar negative appendectomy rate (15%) and appendiceal perforation rate (25%), between 1987 and 1998, despite a supposed, though not evaluated, wider use of preoperative imaging in an epidemiological series including more than 63,000 patients.

A study by Raman et al. (2008) added to, if still needed, the utility of systematic imaging in acute appendicitis management. Their retrospective study reported appendectomies performed over a 10 years period, analyzing them year by year; 1,081 consecutive patients who had undergone appendectomy from 1996 to 2006 were included. The rate of CT use, the rate of unnecessary appendectomy, the rate of perforation, and the relationship between CT and ultrasonography use were analyzed. The rate of CT use steadily increased from 20% in 1996 to 85% in 2006, reaching a maximum of 93% in 2005, whereas the use of ultrasonography decreased from 24% in 1996 to 9% in 2006. In the meantime, the rate of both unnecessary appendectomy and appendiceal perforation decreased from 24% to 3% and from 18% to 5%, respectively.

Although these data substantially demonstrate the positive impact of CT in acute appendicitis management, with a concomitant decrease in the rate of unnecessary appendectomy and appendiceal perforation, the substitution of ultrasonography by CT is worth considering. Whereas from 1996 to 2006, one CT examination was performed for one ultrasonography examination, 8 years later, from 2004 to 2006, ten CT examinations were performed for one ultrasonography examination. This shift toward the use of CT may be explained by the slightly better performance of CT for the diagnosis of acute appendicitis, in terms of sensitivity and specificity, the best visualization of appendiceal perforations, the better diagnostic confidence in excluding acute appendicitis by easier identification of a normal appendix on CT, the faster learning curve for CT, the possible reviewing a posteriori of scan examinations on CT, and the shorter duration of a CT examination. Nevertheless, this shift toward the use of CT raises the problem of exposure to ionizing radiation, especially in young patients, for which ultrasonography should be preferred as the primary imaging modality. But, when a scan is necessary, the radiologist is responsible for optimizing the scanning parameters to minimize the dose delivered to the patient, while retaining proper image quality warranting interpretation (Taourel 2008).

References

Abdullgaffar B (2009) Diverticulosis and diverticulitis of the appendix. Int J Surg Pathol 17(3):231–237

Addiss DG, Shaffer N, Fowler BS, Tauxe RV (1990) The epidemiology of appendicitis and appendectomy in the United States. Am J Epidemiol 132(5):910–925

Agha FP, Ghahremani GG, Panella JS, Kaufman MW (1987) Appendicitis as the initial manifestation of Crohn's disease: radiologic features and prognosis. AJR Am J Roentgenol 149(3):515–518

Akbulut S, Dursun P, Kocbiyik A, Harman A, Sevmis S (2009) Appendiceal endometriosis presenting as perforated appendicitis: report of a case and review of the literature. Arch Gynecol Obstet 280(3):495–497

Almeida AT, Melao L, Viamonte B, Cunha R, Pereira JM (2009) Epiploic appendagitis: an entity frequently unknown to clinicians—diagnostic imaging, pitfalls, and look-alikes. AJR Am J Roentgenol 193(5):1243–1251

Alobaidi M, Shirkhoda A (2003) Value of bone window settings on CT for revealing appendicoliths in patients with appendicitis. AJR Am J Roentgenol 180(1):201–205

Alvarado A (1986) A practical score for the early diagnosis of acute appendicitis. Ann Emerg Med 15(5):557–564

Anderson SW, Soto JA, Lucey BC, Ozonoff A, Jordan JD, Ratevosian J, Ulrich AS, Rathlev NK, Mitchell PM, Rebholz C, Feldman JA, Rhea JT (2009) Abdominal 64-MDCT for suspected appendicitis: the use of oral and IV contrast material versus IV contrast material only. AJR Am J Roentgenol 193(5):1282–1288

Andersson RE, Petzold MG (2007) Nonsurgical treatment of appendiceal abscess or phlegmon: a systematic review and meta-analysis. Ann Surg 246(5):741–748

Athanassopoulos A, Speakman MJ (1995) Appendicovesical fistula. Int Urol Nephrol 27(6):705–708

Baek SK, Kim MS, Kim YH, Chung WJ, Kwon JH (2008) A case of stump appendicitis after appendectomy. Korean J Gastroenterol 51(1):45–47

Balthazar EJ, Gollapudi P (2000) Septic thrombophlebitis of the mesenteric and portal veins: CT imaging. J Comput Assist Tomogr 24(5):755–760

Balthazar EJ, Megibow AJ, Gordon RB, Hulnick D (1987) Cecal diverticulitis: evaluation with CT. Radiology 162(1 Pt 1):79–81

Balthazar EJ, Megibow AJ, Siegel SE, Birnbaum BA (1991) Appendicitis: prospective evaluation with high-resolution CT. Radiology 180(1):21–24

Balthazar EJ, Birnbaum BA, Yee J, Megibow AJ, Roshkow J, Gray C (1994) Acute appendicitis: CT and US correlation in 100 patients. Radiology 190(1):31–35

Barker DJ (1989) Rise and fall of Western diseases. Nature 338(6214):371–372

Basu NN, Doddi S, Turner L, Sinha PS (2009) Tooth crown foreign body appendicitis. Dig Surg 26(1):22–23

Bendeck SE, Nino-Murcia M, Berry GJ, Jeffrey RB Jr (2002) Imaging for suspected appendicitis: negative appendectomy and perforation rates. Radiology 225(1):131–136

Benjaminov O, Atri M, Hamilton P, Rappaport D (2002) Frequency of visualization and thickness of normal appendix at nonenhanced helical CT. Radiology 225(2):400–406

Bennett GL, Birnbaum BA, Balthazar EJ (2004) CT of Meckel's diverticulitis in 11 patients. AJR Am J Roentgenol 182(3):625–629

Bennett GL, Tanpitukpongse TP, Macari M, Cho KC, Babb JS (2009) CT diagnosis of mucocele of the appendix in patients with acute appendicitis. AJR Am J Roentgenol 192(3):W103–W110

Bingol-Kologlu M, Fedakar M, Yagmurlu A, Dindar H, Gokcora IH (2006) An exceptional complication following appendectomy: acute inguinal and scrotal suppuration. Int Urol Nephrol 38(3–4):663–665

Birnbaum BA, Wilson SR (2000) Appendicitis at the millennium. Radiology 215(2):337–348

Biscaldi E, Ferrero S, Fulcheri E, Ragni N, Remorgida V, Rollandi GA (2007a) Multislice CT enteroclysis in the diagnosis of bowel endometriosis. Eur Radiol 17(1):211–219

Biscaldi E, Ferrero S, Remorgida V, Rollandi GA (2007b) Bowel endometriosis: CT-enteroclysis. Abdom Imaging 32(4):441–450

Boudiaf M, Zidi SH, Soyer P, Hamidou Z, Panis Y, Pelage JP, Rymer R (2000) Primary epiploic appendicitis: CT diagnosis for conservative treatment. Presse Med 29(5):231–236

Brenner DJ, Hall EJ (2007) Computed tomography—an increasing source of radiation exposure. N Engl J Med 357(22):2277–2284

Chang CC, Wang SS (2007) Acute abdominal pain in the elderly. Int J Gerontol 1(2):77–82

Chang YS, Min SY, Joo SH, Lee SH (2008) Septic thrombophlebitis of the porto-mesenteric veins as a complication of acute appendicitis. World J Gastroenterol 14(28):4580–4582

Checkoff JL, Wechsler RJ, Nazarian LN (2002) Chronic inflammatory appendiceal conditions that mimic acute appendicitis on helical CT. AJR Am J Roentgenol 179(3):731–734

Chen MM, Coakley FV, Kaimal A, Laros RK, Laros RK Jr (2008) Guidelines for computed tomography and magnetic resonance imaging use during pregnancy and lactation. Obstet Gynecol 112(2 Pt 1):333–340

Chen CW, Hsiao CW, Wu CC, Jao SW, Lee TY, Kang JC (2010) Necrotizing fasciitis due to acute perforated appendicitis: case report. J Emerg Med 39(2):178–180

Cianci R, Filippone A, Basilico R, Storto ML (2008) Idiopathic segmental infarction of the greater omentum diagnosed by unenhanced multidetector-row CT and treated successfully by laparoscopy. Emerg Radiol 15(1):51–56

Clarke PD (1987) Computed tomography of gangrenous appendicitis. J Comput Assist Tomogr 11(6):1081–1082

Cobben L, Groot I, Kingma L, Coerkamp E, Puylaert J, Blickman J (2009) A simple MRI protocol in patients with clinically suspected appendicitis: results in 138 patients and effect on outcome of appendectomy. Eur Radiol 19(5):1175–1183

Coulier B, Maldague P, Bourgeois A, Broze B (2007) Diverticulitis of the small bowel: CT diagnosis. Abdom Imaging 32(2):228–233

D'Acremont B, Bonnichon J, Sarfati E (1995) Appendicite aiguë. In: Ellipses (ed) Hépatogastroentérologie. Broché, Paris, pp 319–324

Dearing DD, Recabaren JA, Alexander M (2008) Can computed tomography scan be performed effectively in the diagnosis of acute appendicitis without the added morbidity of rectal contrast? Am Surg 74(10):917–920

Delabrousse E (2009) TDM des urgences abdominales. Masson, Paris

Deorah S, Seenu V, Pradeep KK, Sharma S (2005) Spontaneous appendico-cutaneous fistula—a rare complication of acute appendicitis. Trop Gastroenterol 26(1):48–50

Ege G, Akman H, Sahin A, Bugra D, Kuzucu K (2002) Diagnostic value of unenhanced helical CT in adult patients with suspected acute appendicitis. Br J Radiol 75(897):721–725

Ein SH, Langer JC, Daneman A (2005) Nonoperative management of pediatric ruptured appendix with inflammatory mass or abscess: presence of an appendicolith predicts recurrent appendicitis. J Pediatr Surg 40(10):1612–1615

Esses D, Birnbaum A, Bijur P, Shah S, Gleyzer A, Gallagher EJ (2004) Ability of CT to alter decision making in elderly patients with acute abdominal pain. Am J Emerg Med 22(4):270–272

Fefferman NR, Roche KJ, Pinkney LP, Ambrosino MM, Genieser NB (2001) Suspected appendicitis in children: focused CT technique for evaluation. Radiology 220(3):691–695

Fitz R (1886) Perforating inflammation of the vermiform appendix with special reference to its early diagnosis and treatment. Trans Assoc Am Physicians 1:107–144

Flum DR, Morris A, Koepsell T, Dellinger EP (2001) Has misdiagnosis of appendicitis decreased over time? A population-based analysis. JAMA 286(14):1748–1753

Foley TA, Earnest Ft, Nathan MA, Hough DM, Schiller HJ, Hoskin TL (2005) Differentiation of nonperforated from perforated appendicitis: accuracy of CT diagnosis and relationship of CT findings to length of hospital stay. Radiology 235(1):89–96

Freeland M, King E, Safcsak K, Durham R (2009) Diagnosis of appendicitis in pregnancy. Am J Surg 198(6):753–758

Funaki B (2000) Nonenhanced CT for suspected appendicitis. Radiology 216(3):916–918

Funaki B, Grosskreutz SR, Funaki CN (1998) Using unenhanced helical CT with enteric contrast material for suspected appendicitis in patients treated at a community hospital. AJR Am J Roentgenol 171(4):997–1001

Ganguli S, Raptopoulos V, Komlos F, Siewert B, Kruskal JB (2006) Right lower quadrant pain: value of the nonvisualized appendix in patients at multidetector CT. Radiology 241(1):175–180

Garcia K, Hernanz-Schulman M, Bennett DL, Morrow SE, Yu C, Kan JH (2009) Suspected appendicitis in children: diagnostic importance of normal abdominopelvic CT findings with nonvisualized appendix. Radiology 250(2): 531–537

Giuliano V, Giuliano C, Pinto F, Scaglione M (2006) Chronic appendicitis "syndrome" manifested by an appendicolith and thickened appendix presenting as chronic right lower abdominal pain in adults. Emerg Radiol 12(3):96–98

Gronroos JM, Gronroos P (2001) Diagnosis of acute appendicitis. Radiology 219(1):297–298

Gronroos P, Huhtinen H, Gronroos JM (2009) Normal leukocyte count and C-reactive protein value do not effectively exclude acute appendicitis in children. Dis Colon Rectum 52(5):1028–1029 author reply 1029

Hermans JJ, Hermans AL, Risseeuw GA, Verhaar JC, Meradji M (1993) Appendicitis caused by carcinoid tumor. Radiology 188(1):71–72

Hoeffel C, Crema MD, Belkacem A, Azizi L, Lewin M, Arrive L, Tubiana JM (2006) Multi-detector row CT: spectrum of diseases involving the ileocecal area. Radiographics 26(5):1373–1390

Holden DM, Einstein DM (2007) Which imaging test for right lower quadrant pain? Cleve Clin J Med 74(1):37–40

Hopkins KL, Patrick LE, Ball TI (2001) Imaging findings of perforative appendicitis: a pictorial review. Pediatr Radiol 31(3):173–179

Horattas MC, Guyton DP, Wu D (1990) A reappraisal of appendicitis in the elderly. Am J Surg 160(3):291–293

Horrow MM, White DS, Horrow JC (2003) Differentiation of perforated from nonperforated appendicitis at CT. Radiology 227(1):46–51

Horton KM, Corl FM, Fishman EK (2000) CT evaluation of the colon: inflammatory disease. Radiographics 20(2):399–418

Huynh LN, Coughlin BF, Wolfe J, Blank F, Lee SY, Smithline HA (2004) Patient encounter time intervals in the evaluation of emergency department patients requiring abdominopelvic CT: oral contrast versus no contrast. Emerg Radiol 10(6):310–313

Irvin TT (1989) Abdominal pain: a surgical audit of 1190 emergency admissions. Br J Surg 76(11):1121–1125

Izawa JI, Taylor BM, Denstedt JD (1998) Appendicovesical fistula: case report and review. Can J Urol 5(2):566–568

Jacobs JE, Birnbaum BA, Macari M, Megibow AJ, Israel G, Maki DD, Aguiar AM, Langlotz CP (2001) Acute appendicitis: comparison of helical CT diagnosis focused technique with oral contrast material versus nonfocused technique with oral and intravenous contrast material. Radiology 220(3):683–690

Jan YT, Yang FS, Huang JK (2005) Visualization rate and pattern of normal appendix on multidetector computed tomography by using multiplanar reformation display. J Comput Assist Tomogr 29(4):446–451

Jeffrey RB Jr, Federle MP, Tolentino CS (1988) Periappendiceal inflammatory masses: CT-directed management and clinical outcome in 70 patients. Radiology 167(1): 13–16

Johnson PT, Horton KM, Mahesh M, Fishman EK (2006) Multidetector computed tomography for suspected appendicitis: multi-institutional survey of 16-MDCT data acquisition protocols and review of pertinent literature. J Comput Assist Tomogr 30(5):758–764

Johnson PT, Horton KM, Kawamoto S, Eng J, Bean MJ, Shan SJ, Fishman EK (2009) MDCT for suspected appendicitis: effect of reconstruction section thickness on diagnostic accuracy, rate of appendiceal visualization, and reader confidence using axial images. AJR Am J Roentgenol 192(4):893–901

Kamel IR, Goldberg SN, Keogan MT, Rosen MP, Raptopoulos V (2000) Right lower quadrant pain and suspected appendicitis: nonfocused appendiceal CT—review of 100 cases. Radiology 217(1):159–163

Karabulut N, Boyaci N, Yagci B, Herek D, Kiroglu Y (2007) Computed tomography evaluation of the normal appendix: comparison of low-dose and standard-dose unenhanced helical computed tomography. J Comput Assist Tomogr 31(5):732–740

Kessler N, Cyteval C, Gallix B, Lesnik A, Blayac PM, Pujol J, Bruel JM, Taourel P (2004) Appendicitis: evaluation of sensitivity, specificity, and predictive values of US, Doppler US, and laboratory findings. Radiology 230(2):472–478

Keyzer C, Tack D, de Maertelaer V, Bohy P, Gevenois PA, Van Gansbeke D (2004) Acute appendicitis: comparison of low-dose and standard-dose unenhanced multi-detector row CT. Radiology 232(1):164–172

Keyzer C, Cullus P, Tack D, De Maertelaer V, Bohy P, Gevenois PA (2009) MDCT for suspected acute appendicitis in adults: impact of oral and IV contrast media at standard-dose and simulated low-dose techniques. AJR Am J Roentgenol 193(5):1272–1281

Kim N, Reed WP Jr, Abbas MA, Katz DS (2004) CT identification of abscesses after dropped appendicoliths during laparoscopic appendectomy. AJR Am J Roentgenol 182(5):1203–1205

Kim HC, Yang DM, Jin W, Kim GY, Choi SI (2008a) Metastasis to the appendix from a hepatocellular carcinoma manifesting as acute appendicitis: CT findings. Br J Radiol 81(967):e194–e196

Kim HC, Yang DM, Jin W, Park SJ (2008b) Added diagnostic value of multiplanar reformation of multidetector CT data in patients with suspected appendicitis. Radiographics 28(2):393–405, discussion 405–396

Kim YJ, Kim JE, Kim HS, Hwang HY (2009) MDCT with coronal reconstruction: clinical benefit in evaluation of suspected acute appendicitis in pediatric patients. AJR Am J Roentgenol 192(1):150–152

Klingler PJ, Seelig MH, DeVault KR, Wetscher GJ, Floch NR, Branton SA, Hinder RA (1998) Ingested foreign bodies within the appendix: a 100-year review of the literature. Dig Dis 16(5):308–314

Lane MJ, Liu DM, Huynh MD, Jeffrey RB Jr, Mindelzun RE, Katz DS (1999) Suspected acute appendicitis: nonenhanced helical CT in 300 consecutive patients. Radiology 213(2):341–346

Lau WY, Fan ST, Yiu TF, Chu KW, Lee JM (1985) Acute appendicitis in the elderly. Surg Gynecol Obstet 161(2):157–160

Lazarus E, Mayo-Smith WW, Mainiero MB, Spencer PK (2007) CT in the evaluation of nontraumatic abdominal pain in pregnant women. Radiology 244(3):784–790

Lee JH, Jeong YK, Park KB, Park JK, Jeong AK, Hwang JC (2005) Operator-dependent techniques for graded compression sonography to detect the appendix and diagnose acute appendicitis. AJR Am J Roentgenol 184(1):91–97

Lee KH, Kim YH, Hahn S, Lee KW, Kim TJ, Kang SB, Shin JH (2006a) Computed tomography diagnosis of acute appendicitis: advantages of reviewing thin-section datasets using sliding slab average intensity projection technique. Invest Radiol 41(7):579–585

Lee KH, Kim YH, Hahn S, Lee KW, Lee HJ, Kim TJ, Kang SB, Shin JH, Park BJ (2006b) Added value of coronal reformations for duty radiologists and for referring physicians or surgeons in the CT diagnosis of acute appendicitis. Korean J Radiol 7(2):87–96

Lee SY, Coughlin B, Wolfe JM, Polino J, Blank FS, Smithline HA (2006c) Prospective comparison of helical CT of the abdomen and pelvis without and with oral contrast in assessing acute abdominal pain in adult Emergency Department patients. Emerg Radiol 12(4):150–157

Lee KH, Hong H, Hahn S, Kim B, Kim KJ, Kim YH (2008) Summation or axial slab average intensity projection of abdominal thin-section CT datasets: can they substitute for the primary reconstruction from raw projection data? J Digit Imaging 21(4):422–432

Levine CD, Aizenstein O, Wachsberg RH (2004) Pitfalls in the CT diagnosis of appendicitis. Br J Radiol 77(921):792–799

Lewis LM, Klippel AP, Bavolek RA, Ross LM, Scherer TM, Banet GA (2007) Quantifying the usefulness of CT in evaluating seniors with abdominal pain. Eur J Radiol 61(2):290–296

Lim HK, Bae SH, Seo GS (1992) Diagnosis of acute appendicitis in pregnant women: value of sonography. AJR Am J Roentgenol 159(3):539–542

Lim HK, Lee WJ, Lee SJ, Namgung S, Lim JH (1996) Focal appendicitis confined to the tip: diagnosis at US. Radiology 200(3):799–801

Lowe LH, Penney MW, Scheker LE, Perez R Jr, Stein SM, Heller RM, Shyr Y, Hernanz-Schulman M (2000) Appendicolith revealed on CT in children with suspected appendicitis: how specific is it in the diagnosis of appendicitis? AJR Am J Roentgenol 175(4):981–984

Ma KW, Chia NH, Yeung HW, Cheung MT (2010) If not appendicitis, then what else can it be? A retrospective review of 1492 appendectomies. Hong Kong Med J 16(1):12–17

Macari M, Balthazar EJ (2003) The acute right lower quadrant: CT evaluation. Radiol Clin North Am 41(6):1117–1136

Macari M, Hines J, Balthazar E, Megibow A (2002) Mesenteric adenitis: CT diagnosis of primary versus secondary causes, incidence, and clinical significance in pediatric and adult patients. AJR Am J Roentgenol 178(4):853–858

Marin D, Ho LM, Barnhart H, Neville AM, White RR, Paulson EK (2010) Percutaneous abscess drainage in patients with perforated acute appendicitis: effectiveness, safety, and prediction of outcome. AJR Am J Roentgenol 194(2):422–429

Mathias J, Bruot O, Ganne P-A, Laurent V, Regent D (2008) Appendicite. In: Encyclopédie Médico Chirurgicale, vol RADIOLOGIE ET IMAGERIE MÉDICALE: Abdominale-Digestive. ElsevierMasson, Paris

McBurney C (1889) Experiences with early operative interference in cases of diseases of the vermiform appendix. N Y Med J 50:676–684

Migraine S, Atri M, Bret PM, Lough JO, Hinchey JE (1997) Spontaneously resolving acute appendicitis: clinical and sonographic documentation. Radiology 205(1):55–58

Misra SP, Dwivedi M, Misra V, Singh PA, Agarwal VK (1999) Preoperative sonographic diagnosis of acute appendicitis caused by *Ascaris lumbricoides*. J Clin Ultrasound 27(2):96–97

Morino M, Pellegrino L, Castagna E, Farinella E, Mao P (2006) Acute nonspecific abdominal pain: a randomized, controlled trial comparing early laparoscopy versus clinical observation. Ann Surg 244(6):881–886; discussion 886–888

Moteki T, Ohya N, Horikoshi H (2009) Prospective examination of patients suspected of having appendicitis using new computed tomography criteria including "maximum depth of intraluminal appendiceal fluid greater than 2.6 mm". J Comput Assist Tomogr 33(3):383–389

Mussack T, Schmidbauer S, Nerlich A, Schmidt W, Hallfeldt KK (2002) Chronic appendicitis as an independent clinical entity. Chirurg 73(7):710–715

Nandipati K, Parithivel V, Niazi M (2008) Schistosomiasis: a rare cause of acute appendicitis in the African American population in the United States. Am Surg 74(3):221–223

Neville AM, Paulson EK (2009) MDCT of acute appendicitis: value of coronal reformations. Abdom Imaging 34(1):42–48

Nikolaidis P, Hwang CM, Miller FH, Papanicolaou N (2004) The nonvisualized appendix: incidence of acute appendicitis when secondary inflammatory changes are absent. AJR Am J Roentgenol 183(4):889–892

O'Shea SJ, Martin DF (2003) Percutaneous removal of retained calculi from the abdomen. Cardiovasc Intervent Radiol 26(1):81–84

Patel SJ, Reede DL, Katz DS, Subramaniam R, Amorosa JK (2007) Imaging the pregnant patient for nonobstetric conditions: algorithms and radiation dose considerations. Radiographics 27(6):1705–1722

Paulson EK, Coursey CA (2009) CT protocols for acute appendicitis: time for change. AJR Am J Roentgenol 193(5):1268–1271

Paulson EK, Harris JP, Jaffe TA, Haugan PA, Nelson RC (2005) Acute appendicitis: added diagnostic value of coronal reformations from isotropic voxels at multi-detector row CT. Radiology 235(3):879–885

Pedrosa I, Lafornara M, Pandharipande PV, Goldsmith JD, Rofsky NM (2009) Pregnant patients suspected of having acute appendicitis: effect of MR imaging on negative laparotomy rate and appendiceal perforation rate. Radiology 250(3):749–757

Pereira JM, Sirlin CB, Pinto PS, Casola G (2005) CT and MR imaging of extrahepatic fatty masses of the abdomen and pelvis: techniques, diagnosis, differential diagnosis, and pitfalls. Radiographics 25(1):69–85

Pickhardt PJ, Levy AD, Rohrmann CA Jr, Abbondanzo SL, Kende AI (2002) Non-Hodgkin's lymphoma of the appendix: clinical and CT findings with pathologic correlation. AJR Am J Roentgenol 178(5):1123–1127

Pickhardt PJ, Levy AD, Rohrmann CA Jr, Kende AI (2003) Primary neoplasms of the appendix: radiologic spectrum of disease with pathologic correlation. Radiographics 23(3):645–662

Pinto Leite N, Pereira JM, Cunha R, Pinto P, Sirlin C (2005) CT evaluation of appendicitis and its complications: imaging techniques and key diagnostic findings. AJR Am J Roentgenol 185(2):406–417

Poortman P, Oostvogel HJ, Bosma E, Lohle PN, Cuesta MA, de Lange-de Klerk ES, Hamming JF (2009) Improving diagnosis of acute appendicitis: results of a diagnostic pathway with standard use of ultrasonography followed by selective use of CT. J Am Coll Surg 208(3):434–441

Prieto-Nieto I, Perez-Robledo JP, Hardisson D, Rodriguez-Montes JA, Larrauri-Martinez J, Garcia-Sancho-Martin L (2001) Crohn's disease limited to the appendix. Am J Surg 182(5):531–533

Rabinowitz CB, Egglin TK, Beland MD, Mayo-Smith WW (2007) Outcomes in 74 patients with an appendicolith who did not undergo surgery: is follow-up imaging necessary? Emerg Radiol 14(3):161–165

Raman SS, Osuagwu FC, Kadell B, Cryer H, Sayre J, Lu DS (2008) Effect of CT on false positive diagnosis of appendicitis and perforation. N Engl J Med 358(9):972–973

Randal Bollinger R, Barbas AS, Bush EL, Lin SS, Parker W (2007) Biofilms in the large bowel suggest an apparent function of the human vermiform appendix. J Theor Biol 249(4):826–831

Rao PM, Mueller PR (1998) Clinical and pathologic variants of appendiceal disease: CT features. AJR Am J Roentgenol 170(5):1335–1340

Rao PM, Rhea JT, Novelline RA (1997a) Appendiceal and peri-appendiceal air at CT: prevalence, appearance and clinical significance. Clin Radiol 52(10):750–754

Rao PM, Rhea JT, Novelline RA (1997b) CT diagnosis of mesenteric adenitis. Radiology 202(1):145–149

Rao PM, Rhea JT, Novelline RA (1997c) Distal appendicitis: CT appearance and diagnosis. Radiology 204(3):709–712

Rao PM, Rhea JT, Novelline RA (1997d) Sensitivity and specificity of the individual CT signs of appendicitis: experience with 200 helical appendiceal CT examinations. J Comput Assist Tomogr 21(5):686–692

Rao PM, Rhea JT, Novelline RA, McCabe CJ, Lawrason JN, Berger DL, Sacknoff R (1997e) Helical CT technique for the diagnosis of appendicitis: prospective evaluation of a focused appendix CT examination. Radiology 202(1):139–144

Rao PM, Rhea JT, Novelline RA, Mostafavi AA, Lawrason JN, McCabe CJ (1997f) Helical CT combined with contrast material administered only through the colon for imaging of suspected appendicitis. AJR Am J Roentgenol 169(5):1275–1280

Rao PM, Wittenberg J, McDowell RK, Rhea JT, Novelline RA (1997g) Appendicitis: use of arrowhead sign for diagnosis at CT. Radiology 202(2):363–366

Rao PM, Rhea JT, Novelline RA, Mostafavi AA, McCabe CJ (1998) Effect of computed tomography of the appendix on treatment of patients and use of hospital resources. N Engl J Med 338(3):141–146

Rettenbacher T, Hollerweger A, Macheiner P, Rettenbacher L, Frass R, Schneider B, Gritzmann N (2000) Presence or absence of gas in the appendix: additional criteria to rule out or confirm acute appendicitis—evaluation with US. Radiology 214(1):183–187

Rhea JT, Rao PM, Novelline RA, McCabe CJ (1997) A focused appendiceal CT technique to reduce the cost of caring for patients with clinically suspected appendicitis. AJR Am J Roentgenol 169(1):113–118

Rioux M (1992) Sonographic detection of the normal and abnormal appendix. AJR Am J Roentgenol 158(4):773–778

Rusnak RA, Borer JM, Fastow JS (1994) Misdiagnosis of acute appendicitis: common features discovered in cases after litigation. Am J Emerg Med 12(4):397–402

Schumpelick V, Dreuw B, Ophoff K, Prescher A (2000) Appendix and cecum. Embryology, anatomy, and surgical applications. Surg Clin North Am 80(1):295–318

Seo H, Lee KH, Kim HJ, Kim K, Kang SB, Kim SY, Kim YH (2009) Diagnosis of acute appendicitis with sliding slab ray-sum interpretation of low-dose unenhanced CT and standard-dose i.v. contrast-enhanced CT scans. AJR Am J Roentgenol 193(1):96–105

Sgourakis G, Sotiropoulos GC, Molmenti EP, Eibl C, Bonticous S, Moege J, Berchtold C (2008) Are acute exacerbations of chronic inflammatory appendicitis triggered by coprostasis and/or coproliths? World J Gastroenterol 14(20):3179–3182

Shapiro MP, Gale ME, Gerzof SG (1989) CT of appendicitis. Diagnosis and treatment. Radiol Clin North Am 27(4):753–762

Sheridan WG, White AT, Havard T, Crosby DL (1992) Nonspecific abdominal pain: the resource implications. Ann R Coll Surg Engl 74(3):181–185

Shetty MK, Garrett NM, Carpenter WS, Shah YP, Roberts C (2010) Abdominal computed tomography during pregnancy for suspected appendicitis: a 5-year experience at a maternity hospital. Semin Ultrasound CT MR 31(1):8–13

Shin LK, Halpern D, Weston SR, Meiner EM, Katz DS (2005) Prospective CT diagnosis of stump appendicitis. AJR Am J Roentgenol 184(3 Suppl):S62–S64

Simillis C, Symeonides P, Shorthouse AJ, Tekkis PP (2010) A meta-analysis comparing conservative treatment versus acute appendectomy for complicated appendicitis (abscess or phlegmon). Surgery. 147(6):818–829

Simon AM, Birnbaum BA, Jacobs JE (2000) Isolated infarction of the cecum: CT findings in two patients. Radiology 214(2):513–516

Singh AK, Gervais DA, Lee P, Westra S, Hahn PF, Novelline RA, Mueller PR (2006) Omental infarct: CT imaging features. Abdom Imaging 31(5):549–554

Singh A, Danrad R, Hahn PF, Blake MA, Mueller PR, Novelline RA (2007) MR imaging of the acute abdomen and pelvis: acute appendicitis and beyond. Radiographics 27(5):1419–1431

Singh AK, Hahn PF, Gervais D, Vijayraghavan G, Mueller PR (2008) Dropped appendicolith: CT findings and implications for management. AJR Am J Roentgenol 190(3):707–711

Sivit CJ (1993) Diagnosis of acute appendicitis in children: spectrum of sonographic findings. AJR Am J Roentgenol 161(1):147–152

Stabile Ianora AA, Moschetta M, Lorusso V, Scardapane A (2010) Atypical appendicitis: diagnostic value of volume-rendered reconstructions obtained with 16-slice multidetector-row CT. Radiol Med 115(1):93–104

Stromberg C, Johansson G, Adolfsson A (2007) Acute abdominal pain: diagnostic impact of immediate CT scanning. World J Surg 31(12):2347–2354 discussion 2355–2348

Tamburrini S, Brunetti A, Brown M, Sirlin CB, Casola G (2005) CT appearance of the normal appendix in adults. Eur Radiol 15(10):2096–2103

Tamburrini S, Brunetti A, Brown M, Sirlin C, Casola G (2007) Acute appendicitis: diagnostic value of nonenhanced CT with selective use of contrast in routine clinical settings. Eur Radiol 17(8):2055–2061

Tamir IL, Bongard FS, Klein SR (1990) Acute appendicitis in the pregnant patient. Am J Surg 160(6):571–575 discussion 575–576

Taourel P (2008) Impact of CT on negative appendectomy and appendiceal perforation rates. J Radiol 89(3 Pt 1):289–290

Taourel P, Aufort S, Merigeaud S, Doyon FC, Hoquet MD, Delabrousse E (2008) Imaging of ischemic colitis. Radiol Clin North Am 46(5):909–924, vi

Tsuboi M, Takase K, Kaneda I, Ishibashi T, Yamada T, Kitami M, Higano S, Takahashi S (2008) Perforated and nonperforated appendicitis: defect in enhancing appendiceal wall–depiction with multi-detector row CT. Radiology 246(1):142–147

Tzovaras G, Liakou P, Makryiannis E, Paroutoglou G (2007) Acute appendicitis due to appendiceal obstruction from a migrated biliary stent. Am J Gastroenterol 102(1): 195–196

Urban BA, Fishman EK (2000a) Tailored helical CT evaluation of acute abdomen. Radiographics 20(3):725–749

Urban BA, Fishman EK (2000b) Targeted helical CT of the acute abdomen: appendicitis, diverticulitis, and small bowel obstruction. Semin Ultrasound CT MR 21(1):20–39

Walker AR, Segal I (1990) What causes appendicitis? J Clin Gastroenterol 12(2):127–129

Walker AR, Segal I (1995) Appendicitis: an African perspective. J R Soc Med 88(11):616–619

Weltman DI, Yu J, Krumenacker J Jr, Huang S, Moh P (2000) Diagnosis of acute appendicitis: comparison of 5- and 10-mm CT sections in the same patient. Radiology 216(1): 172–177

Whitley S, Sookur P, McLean A, Power N (2009) The appendix on CT. Clin Radiol 64(2):190–199

Wilharm A, Gras F, Muckley T, Hofmann GO (2010) Necrotizing fasciitis after "banal" back pain: an unusual course of a retrocoecal appendicitis and its sequellae. Chirurg 81(5):472–476

York GL (2003) A unique case of foreign-body appendicitis. AJR Am J Roentgenol 181(5):1431–1432

Ischemia (Acute Mesenteric Ischemia and Ischemic Colitis)

Stefania Romano and Luigia Romano

Contents

1	**Epidemiology**	184
2	**Physiopathology**	184
3	**Clinical Findings**	185
4	**CT Findings**	186
4.1	Small Intestine Vascular Disease from Arterial Supply Deficiency	186
4.2	Small Intestine Vascular Disease from Impaired Venous Drainage	188
4.3	Colonic Ischemia	191
4.4	CT Pitfalls	193
5	**CT Impact on Management**	195
6	**Diagnostic Strategy**	195
	References	196

S. Romano (✉) · L. Romano
Department of Diagnostic Imaging,
Section of General and Emergency Radiology,
"A.Cardarelli" Hospital, Viale Cardarelli, 9,
80131 Napoli, Italy
e-mail: stefromano@libero.it

Abstract

Diagnosis of intestinal disease related to vascular disorders could represent a critical diagnostic challenge for the emergency radiologist. Terms such as "ischemia" and "infarction" of the intestine are often used erroneously as synonyms: however, whereas the ischemia could be a totally reversible event, the infarction corresponds to a tissue death with no chance for the tissue to heal. Both terms indicate as different degrees or stages of disease an injury caused by interruption of the blood supply to the intestinal tissue. It is possible to distinguish three main different conditions underlying an intestinal ischemic event: arterial blood supply deficiency mainly related to embolism or thrombosis; impaired venous drainage; decreased mesenteric blood flow or low-flow state. Acute mesenteric ischemia can be considered a real, true emergency because of the associated significant mortality rate, which can be extremely high. A prompt diagnosis of any intestinal ischemic disorder of the intestine is imperative. However, because most patients affected by bowel ischemia can present with nonspecific signs and symptoms, it could be difficult to diagnose intestinal ischemia or infarction. Diagnostic imaging and especially multidetector computed tomography (MDCT) could be of great help in the management of patients with acute abdomen related to suspected acute mesenteric ischemia. Knowledge of the pathophysiology of the intestine is essential in order to recognize findings related to pathologic changes of the intestine affected by vascular disorders in different stages of disease

P. Taourel (ed.), *CT of the Acute Abdomen,* Medical Radiology. Diagnostic Imaging,
DOI: 10.1007/174_2010_82, © Springer-Verlag Berlin Heidelberg 2011

from different causes. In this chapter, MDCT findings of disorders from impaired venous drainage and from arterial blood flow insufficiency involving the small and the large intestine will be considered, considering also criteria for differential diagnosis.

1 Epidemiology

In patients with acute abdominal syndrome, diagnosis of intestinal disease related to vascular disorders could represent a critical diagnostic challenge for the emergency radiologist. Terms such as "ischemia" and "infarction" of the intestine are often used erroneously as synonyms; however, whereas the *ischemia* could be a totally reversible event, the *infarction* corresponds to a tissue death with no chance for the tissue to heal. Both terms indicate as different degrees or stages of disease an injury caused by interruption of the blood supply to the intestinal tissue (Fenoglio-Preiser et al. 2008). It is possible to distinguish three main different conditions underlying an intestinal ischemic event (Paterno and Longo 2008; Klatte et al. 1982): arterial blood supply deficiency mainly related to embolism or thrombosis (splanchnic); impaired venous drainage (postsplanchnic); decreased mesenteric blood flow or low-flow state (i.e., cardiac failure, myocardial infarction, bleeding, and hypovolemia) (presplanchnic). Acute mesenteric ischemia can be considered a real, true emergency because of the associated significant mortality rate, which can range between 30 and 90% (Paterno and Longo 2008; Herbert and Steele 2007; Martinez and Hogan 2004). The incidence of this pathologic entity was estimated in a large study based on either autopsies or operations as 12.9 per 100,000 persons per year, increasing with age and equally distributed among males and females (Acosta 2010). The same study reported the incidence of superior mesenteric artery occlusion, nonocclusive mesenteric ischemia, and mesenteric vein thrombosis as 68, 16, and 16%, respectively. It is obvious that a prompt diagnosis of any intestinal ischemic disorder of the intestine is imperative. However, because most patients affected by bowel ischemia can present with nonspecific signs and symptoms, especially those who have other pressing clinical issues, it could be difficult to recognize ischemia or infarction of the bowel (Gore et al. 2008).

Clinical questions in patients with acute abdomen from intestinal ischemia are different in most cases. Often other diseases (appendicitis, diverticulitis, bowel obstruction, peptic ulcer disease, gastroenteritis, infectious ileocolitis, inflammatory bowel disease, pancreatitis, cholecystitis, and rupture of an aortic aneurysm) enter the clinician's mind as the most likely diagnosis, with ischemia placed at the bottom of the differential diagnosis (Gore et al. 2008). Diagnostic imaging and especially multidetector computed tomography (CT) could be of great help in the management of patients with acute abdomen related to suspected acute mesenteric ischemia; however, in order to acquire important information for an efficient radiologic diagnosis, knowledge of the pathophysiology of the intestine is essential.

2 Physiopathology

In the acute ischemic disease of the intestine, multiple factors and processes contribute to develop bowel wall damage: cellular dysfunction, edema, and death caused by the interruption of a normal blood supply to the intestinal tissue; subsequent anoxia leads to lactic acidosis and anaerobic metabolism (Fenoglio-Preiser et al. 2008). It has been reported that to cause a tissue injury, the overall hematic supply to the small intestine has to be reduced by more than 50% (Fenoglio-Preiser et al. 2008; Bulkley et al.1985). The first sign of damage from ischemia is represented by increased capillary permeability, followed by epithelial cell injury if the ischemic event continues and persists (Fenoglio-Preiser et al. 2008). Mucosal damage then proceeds with coagulative necrosis development (Fenoglio-Preiser et al. 2008). If after an ischemic event reperfusion occurs, a reverse process could allow regeneration of the cells and washout of the toxic metabolites (Fenoglio-Preiser et al. 2008). The correlated acute inflammation status of the reperfused intestine is due to the production of reactive molecules caused by activation of the inflammatory cells (Fenoglio-Preiser et al. 2008). The reperfusion process with oxygen into anoxic tissue causes oxygen free radical cascades that secondarily increase mucosal and vascular permeability, with consequent potential mucosal damage that could also lead to bacterial sepsis (Fenoglio-Preiser et al. 2008). The microvascular injury from ischemia can result in a mucosal influx of neutrophil cells that also represents a source of reactive oxygen metabolites (Fenoglio-Preiser et al. 2008).

The small intestinal vasculature can respond to reduction of blood flow and of the oxygen content: occlusive arterial disease or significant reduction of inhaled oxygen causes a prompt but transient increase in spike potentials and contractions (Fondacaro 1984; Gilsdorf et al. 1983; Granger and Barrowman 1983; Kvietys et al. 1980; Wheaton et al. 1981). Quiescence of the musculature usually follows this intestinal hypermotility; segmental ischemia can cause alterations in motility of the entire small intestine through a reflex activity (Fondacaro 1984). In animal experimental data, it has been found that moderate ischemia can cause increased gastric emptying and decreased intestinal transit, however, 1 day later an active inflammation can occur at the ischemic site, with marked reduced motility of the entire intestine (Fondacaro 1984; Nylander and Wikstrom 1968). On the other hand, high-grade ischemia seems to stop the gastric emptying activity, with slowing of wave propagation in the visceral muscle (Fondacaro 1984). Restoration of a normal motor activity of the intestine after an ischemic event and reperfusion seems to be correlated with the temporal extent of the ischemia itself (Fondacaro 1984): the intestinal musculature seems to be less sensitive than the mucosa to ischemia, but if the ischemia is prolonged and severe, relevant damage to motility could occur (Fondacaro 1984).

In the large bowel, there is a complex network of intramural and extramural plexus of vascular supply from the superior and the inferior mesenteric arteries that can play an important role acting as collateral perfusion in the case of occlusion of an arterial major branch (Kvietys and Granger 1984). A lesser amount of epithelial desquamation and mild dilatation of blood vessels in the mucosa during the ischemic event represent damage to the colonic wall; after reperfusion, desquamation of the epithelium, cell necrosis, edema, and vascular dilatation can be observed (Kvietys and Granger 1984).

3 Clinical Findings

Abdominal pain represents the "core" symptoms underlying the acute disease caused by vascular disorder of the intestine. However, in the early phase of the disease severe pain could have no proportionate relationship to the physical signs, being due to an intense muscular spasm representing the immediate consequence of a decreased blood supply (Perko et al. 2002). Sudden symptoms of acute abdomen from mesenteric ischemia in patients apparently in good health is more frequently observed if the vascular disorder is related to embolism; in nonocclusive low-flow-state ischemia or in the case of mesenteric venous thrombosis, a gradual onset of symptoms with a more prolonged clinical course can be observed (Bartone et al. 2008). Typically, the mesenteric arterial embolism can clinically present different signs such as sudden abdominal pain, nausea, vomiting, hematochezia or melena, hypotension, peritonitis, whereas in the case of mesenteric arterial thrombosis it is usually evidenced as an insidious onset with progression of constant abdominal pain (Bartone et al. 2008). Nonocclusive ischemia can be correlated with acute or subacute symptoms, with abdominal tenderness and distension, muscular defense, hypotension, fever, decreased bowel sounds, nausea, and anorexia (Bartone et al. 2008). Patients with vascular disorders of the intestine related to impaired venous drainage from mesenteric vein thrombosis complain of a diffuse or localized long-standing abdominal pain associated with anorexia and diarrhea, or sometimes also fever and abdominal distension (Bartone et al. 2008). Patients with ischemic disease of the colon often present with left lower abdominal quadrant pain, with the descending colon being more commonly involved; a sudden, crampy abdominal pain is usually mentioned by the patient, accompanied by urgency to defecate; mild bleeding is common; abdominal distension, anorexia, nausea, and vomiting could also be present (Taourel et al. 2008). No specific laboratory parameter or biochemical or hematological combined marker seems to present sufficient sensitivity and specificity to allow diagnosis of acute mesenteric ischemia (Perko et al. 2002). The main laboratory findings correlated with mesenteric ischemia are hemoconcentration, acidosis with high anion gap, and alterations in the leukocyte count and lactate concentration (Bartone et al. 2008; Oldenburg et al. 2004). A diagnostic triad of acidosis, leukocytosis, and hyperphosphatemia has been reported as a useful tool in the clinical setting of a patient with acute mesenteric ischemia (Jamieson et al. 1982). Earlier, altered nonspecific laboratory parameters are high

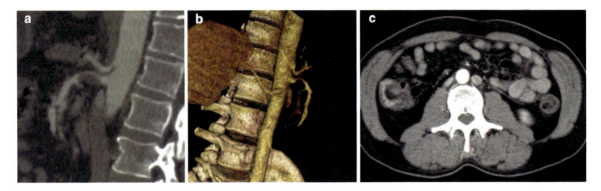

Fig. 1 Endoluminal defect of opacification from a thrombus in the superior mesenteric artery at the origin is appreciable on CT sagittal (**a**) and 3D (**b**) reconstructions. Signs of a spastic reflex ileus are evident, with normal enhanced and collapsed small bowel loops: this finding could represent the very early stage of ischemia, which requires accurate monitoring (**c**)

levels of serum amylase, aspartate aminotransferase, lactate dehydrogenate, and creatine phosphokinase; hyperphosphatemia and hyperkalemia are usually present at the late stage of ischemia, often associated with intestinal infarction and wall necrosis (Bartone et al. 2008; Oldenburg et al. 2004).

4 CT Findings

4.1 Small Intestine Vascular Disease from Arterial Supply Deficiency

The added value of the CT examination in a patient with acute abdomen related to mesenteric ischemia has been well established. This imaging method allows an efficient evaluation of the mesenteric vasculature as well as of the intestinal wall and other abdominal hollow and solid structures and related findings. The main problem in the imaging of the patient suspected of having an "intestinal ischemia" is related, on one hand, to "what" the CT findings are able to offer to us in term of diagnostic "specificity" and "sensitivity". On the other hand, problems in interpretation of the imaging findings are due in most cases to the lack of knowledge of the ischemic disease progression and pathologic changes of the intestinal wall with respect to the timing of the disease itself. Common mistakes could also be represented by the confusion between ischemia (potentially reversible injury) and infarction (not-reversible injury with death of the intestinal segment involved) and errors in reporting the salient imaging findings that could help surgeons and clinicians in the management of the patient with acute disease. To support this process, it is imperative to be able to evaluate the endoluminal opacification and caliber of the superior mesenteric arterial district, to diagnose the ischemic disease when at early stage, to make a correct diagnosis of damage from reperfusion, to suggest a correct follow-up in terms of diagnostic imaging or interventional procedures, and to note the intestinal infarction signs, giving a comprehensive evaluation of the extent of damage. At the basis of interpreting the CT images of acute disease of the small intestine due to arterial supply deficiency is the knowledge of the early morphologic changes of the intestine due to the acute injury. It is important to note that the intestine is an "alive" structure able to react to injury, firstly with a neurogenic response by the spastic reflex ileus, in which the intestinal loops are collapsed with no endoluminal content, followed by the hypotonic state, in which the loops are distended by air (Romano et al. 2008). In these stages, the superior mesenteric artery can show defects in the endoluminal opacification by thrombosis or embolism or have a caliber reduction from low-flow nonocclusive disease. Parietal enhancement of the small bowel could be normal or in some cases it can appear higher and brighter than usual (Fig. 1). In the following stage, characterized by predominantly air distension of the small intestine, the wall could appear thinner than normal and an accurate evaluation of the parietal enhancement is mandatory. From this stage, in the absence of reperfusion, intestinal ischemia can progress to infarction (Fig. 2). When on CT examination in a patient with acute abdomen the presence of air-dilated small bowel loops is evident, occlusion of the superior

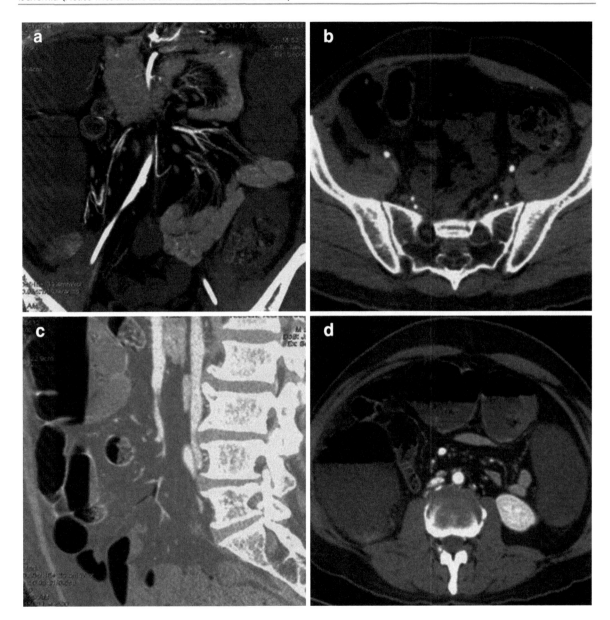

Fig. 2 Extensive defects of endoluminal opacification from thrombosis were found in the inferior mesenteric artery and its aberrant branches that supply the distal ileum (*arrow* in **a**). Consequentely, small intestine ileal segmental infarction can be noted, with loops distended by gas and fluid, with thin nonenhanced wall with little air bubbles either in the wall (**b**) or in small venous mesenteric vessels (**c**); the colon shows extensive signs of infarction, with absence of enhancement of the wall, which appears not thickened, with evidence also of some little air bubbles from parietal pneumatosis (**c**, **d**). The intestinal wall feature could be related to the absence of reperfusion after ischemia, the fluid filling the lumen attesting also to a subsequent stasis to the intestinal transit

mesenteric artery or a diminished caliber of the opacified vessel, in patients with suggestive clinical history for mesenteric vascular disorders, could be suggestive of intestinal ischemia. However, in the absence of vessel abnormalities and nonspecific clinical data, an alternative diagnostic hypothesis should be considered, with reflex spastic ileus and hypotonic ileus findings being nonspecific for intestinal ischemia but common as early reactions of different intestinal injuries (Romano et al. 2008). When the appearance of the small intestine is altered and the clinical symptoms are suggestive of intestinal

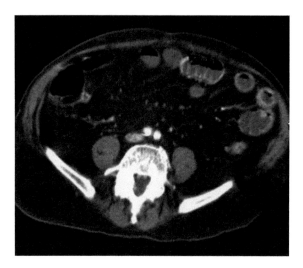

Fig. 3 In a patient affected by cardiopathy, the acute abdominal pain occurred suddenly after an atrial fibrillation episode. Nonsignificant reduction of the caliber of the superior mesenteric artery and secondary branches could be observed, neither an endoluminal defect of opacification from embolism; however, some of the intestinal loop had parietal hyperemia from ischemic injury. The patient recovered without the need for surgical intervention

ischemia in the absence of endoluminal vascular defects of opacification, low-flow-state conditions could be strongly considered (Romano et al. 2008). After an ischemic injury to the small intestine, when reperfusion occurs, blood plasma, contrast medium, or erythrocytes may extravasate through the disrupted vascular wall and mucosa, causing wall thickening and fluid filling of the lumen (Chou et al. 2004). CT findings in this stage of vascular disease of the small intestine could give us important information regarding the mesenteric arterial vasculature as well as the small bowel wall appearance, especially the presence of submucosa edema and possible moderate hyperdensity of the mucosa (Romano et al. 2008). In this stage it is important to differentiate between normal enhancement of the bowel wall and abnormal hyperdensity from mural hemorrhage. In fact, imaging findings on CT examination could be correlated with the histopathologic changes that occur in the intestine after an ischemic event, from the damage to the epithelium to inflammation, edema, and hemorrhage into the submucosa from reperfusion injuries (Romano et al. 2006) (Figs. 3, 4, 5, 6). At the same time, evidence from the CT findings of the late stage of intestinal vascular disease (intestinal infarction) with death, necrosis of the involved bowel, is correlated with the evidence of absent enhancement of the intestinal wall and the presence of pneumatosis (parietal, mesenteric, and portal) and free peritoneal air if perforation of the bowel has occurred (Romano et al. 2008). In this stage, attention to the endoluminal opacification of the mesenteric vessels could not be primary than a correct interpretation of the signs of intestinal necrosis (Romano et al. 2008).

4.2 Small Intestine Vascular Disease from Impaired Venous Drainage

Vascular disorders of the intestine due to mesenteric venous thrombosis in the acute forms differ from the acute conditions in terms of arterial origin, presenting a slow evolution on the order of days or weeks before an increased and persistent abdominal pain occurs (Laureano and Wade 1998). Frequently observed in patients with hepatopathy, cirrhosis, and/or portal hypertension (Fig. 7), thrombosis of the superior mesenteric vein can be also primary; however, other conditions such as polycytemia, systemic diseases, high level of plasmatic platelets, and an estrogen–progesterone therapy may all represent potential risk factors for mesenteric thrombosis (Jost and Gloviczki 2002; Kitchens 1992; Romano et al. 2006). CT examination to observe imaging findings of intestinal disorders related to mesenteric thrombosis is not rare (i.e., patients affected by chronic liver disease): difficulties can occur in discriminating between intestinal segments affected by injury from impaired venous drainage of medium–high stage and in diagnosing an intestinal infarction from venous origin. CT findings of vascular disorder due to impaired venous drainage from venous occlusions are related to the pathologic changes in the bowel wall, ranging from congestion and swelling of the bowel wall with edema to hemorrhage, with fluid flowing out from the bowel and the mesentery into the peritoneal cavity, as observed in animal experimental models (Friedberg 1965; Noer 1943; Polk 1966; Laureano and Wade 1998). Whereas in these models progression to infarction with bowel necrosis occurred in a few hours, in human clinical observations the entire process is longer, owing to the differences in collateral circulation (Laureano and Wade 1998). In radiologic clinical practice, on diagnostic imaging visualization of findings related to an early stage of intestinal disease from impaired venous

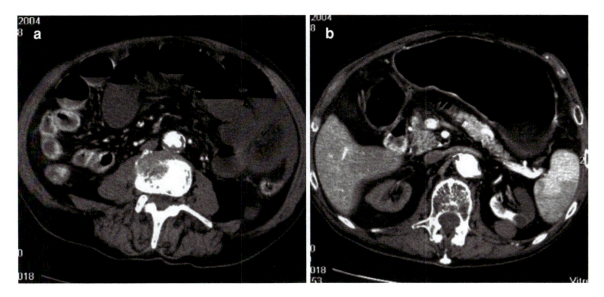

Fig. 4 This case of a small endoluminal defect of opacification in the secondary branches of the superior mesenteric artery shows different stages of ischemic disease affecting the small intestine, with some segments characterized by parietal hyperdensity from an intermediate degree of ischemia, whereas others are in the late stage, infarcted, with no enhancement of the wall, which appears thin with fluid filling the lumen (**a**). The loops with infarction did not show signs of damage from reperfusion. The superior mesenteric artery at the origin was well opacified (**b**)

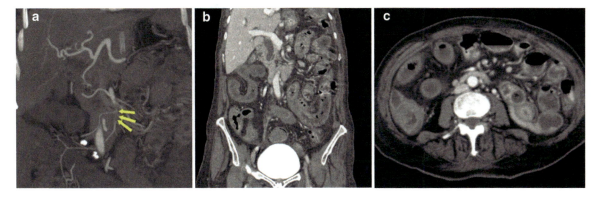

Fig. 5 The extensive defect of endoluminal opacification of the superior mesenteric artery (**a**) caused ischemic damage to the intestine with evidence of most small bowel loops as well as the ascending colon showing submucosa edema as a sign of reperfusion (**b**), whereas other small intestinal segments show hyperdensity from transmural hemorrhagic phenomena (**c**)

drainage may be rare: although if the initial reaction of the small intestine to a superior mesenteric vein occlusion could be done by spasticity of the loops, due to the underlying slow pathophysiologic process related to thrombosis, a following progression of the disease with air distension of the involved intestine could be masked by intramural and mesenteric edema (Romano et al. 2006). In terms of CT findings, in a patient with acute abdomen and evidence of mesenteric venous thrombosis, the evidence of spastic intestine with a collapsed lumen or distended by air could be considered as an early stage of vascular disease of the bowel. However, in most cases it is common to find imaging signs of more advanced disease (Romano et al. 2008). With progression of mesenteric venous occlusion, the intravascular volume and the hydrostatic pressure increase and the arterial blood flows into capillaries and venules of the

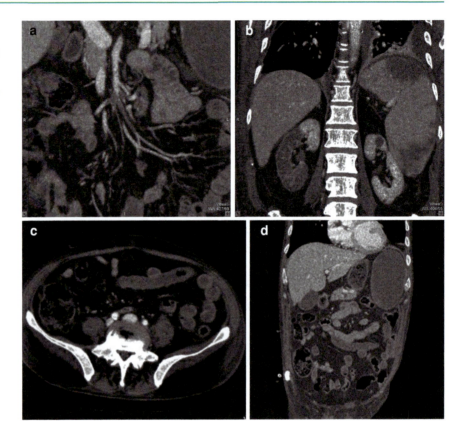

Fig. 6 Thrombosis of superior mesenteric artery branches (**a**) caused ischemic injury of the small intestine; ischemic area of the right kidney and spleen could also be noted (**b**). Reperfusion damage in the phase of healing could be observed with weak thickening and hypodensity of some intestinal segments, whereas others appear completely normal in features and wall enhancement (**c**, **d**)

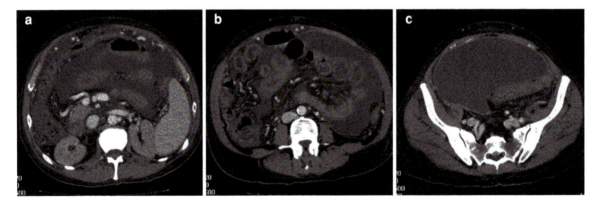

Fig. 7 Bowel wall alteration from portal hypertension in a patient with liver cirrhosis and ascites. Parietal thickening of the intestine characterized either by submucosal edema, particularly at the level of the ascending colon (**a**), or by diffuse hyperdensity from submucosal hemorrhage (**b**, **c**)

bowel and the mesentery, causing extravasation of plasma, red blood cells, and contrast material in the fenestrations of the arteriocapillary endothelium into the submucosa (Chou 2002, 2004). CT findings at this stage of disease are the evidence of mesenteric venous thrombosis, small bowel thickening, higher enhancement from intramural hemorrhage, and evidence of submucosa edema, with alternation of layers of different density, with hypodense submucosa (Romano et al. 2006) (Figs. 8, 9). From this stage, healing of the intestinal injury related to impaired venous drainage can be often achieved with a medical

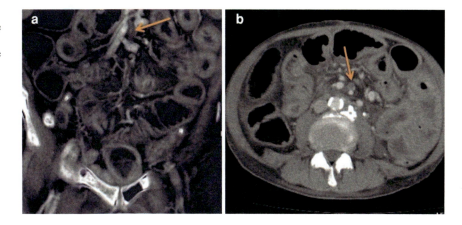

Fig. 8 Extensive thrombosis of the secondary branch of the superior mesenteric vein (*arrow* in **a**, **b**) with evidence of small intestinal wall thickening with edema; note the diffuse hyperdensity not limited to mucosa

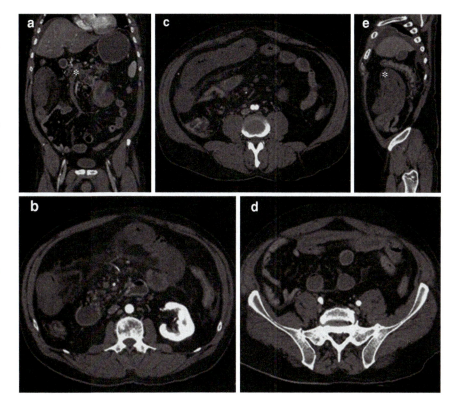

Fig. 9 Extensive splenic-portal venous thrombosis (*asterisk* in **a**), with infarction of some jejunal loops (**b**, **c**). Note the feature of the distal jejunum, presenting parietal enhancement and damage from impaired venous drainage; note the appearance of the ileum, with most loops collapsed, spastic (**d**). Different appearance of the intestine with the presence of infarcted segments (*asterisk* in **e**) and damage from impaired venous drainage in the following tract; ileum is collapsed. Note also the appearance of the large intestine, with tristratification of the wall and hyperenhanced mucosa

therapy; however, persistence of the disease causes a chronic alteration in the intestinal wall, and rarely progresses to intestinal infarction (Romano et al. 2006). In this case, the CT findings of intestinal infarction as the late stage of injury from impaired venous drainage (Fig. 9) are related to the evidence of mesenteric vein occlusion, peritoneal fluid, marked wall thickening, absence of parietal enhancement, and intramural and/or portal-mesenteric pneumatosis (Romano et al. 2008).

4.3 Colonic Ischemia

Vascular disorders of the colon include various pathologic and clinical findings of different grades of severity from self-limiting and transient ischemia to bowel infarction (Marston 1986; Robert et al. 1993; Balthazar et al. 1999; Romano et al. 2006). Ischemic colitis was considered as a form of nonocclusive ischemic disease, with no correlations between the site and extension of the intestinal involvement and the distribution of the superior or inferior mesentery artery or vein (Eisenberg et al. 1979; Brandt and Boley 1993; Balthazar et al. 1999; Zimmermann and Granger 1992; Romano et al. 2006). The colonic regions pertinent to Griffith's point (the junction between the distribution of the superior and inferior mesenteric arteries closed to the colonic splenic flexure) and Sudeck's point (the anastomotic plexus between the inferior mesenteric and the hypogastric arteries at the rectosigmoid junction) have been reported as most commonly involved by ischemic injuries (Balthazar et al. 1999; Rogers and David 1995; Romano et al. 2006). Regarding the various degrees of injury from ischemia affecting the colon, the damage could range from mucosal ulcerations to submucosa edema and hemorrhage to transmural infarction (Balthazar et al. 1999). CT findings of ischemic disease of the colon could be considered in a disease–progression grading scale (Romano et al. 2006), from early injury to late evidence of infarction. Acute ischemic damage to the colon can be segmental or diffuse, with the typical pattern consisting in hemorrhage in the lamina propria associated with superficial epithelial necrosis (Whitehead 1972; Petras 2004) that could progress to full-thickness ulceration of the mucosa (Petras 2004). At this stage CT could be a useful tool to evaluate the colonic wall feature and injury: mural thickening with hyperdensity of the mucosa from hemorrhage associated with submucosal edema has the typical sign of the "little rose" (Romano et al. 2006, 2007), appreciable on the axial scan especially at the level of the descending colon (Fig. 10). A small amount of peritoneal fluid with evidence of pericolic streakiness and shaggy contour of the involved intestine are additional findings to note (Romano et al. 2006). The inferior artery vascular tree could be easily evaluated on the multiplanar reformation in the arterial phase of the study. Persistence of the ischemic injury without reperfusion causes a concentric, symmetric, mild mural thickening with homogeneous density of the large bowel wall, offering a well-defined edge (Fig. 11); pericolic streakiness could be present as well as a moderate amount of peritoneal fluid (Romano et al. 2006). If the ischemia persists longer, infarction could develop, with necrosis of the involved colonic segment. Reperfusion after the ischemic event causes marked submucosal edema (Fig. 12), wall thickening and inhomogeneous parietal enhancement, loss of colonic haustra, and pericolic streakiness of different degrees (Romano et al. 2006).

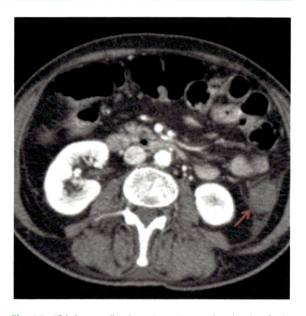

Fig. 10 "Little rose" sign (*arrow*) at the level of the descending colon from the early stage of large bowel ischemia due to parietal thickening with mucosal hyperdensity and submucosal hypodensity from edema. Note the small amount of perivisceral fluid

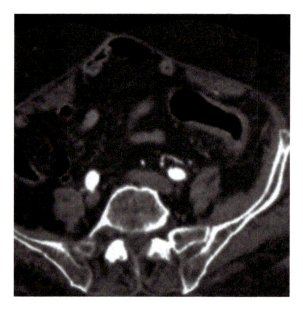

Fig. 11 Descending colon ischemia at the second stage without reperfusion showing symmetric thickening of the wall

Progression of the colonic ischemia to infarction leads to imaging findings related to bowel necrosis with the absence of enhancement and the presence of parietal pneumatosis and free peritoneal or retroperitoneal air if perforation occurs (Fig. 2, 13).

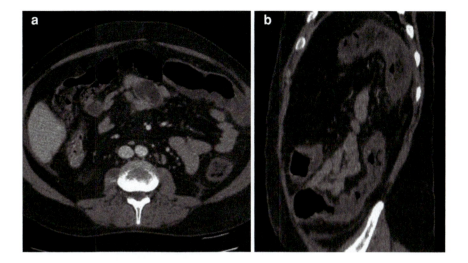

Fig. 12 Ischemia of the colon with reperfusion signs (**a**, **b**): parietal thickening with submucosal edema

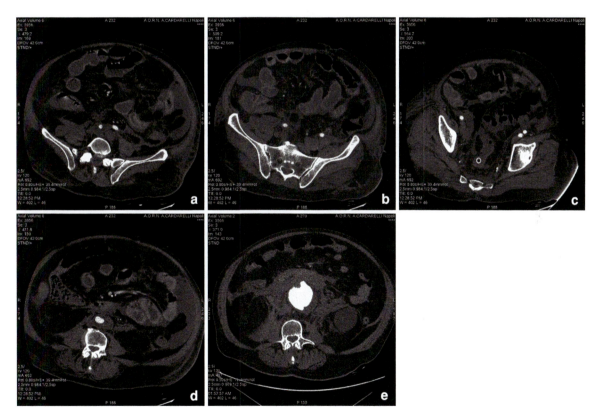

Fig. 13 Infarction of the distal descending and sigmoid colon infarction (**a–c**) in a patient submitted to abdominal aortic surgery (**d**) after rupture of an aneurysm (**e**). Note the complete absence of enhancement of the involved colonic segment and the presence of a bubble of gas from parietal pneumatosis due to the late stage of ischemia with infarction

4.4 CT Pitfalls

Diagnosis of intestinal ischemia is not easy, especially if the CT examination is not performed adequately (i.e., administration of intravenous contrast medium, multiphase examination, thin slice thickness with back reconstructions less than 1 mm). Evaluation of the intestinal trophism is not easy without knowledge of the physiopathologic changes that occur in the bowel wall as a consequence of deficiency in blood supply or

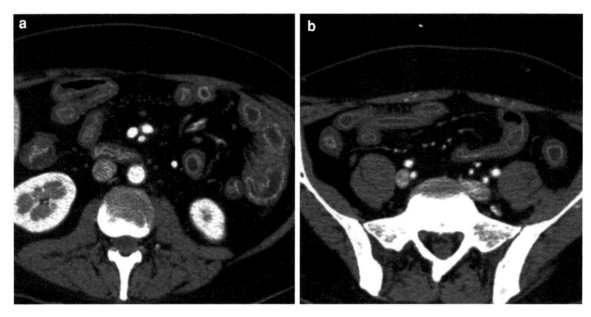

Fig. 14 Intestinal ischemia has to be differentiated from other findings of intestinal wall abnormality. In this case a diffuse enteritis in a young patient with bone marrow transplant is shown (**a**, **b**). Note the diffuse "target sign" with hyperenhancement of the mucosa and stratification of the wall. Mesenteric vessels were well opacified

Fig. 15 Small intestine segmental thickening with mucosal and serosal hemorrhage and mesenteric engorgement in a patient affected by coagulopathy (**a**, **b**)

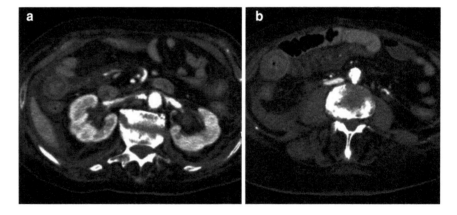

impaired venous drainage. Reperfusion damage to the intestine from an arterial cause, mainly represented on CT by evidence of submucosal hypodensity from edema, has to be differentiated with the target sign from venous occlusive disease or stratification of the bowel from inflammation related to enteritis of other origin (Figs. 14, 15). Again, evaluation of parietal enhancement of a segment affected by disease from impaired venous drainage is not easy in some cases for experienced radiologists not well trained in emergency intestinal disease imaging. Other aspects to consider as potential pitfalls are the enhancement and features of the colon in ischemic injury: weak hyperdensity of the bowel wall from hemorrhage could be erroneously considered a "normal finding," or a mistake could be made in evaluating a thin colonic segment from infarction, described as "ischemic" and not irreversible death. Appropriate definition of "pneumatosis" and evaluation of any eventual different benign cause of this findings (such as the presence of parietal air from damage related to overdistension of the lumen, not related to wall infarction) is mandatory (Fig. 16). To limit any potential error in diagnosis in the case of CT examination for clinical suspicion of vascular intestinal disorder, it should be mandatory to evaluate the imaging findings related to the bowel wall and to

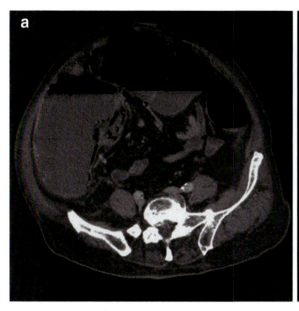 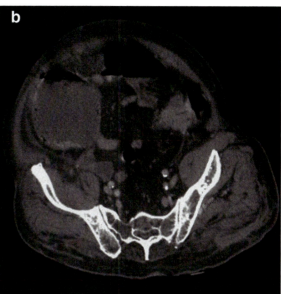

Fig. 16 Parietal pneumatosis is not related to intestinal infarction. Presence of gas in the wall of the ascending colon (**a**, **b**) distended by fluid in a patient with large bowel obstruction caused by a proximal sigmoid colon neoplasm (**b**). The wall of the ascending colon shows normal parietal enhancement with no sign of infarction. The concept of "benign" pneumatosis is related to the presence of this finding in conditions other than intestinal ischemia; in this case the parietal pneumatosis was caused by overdistension of the gut with damage to the mucosa and spread in the wall of some amount of gas

other abdominal structures considering the clinical history of the patient, the laboratory parameters, the type of abdominal pain, and the results of any eventual recent diagnostic imaging examination performed.

5 CT Impact on Management

Advances in technology of the CT equipment with the introduction of multidetector-row machines contributed to improvement in the diagnostic imaging using CT, with a positive gain in time needed and efficacy in response to clinical questions, especially in emergency patients. The use of multiphasic evaluation of anatomic structures with the added value of some software to reduce the overall radiation doses administered to patients during examinations improved the number and type of clinical requests for this imaging method. Actually, the use of CT is widespread in the main emergency department and diagnostic efficacy in numerous and different diseases, traumatic and nontraumatic, is attested by multiple scientific publications from large series of patients. The impact of CT on the management of the acute abdominal pain from mesenteric ischemic affection is high: the use of this method as a first-line or immediate second-line examination, because of the diagnostic support provided by the imaging findings, could be of extreme importance either to indicate in what phase or stage of ischemic disease (if any) the patient is or to allow a prompt diagnosis of vascular disease of the intestine that could require interventional procedures or surgery.

6 Diagnostic Strategy

Despite the current widespread use of CT as the first-line examination in patients with acute abdominal pain, there is still a role for the basic imaging methods (conventional radiograph and ultrasonography), represented by detection of gross abdominal findings underlying an acute disease, such as the evidence on conventional radiography of fluid or gaseous distension of the intestine and bowel loop features or the presence of free peritoneal air. Using ultrasonography of the abdomen it is possible to document the presence of peritoneal fluid as well as the evaluation of the intestinal peristalsis, the fluid-filled lumen, and the features of the bowel wall and plicae. Findings from basic imaging methods could help in selecting patients who could benefit from an immediate CT examination, evaluating firstly the cause and potential stage of the disease. Detection of an endoluminal defect of opacification of mesenteric vessels by CT could suggest the type of disease to be subjected to angiographic procedures or to be clinically treated with medical therapy. The most important role of CT is to provide diagnostic information for a correct interpretation of the findings in order to select patients who require immediate surgical intervention. Follow-up examination of the intermediate stage of ischemia could be done with CT if no specific radiation risks are present. Serial ultrasonography examination could help in monitoring any abnormality in the bowel wall detected by CT, especially the damage from reperfusion characterized by parietal thickening and edema, suggesting a relapse in injury or recovery from an ischemic event. The combination of findings from different imaging methods could be added value for an efficient diagnostic strategy for patients affected by vascular disorders of the intestine.

References

Acosta S (2010) Epidemiology of mesenteric vascular disease: clinical implications. Semin Vasc Surg 23(1):4–8

Balthazar EJ, Yen BC, Gordon RB (1999) Ischemic colitis: CT evaluation of 54 cases. Radiology 211:381–388

Bartone G et al (2008) Clinical symptoms of intestinal vascular disorders. Radiol Clin North Am 46:887–889

Brandt LJ, Boley SJ (1993) Ischemic and vascular lesions of the bowel. In: Sleisenger MH, Fordtran JS (eds) Gastrointestinal disease: pathophysiology, diagnosis, management, 5th edn. Saunders, Philadelphia, pp 1940–1945

Bulkley GB et al (1985) Relationship of blood flow and oxygen consumption to ischemic injury in the canine small intestine. Gastroenterology 89:852–857

Chou CK (2002) CT manifestation of bowel ischemia. AJR Am J Roentgenol 178:87–91

Chou CK et al (2004) CT of small bowel ischemia. Abdom Imaging 29:18–22

Eisenberg RL, Montgomery CK, Margulis AR (1979) Coltis in the elderly: ischemic colitis mimicking ulcerative and granulomatous colitis. AJR Am J Roentgenol 133:1113–1118

Fenoglio-Preiser CM et al (2008) The nonneoplastic small intestine. In: Fenoglio-Preiser CM (ed) Gastrointestinal pathology. An atlas and text, 3rd edn. Wolters Kluwer, Lippincott, Williams & Wilkins, Philadelphia, pp 326–339

Fondacaro JD (1984) Intestinal blood flow and motility. In: Shepherd AP, Granger DN (eds) Physiology of the intestinal circulation. Raven Press, New York, pp 107–119

Friedberg MJ, Polk HC Jr (1965) Superior mesenteric arteriography in experimental mesenteric venous thrombosis. Radiology 85:38–45

Gilsdorf RB et al (1983) Posterior hypothalamic effects on gastrointestinal blood flow in the conscious cat. Proc Soc Exp Biol Med 143:329–334

Gore RM et al (2008) Imaging in intestinal ischemic disorders. Radiol Clin North Am 46:845–875

Granger DN, Barrowman JA (1983) Microcirculation of the alimentary tract. II. Pathophysiology of edema. Gastroenterology 84:1035–1049

Herbert GS, Steele SR (2007) Acute and chronic mesenteric ischemia. Surg Clin North Am 87:1115–1134

Jamieson WG et al (1982) The early diagnosis of massive acute intestinal ischemia. Br J Surg 69(Suppl):552–553

Jost CJ, Gloviczki P (2002) Mesenteric vein thrombosis. In: Geroulakos G, Cherry KJ (eds) Disease of the visceral circulation. Arnold, London, pp 145–157

Klatte EC et al (1982) Angiographic studies of the upper gastrointestinal tract. In: Scott HW, Sawyers JL (eds) Surgery of the stomach, duodenum and small intestine. pp 194–197

Kitchens CS (1992) Evolution of our understanding of the pathophysiology of primary mesenteric venous thrombosis. Am J Surg 163:346–348

Kvietys PR, Granger DN (1984) Physiology, pharmacology and pathology of the colonic circulation. In: Shepherd AP, Granger DN (eds) Physiology of the intestinal circulation. Raven Press, New York, pp 131–142

Kvietys PR et al (1980) Intrinsic control of colonic blood flow and oxygenation. Am J Physiol 238:478–484

Laureano BA, Wade TP (1998) Mesenteric venous disease. In: Longo WE, Peterson GJ, Jacobs DL (eds) Intestinal ischemia disorders. Quality Medical Publishing, St Louis, pp 207–219

Martinez JP, Hogan GJ (2004) Mesenteric ischemia. Emerg Med Clin North Am 22(4):909–928

Marston A (1986) Vasular disease of the gastrointestinal tract. William and Wilkins, Baltimore, pp 152–173

Noer RJ (1943) The blood vessels of the jejunum and ileum: a comparative study of man and certain laboratory animals. Am J Anat 73:293–334

Nylander G, Wikstrom S (1968) Propulsive gastrointestinal motility in regional and graded ischemia of the small bowel. An experimental study in rats. I. Immediate results. Acta Chir Scand 385(Suppl):1–67

Oldenburg WA et al (2004) Acute mesenteric ischemia: a clinical review. Arch Intern Med 164(10):1054–1062

Paterno F, Longo WE (2008) The etiology and pathogenesis of vascular disorders of the intestine. Radiol Clin North Am 46:877–885

Perko MJ et al (2002) Management of acute visceral ischemia. In: Geroulakos G, Cherry KJ (eds) Diseases of the visceral circulation. Arnold, London, pp 80–87

Petras RE (2004) Acute ischemic colitis. In: Mills SE (ed) Sternberg's diagnostic surgical pathology. Lippincott Williams & Wilkins, Philadelphia, p 1495

Polk HC Jr (1966) Experimental mesenteric venous occlusion. III. Diagnosis and treatment of induced mesenteric venous thrombosis. Ann Surg 163:432–444

Robert JH, Mentha G, Rohner A (1993) Ischaemic colitis: two distinct patterns of severity. Gut 34:4–6

Rogers AI, David S (1995) Intestinal blood flow and diseases of vascular impairement. In: Haubrich WS, Schaffner F, Berck JE (eds) Gastroenterology, 5th edn. Saunders, Philadelphia, pp 1212–1234

Romano S et al (2006) Ischemia and infarction of the small bowel and colon: spectrum of imaging findings. Abdom Imaging 31(3):277–292

Romano S et al (2007) Multidetector row computed tomography findings from ischemia to infarction of the large bowel. Eur J Rad 61(3):433–441

Romano S et al (2008) Small bowel vascular disorders from arterial etiology and impaired venous drainage. Radiol Clin North Am 46:891–908

Taourel P et al (2008) Imaging of ischemic colitis. Radiol Clin North Am 46:909–924

Wheaton GB et al (1981) Gross anatomy of the splanchnic vasculature. In: Granger DN, Bulkley GB (ed) Measurement of blood flow: applications to the splanchnic circulation. Williams and Wilkins, Baltimore, pp 9–45

Whitehead R (1972) The pathology of intestinal ischemia. Clin Gastroenterol 1:613–637

Zimmermann BJ, Granger DN (1992) Reperfusion injury. Surg Clin North Am 72:65–83

Diverticulitis

Jean-Michel Bruel and Patrice Taourel

Contents

1	**Introduction**	200
2	**Epidemiology**	200
3	**Physiopathology**	200
4	**Clinical Findings**	200
5	**CT Findings**	201
6	**CT Pitfalls and Limits**	204
6.1	Epiploic Appendagitis	205
6.2	Differentiation of Diverticulitis from Carcinoma	205
6.3	Right-Sided Colonic Diverticulitis	207
6.4	Delayed Diagnosis of Diverticulitis	208
7	**CT Impact on the Management**	208
7.1	CT Confirms the Diagnosis of Diverticulitis	209
7.2	CT Evaluates the Severity and Extent of Diverticulitis	209
7.3	CT Assists the Treatment Planning of Abscesses	214
7.4	CT Demonstrates Other Causes of Abdominal Pain	214
8	**Diagnostic Strategy**	214
8.1	CT: The Imaging Test of Choice for the Diagnosis and Management	214
8.2	Plain Films of the Abdomen	216
8.3	Contrast Enema	216
8.4	Ultrasonography	217
8.5	Magnetic Resonance Imaging	217
8.6	Colonoscopy	217
9	**Conclusion**	218
References		218

J.-M. Bruel (✉)
Department of Medical Imaging, Hôpital Saint-Eloi,
CHRU of Montpellier, 80 avenue Augustin Fliche,
34295 Montpellier Cedex 5, France
e-mail: chujmbruel@gmail.com

P. Taourel
Department of Medical Imaging,
Hôpital Lapeyronie, CHRU of Montpellier,
191 Avenue du Doyen Gaston Giraud,
34295 Montpellier Cedex 5, France

Abstract

Colonic diverticulosis, defined as a symptomless acquired disease resulting from the development of multiple diverticula on the colonic wall, is the most common colonic disease in Western industrial countries. The spectrum of acute diverticulitis, resulting from acute inflammation and infection of these diverticula, ranges from localized microperforation with a focal diverticulitis to life-threatening free perforation with generalized purulent or fecal peritonitis. After the initial clinical attack, recurrent episodes are frequently observed. The most common complication of diverticulitis is diverticular abscesses, much more severe when they are not confined to the mesocolon. The severity of a clinical episode of acute colonic diverticulitis is related to the development of pericolic lesions (abscess, fistula, peritonitis). In these conditions, computed tomography is now the diagnostic radiological examination of choice in patients with suspected acute diverticulitis, and should be used without delay in every patient in every clinical episode of acute diverticulitis (1) to confirm the diagnosis of acute diverticulitis, (2) to identify or exclude other causes of abdominal pain, (3) to evaluate the severity and the extent of the acute disease, and (4) to assist the decision management.

P. Taourel (ed.), *CT of the Acute Abdomen,* Medical Radiology. Diagnostic Imaging,
DOI: 10.1007/174_2010_83, © Springer-Verlag Berlin Heidelberg 2011

1 Introduction

Diverticulitis is defined as inflammation of diverticula, or small outpouchings, of the digestive tract (Balthazar 1994; Ferzoco et al. 1998; Lawrimore and Rhea 2004; DeStigter and Keating 2009). Even though such an inflammation may occur in diverticula everywhere in the digestive tract (such as in the esophagus, stomach, duodenum, jejunum, or ileum), the term "diverticulitis" usually refers to the inflammation of colonic diverticula, and only this part will be discussed in this chapter.

Colonic diverticula are acquired herniations of the mucosa and of parts of the submucosa through the muscularis propria. Colonic diverticulosis is a clinically silent (symptomless) disease resulting from the development of multiple diverticula on the colonic wall. "Diverticular disease" includes the diverticulitis and its complications, and the diverticular hemorrhage. Diverticular hemorrhage is a complication of diverticulosis, but is not related to a clinical attack of diverticulitis, and therefore is discussed not in this chapter but in the chapter "Gastrointestinal Bleeding". "Colonic diverticulitis" refers to the acute inflammation and/or infection of diverticula. "Complicated diverticulitis" corresponds to the development of severe complications such as abscesses, fistula, peritonitis, and digestive stenoses resulting in bowel obstruction. The scheme devised by Hinchey et al. (1978) is a useful tool to classify the variety of inflammatory conditions encountered in patients with acute colonic diverticulitis according to the severity of the disease. This Hinchey scheme separates acute colonic diverticulitis into four stages: stage I pericolic abscess or phlegmon; stage II pelvic, intra-abdominal, or retroperitoneal abscess; stage III generalized purulent peritonitis; and stage IV generalized fecal peritonitis. It has good correlation with the morbidity and mortality of the disease.

2 Epidemiology

Colonic diverticulosis is the most common colonic disease in Western industrial nations, with an estimated incidence of 30% in individuals over 50 years old and up to 50% in individuals over the age of 70 and 66% in individuals over the age of 85 (Ferzoco et al. 1998). The acquired herniations of the colonic mucosa through weak spots of the muscularis propria (mostly at sites where the vasa recta perforate the muscularis propria and penetrate the submucosa) commonly result in multiple diverticula. The diverticular wall is therefore thin, including the mucosa and portions of the submucosa, but not the muscularis propria. The size of the diverticula ranges from tiny spikes to larger spheres up to 2 cm in diameter. Diverticula are found in all parts of the colon, although by far the most common location is the sigmoid, where the intraluminal pressure is the highest, particularly as a response to a lifelong consumption of a low-residue diet (producing low-volume stools that require a high degree of propulsive effort for expulsion). The colonic wall of patients with diverticulosis is markedly thickened by "myochosis" (Balthazar 1994; Ferzoco et al. 1998; Lawrimore and Rhea 2004).

3 Physiopathology

Diverticulitis occurs in 10–35% of patients with diverticulosis. The pathological basis is an infection and inflammation of the apex of a diverticulum, resulting in a microperforation of the diverticulum wall and spreading rapidly into the surrounding pericolic and mesocolic fat inflammation. Consequently, the pivotal lesions of the disease may be better described as "peridiverticulitis" or pericolitis, and the severity of a clinical attack of the disease is related to the development of the pericolic lesions (abscess, fistula, and peritonitis) (Balthazar 1994; Ferzoco et al. 1998; Lawrimore and Rhea 2004). However, the terms "perforated diverticulitis" and "perforated diverticulum" should be reserved for free (not-walled-off) perforation into the peritoneal cavity, resulting in purulent or fecal peritonitis (Ferzoco et al. 1998). These physiopathological data stress the importance of the use of cross-sectional imaging for direct visualization of both the intramural component (diverticula and colonic wall thickening) and the extramural component (inflammatory changes in the pericolic fat and advanced complications) of diverticular disease.

4 Clinical Findings

The clinical diagnosis of acute colonic diverticulitis may be difficult. The classic pattern of left lower quadrant pain, tenderness, fever, and leukocytosis is theoretically suggestive of acute colonic diverticulitis (Balthazar 1994; Ferzoco et al. 1998; Lawrimore and Rhea 2004; DeStigter and Keating 2009) but the complete combination of these signs is actually seldom found. In a large prospective study including 542 patients with acute diverticulitis of the descending or sigmoid colon, a temperature of more than 99.5°F was found in only 77% of patients and leukocytosis of more than 11,000/mL was found in 54% of patients (Ambrosetti et al. 2002). Moreover numerous acute abdominal conditions can mimic the classic pattern of a diverticulitis, and a final diagnosis of acute colonic diverticulitis is assessed in less than 50% of patients with clinically suspected diverticulitis. Finally, even though clinical and biological findings can indicate the diagnosis of acute colonic diverticulitis, they may fail to assess the site and the severity of the pericolic extension of the lesions. Severe diverticulitis can occur in certain groups of patients with altered immunity response; these risk factors include debilitated elderly patients, patients with renal disorders, and patients receiving corticosteroids or nonsteroidal anti-inflammatory drugs. It has been reported that the initial attack is frequently more severe and that recurrent episodes of diverticulitis do not lead to more complications and more conservative treatment failure (Pittet et al. 2009). Several observers have emphasized that the frequency of acute colonic diverticulitis is increasing in young people (less than 40 years old), particularly with obesity (Shah et al. 2010), and that young patients often develop more severe forms of diverticulitis (Simonowitz and Paloyan 1977; Chodak et al. 1981; Ouriel and Schwartz 1983; Freischlag et al. 1986; Ambrosetti et al. 1994; Hall et al. 2010), but this last issue remains controversial (Zaidi and Daly 2006).

Thus the systematic use of a technique assessing the diagnosis accurately and evaluating the severity of the disease is of outstanding importance. This technique used today is computed tomography (CT).

5   CT Findings

The use of CT for evaluation of acute colonic diverticulitis was initially reported more than 25 years ago (Hulnick et al. 1984; Cho et al. 1990; Balthazar et al. 1990; Pradel et al. 1997) but the diagnosis and management of patients with diverticulitis was dramatically improved with the development of multidetector CT at the beginning of the twenty-first century and CT is nowadays the method of choice. Multidetector CT scanners allow thinner section slices, and a shorter examination time, resulting in images with better resolution and high-quality coronal and sagittal images (Kircher et al. 2002 ; Werner et al. 2003). Moreover, the prospective study by Ambrosetti et al. (2000), demonstrating the higher accuracy of CT versus contrast enema (CE), is of outstanding importance for the definitive acceptance of CT as the method of choice.

The use of CT in patients with suspected diverticulitis requires careful attention to the CT protocol.

The multidetector CT image data volume should be obtained from the dome of the diaphragm to the inferior aspect of the pubic symphysis (with thin collimation and a short acquisition time); CT data are reconstructed with thin, overlapped slices for multiplanar (coronal and sagittal planes) reformation and 3–5-mm-thick contiguous axial slices; the image series are sent to a dedicated workstation and/or a picture archiving and communication system.

Vascular enhancement by iodinated contrast material is mandatory in most cases, unless it is contraindicated; special attention should be paid to older patients and those with metabolic disorders in assessing the renal impact of contrast material administration. In general, the most helpful scanning phase is the late portal phase (70 s) for a better delineation of the colonic wall and the enhanced wall of small pericolic abscesses, but also for evaluating the mesenteric vessels by systematically looking for inferior mesenteric and portal vein thrombosis, and hepatic abscesses, acute colonic diverticulitis being the main cause of the septic thrombosis of the portal vein. Multiphasic scanning should be used only for specific indications to limit the radiation dose particularly in young patients with colonic diverticular disease that may lead to recurrent acute episodes. This stresses the development of CT protocols with a low radiation dose (Tack et al. 2005).

Changes in the CT protocol should be decided on according to the clinical conditions and/or the preliminary results of the CT examination. In selected cases, colorectal opacification (Figs. 1, 2) and/or acquisition of images with the patient in the prone position may be helpful to clarify equivocal findings, particularly for assessing the extradigestive

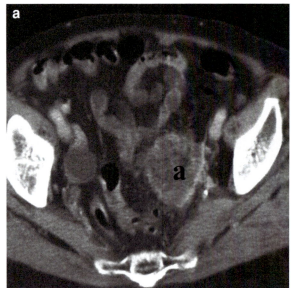
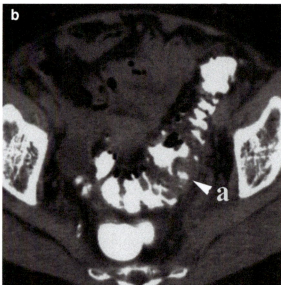

Fig. 1 Acute diverticulitis of the sigmoid colon (complicated by a large abscess). Technical protocol of computed tomography (CT) examination: axial CT slices before (a) and after (b) colonic contrast material administration through a rectal tube. a The heterogeneous content of the abscess (*a*). b After colonic contrast material administration, spread of the colonic contrast material into the abscess's cavity is clearly visible (*arrowhead a*)

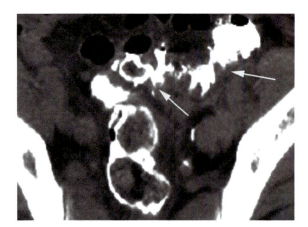

Fig. 2 Acute diverticulitis of the sigmoid colon. Technical protocol of CT examination: multidetector CT (MDCT) examination after rectal administration of colonic contrast material. The coronal reformat shows several "arrowhead sign" patterns (*arrows*), defined by an arrowhead-shaped configuration of contrast material found at the narrowed neck of a diverticulum

location of a small amount of gas and/or the route of a sinus tract or a complex fistula, and to demonstrate the "arrowhead sign," defined as an arrowhead-shaped configuration of contrast material found at the narrowed neck of a diverticulum (Rao and Rhea 1998;

Kircher et al. 2002). As many authors, we do not use oral contrast material.

The method of image evaluation is critical to optimize interpretation; additional window level and width settings are mandatory to identify tiny bubbles of extraluminal gas (CT lung windows); the systematic use of multiplanar reformation, particularly in the coronal plane, is recommended (Paulson et al. 2004; Ghekiere et al. 2007).

The main CT findings for the diagnosis of acute colonic diverticulitis are nowadays well established (Pradel et al. 1997; Lefèvre et al. 1999; Horton et al. 2000; Kircher et al. 2002; Werner et al. 2003) and associate both the intramural patterns (diverticula and bowel wall thickening) and the extramural patterns consisting in inflammatory changes in the pericolic and mesocolic fat (Fig. 3).

Thickening of the bowel wall should be considered as present when the thickness of the colonic wall, evaluated in a colonic segment with a slightly distended lumen, exceeds 4 mm. Diverticula are easily identified as flask-shaped outpouchings from the colonic wall, filled with air or residues of fecal or contrast material. Actually, the hallmark of acute diverticulitis on CT scans is the alteration of the pericolic fat (Balthazar 1994; Kircher et al. 2002;

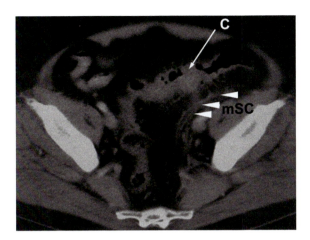

Fig. 3 Nonsevere acute colonic diverticulitis, without any abscess. Characteristic patterns combine intramural patterns—note the thickening of the colonic wall with progressive transition (*arrow C*) and the numerous small air-filled diverticula—and extramural patterns with thickening of the root of the sigmoid mesocolon (*arrowheads mSC*) and the pericolic fat stranding within the mesocolon

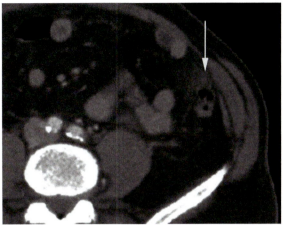

Fig. 5 Focal acute diverticulitis at the descending–sigmoid colon transition. The MDCT axial slice depicts linear or inhomogeneous soft-tissue attenuation interspersed in the pericolic fat, and defined as "fat stranding". Note the diverticulum located in the center of fat stranding, representing the sign of "inflamed diverticulum"

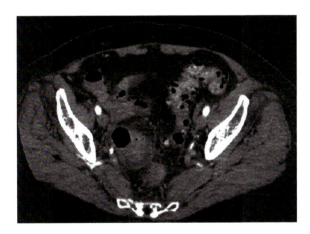

Fig. 4 Diverticulosis without any patterns indicating acute diverticulitis. Note the thickening of the wall of the sigmoid colon and the numerous diverticula of various sizes, filled with air and/or residues of fecal or colonic contrast material

Pereira et al. 2004) because the intramural patterns such as diverticula and bowel wall thickening related to myochosis, even in combination, can be observed in diverticulosis, from any acute disease, as demonstrated in Fig. 4.

The basic alteration of the pericolic fat is the fat stranding, which is defined as a linear or inhomogeneous soft-tissue density interspersed in the fat. The degree of the extracolic inflammatory reaction varies depending on the size of perforation, bacterial contamination, and host response. In focal diverticulitis only a slight increase in the attenuation of fat adjacent to a single diverticulum may be present, and the "inflamed diverticulum" pattern has been defined as a diverticulum located in the center of fat stranding (Kircher et al. 2002) (Figs. 5, 6).

In mild cases with a walled-off perforation into the mesocolon, thickening of the root of the sigmoid mesocolon, fine linear strands, and tiny bubbles of extraluminal gas within the mesocolon can be seen (Fig. 7). In severer cases, heterogeneous soft-tissue densities representing phlegmons and/or partially loculated fluid collections (that may or may not contain tiny bubbles of gas and/or air–fluid level) representing abscesses can develop in the mesocolon (Figs. 8, 9, 10) or more distantly in the peritoneal cavity (Fig. 11) or the retroperitoneum (Fig. 12).

Blind sinus tracts and fistulas are depicted as linear or tubular branching structures within the pericolic tissues. They may contain bubbles of gas and/or colonic contrast material. They can terminate in an abscess (sinus tract) or communicate with adjacent organs (fistulas). The presence of free fluid, depicted as water density fluid within the inferior peritoneal spaces (pelvic peritoneal recesses particularly), may be related to a nonspecific inflammatory reaction of the peritoneum. Instead, free peritoneal air, depicted as a large amount of gas or tiny bubbles of gas free in

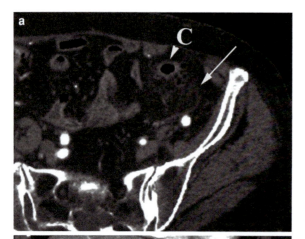

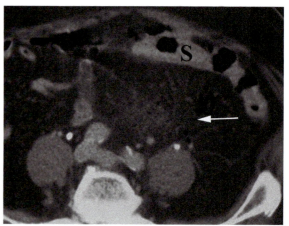

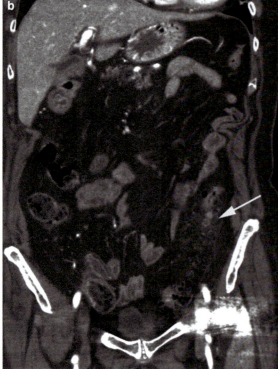

Fig. 6 Focal acute diverticulitis of the descending colon. MDCT examination with axial slice (**a**) and coronal reformat (**b**). **a** The CT axial slice depicts the thickening of the colonic wall (*arrowhead C*), numerous air-filled diverticula, and typical pericolic fat stranding with a slight thickening of the root of the mesocolon (*arrow*). **b** The coronal reformat shows the extent of the fat stranding and mesocolon thickening. Inflamed diverticula slightly thickened and enhanced are clearly visible (*arrow*). Note the punctiform and linear patterns of the pericolic fat alteration and the absence of extradigestive gas

the peritoneal cavity, indicates a free perforation rapidly resulting in generalized purulent peritonitis (Fig. 11). In fecal peritonitis, consisting in the most

Fig. 7 Acute colonic diverticulitis. Mild form of the disease with a walled-off perforation resulting in an inflammatory lesion confined within the sigmoid mesocolon. The CT axial slice demonstrates the fat stranding of the sigmoid mesocolon. Within this lesion, tiny bubbles, and a slightly larger pocket, of extradigestive gas (*arrow*) are clearly visible

severe complication of acute colonic diverticulitis, fecal material spreads out of the colonic lumen, through a wide perforation of the colonic wall, into the peritoneal cavity.

6 CT Pitfalls and Limits

In 50–70% of patients with clinically suspected diverticulitis this disease is not confirmed as the final diagnosis (Cho et al. 1990; Pradel et al. 1997; Rao et al. 1998; Ambrosetti et al. 2000; Kircher et al. 2002).

Currently CT is the imaging test of choice to identify or exclude other causes of left lower quadrant pain mimicking sigmoid diverticulitis. In patients with left lower quadrant pain, alternative diagnoses that should be considered (Table 1) include colitis (infectious/inflammatory or ischemic), colonic carcinoma, epiploic appendagitis, neutropenic colitis, functional colonic disorders, and extragastrointestinal disorders (pyelonephritis or gynecologic diseases), but differentiating sigmoid diverticulitis from carcinoma remains the major differential diagnostic consideration.

Special attention should be paid to epiploic appendagitis, differentiation of diverticulitis from carcinoma, right-sided colonic diverticulitis, and the limits resulting from delayed CT diagnosis of acute diverticulitis.

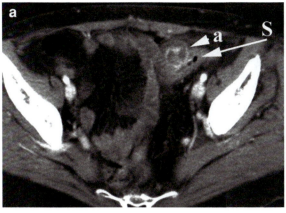 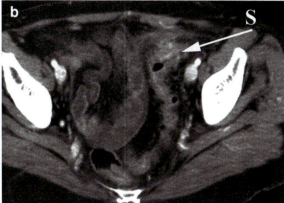

Fig. 8 Acute colonic diverticulitis. Severer form (Hinchey stage I) of the disease. CT axial slices demonstrate a small (less than 3 cm in diameter) fluid-filled abscess, partially loculated (**a**), with an enhanced thickened wall (*arrowhead a*). This lesion is abutting the sigmoid colon (*arrow S*) altered by numerous diverticula spreading distally (**b**), remains confined to the sigmoid mesocolon, and should be described as stage I in the Hinchey scheme

Table 1 Alternative causes of left lower quadrant pain mimicking acute colonic diverticulitis

Colitides
Ischemic colitis
Infectious colitis
Granulomatous colitis
Ulcerative colitis
Neutropenic colitis
Colonic carcinoma
Epiploic appendagitis[a] (Jalaguier et al. 2010)
Bowel obstruction[a] (Kim et al. 1998)
Functional colonic disorders
Extragastrointestinal disorders
Renal colic
Pyelonephritis
Gynecologic diseases[a] (Panghaal et al. 2009)

[a] May also occur as a complication of acute colonic diverticulitis, as reported in the literature and shown on the chapter dealing with acute gynecological disease

6.1 Epiploic Appendagitis

Epiploic appendagitis can be primary or secondary. Primary epiploic appendagitis develops secondary to acute inflammation resulting from the torsion of epiploic appendices (Rioux and Langis 1994; Singh et al. 2005; de Brito et al. 2008) and ischemia by obstruction and/or thrombosis of appendiceal drainage veins. The most common sites of acute epiploic appendagitis are areas adjacent to the sigmoid colon and the descending colon. Primary epiploic appendagitis results in a clinical condition mimicking acute colonic diverticulitis with focal exquisite lower abdominal pain, diagnosed with CT (or ultrasonography) by the demonstration of an ovoid lesion within the pericolic fat, surrounded by inflammatory changes and abutting the colonic wall (Fig. 13). Epiploic appendagitis is usually a self-limiting condition that can be managed conservatively with oral anti-inflammatory medications and resolves spontaneously within a few days. It is important to correctly diagnose acute epiploic appendagitis on CT images to avoid unnecessary hospital admission, antibiotic therapy, laboratory testing, dietary restrictions (Singh et al. 2005), and/or, moreover, unnecessary surgery. Secondary epiploic appendagitis can occur in patients with pericolic inflammatory changes, as in acute diverticulitis or other colitides, from spreading inflammatory process to the local epiploic appendages, and a resultant difficulty of diagnosis on the basis of CT images (Jalaguier et al. 2010).

6.2 Differentiation of Diverticulitis from Carcinoma

Colonic carcinoma is the main consideration in the differential diagnosis for the findings on CT. The presence of diverticula in an involved colonic

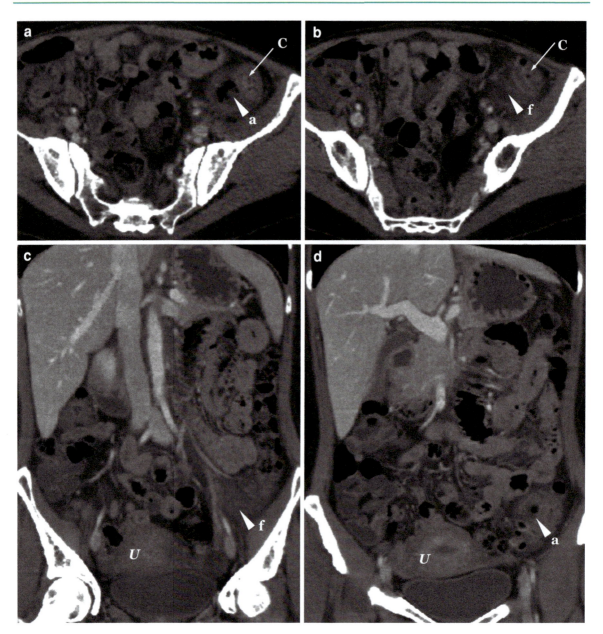

Fig. 9 Left lower quadrant pain with fever occurring in a young female patient in the postpartum period. Acute colonic diverticulitis of the junction of the descending colon with the sigmoid colon is easily confirmed by MDCT with axial slices (**a**, **b**) and coronal reformats (**c**, **d**) demonstrating a collection (*arrowhead a*), with a thickened wall and air content, developed close to the colon (*arrow C*) and confined within the altered fat (*arrowhead f*) of the mesocolon. Coronal reformats evaluate the extent of the lesion clearly within the mesocolon; note the postpartum enlarged uterus (*U*)

segment cannot be used to exclude neoplasm because of the high prevalence of diverticulosis in the general population. In general, pericolic fat stranding with fluid at the root of the mesocolon and engorgement of blood vessels is more suggestive of diverticulitis than of neoplasm. Instead, colonic wall thickening is usually greater (more than 2 cm), more focal, more eccentric, and with a more abrupt zone of transition with overhanging edges (Fig. 14) in neoplasm than in diverticulitis. But a colonic carcinoma, particularly

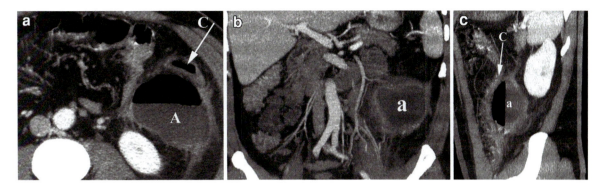

Fig. 10 Acute diverticulitis of the descending colon complicated by a large, but confined abscess, without any spread into the peritoneal cavity. The CT axial slice (**a**) shows a large abscess (*A*) containing an air–fluid level. The coronal reformat (**b**) according to a posterior plane (through the purulent content *a* of the abscess) demonstrates the anatomical relationships between the abscess and the inferior mesenteric vessels. The sagittal reformat (**c**) evaluates the displacement of the descending colon anteriorly (*arrow C*). (Courtesy of D. Regent, Nancy, France)

when the tumor is perforated and or altered by inflammatory reaction, may mimic diverticulitis. Several studies have stressed both the difficulties and limits of this differential diagnosis and have tried to assess specific signs of diverticulitis versus carcinoma (Balthazar et al. 1990; Padidar et al. 1994; Chintapalli et al. 1999). The most helpful issues are the following: (1) the presence of numerous pericolic lymph nodes (measuring 1 cm or more in the short axis) is more frequent in carcinoma, (2) the combination of a mild circumferential thickening of the colonic wall longer than 10 cm with a progressive transition with the nonnarrowed proximal and distal colon, and inflammatory changes of the mesocolon are suggestive of diverticulitis, and (3) none of these CT signs, isolated or in combination, have sufficient specificity for a definitively correct diagnosis.

Goh et al. (2007) reported that CT perfusion measurements enable differentiation and better discrimination, in comparison with morphologic criteria, between cancer and diverticulitis. However, in every patient medically managed for acute diverticulitis, it is crucial to perform colonoscopy 4–6 weeks after the onset of acute diverticulitis to rule out a colonic carcinoma (Haute Autorité de Santé 2006; Zins et al. 2007). If videocolonoscopy is contraindicated or not accepted, a CT examination dedicated to the precise analysis of the colon such as virtual colonoscopy (Hjern et al. 2007; Laurent 2007) or colo-CT examination after water enema (Pilleul et al. 2006) may be used.

6.3 Right-Sided Colonic Diverticulitis

Cecal diverticulitis is a relatively rare pathologic entity in Western countries. Cecal diverticula are classified as true (congenital) or false (acquired). The congenital variety is usually larger and solitary and occurs more frequently in Asian individuals, and is characterized by a fully developed digestive wall, including the different layers of the digestive wall, and particularly the muscularis propria. Most diverticula of the cecum and the ascending colon are acquired and are similar to diverticula currently found in the remainder of the colon (sigmoid, descending, and transverse colon).

Right-sided acute diverticulitis is often clinically misdiagnosed regarding the numerous alternative diagnoses possible in a patient with right lower quadrant pain (Jang et al. 2000; Lee et al. 2008).

The main consideration in the differential diagnosis is acute appendicitis but other diseases that can present with acute right lower quadrant pain, including acute terminal ileitis (Crohn's disease), typhlitis, and, in women, pelvic inflammatory disease, complications of ovarian cyst (hemorrhage, torsion, and leak), endometriosis, and ectopic pregnancy. Less common causes of right lower quadrant pain include segmental infarction of the greater omentum, mesenteric adenitis, epiploic appendagitis, perforated cancer, and ileal or Meckel's diverticulitis.

CT findings in right-sided acute diverticulitis are similar to those depicted in the sigmoid colon:

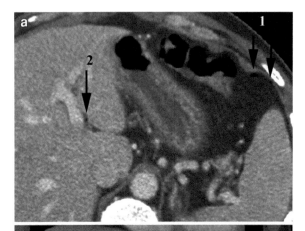

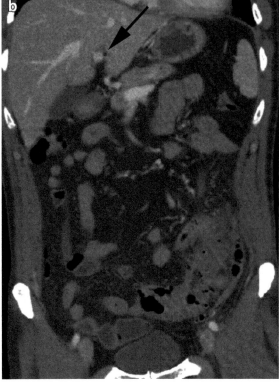

Fig. 11 Severe acute colonic diverticulitis of the junction of the descending colon with the sigmoid colon. Free perforation into the peritoneal cavity is confirmed by MDCT axial slices (**a**) and coronal reformat (**b**). The CT demonstration of tiny bubbles of extraluminal gas within the left side of the subphrenic space (*arrows* 1) and hepatic pedicle (arrow 2), indicating a pneumoperitoneum from the perforated sigmoid diverticulitis (**b**), requires dedicated window settings. Note the regional pericolic spread of the disease with badly limited inflammatory mass and multiple pockets of extradigestive gas. This acute colonic diverticulitis should be described as stage III in the Hinchey scheme (generalized purulent peritonitis), and requires emergency surgery

diverticulum (with or without a high-attenuation value stercolith), bowel wall thickening, and changes of the pericolic fat (with fat stranding, and abscess in severer forms). CT may be helpful by demonstrating a normal entire appendix and ruling out appendicitis. Other CT findings may be the inflamed diverticulum sign (Fig. 15) and the depiction of a stercolith within the diverticulum. Currently it is difficult to differentiate advanced cecal diverticulitis from cecal neoplasm; the precise preoperative diagnosis is difficult and the most helpful patterns for the diagnosis of diverticulitis may be the inflamed diverticulum sign and the depiction of a multilayered diverticulum wall on a high-resolution enhanced CT scan (Jang et al. 2000).

6.4 Delayed Diagnosis of Diverticulitis

One of the main difficulties of CT in diverticulitis is a too long interval between the clinical onset of the acute episode and the time when the CT examination is performed. Too many patients with likely nonsevere clinical forms of acute diverticulitis are medically managed, particularly as outpatients, without any morphological evidence, and the CT examination is finally performed several days (or weeks) after the medical treatment starts; in such a condition, the CT examination may show few signs, limited to the depiction of diverticula and bowel wall thickening, which may indicate only a diverticulosis, and the significant patterns, indicating the acute episode and its severity, may have disappeared. Moreover, this lack of evidence is critical: the choice of the correct management of a patient who has likely had several recurrent episodes and for whom there is indication for elective surgical resection of the sigmoid colon should be discussed as a function of the evidence and the severity of the acute episodes of diverticulitis (Haute Autorité de Santé 2006).

7 CT Impact on the Management

The recommendation to perform a nondelayed CT scan in every patient when acute diverticulitis is clinically suspected serves the following functions: (1) to confirm the diagnosis of diverticulitis, (2) to evaluate the severity and extent of disease, (3) to

Diverticulitis

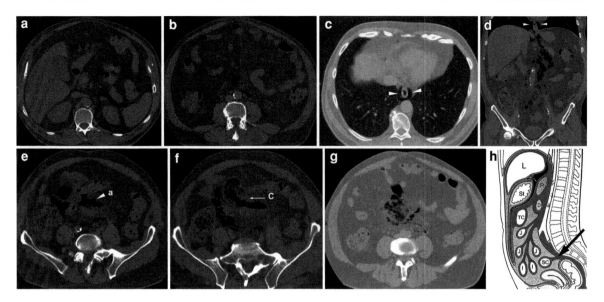

Fig. 12 Severe acute sigmoid diverticulitis. Free perforation into the retroperitoneum. Perforation of the diverticulitis into the subperitoneal space is not confined to the sigmoid mesocolon. Extradigestive air spreads to the retroperitoneal space, resulting in retroperitoneal emphysema ("pneumoretroperitoneum") dissecting the fatty retroperitoneal content, and depicted as linear tracts and/or small rounded pockets of air-attenuation values (**a**, **b**). This retroperitoneal emphysema spreads to the inferior mediastinum (*arrowheads* in **c**, **d**). On the inferior MDCT slices (**e**, **f**), note that retroperitoneal gas is abutting a juxtacolic abscess (*arrowhead a*) and inflamed sigmoid colon (*arrow C*) with thickened wall and air-filled diverticula. **g** The axial CT slice with dedicated settings of the window level and width (CT lung windows) demonstrates clearly the patterns of extradigestive gas spreading into the retroperitoneal spaces. **h** The sagittal view drawing demonstrates the continuity of the subperitoneal space of the sigmoid mesocolon with retroperitoneum (in *gray*); the *black arrow* points to the continuity of the sigmoid mesocolon with retroperitoneum. *D* duodenum, *I* ileum, *J* jejunum, *L* liver, *P* pancreas, *SC* sigmoid colon, *St* stomach, *TC* transverse colon. (**h** From Ragu 2010)

assist the treatment planning of complications such as abscess, and (4) to demonstrate other causes of abdominal pain that may mimic diverticulitis.

7.1 CT Confirms the Diagnosis of Diverticulitis

The initially reported sensitivities of CT for the diagnosis of acute diverticulitis ranged from 69 to 95%. With the advancement of CT scan technology, the improving technique of CT examination, the more precise CT criteria, and the greater experience in the interpretation of these CT findings, the reported sensitivities for the diagnosis of diverticulitis have progressively increased up to 98–99% (Table 2).

In a study including 312 patients and with the use of thin-section helical CT with colonic contrast material, the overall CT interpretation had sensitivity, specificity, positive and negative predictive values, and overall accuracy of 99% (Kircher et al. 2002).

7.2 CT Evaluates the Severity and Extent of Diverticulitis

The severity of a clinical attack of the disease (initial or recurrent episode) is related to the development of the extracolic lesions (abscess, peritonitis, fistula, and portal septic thrombosis). CT can evaluate the locoregional and distant spread of the infection accurately, and CT findings correlate with the surgical staging scheme reported by Hinchey et al. (1978) and its adaptation by Wasvary et al. (1999). Moreover the Hinchey scheme correlates with the mortality of the disease: 0, 4, 20, and 45% in Hinchey stages I, II, II, and IV, respectively (Nespoli et al. 1993) (Table 3).

CT is also known to be a helpful method to investigate patients with bowel obstruction (Taourel

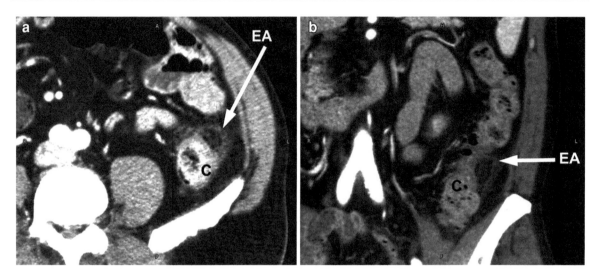

Fig. 13 Epiploic appendagitis depicted on MDCT axial slice (**a**) and coronal reformat (**b**) of the left iliac fossa. CT images demonstrate an ovoid lesion (*arrow EA*) within the pericolic fat, abutting the wall of the descending colon (*C*)

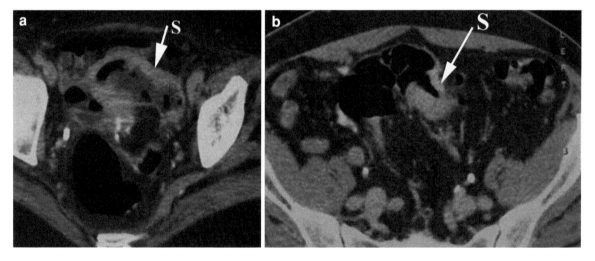

Fig. 14 Perforated carcinoma of the sigmoid colon (*arrow S*). CT axial images demonstrate a 4-cm-long thickening of the colonic wall and inflammatory changes of the pericolic fat (**a**). The abruptly altered caliber of the colonic lumen with overhanging-edge thickening of the bowel wall should suggest a carcinoma rather than a diverticulitis (**b**)

et al. 1995), particularly complicating acute colonic diverticulitis.

7.2.1 Diverticular Abscesses

Abscess formation occurs in 16–35% of patients with acute diverticulitis, and the severity of this complication depends on the size, number, and mainly location of the abscess.

Hinchey stage I denotes a phlegmon or abscess confined to the mesocolon and that is commonly less than 3 cm in diameter. These patients are currently managed with antibiotics and dietary restrictions. A follow-up CT examination is recommended, depending on the clinical condition, to rule out progression to a severer stage of the disease. In the case of unsuccessful medical management, surgical resection by open laparotomy or laparoscopy is indicated, with or without the protection of a proximal diverting colostomy.

In Hinchey stage II, a pericolic abscess spreads to the pelvic and/or abdominal peritoneal recesses, or to the retroperitoneum, but remains contained by an

Table 2 Diagnostic value of computed tomography for suspected acute colonic diverticulitis

Investigation	No. of patients	Sensitivity (%)	Specificity (%)	Positive predictive value (%)	Negative predictive value (%)	Accuracy (%)	Alternative diagnosis seen (%)
Cho et al. (1990)	56	93	100	NA	NA	NA	69
Stefánsson et al. (1997)	88	69	100	NA	NA	NA	NA
Pradel et al. (1997)	64	91	77	81	88	84	50
Rao et al. (1998)	150	97	100	100	98	98	58
Ambrosetti et al. (2000)	420	98	NA	97	NA	NA	NA
Kircher et al. (2002)	312	99	99	99	99	99	70

NA not applicable

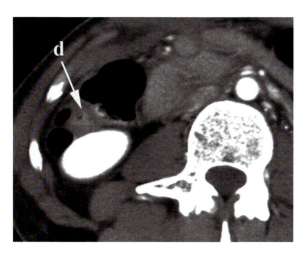

Fig. 15 Right-sided diverticulitis. The CT axial image demonstrates a slightly enhanced diverticulum (*arrow d*) wall within the altered pericolic fat, close to the descending colon

Table 3 Hinchey's surgical scheme of acute diverticulitis and correlation to mortality

Stage	Surgical criteria	Mortality (%)
I	Phlegmon or abscess confined to the mesocolon	0
II	Abscess within the pelvis, abdomen, or retroperitoneum	4
III	Generalized purulent peritonitis	20
IV	Fecal peritonitis	45

From Hinchey et al. (1978) and Nespoli et al. (1993)

abscess wall and the surrounding peritoneal or retroperitoneal structures. Large abscesses (5 cm in diameter) are treated with antibiotics, but a complementary interventional procedure by percutaneous drainage may be indicated. Large pericolic abscess may be difficult to differentiate from a giant colonic diverticulum (Steenvoorde et al. 2004; Thomas et al. 2006; Chatora and Kumaran 2009).

7.2.2 Peritonitis

Hinchey stage III corresponds to a generalized purulent peritonitis. More than the clinical findings (diffuse abdominal guarding and other clinical signs of peritonitis), sometimes masked by the immunoreactive behavior of the patient, the presence of free peritoneal gas, even as very tiny bubbles trapped in peritoneal recesses or within the subphrenic spaces (Fig. 11), is diagnostic of generalized peritonitis and indicates emergency surgery. The indication for a single-stage colonic resection versus resection with anastomosis protected by a proximal lateral diverting colostomy versus Hartman's procedure depends on the operative findings and general condition of the patient.

Hinchey stage IV is defined by a fecal spread into the peritoneal cavity, through a large perforation of the bowel wall, resulting in fecal peritonitis with life-threatening sepsis. Patients with this most severe complication of colonic diverticulitis should undergo immediate laparotomy.

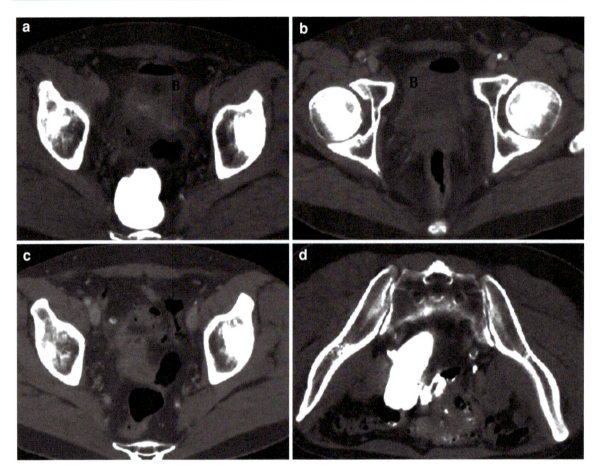

Fig. 16 Severe acute sigmoid diverticulitis with colovesical fistula. CT axial slices easily demonstrate gas within the urinary bladder; note the thickening of the bladder wall (*B*) and the air–fluid level in the anterior part of the bladder (**a**). The sigmoid colon is altered by an inflammatory process, with an inflammatory mass abutting the bladder wall (**b**) but the full assessment of the fistula route remains difficult (**c**), even after administration of colonic iodinated contrast rectally and CT scanning with the patient in the prone position (**d**)

7.2.3 Fistulas

Five percent to 9% of surgical operations for complicated diverticulitis are related to fistula. Colovesical fistulas are the most frequent fistulas complicating acute colonic diverticulitis and should be suspected in patients with urinary infection and pneumaturia. They are less common in women than in men, probably because of the interposition of the uterus between the sigmoid colon and the urinary bladder; and are often easily demonstrated by CT scans, with a perisigmoid inflammatory mass abutting or immediately adjacent to the urinary bladder wall, and a variable amount of air over an air–fluid level within the lumen of the bladder (Fig. 16). These patterns have a high specificity value when there is no history of prior urinary instrumentation. Other types of fistulas can communicate with a small bowel loop, salpinx, uterus, vagina, or abdominal wall, and the route of the fistulas may be highly complex, and not or only partially demonstrated by CT examination (Cho et al. 1990; Werner et al. 2003, Panghaal et al. 2009) even when using iodinated contrast material injected anorectally (Fig. 17) or through the external orifice of a colocutaneous fistula, and dedicated changes of the position of the patient.

7.2.4 Portomesenteric Veins Septic Thrombosis and Liver Abscesses

Septic thrombosis of the inferior mesenteric vein is a rare complication of acute colonic diverticulitis (Balthazar and Gollapudi 2000; Sebastià et al. 2000; Bekkhoucha et al. 2008). The spread of septic

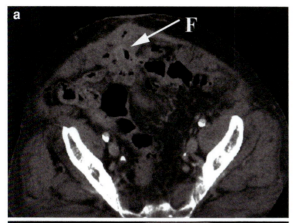
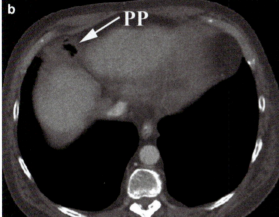
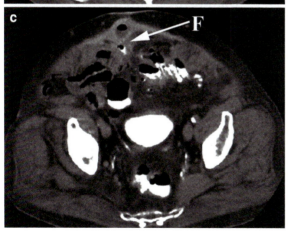

Fig. 17 Severe acute sigmoid diverticulitis with complex colovesical fistula and perforation into the peritoneal cavity. Axial CT slices. CT demonstrates a complex fistula route partially marked by gas bubbles (*arrow F*), spreading into the anterior abdominal wall (**a**). On a CT slice of the upper abdomen (**b**), note the clear CT depiction of a small gas pocket (*arrow PP*), within the right side of the subphrenic space, indicative of pneumoperitoneum and diagnostic of generalized peritonitis. The anterior route of this complex colocutaneous fistula is better analyzed (**c**) after administration of colonic iodinated contrast rectally (*arrow F*)

thrombosis to the portal vein and its intrahepatic branches can lead to pyogenic abscess of the liver (Fig. 18). Systematic attention should be paid to the inferior mesenteric vein, portal vein, and liver when analyzing CT images. The diagnosis of this complication advocates the use of enhanced CT examination and careful display of the windowing settings (see "Sect. 5"). Thrombosis, with or without intravascular gas, of the inferior mesenteric and portal veins can easily be demonstrated with contrast-enhanced CT. Gas in the mesentericoportal veins appears as tubular areas—or linear-branching images within the liver—of air-attenuation values (Fig. 19). On contrast-enhanced CT, these abscesses are generally large hypoattenuating lesions, with well-defined outlines, and may contain gas (Mortelé et al. 2004).

Treatment consists of anticoagulation plus antibiotic therapy. Elective sigmoid colectomy is indicated but an emergency colectomy may be required in the cases of failure of medical therapy (Bekkhoucha et al. 2008).

7.2.5 Colonic Stenoses and Bowel Obstruction

Bowel obstruction can occur in patients with colonic diverticulitis, either as small bowel obstruction related to a diverticular abscess (Kim et al. 1998) or by direct obstruction of the colonic lumen by narrowing inflammatory diverticular disease, resulting in large bowel obstruction, mostly of the sigmoid loop (Taourel et al. 2003).

Acute colonic diverticulitis is an uncommon cause of small bowel obstruction and may be overlooked as a cause. Clinically the diverticulitis may be masked by the clinical symptoms of small bowel obstruction and the diagnosis is doubtful when the patient suffers the first attack of diverticulitis. Anatomic proximity of the distal jejunum and the proximal ileum to the sigmoid colon explains why small bowel loops can be trapped in the pericolic inflammatory process, resulting in fixation, narrowing, and finally obstruction. When diverticulitis is correctly diagnosed as the cause of the small bowel obstruction, the patient can be initially managed medically, immediate surgery may be avoided, and elective sigmoid colectomy may be planned as a safe one-stage surgical procedure (Kim et al. 1998). Obstructing colonic stenoses resulting from diverticulitis may be difficult to differentiate from obstructing colonic carcinoma.

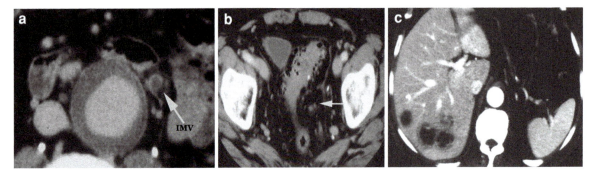

Fig. 18 Severe acute colonic diverticulitis with portomesenteric vein septic thrombosis and hepatic abscesses. CT axial images demonstrate the enlargement of the inferior mesenteric vein with an enhanced vascular wall and unenhanced lumen (**a**, *arrow IMV*). More proximally, the inferior mesenteric pedicle is seen on the inferior CT slice (**b**, *arrow*), close to a slightly changed sigmoid colon, with diverticula and thickening of the root of the sigmoid mesocolon. Septic thrombosis spreads to the portal vein and results in the development of right-sided hepatic abscesses (**c**). (Courtesy of D. Regent, Nancy, France)

7.3 CT Assists the Treatment Planning of Abscesses

A number of studies evaluating percutaneous CT-guided catheter drainage of diverticular abscesses as an adjunct to surgical therapy have been reported (Neff et al. 1987; Mueller et al. 1987; Stabile et al. 1990; Ambrosetti et al. 2005). Patients with abscesses of 4–5 cm or larger can be managed with CT-guided abscess drainage (Fig. 20) followed by secondary colectomy. This type of management obviates surgical abscess drainage and results in rapid resolution of clinical sepsis and stabilization of the patients. Once the abscesses are resolved, a single-stage surgical operation, by sigmoid resection and closure, can be performed safely. The benefit of CT scan-guided percutaneous abscess drainage and the size of the abscesses to be drained (vs. dedicated antibiotherapy alone) remain controversial (Siewert et al. 2006; Brandt et al. 2006), and the criteria for successful management are actually based on the clinical outcome and the laboratory test results. In the case of successful management, the indication for an elective sigmoid resection is still debated (Pessaux et al. 2004; Klarenbeek et al. 2010).

7.4 CT Demonstrates Other Causes of Abdominal Pain

CT is the imaging test of choice to identify or exclude other causes of abdominal pain that may mimic diverticulitis. Numerous alternative diagnoses may be discussed in a patient with left lower quadrant pain as previously shown. Given the epidemiological factors and clinical expression of diverticular disease in the aging population, differentiation of colonic carcinoma from diverticulitis should be stressed again as one of the major concerns; it should be also remembered that this differentiation on the basis of only CT findings is very difficult, not to say hazardous.

8 Diagnostic Strategy

CT is now widely accepted as the diagnostic radiological examination of choice in patients with suspected acute diverticulitis (Haute Autorité de Santé 2006; Zins et al. 2007; American College of Radiology 2008).

8.1 CT: The Imaging Test of Choice for the Diagnosis and Management

It is recommended to perform a CT examination in every patient every time an acute diverticulitis is clinically suspected. This CT examination should be performed within 24 h of the patient being admitted to hospital or within 72 h after acute diverticulitis is suspected and the medical treatment is initialized in an outpatient setting (Zins et al. 2007).

For the diagnosis and the management of colonic diverticular disease, in most cases CT, as the safest and most cost-effective method of diagnosis, should replace the other imaging modalities such as plain

Diverticulitis

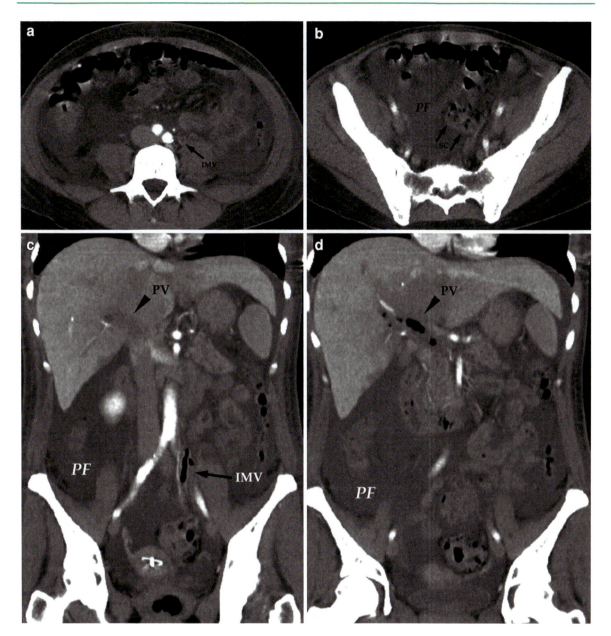

Fig. 19 Severe acute colonic diverticulitis with portomesenteric vein septic thrombosis. CT axial slices depict a thrombosis of the inferior mesenteric vein (**a**, *arrow IMV*) with enhanced vascular wall and unenhanced lumen. On inferior CT slices (**b**) the inferior mesenteric vein is abutting the sigmoid colon (*arrows SC*), with diverticula but without any pericolic abscess. In this patient, peritoneal effusion (*PF*) is related to a rapidly extensive portal vein full thrombosis. On CT coronal reformats (**c, d**) tubular images of air-attenuation values are seen within both the inferior mesenteric vein (*arrow IMV*) and the portal vein (*arrowhead PV*)

films of the abdomen (PFA), CE, ultrasonography, magnetic resonance imaging, and colonoscopy.

CT has a clinical impact both on the diagnosis and on the management of patients with acute colonic diverticulitis and has been demonstrated as a valuable tool for determining prognosis factors.

Ambrosetti et al. (2002) reported that abdominal CT findings such as abscess, extradigestive gas, and extradigestive colonic contrast are indicators of severe forms of acute diverticulitis. In this same prospective study including 542 patients, by comparing severe acute colonic diverticulitis and nonsevere forms, these

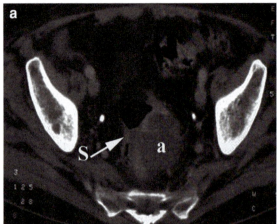 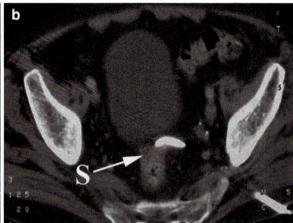

Fig. 20 Severe acute sigmoid diverticulitis with pelvic abscess. Percutaneous abscess drainage under CT guidance. a The CT axial slice demonstrates a large abscess (*a*) abutting the wall of the sigmoid colon (*arrow S*) and spreading down in the presacral region on the left side of the rectum. b This abscess is drained percutaneously, via a transgluteal approach. Note the location of the tip of the draining catheter, close to the rectosigmoid junction (*arrow S*) and the emptying of the abscess cavity

authors reported a higher risk of unsuccessful medical management of the acute phase and a higher risk of recurrence (26% vs. 4% with $p < 0.0001$ and 36% vs. 17% with $p < 0.0001$, respectively). Moreover, in a more recent prospective study, Poletti et al. (2004) reported that the CT findings significantly correlating with an unsuccessful medical management were abscess and/or tiny bubbles of extradigestive gas more than 5 mm in diameter. These data should be considered when transcutaneous drainage and/or surgical operation are discussed, but this issue and the actual indications for elective sigmoid resection in diverticular disease are still debated (Klarenbeek et al. 2010).

8.2 Plain Films of the Abdomen

The plain films of the abdomen (PFA) cannot assess the diagnosis of acute colonic diverticulitis. In a retrospective study including 1,000 consecutive patients with acute abdominal pain, the sensitivity of PFA for the diagnosis of acute colonic diverticulitis was 0% (Ahn et al. 2002). The role of PFA for diagnosing a free perforation, either in the peritoneal cavity or in the retroperitoneum, is uncertain. The sensitivity of PFA for the diagnosis of a suspected pneumoperitoneum in patients with diverticulitis is much lower than that of CT, because tiny bubbles of distant intraperitoneal gas, which have the same clinical significance of generalized peritonitis in this condition as a large pneumoperitoneum, are easily demonstrated by CT and are overlooked by PFA. Therefore, in patients with suspected acute colonic diverticulitis, CT rather than PFA should be used.

8.3 Contrast Enema

Traditionally, the contrast enema (CE) examination has been the primary method for examining patients suspected of having acute colonic diverticulitis. The classic findings are sigmoid narrowing (typically long, symmetric, and with a gradual zone of transition), muscle hypertrophy with sacculations, and diverticula. But these patterns may be seen in patients with chronic diverticular disease and may not be diagnostic of acute diverticulitis. A specific diagnosis can be made only when there is extravasation of contrast material from a diverticulum. The contrast material may extravasate into the peritoneal cavity, a walled-off abscess, a sinus tract, or a fistula. The main limit of CE examination is not depicting the pericolic lesions directly, and a large pericolic abscess can only be indirectly inferred mainly from compression and displacement of the colonic wall. Instead, CE may be helpful for differentiating diverticulitis from carcinoma. As early as 1984, a study by Hulnick et al. (1984) showed that, compared with CT, CE underestimated the severity of the diverticulitis in 41% of patients. In 1990 Cho et al. (1990) reported a better diagnostic accuracy with CT (93%) than with CE (80%). Finally, in 2000 Ambrosetti et al. (2000), in the main prospective study comparing CE and CT and including 420 patients, demonstrated the superiority of CT for both the diagnosis of acute colonic diverticulitis and the precise assessment of the severity of the disease. Even though use of CE is still proposed in a few selected patients with colonic diverticulitis (for evaluating the route of a complex fistula or differentiating diverticulitis from colonic carcinoma), CE has less and less of a significant role in acute colonic diverticulitis and should be replaced by CT as the first-step imaging method for the diagnosis of acute colonic diverticulitis.

8.4 Ultrasonography

The ultrasonography findings in acute colonic diverticulitis have been reported for15–20 years and are similar to the CT findings: hypoechoic thickening of the colonic wall, alterations of the pericolic fat depicted as hyperechoic, and diverticula (Pradel et al. 1997; Puylaert 2001; Ripollés et al. 2003). The reported sensitivity and specificity of ultrasonography for the diagnosis of acute colonic diverticulitis are 84–98% and 80–98%, respectively. This high accuracy has been reported mainly for nonsevere acute colonic diverticulitis and requires a rigorous examination technique and great experience of the investigator in ultrasonography examination of the gastrointestinal tract. Ultrasonography examination may be sufficient for the diagnosis of either nonsevere diverticulitis (focal diverticulitis with limited changes of the pericolic fat) or several alternative diagnoses (epiploic appendagitis). However a recent meta-analysis showed no statistically significant difference in the accuracy of ultrasonography and CT in diagnosing acute colonic diverticulitis (Laméris et al. 2008). CT examination is considered more useful for precise determination of alternative diagnoses, but transabdominal ultrasonography complemented by an endovaginal ultrasonography examination should be the initial preferred modality in women of child-bearing age. However, ultrasonography examination should likely have a more prominent place in the initial setting of acute abdominal pain: in a fully

paired multicenter diagnostic accuracy study with prospective data collection, including 1,021 patients, 665 (25%) having a final diagnosis classified as urgent, Laméris et al. (2009) evaluated the added value of plain radiographs, ultrasonography, and CT after clinical evaluation for making urgent diagnoses in patients presenting with abdominal pain. The main objective of the study was to identify an optimal imaging strategy for the accurate detection of urgent conditions in patients with acute abdominal pain. Although CT was the most sensitive imaging method for detecting urgent conditions in these patients with acute abdominal pain, using ultrasonography first and CT only in those patients with negative or inconclusive ultrasonography findings resulted in the best sensitivity and lowered exposure to radiation.

8.5 Magnetic Resonance Imaging

Even though magnetic resonance imaging may be considered to provide patterns similar to the CT ones (Buckley et al. 2007), it has several limitations for its use in patients with suspected acute colonic diverticulitis: limited accessibility and longer examination time, and moreover lack of sensitivity to depict a pneumoperitoneum, particularly for tiny bubbles of extraluminal gas.

8.6 Colonoscopy

Colonoscopy is strictly contraindicated in the acute phase of an onset of suspected colonic diverticulitis. Virtual colonoscopy, with CT or magnetic resonance imaging, requires a high degree of colonic distension after anorectal insufflation and is, therefore, contraindicated in the acute phase of an onset of suspected colonic diverticulitis. Instead, 4–6 weeks after the acute diverticulitis resolves, it is mandatory to rule out a colonic carcinoma and colonoscopy should be performed particularly in patients with a doubtful narrowing of the colonic lumen, and for many authors as a systematic test in all patients over 50 years old or with risk factors for colonic carcinoma; virtual colonoscopy (Hjern et al. 2007; Laurent 2007) or colo-CT examination after water enema (Pilleul et al. 2006; Ridereau-Zins et al. 2009) has been performed may be used as an alternative for ruling out a colonic carcinoma, if videocolonoscopy is not accepted or is contraindicated.

9 Conclusion

CT is now widely accepted as the diagnostic radiological examination of choice in patients with suspected acute diverticulitis.

CT examination should be performed in every patient every time an acute diverticulitis is clinically suspected to serve the following functions: (1) to confirm the diagnosis of acute diverticulitis by demonstrating inflammatory pericolic changes associated with colonic diverticula, (2) to identify or exclude other causes of abdominal pain that may mimic diverticulitis, (3) to evaluate the severity and the extent of the acute disease, and (4) to assist the decision management not only in emergency conditions by evaluating the complications accurately and in selective (but still debated) conditions by guiding a percutaneous drainage, but also in discussing the actual need for an elective sigmoid colectomy.

This CT examination should be performed within 24 h of the patient being admitted to hospital or within 72 h after acute diverticulitis is suspected and the medical treatment is initialized in an outpatient setting.

Ultrasonography should be considered as a helpful imaging method for the diagnosis of unexplained acute abdominal pain when performed by an experimented observer familiar with the ultrasonographic evaluation of the gastrointestinal tract, but is of more limited value in severe diverticulitis. However, ultrasonography examination should be the initial preferred imaging modality in the setting of left lower quadrant pain with or without fever in women of childbearing age.

References

Ahn SH, Mayo-Smith WW, Murphy BL et al (2002) Acute non traumatic abdominal pain in adult patients: abdominal radiography compared with CT evaluation. Radiology 225:159–164

Ambrosetti P, Robert JH, Witzig JA et al (1994) Acute left colonic diverticulitis: a prospective analysis of 226 consecutive cases. Surgery 115:546–550

Ambrosetti P, Jenny A, Becker C et al (2000) Acute left colonic diverticulitis: compared performance of computed tomography and water-soluble contrast enema. Prospective evaluation of 420 patients. Dis Colon Rectum 43:1363–1367

Ambrosetti P, Becker C, Terrier F (2002) Colonic diverticulitis: impact of imaging on surgical management—a prospective study of 542 patients. Eur Radiol 12:1145–1149

Ambrosetti P, Chautems R, Soravia C et al (2005) Long-term outcome of mesocolic and pelvic diverticular abscesses of the left colon: a prospective study of 73 cases. Dis Colon Rectum 48:787–791

American College of Radiology (2008) ACR appropriateness criteria. http://www.acr.org/SecondaryMainMenuCategories/quality_safety/app_criteria/pdf/ExpertPanelonGastrointestinalImaging/AcuteAbdominalPainandFeverorSuspectedAbdominalAbscessDoc1.aspx. Accessed 28 Aug 2010

Balthazar EJ (1994) Diverticular disease. In: Gore RM, Levine SM, Laufer I (eds) Textbook of gastrointestinal radiology. Saunders, Philadelphia, pp 1072–1097

Balthazar EJ, Gollapudi P (2000) Septic thrombophlebitis of the mesenteric and portal veins: CT imaging. J Comput Assist Tomogr 24:755–760

Balthazar EJ, Megibow A, Schinella RA et al (1990) Limitations in the CT diagnosis of acute diverticulitis: comparison of CT, contrast enema, and pathologic findings in 16 patients. Am J Roentgenol 154:281–285

Bekkhoucha S, Boulay-Colleta I, Turner L et al (2008) Pylephlebitis in the course of diverticulitis. J Chir 145:284–286

Brandt D, Gervaz P, Durmishi Y et al (2006) Percutaneous CT scan-guided drainage vs. antibiotherapy alone for Hinchey II diverticulitis: a case-control study. Dis Colon Rectum 49:1533–1538

Buckley O, Geoghegan T, McAuley G et al (2007) Pictorial review: magnetic resonance imaging of colonic diverticulitis. Eur Radiol 17:221–227

Chatora GT, Kumaran M (2009) Giant colonic pseudo-diverticula importance of and aids to radiological diagnosis: a case series. Cases J 2:9314

Chintapalli KN, Chopra S, Ghiatas AA et al (1999) Diverticulitis versus colon cancer: differentiation with helical CT findings. Radiology 210:429–435

Cho KC, Morehouse HT, Alterman DD (1990) Sigmoid diverticulitis: diagnostic role of CT-comparison with barium enema studies. Radiology 176:111–115

Chodak GW, Rangel DM, Passaro E Jr (1981) Colonic diverticulitis in patients under age 40: need for earlier diagnosis. Am J Surg 141:699–702

de Brito P, Gomez MA, Besson M et al (2008) Frequency and epidemiology of primary epiploic appendagitis on CT in adults with abdominal pain. J Radiol 89:235–243

DeStigter KK, Keating DP (2009) Acute colonic diverticulitis. Clin Colon Rectal Surg 22:147–155

Ferzoco LB, Raptopoulos V, Silen W (1998) Acute diverticulitis. N Engl J Med 338:1521–1526

Freischlag J, Bennion RS, Thompson JE Jr (1986) Complications of diverticular disease of the colon in young people. Dis Colon Rectum 29:639–643

Ghekiere O, Lesnik A, Millet I et al (2007) Direct visualization of perforation sites in patients with a non-traumatic free pneumoperitoneum: added diagnostic value of thin transverse slices and coronal and sagittal reformations for multi-detector CT. Eur Radiol 17:2302–2309

Goh V, Halligan S, Taylor SA et al (2007) Differentiation between diverticulitis and colorectal cancer: quantitative CT perfusion measurements versus morphologic criteria–initial experience. Radiology 242:456–462

Hall JF, Roberts PL, Ricciardi R et al (2010) Colonic diverticulitis: does age predict severity of disease on CT imaging? Dis Colon Rectum 53:121–125

Haute Autorité de Santé (2006) Complications of colonic diverticulosis. Clinical practice guidelines. http://www.has-sante.fr/portail/upload/docs/application/pdf/2008-08/complications_diverticulose_colique_-_recommandations.pdf. Accessed 28 August 2010

Hinchey EJ, Schaal PG, Richards GK et al (1978) Treatment of perforated diverticular disease of the colon. Adv Surg 12:85–109

Hjern F, Jonas E, Holmström B et al (2007) CT colonography versus colonoscopy in the follow-up of patients after diverticulitis—a prospective, comparative study. Clin Radiol 62:645–650

Horton KM, Corl FM, Fishman EK (2000) CT evaluation of the colon: inflammatory disease. Radiographics 20:399–418

Hulnick DH, Megibow AJ, Balthazar EJ et al (1984) Computed tomography in the evaluation of diverticulitis. Radiology 152:491–495

Jalaguier A, Zins M, Rodallec M et al (2010) Accuracy of multidetector computed tomography in differentiating primary epiploic appendagitis from left acute colonic diverticulitis associated with secondary epiploic appendagitis. Emerg Radiol 17:51–56

Jang HJ, Lim HK, Lee SJ et al (2000) Acute diverticulitis of the cecum and ascending colon : the value of thin-section helical CT findings in excluding colonic carcinoma. Am J Roentgenol 174:1397–1402

Kim AY, Bennett GL, Bashist B et al (1998) Small-bowel obstruction associated with sigmoid diverticulitis: CT evaluation in 16 patients. Am J Roentgenol 170:1311–1313

Kircher MF, Rhea JT, Kihiczak D et al (2002) Frequency, sensitivity, and specificity of individual signs of diverticulitis on thin-section helical CT with colonic contrast material: experience with 312 cases. Am J Roentgenol 178:1313–1318

Klarenbeek BR, Samuels M, van der Wal MA et al (2010) Indications for elective sigmoid resection in diverticular disease. Ann Surg 251:670–674

Laméris W, van Randen A, van Es HW et al OPTIMA study group (2009) Imaging strategies for detection of urgent conditions in patients with acute abdominal pain: diagnostic accuracy study. BMJ 338:b2431. doi:10.1136/bmj.b2431

Laméris W, van Randen A, Bipat S et al (2008) Graded compression ultrasonography and computed tomography in acute colonic diverticulitis: meta-analysis of test accuracy. Eur Radiol 18:2498–2511

Laurent V (2007) Colon examinations in 2007: new horizons opened by the CT and MRI. Colon Rectum 1:157–165

Lawrimore T, Rhea JT (2004) Computed tomography evaluation of diverticulitis. J Intensive Care Med 19:194–204

Lee IK, Jung SE, Gorden DL et al (2008) The diagnostic criteria for right colonic diverticulitis: prospective evaluation of 100 patients. Int J Colorectal Dis 23:1151–1157

Lefèvre F, Béot S, Chapuis F et al (1999) Computed tomography study of the sigmoid colon: discriminating diagnostic criteria and interobserver correlations. J Radiol 80:447–456

Mortelé KJ, Segatto E, Ros PR (2004) The infected liver: radiologic-pathologic correlation. Radiographics 24:937–955

Mueller PR, Saini S, Wittenburg J et al (1987) Sigmoid diverticular abscesses: percutaneous drainage as an adjunct to surgical resection in 24 cases. Radiology 164:321–325

Neff CC, van Sonnenberg E, Casola G et al (1987) Diverticular abscesses: percutaneous drainage. Radiology 163:15–18

Nespoli A, Ravizzini C, Trivella M et al (1993) The choice of surgical procedure for peritonitis due to colonic perforation. Arch Surg 128:814–818

Ouriel K, Schwartz SI (1983) Diverticular disease in the young patient. Surg Gynecol Obstet 156:1–5

Padidar AM, Jeffrey RB Jr, Mindelzun RE et al (1994) Differentiating sigmoid diverticulitis from carcinoma on CT scans: mesenteric inflammation suggests diverticulitis. Am J Roentgenol 163:81–83

Panghaal VS, Chernyak V, Patlas M et al (2009) CT features of adnexal involvement in patients with diverticulitis. Am J Roentgenol 192:963–966

Paulson EK, Jaffe TA, Thomas J et al (2004) MDCT of patients with acute abdominal pain: a new perspective using coronal reformations from submillimeter isotropic voxels. Am J Roentgenol 183:899–906

Pereira JM, Sirlin CB, Pinto PS et al (2004) Disproportionate fat stranding: a helpful CT sign in patients with acute abdominal pain. Radiographics 24:703–715

Pessaux P, Muscari F, Ouellet JF et al (2004) Risk factors for mortality and morbidity after elective sigmoid resection for diverticulitis: prospective multicenter multivariate analysis of 582 patients. World J Surg 28:92–96

Pilleul F, Bansac-Lamblin A, Monneuse O et al (2006) Water enema computed tomography: diagnostic tool in suspicion of colorectal tumor. Gastroenterol Clin Biol 30:231–234

Pittet O, Kotzampassakis N, Schmidt S et al (2009) Recurrent left colonic diverticulitis episodes: more severe than the initial diverticulitis? World J Surg 33:547–552

Poletti PA, Platon A, Rutschmann O et al (2004) Acute left colonic diverticulitis: can CT findings be used to predict recurrence? Am J Roentgenol 182:1159–1165

Pradel JA, Adell JF, Taourel P et al (1997) Acute colonic diverticulitis: prospective comparative evaluation with US and CT. Radiology 205:503–512

Puylaert JBCM (2001) Ultrasound of acute GI tract conditions. Eur Radiol 11:1867–1877

Ragu N (2010) Embryologie, anatomie et techniques d'imagerie du péritoine. In: Régent D, Vilgrain V (eds) Imagerie de l'abdomen. Lavoisier, Paris, pp 623–654

Rao PM, Rhea JT (1998) Colonic diverticulitis: evaluation of the arrowhead sign and the inflamed diverticulum for CT diagnosis. Radiology 209:775–779

Rao PM, Rhea JT, Novelline RA et al (1998) Helical CT with only colonic contrast material for diagnosing diverticulitis: prospective evaluation of 150 patients. Am J Roentgenol 170:1445–1449

Ridereau-Zins C, Aubé C, Luet D et al (2009) Assessment of water enema computed tomography: an effective imaging technique for the diagnosis of colon cancer. Abdom Imaging 35:407–413

Rioux M, Langis P (1994) Primary epiploic appendagitis: clinical, US, and CT findings in 14 cases. Radiology 191:523–526

Ripollés T, Agramunt M, Martínez MJ et al (2003) The role of ultrasound in the diagnosis, management and evolutive prognosis of acute left-sided colonic diverticulitis: a review of 208 patients. Eur Radiol 13:2587–2595

Sebastià C, Quiroga S, Espin E et al (2000) Portomesenteric vein gas: pathologic mechanisms, CT findings, and prognosis. Radiographics 20:1213–1224

Shah AM, Malhotra A, Patel B et al (2010) Acute diverticulitis in the young: a 5-year retrospective study of risk factors, clinical presentation and complications. Colorectal Dis. doi: 10.1111/j.1463-1318.2010.02372.x

Siewert B, Tye G, Kruskal J et al (2006) Impact of CT-guided drainage in the treatment of diverticular abscesses: size matters. Am J Roentgenol 186:680–686

Simonowitz D, Paloyan D (1977) Diverticular disease of the colon in patients under 40 years of age. Am J Gastroenterol 67:69–72

Singh AK, Gervais DA, Hahn PF et al (2005) Acute epiploic appendagitis and its mimics. Radiographics 25:1521–1534

Stabile BE, Puccio E, van Sonnenberg E et al (1990) Preoperative percutaneous drainage of diverticular abscesses. Am J Surg 159:99–104

Steenvoorde P, Vogelaar FJ, Oskam J et al (2004) Giant colonic diverticula. Review of diagnostic and therapeutic options. Dig Surg 21:1–6

Stefánsson T, Nyman R, Nilsson S et al (1997) Diverticulitis of the sigmoid colon. A comparison of CT, colonic enema and laparoscopy. Acta Radiol 38:313–319

Tack D, Bohy P, Perlot I et al (2005) Suspected acute colon diverticulitis: imaging with low-dose unenhanced multi-detector row CT. Radiology 237:189–196

Taourel PG, Fabre JM, Pradel JA et al (1995) Value of CT in the diagnosis and management of patients with suspected acute small-bowel obstruction. Am J Roentgenol 165:1187–1192

Taourel P, Kessler N, Lesnik A et al (2003) Helical CT of large bowel obstruction. Abdom Imaging 28:267–275

Thomas S, Peel RL, Evans LE et al (2006) Best cases from the AFIP: giant colonic diverticulum. Radiographics 26:1869–1872

Wasvary H, Turfah F, Kadro O, Beauregard W (1999) Same hospitalization resection for acute diverticulitis. Am Surg 65:632–635

Werner A, Diehl SJ, Farag-Soliman M et al (2003) Multi-slice spiral CT in routine diagnosis of suspected acute left-sided colonic diverticulitis: a prospective study of 120 patients. Eur Radiol 13:2596–2603

Zaidi E, Daly B (2006) CT and clinical features of acute diverticulitis in an urban U.S. population rising frequency in young, obese adults. Am J Roentgenol 187:689–694

Zins M, Bruel JM, Pochet P et al (2007) Question 1. What is the diagnostic value of the different tests for simple and complicated diverticulitis? What diagnostic strategy should be used? Gastroenterol Clin Biol 31:3S15–3S19

Nonischemic Colitis

Philippe Soyer, Mourad Boudiaf, Youcef Guerrache,
Christine Hoeffel, Xavier Dray, and Patrice Taourel

Contents

1	**Introduction**	222
2	**CT Technique**	222
3	**Idiopathic Inflammatory Colon Diseases**	223
3.1	Clinical Considerations	223
3.2	MDCT Presentation	224
3.3	Differential Diagnosis	227
4	**Nontuberculous Infectious Colitis**	227
4.1	General Considerations	227
4.2	MDCT Presentation	229
4.3	Differential Diagnosis	229
5	**Pseudomembranous Colitis**	229
5.1	Clinical Considerations	229
5.2	MDCT Presentation	230
5.3	Differential Diagnosis	231
6	**Tuberculosis**	232
6.1	Clinical Considerations	232
6.2	MDCT Presentation	232
6.3	Differential Diagnosis	233

7	**Typhlitis**	233
7.1	Clinical Considerations	233
7.2	MDCT Presentation	233
7.3	Differential Diagnosis	234
8	**Radiation Colitis**	234
8.1	Clinical Considerations	234
8.2	MDCT Presentation	234
8.3	Differential Diagnosis	234
9	**Graft-Versus-Host Disease**	235
9.1	Clinical Considerations	235
9.2	MDCT Presentation	235
9.3	Differential Diagnosis	235
References		235

P. Soyer (✉) · M. Boudiaf · Y. Guerrache
Department of Abdominal Imaging,
Hôpital Lariboisière-AP-HP, Université Diderot-Paris 7,
2, rue Ambroise Paré, 75475 Paris Cedex 10, France
e-mail: philippe.soyer@lrb.aphp.fr

C. Hoeffel
Department of Radiology, Hôpital Robert Debré,
11, boulevard Pasteur, 51092 Reims Cedex, France

X. Dray
Department of Digestive Diseases,
Hôpital Lariboisière-AP-HP, Université Diderot-Paris 7,
2, rue Ambroise Paré, 75475 Paris Cedex 10, France

P. Taourel
Department of Medical Imaging, Hôpital Lapeyronie,
371, avenue du Doyen Gaston Giraud,
34295 Montpellier Cedex 5, France

Abstract

Many patients with acute colitis present with abdominal pain or other nonspecific symptoms. In these patients, multidetector row CT is often used as the initial diagnostic test, which plays a pivotal role. This imaging technique can demonstrate inflammatory changes in the colonic wall, determine the extent of the disease, and detect the potential complications. In addition, multidetector row CT helps identify myriad extracolonic conditions that are responsible for the nonspecific symptoms should the patients have a cause of symptoms other than colitis. In most cases, the specific cause of colitis is determined on the basis of the results of clinical examination, laboratory tests, optical colonoscopy, and colonic biopsy. However, in equivocal cases or emergency situations, multidetector row CT findings help narrow the differential diagnosis. Many multidetector row CT features or patterns are helpful in distinguishing between the various types of colitis. They include the degree of wall thickening

P. Taourel (ed.), *CT of the Acute Abdomen*, Medical Radiology. Diagnostic Imaging,
DOI: 10.1007/174_2011_159, © Springer-Verlag Berlin Heidelberg 2011

and colonic edema, the extent and location of the disease, extraluminal manifestations, and types of complication. Multidetector row CT has a critical role in determining the most appropriate therapeutic approach in a substantial number of cases.

1 Introduction

"Colitis" is a comprehensive term that corresponds to an acute or chronic inflammatory process that involves the whole colon or that is restricted to some portions. The critical role of multidetector row CT (MDCT) in patients with suspected colitis is well established. This technique is considered the primary imaging test for the evaluation of patients suspected of having such a condition. This is because MDCT is available at virtually all institutions, and also because MDCT is able to accurately demonstrate the colonic wall as well as the pericolic fatty tissues, and adjacent structures. As a consequence, MDCT is a highly sensitive imaging technique for the detection of intramural inflammatory conditions as well as extraluminal consequences of colitis (Horton et al. 2000; Thoeni and Cello 2006).

Patients with colitis frequently present with abdominal pain, so a specific diagnosis is often difficult on the basis of clinical symptoms only. Conversely, MDCT is particularly valuable for the detection and characterization of many conditions that may cause colitis, including idiopathic inflammatory colon disease (i.e., Crohn's disease and ulcerative colitis), infectious colitis, which may be due to bacterial, viral, fungal, and parasitic organisms, typhlitis, radiation colitis, graft-versus-host disease, and pseudomembranous colitis.

This chapter describes the MDCT technique that is best suited for the investigation of patients with suspected colitis and reviews the MDCT features of the most frequent inflammatory conditions that affect the colon, with particular emphasis on suggestive features that may help radiologists distinguish between specific diseases.

2 CT Technique

Many patients presenting with clinical suspicion of acute colitis often have nonspecific symptoms. Therefore, MDCT of the abdomen and pelvis should be performed with a general protocol that works for most cases, unless the patient has a prior history of documented inflammatory bowel disease such as Crohn's disease or ulcerative colitis.

At our institution and at that of others, when MDCT is performed for possible acute colitis, a water enema is preferably used. Water enema distends the rectum and colon and helps discriminate between collapsed bowel wall and mural thickening due to an inflammatory condition. Water enema helps better demonstrate the status of the colonic wall, determine the degree of wall thickening, and detect increased enhancement by comparison with positive contrast material enema. In addition, unlike positive contrast materials, water does not interfere with three-dimensional MDCT reconstructions (Horton et al. 2000). This approach for colon tagging is our favored one, unless colonic perforation or anastomotic dehiscence after surgery is suspected. In this regard, in patients with known colonic disease who are prone to generate perforation, fistula, and abscess, enema is obtained with diluted iodinated contrast material at a concentration of 0.1%. After anal insertion of a lubricated enema tube, the tube is connected to a bag that contains 1–2 L of lukewarm plain water. Water is gently infused through gravity in 2–3 min. In some cases, particularly in elderly patients, a tube equipped with a small latex-free inflatable balloon can be used. A scout view or limited volume acquisition at the level of the pelvis is obtained to make sure that adequate colonic distension is achieved before the start of the MDCT study (Horton et al. 2000; Thoeni and Cello 2006). The use of plain water is the best option and, when possible, it is our preferred one. However, in some instances, patients presenting with acute colitis have symptoms similar to those observed in acute colonic diverticulitis, so a positive contrast material is used to fill the colon.

Intravenous administration of iodinated contrast material is not mandatory for a correct diagnosis in many instances. However, it is helpful for depicting extracolonic disease. In addition, the analysis of patterns of enhancement may provide suggestive clues to the specific diagnosis, as discussed below. We routinely administer 120 mL of nonionic iodinated contrast material at a concentration of 30 g of iodine per 100 mL at a rate of 3 mL/s through a 20-gauge venous catheter. However, the total volume should ideally be adapted to the patient's weight, with

1.5 mL of contrast material for 1 kg of body weight. Helical scanning starts 50 s after the beginning of contrast material injection. This delay corresponds to the mesenteric phase of abdominal imaging (Schindera et al. 2007), which allows detection of subtle colonic wall abnormalities. This phase provides a comprehensive evaluation of the abdomen and pelvis, including abdominal vessels that may be abnormal because of the underlying disease.

Currently, MDCT of the colon is routinely performed with 64-slice or more helical CT scanners but the use of equipment yielding a lower number of slices is still possible. Patients are positioned head first with respect to the scanner gantry and in the supine position. Several scanning protocols with different parameters can be used, but there is a trend toward obtaining a collimation thickness less than 1 mm, so that submillimeter voxel reconstruction can be obtained. An online, real-time, anatomy-adapted, attenuation-based tube current modulation technique is generally used to decrease the radiation dose given to the patient by up to 30% (Kalra et al. 2004). Scanning is performed from the dome of the liver to the symphysis pubis, using a cephalocaudad direction, after breath-hold instruction has been given. Typically, the radiation dose given to the patient is around 6.2 mSv when one single imaging pass during the mesenteric phase is performed and can reach up to 13 mSv when two imaging passes are performed.

After acquisition, MDCT data are reconstructed twice using a soft tissue reconstruction kernel in the axial plane. A first set is obtained with a thickness of 2–3-mm at 2–3-mm intervals for analysis of axial images. A second set is obtained at 0.6-mm thickness at 0.5-mm intervals for multiplanar reconstructions as well as for maximum intensity projection (MIP) views. The advantage of MDCT is that data can be used to obtain multiple reformations in different planes, on the basis of isotropic voxels. Multiplanar reconstructions and MIP views are interpreted along with axial images to better understand the distribution of colonic segments, improve localization of colonic abnormalities, and analyze the colonic vascularization. In this regard, it is crucial to understand that MIP images should complement and not replace careful analysis of the axial images because interpretation of MIP images alone could result in misdiagnosis. In most institutions, images are subsequently sent to a picture archiving and communication system workstation for further analysis. The outstanding quality of reformatted images provides improved visualization of the extent of inflammatory changes of the colon and makes treatment planning easier. The added benefit of multiplanar reformations is especially evident for effective assessment of the ileocecal area (Hoeffel et al. 2006). In addition, it has been demonstrated that the routine use of coronal reformations markedly reduces the number of images required for viewing by the referring physician to a minimum (Horton et al. 2000). Therefore, MDCT has a pivotal role in the routine diagnostic workup of patients with suspected colitis, but all pertinent information must be integrated into the final diagnosis.

3 Idiopathic Inflammatory Colon Diseases

3.1 Clinical Considerations

Patients with Crohn's disease and patients with ulcerative colitis usually present with similar symptoms, including nonspecific abdominal pain, cramping, tenesmus, and hematochezia. In the case of rectal involvement, patients have frequent but small-volume stools with a sensation of incomplete evacuation. Patients with Crohn's disease frequently complain of acute pain in the ileocecal area and fever that mimic acute appendicitis. Although clinical history and endoscopic findings are the bases for differentiating between Crohn's disease and ulcerative colitis, MDCT may help differentiate between these two entities when clinical, endoscopic, and histopathological findings are equivocal. In addition, MDCT provides visualization of the bowel wall and adjacent structures such that it plays an important role in the detection of a variety of complications of inflammatory bowel diseases.

Extraintestinal manifestations are common with Crohn's disease and ulcerative colitis, particularly large-joint nondestructive arthritis, spondylitis, and erythema nodosum.

Ulcerative colitis is associated with an increased risk of venous and arterial thrombosis due to increased coagulability. Vascular manifestations of ulcerative colitis account for 2% of all extraintestinal manifestations (Lefèvre et al. 2010). More than 60%

Table 1 CT distinction between ulcerative colitis and Crohn's disease (adapted from Thoeni and Cello 2006)

Feature	Ulcerative colitis	Crohn's disease
Distribution	Continuous	Skip
Symmetry	Symmetric	Asymmetric
Location	From the rectum to other colonic segments	Right-sided or most extensive
Small bowel involvement	Rare (only terminal ileum)	Common
Fat	Perirectal fat increased	Mesenteric fat increased
Pericolic stranding	Rare	++
Lymph nodes	Not enlarged	Enlarged
Main complications	Toxic megacolon, mesenteric thrombosis	Fistula, phlegmon, abscess, bowel obstruction

of the vascular complications consist of peripheral venous thrombosis or pulmonary embolism. Unusual sites of thrombosis include mesenteric, portal, hepatic, and cerebral veins (Papa et al. 2008; Lefèvre et al. 2010). In one large study, over an 11-year period, thromboembolic complications occurred in 1.3% of patients with ulcerative colitis (Talbot et al. 1986). Sixty-six percent of them had either deep vein thrombosis or pulmonary embolism, with a mortality rate as high as 25% (Talbot et al. 1986). Accurate identification of complications is important because they influence the patient's treatment, have an impact on the outcome, and undetected complications may have severe consequences.

3.2 MDCT Presentation

Considerable overlap exists between the MDCT findings in Crohn's disease and in ulcerative colitis summarized in Table 1. However, some features may help distinguish between the two conditions. Crohn's disease that affects the colon results in extensive involvement of the ascending colon and terminal ileum, which both exhibit marked mural thickening and narrowing. Severe involvement with marked inflammation results in stenosis of the ileocecal valve and proximal dilatation of the ileum. Diffuse involvement of the colon may occur in Crohn's disease but involvement of the descending colon as the single location is rare. By contrast, ulcerative colitis is typically left-sided or diffuse, and rarely involves the ascending colon exclusively (Philpotts et al. 1994). In addition, in ulcerative colitis, the rectum is virtually always abnormal, whereas in Crohn's disease, the

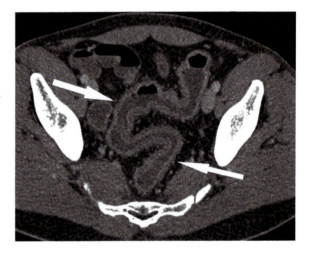

Fig. 1 A 28-year-old man with Crohn's disease limited to the colon. Multidetector CT (MDCT) shows moderate thickening of the rectosigmoid colon (*arrows*). There are no signs suggestive of marked inflammation, and colonic wall enhancement is homogeneous

rectum may be spared although other colonic segments are involved. Luminal narrowing along with mural thickening of the rectum is often associated with perirectal fatty proliferation. This association of the findings is very suggestive of the diagnosis of ulcerative colitis. This association is often found with enlargement of the presacral space which is due to proliferation of perirectal fat.

The most frequent MDCT finding in Crohn's disease and ulcerative colitis is wall thickening (Fig. 1) (Frager et al. 1983; Gore et al. 1996; Macari and Balthazar 2001). The mean wall thickness in Crohn's disease is usually greater (11 mm) than that in ulcerative colitis (7.8 mm) (Philpotts et al. 1994;

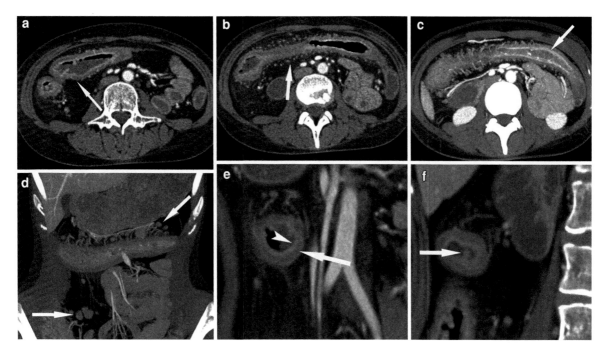

Fig. 2 An 18-year-old woman with Crohn's disease limited to the colon. The patient was receiving steroids when she was admitted for recurrent clinical symptoms that included abdominal pain, hematochezia, and fever. MDCT was performed to confirm the cause of the symptoms and exclude possible extracolonic complications. a The MDCT image in the axial plane shows marked wall thickening (*arrow*) with stratification. b Pericolic increased vascularity (*arrow*) with severe luminal narrowing is noticed. c The maximum intensity projection (MIP) reformatted image in the axial plane better demonstrates increased enhancement of the mucosa and submucosa (*arrow*). d The three-dimensional image in the coronal plane allows comprehensive assessment of the disease and shows markedly enlarged lymph nodes (*arrow*). e Reformatted image in the coronal plane showing stratification of the colonic wall, a finding suggestive for the diagnosis of acute inflammation. Stratification is due to increased enhancement of the mucosa and submucosa (*arrowhead*) and edema of the muscularis propia (*arrow*). f Reformatted image in the coronal plane showing a pseudopolyp (*arrow*) in the colon, a finding suggestive for the diagnosis of Crohn's disease

Fishman et al. 1987). Wall thickening in ulcerative colitis is typically diffuse, symmetric, and continuous, whereas wall thickening in Crohn's disease is typically eccentric, asymmetric, and segmental with apparently disease-free areas (the so-called skip regions) (Table 1). The asymmetric pattern, which typically occurs along the mesenteric border of the intestine, can result in the formation of pseudodiverticula along the antimesenteric border.

In patients with idiopathic inflammatory bowel diseases, thickening of the colonic wall is found in association with mural stratification (Figs. 2, 3, 4). Mural stratification is defined by the presence of two (halo sign) or three (target sign) layers of different attenuation values within the colonic wall (Balthazar 1991). This feature can be observed after intravenous administration of iodinated contrast material and is best depicted when enema has been administered using a neutral contrast material. The halo and target signs most often indicate an acute stage of a colonic disease, but are not specific. By contrast, homogeneous enhancement is consistent with an inactive or a chronic fibrous disease (Choi et al. 2003).

The halo sign corresponds to the combination of hyperenhancement of the muscularis propria with a submucosal low-attenuation ring in the colonic wall that is either due to submucosal deposition of fat (fatty halo sign) or submucosal edema (water halo sign). Discriminating between these two phenotypes of the halo sign is important. The water halo sign indicates acute disease and can be observed in both Crohn's disease and ulcerative colitis. The fatty halo sign indicates chronic disease and is more frequent in ulcerative colitis (Jones et al. 1986a). Other features must be searched for to heighten confidence in diagnosing acute disease. In this regard, enlarged or

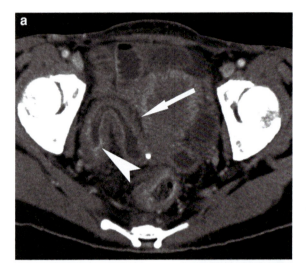

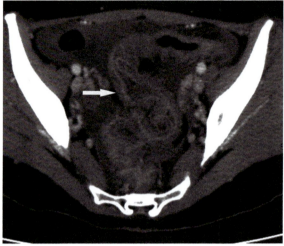

Fig. 4 A 28-year-old woman with known ulcerative colitis. The patient was receiving steroids when she was admitted for abdominal pain and bloody diarrhea. MDCT shows thickening of the rectum and sigmoid colon (*arrow*) with hyperenhancement of the mucosal and submucosal layers. Ascites, indicating acute disease, is present

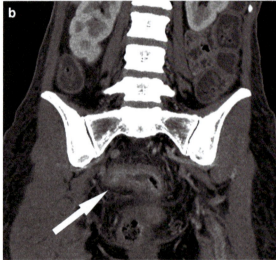

Fig. 3 A 43-year-old woman with known Crohn's disease treated with infliximab and methotrexate, presenting with abdominal pain and tenesmus. **a** MDCT in the axial plane shows marked thickening of the sigmoid colon and rectum (*arrow*), with stratification (*arrowhead*) corresponding to active and severe disease. **b** The coronal image shows pericolic stranding (*arrow*)

engorged pericolic vessels strongly suggest active disease (Fig. 5) (Lee et al. 2002).

Proliferation of mesenteric fat is very suggestive of Crohn's disease (Herlinger et al. 1998; Yamamoto et al. 2005). By contrast, proliferation of perirectal fat is less specific, and can be observed in both Crohn's disease and ulcerative colitis (Philpotts et al. 1994). Mesenteric lymphadenopathy suggests Crohn's disease rather than ulcerative colitis, although this finding is certainly not specific to inflammatory bowel disease (Figs. 2, 3).

Complications of idiopathic inflammatory colon diseases are well depicted with MDCT (Furukawa et al. 2004). It is important to understand that symptomatic patients may have a variety of severe complications that must be depicted rapidly to prompt physicians to start the most appropriate therapy (Fishman et al. 1987; Gossios and Tsianos 1997). In this regard, toxic megacolon is a severe complication of ulcerative colitis which must be ruled out. MDCT is helpful in this task because patients with toxic megacolon present with typical findings which include marked colonic dilatation with large amounts of intraluminal gas and fluid accumulation, along with loss of haustra. The colonic wall is thin and intra-abdominal free fluid effusion is usually present. When present, pneumatosis intestinalis suggests an extremely severe form of disease. Prompt therapy is mandatory to avoid severe or even life-threatening complications such as colonic perforation and peritonitis (Imbriaco and Balthazar 2001; Latella et al. 2002). Other complications can be observed in patients with Crohn's disease. They include pericolic phlegmon and abscess (Casola et al. 1987; Funayama et al. 1996). MDCT allows one to differentiate phlegmon, which is an ill-defined inflammatory mass

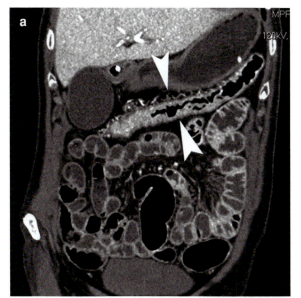

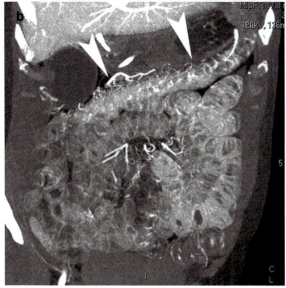

Fig. 5 A 55-year-old woman with Crohn's disease limited to the colon. The patient presented with abdominal pain and bloody diarrhea. **a** MDCT of the colon shows moderate thickening of the colonic wall along with markedly increased pericolic vascularity (*arrowheads*). **b** Increased vascularity (*arrowheads*) is dramatically better assessed using the MIP image

that usually requires treatment with antibiotics only, from abscess, which is a well-defined collection with a peripheral rim that often requires a more aggressive treatment such as percutaneous drainage or surgery, depending on the abscess diameter and location. Abscesses are present in 15–20% of symptomatic patients with Crohn's disease (Ribeiro et al. 1991). Abscesses are detected almost exclusively in Crohn's disease and are not detected in ulcerative colitis (Gore et al. 1984; Philpotts et al. 1994). They are usually the result of a sinus tract fistula or perforation. They are often confined to the bowel wall although they may involve adjacent structures such as the bladder, psoas muscle, and pelvic wall. MDCT can also be used for image guidance when percutaneous drainage of intra-abdominal abscess is required.

Fistulas are frequent complications of Crohn's disease. They most often originate from the rectum rather than the small bowel and the colon. Perianal and rectovaginal fistulas can be detected with MDCT but magnetic resonance imaging is more effective for their depiction.

Because of a possible association between multiple thrombotic sites and ulcerative colitis, MDCT images, which provide a comprehensive evaluation of intra-abdominal veins, including portal and hepatic veins, should be analyzed with particular attention to the status of the portal and hepatic veins in this specific population. It has also been shown that MDCT helps detect unsuspected thrombi (Lefèvre et al. 2010).

3.3 Differential Diagnosis

Proliferation of perirectal fat can be observed in Crohn's disease, ulcerative colitis, pseudomembranous colitis, and radiation colitis (Philpotts et al. 1994). The fatty halo sign can be observed in patients who have received external radiation therapy. Intramural fat can also be present in patients who are free of colonic disease, but in such cases the fatty layer is thinner by comparison with the thickness observed in patients with inflammatory colon disease (Jones et al. 1986a). Toxic megacolon can be observed in infectious colitis. Fistulas can be due to infectious diseases such as tuberculosis and actinomycosis.

4 Nontuberculous Infectious Colitis

4.1 General Considerations

In general, the diagnosis of infectious colitis is based on clinical symptoms and does not require MDCT for detection or differential diagnosis. Patients with

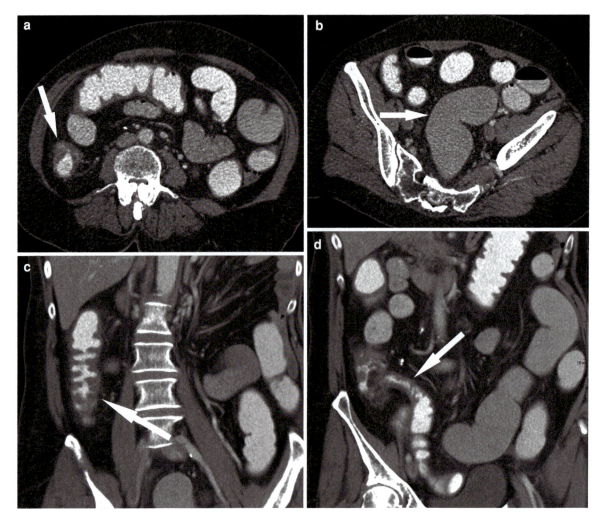

Fig. 6 A 72-year-old woman with abdominal pain, fever, and mild diarrhea. **a** MDCT performed after enema with positive contrast material shows mild thickening of the ascending colon (*arrow*). **b** On MDCT, no abnormalities of the descending colon and sigmoid colon (*arrow*) are visible. **c** Coronal MDCT image showing thickening of haustra in the ascending colon (*arrow*), consistent with inflammation. **d** Coronal MDCT image showing parietal thickening of the terminal ileum (*arrow*). This elective location of the disease suggests infectious colitis secondary to *Salmonella* infection. This was confirmed by the results of fecal cultures

infectious colitis present with an acute onset of dysenteric symptoms, consisting of fever, crampy abdominal pain, abdominal tenderness, tenesmus, and diarrhea. However, infectious colitis may be detected incidentally on MDCT or in patients for whom the clinical symptoms are equivocal.

The diagnosis of infectious colitis may be difficult with MDCT. One reason is that infectious colitis can be due to myriad causes. Another reason is that considerable overlap exists in MDCT presentation of infectious types of colitis. Bacterial causes include *Shigella*, *Salmonella*, *Yersinia*, *Campylobacter*, *Staphylococcus*, and *Chlamydia trachomatis*. Viral causes include cytomegalovirus and rotavirus (Horton et al. 2000). In immunodeficient patients, cytomegalovirus more often generates colitis than ileitis.

Infectious colitis is confirmed clinically on the basis of stool analysis and/or optical colonoscopy findings, and the results of colonic biopsy. The epidemiological context may help determine the cause in the clinical setting of infectious colitis. In homosexual patients, herpes virus and chlamydiae may be responsible for procto-colitis. In immunosuppressed patients, cytomegalovirus is often responsible for colitis, whereas it is rare in immunocompetent patients. In the context of alimentary intoxication involving a whole group of patients, *Escherichia coli* is a common cause. For patients being treated with broad-spectrum antibiotics or chemotherapeutic agents, *Clostridium difficile* must be looked for. This latter organism is responsible for pseudomenbranous colitis, considered later.

On MDCT, all cases of infectious colitis have in common wall thickening, pericolic stranding, and free fluid effusion. Most patients with infectious colitis present with pancolitis, but when restricted to the ascending colon, infectious colitis is most often due to *Salmonella* and *Yersinia*. When restricted to the descending colon, infectious colitis is most often due to *Shigella* or schistosomiasis. When a diffuse involvement is seen, infectious colitis is most often due to cytomegalovirus and *E. coli*.

4.2 MDCT Presentation

In patients with infectious colitis, MDCT uniformly shows colonic wall thickening in association with mucosal and submucosal enhancement. A low-attenuating layer that represents edema may be present within the wall. Free fluid effusion or inflammation of the pericolic fat may also be observed (Philpotts et al. 1994). Multiple air–fluid levels may be seen in the colon owing to increased fluid production and accumulation as well as spontaneous colonic distension. Depending on the portion of abnormal colon, a specific cause may be suggested. In most cases abnormalities are limited to the ascending colon (*Yersinia, Salmonella*) (Fig. 6), although diffuse involvement also occurs (cytomegalovirus, *E. coli*) (Wall and Jones 1992). In contrast, gonorrhea, herpesvirus, and *C. trachomatis* typically involve the rectosigmoid. In schistosomiasis, inflammation is confined to the descending colon or rectosigmoid in 85% of cases, but involvement of the ascending colon can be observed in 9% of cases (Cao et al. 2010).

In the case of colitis due to cytomegalovirus, MDCT shows nonspecific edema with diffuse mucosal ulceration or aphthous ulceration and skip areas. The terminal ileum is rarely involved and the disease most often manifests itself as a diffuse pancolitis with a thickening, which is more prominent at the level of the cecum.

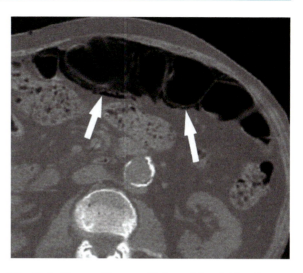

Fig. 7 A 67-year-old man with bacterial arthritis who presented with abdominal pain. MDCT shows cystic pneumatosis (*arrows*) of the wall of the transverse colon. Optical endoscopy findings suggested infectious colitis and stool assay disclosed *Escherichia coli*. The outcome was uneventful after treatment with antibiotics. (Reprinted with permission from Soyer et al. 2008)

4.3 Differential Diagnosis

Colitis due to cytomegalovirus usually mimics ulcerative colitis with diffuse mucosal ulceration or Crohn's colitis with aphthous ulcerations and skip areas (Frager et al. 1986). Pneumatosis intestinalis can be observed in colitis due to *E. coli*, so it may mimic a severe form of ischemic colitis (Fig. 7).

5 Pseudomembranous Colitis

5.1 Clinical Considerations

Pseudomembranous colitis is due to toxins produced by an overgrowth of *C. difficile*, which is a strictly anaerobic organism. During infection, *C. difficile* produces two key virulence determinants, toxin A and toxin B (Kuehne et al. 2010). Over the last decade, the incidence of *C. difficile*-associated disease has progressively increased and this disease is now a frequent clinical problem in North America and Europe. This disease is clinically associated with a profuse watery diarrhea along with abdominal pain and fever (Kelly et al. 1994). This colitis is a complication of broad-spectrum antibiotic therapy and is commonly observed in neutropenic patients. Alteration of normal gut flora by the medications allows colonization by *C. difficile* and production of enterotoxins, resulting in inflammation of the colon, diarrhea, and pseudo-membranous exudates (Kirkpatrick and Greenberg 2001).

Histologically, pseudomembranous colitis is characterized by pseudomembranes, which are made of necrotic mucosal cells. The diagnosis is usually based on clinical history that includes a recent treatment with antibiotics and confirmed by the results of stool assay for the *C. difficile* toxin. However, the clinical presentation can be misleading and a suspected diagnosis may not be made. In addition, stool assays for *C. difficile* toxin have a substantial rate of false negatives, so optical sigmoidoscopy is required for rapid identification of *C. difficile*-associated pseudo-membranous colitis. As a consequence, radiologists should be familiar with the MDCT findings of pseu-domembranous colitis because if it is not treated appropriately, this condition may evolve to toxic megacolon and perforation, and result in a fatal out-come (Morris et al. 1990; Jobe et al. 1995). Oral administration of metronidazole is the first-line ther-apy and oral administration of vancomycin is more often reserved for patients who have experienced a relapse after a course of metronidazole. Probiotic therapies based on administration of *Saccharomyces boulardii* represent another treatment approach. However, some patients with a fulminant form do not respond favorably to medical treatment and need emergency colectomy for cure (Bradley et al. 1988; Kelly et al. 1994; Klingler et al. 2000). In addition, in patients with pseudomembranous colitis, MDCT shows the extent and severity of the disease and potential complications. As a limitation, however, MDCT findings alone do not help predict which patients with pseudomembranous colitis require sur-gery (Kawamoto et al. 1999).

5.2 MDCT Presentation

Thickening of the colonic wall, which may be cir-cumferential or eccentric, is the most common CT finding in pseudomembranous colitis (Hoeffel et al. 2006). The colonic wall thickness ranges from 3 to 32 mm, with a mean value between 10.7 and 14.7 mm (Fishman et al. 1991; Philpotts et al. 1994).

In general, the degree of thickening in pseudomem-branous colitis is greater than that observed in any other inflammatory or infectious disease of the colon except Crohn's disease, so thickening is a helpful differential feature (Ros et al. 1996). On MDCT, the wall thickening in pseudomembranous colitis is often more irregular and shaggy than in Crohn's disease (Fig. 8), in which it is usually symmetric and homo-geneous (Fishman et al. 1991). In patients with pseudomembranous colitis, the bowel wall may be hypoattenuating depending on the amount of edema present or may show prominent enhancement after intravenous administration of iodinated contrast material secondary when marked inflammation is present.

In addition to wall thickening, the colon is often dilated. The dilatation is thought to be secondary to transmural inflammation. Mild pericolic stranding may also be observed. However, the pericolic stranding in pseudomembranous colitis is mild and contrasts with the relatively marked colonic wall thickening. This is because the condition predomi-nantly affects the mucosal and submucosal layers of the colon (Merine et al. 1987a, b).

The target sign, which was originally described in patients with ulcerative colitis and Crohn's disease, has also been reported in association with pseudo-membranous colitis. However, the most famous fea-ture is the accordion sign, which is due to marked thickening of haustral folds. This sign appears as broad transverse bands that may trap oral contrast material (Fishman et al. 1991). The accordion sign (Fig. 9) is very well known and very suggestive for the diagnosis of pseudomembranous colitis. As a limitation, this sign has been reported only in severe cases and is relatively rare. This sign in theory should be present only when oral contrast material has been given to the patient before MDCT examination. However, it has been described in the absence of oral contrast material because it can be due to increased mucosal enhancement after intravenous administra-tion of iodinated contrast material (Macari et al. 1999). The accordion sign can be observed in asso-ciation with acute colitis from other causes (Macari et al. 1999). The sensitivity and specificity of *C. dif-ficile* as the cause of the accordion sign are 38 and 61%, respectively (Macari et al. 1999).

In most cases, pseudomembranous colitis is a dif-fuse disease, such that it is considered a pancolitis.

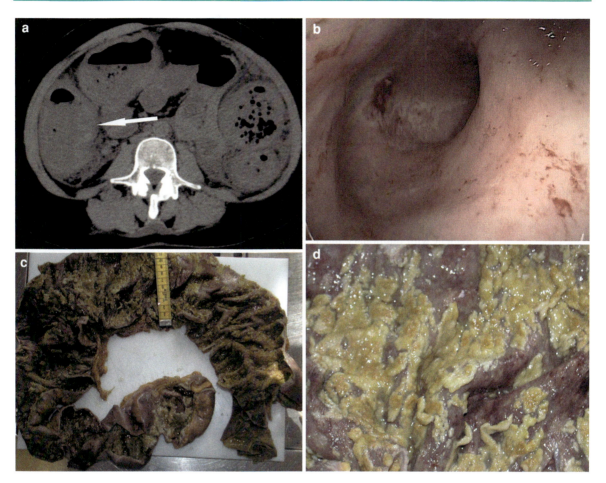

Fig. 8 A 55-year-old woman with abdominal pain and severe diarrhea. The clinical history revealed prior treatment with antibiotics, which is strongly suggestive for the diagnosis of pseudomembranous colitis. **a** MDCT shows spontaneously hyperattenuating mucosa and submucosa (*arrow*) with an enlarged colon. **b** Optical endoscopy shows erythematous, friable mucosa and adherent plaques. **c** Gross specimen after total colectomy showing multiple yellowish pseudomembranes adhering to the mucosa. **d** Magnified view showing typical pseudomembranes

However, in some cases, it may start as a proctitis and progress to the descending colon. It can also be limited to the ascending colon with sparing of the descending colon in up to 30–40% of cases (Ros et al. 1996). Involvement of portions of the colon and rectum has also been reported (Fishman et al. 1991). In addition, pseudomembranous colitis has been reported in patients with ileostomies or defunctionalized loops of the small bowel (Kralovich et al. 1997). Ascites can be observed in approximately one third of patients with pseudomembranous colitis, either as a complication of the infection or because of underlying conditions such as portal hypertension (Ros et al. 1996; Jafri and Marshall 1996).

5.3 Differential Diagnosis

Pericolic stranding is a nonspecific finding, because it can be observed in many other inflammatory and infectious diseases of the colon. However, the pericolic stranding in pseudomembranous colitis is mild and contrasts with the relatively marked colonic wall thickening, since the condition predominantly affects the mucosa and submucosa (Merine et al. 1987a, b).

The accordion sign can be found in cryptosporidiosis, ischemic colitis, lupus vasculitis, ulcerative colitis, Crohn's disease, and infectious colitis due to *Salmonella* or cytomegalovirus (Macari et al. 1999). Ascites may be a helpful feature for differentiating between pseudomembranous colitis and Crohn's disease. However, ascites can also be present in ischemic and infectious colitis.

6 Tuberculosis

6.1 Clinical Considerations

Tuberculous colitis is a rare disorder in Western countries, and its diagnosis may be difficult because it can mimic virtually any other disease. Colonic tuberculosis is usually acquired by ingesting contaminated milk products or, in a patient with pulmonary tuberculosis, by swallowing tracheobronchial secretions. Optical colonoscopy features in colonic tuberculosis include mucosal nodules and ulcers, which may be occasionally associated with strictures, pseudopolypoid folds, or fibrous bands (Boudiaf et al. 1998). Pathological analysis of tissue samples obtained during colonoscopy can show caseating granulomas. However, caseating granulomas are the hallmark of tuberculosis in only one third of cases. The ileocecal valve is often involved. The lesions tend to be transmural with marked desmoplastic reaction and a large amount of fibrous tissue. Inflammation may produce a masslike lesion called "tuberculoma," which mimics colon cancer. The lesions characteristically produce deep transverse ulceration of an irregular or "geographic" contour. Occasionally, enteroenteric fistulae or mixed tuberculous and bacterial abscesses are encountered. The diagnosis is usually established by positive cultures for acid-fast bacillus and acid-fast bacilli staining. Endoscopic and sometimes laparoscopic specimens may be needed for a definitive diagnosis. However, an MDCT scan can be helpful for the diagnosis and may avoid an unnecessary exploratory laparotomy.

6.2 MDCT Presentation

The ileocecal area is the portion of the gastrointestinal tract that is most commonly involved in tuberculosis. Characteristic MDCT features include asymmetric thickening of the ileocecal valve and medial wall of the cecum, exophytic extension engulfing the terminal ileum, and large lymph nodes with central, low-attenuating portions (Hoeffel et al.

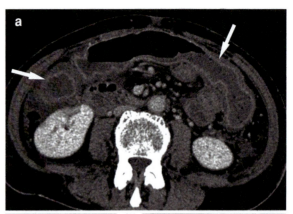

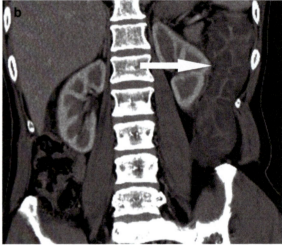

Fig. 9 A 57-year-old man with B-cell lymphoma who was receiving chemotherapy and broad-spectrum antibiotics. The patient was admitted for abdominal pain and bloody diarrhea, with a strong suspicion of pseudomembranous colitis but because of neutropenia, typhlitis could not be excluded. MDCT was thus performed to elucidate the cause of the clinical symptoms. **a** The MDCT image shows marked enhancement of the mucosa and submucosa (*arrows*), with thickening of all colonic portions and distension of the colon due to increased fluid production. **b** Coronal reformation of MDCT images shows thickening of the descending colon and mucosal enhancement resulting in the accordion sign (*arrow*), whereas the ascending colon is relatively normal. These findings are consistent with *Clostridium difficile* colitis

2006). On MDCT, lymph nodes are markedly enlarged and often hypoattenuating with a peripheral rim of enhancement. They may contain calcifications. Fistulae and sinus tracts can be seen, but are less common than in Crohn's disease. Segmental colitis, diffuse colitis, and short strictures that mimic carcinoma may be seen (Thoeni and Cello 2006). A cone-shaped cecum caused by scarring, as well as hypertrophy of the ileocecal valve (Fleischner sign), can be seen on rare occasions (Thoeni and Cello 2006). At an advanced stage, MDCT demonstrates peritoneal thickening, ascites, enlarged abdominal lymph nodes, and thickened intestinal walls (Yilmaz et al. 2002). Coronal reformations show a retracted cecum together with smooth symmetric stenosis of the transverse colon.

6.3 Differential Diagnosis

The most important differential diagnosis of tuberculous colitis is Crohn's disease because of differences in treatment strategies. Distinction between these two entities can be problematic without a laparotomy (Boudiaf et al. 1998). Thickening of the colonic wall may be more prominent in tuberculous colitis than in Crohn's disease. Another helpful clue is that in tuberculous colitis, lymph nodes, when present, are found adjacent to the colon. In Crohn's disease, pericolic fibrofatty proliferation is visible. In addition, in tuberculous colitis, lymph nodes are larger and mural stratification is absent (Makanjuola 1998). Occasionally, a short thick-walled stricture due to tuberculoma may be seen on MDCT and can be mistaken for colonic adenocarcinoma (McDonald and Middleton 1976).

In the case of tuberculous involvement, the cecum is usually retracted and the ileocecal valve is rigid and incompetent. In Crohn's disease, a longer length of the ileum is involved in comparison with tuberculosis (Boudiaf et al. 1998). In addition, in Crohn's disease, lymph nodes often show homogeneous, increased enhancement after intravenous administration of iodinated contrast material when the patient is seen when the disease is acute.

7 Typhlitis

7.1 Clinical Considerations

Typhlitis, which is also called "neutropenic enterocolitis," occurs in neutropenic patients who are receiving treatment for a malignancy, most frequently patients with acute leukemia who are receiving chemotherapy (Wagner et al. 1970). However, typhlitis

has also been reported after bone marrow transplantation (Jones et al. 1986a) and in patients with aplastic anemia, lymphoma, or acquired immunodeficiency syndrome (Wall and Jones 1992). Patients present with fever, watery or bloody diarrhea, gastrointestinal bleeding, and abdominal pain in the right lower quadrant.

Typhlitis is characterized by marked edema and inflammation of the cecum, the ascending colon, and rarely the terminal ileum. The inflammation can lead to transmural necrosis and perforation. In addition, some patients may experience severe or even life-threatening hemorrhage (Gomez et al. 1998). The exact mechanism of this condition has not been fully elucidated, but it is hypothesized that it is the result of a complex combination, which includes neutropenia, ischemia, infection with cytomegalovirus, mucosal hemorrhage, and to some degree neoplastic infiltration (Wall and Jones 1992). Neutropenia is considered the main factor because it generates an overgrowth of colonic germs. Treatment consists of bowel rest, total parenteral nutrition, broad-spectrum antibiotics, and massive fluid and electrolyte replacement. Surgery may be needed in patients with transmural necrosis, perforation, or uncontrolled sepsis. During surgery, all necrotic colonic tissues must be resected (Moir et al. 1986; Schlatter et al. 2002; Otaibi et al. 2002).

7.2 MDCT Presentation

MDCT is the best examination in patients with typhlitis because of the risk of bowel perforation and severe bleeding with optical colonoscopy. MDCT demonstrates cecal distention and marked circumferential thickening of the cecal wall, which may be hypoattenuating when edema is present (Fig. 10) (Adams et al. 1985). The terminal ileum can be involved and free fluid effusion can be present (Frick et al. 1984; Wagner et al. 1970). Pneumatosis of the cecal wall is a very specific sign although it is rarely visible (Kirkpatrick and Greenberg 2003). Although typhlitis has often been described as a disease of the ascending colon, other portions of the colon can also be involved (Connor et al. 1984; Wood et al. 1995; Kirkpatrick and Greenberg 2003; Soyer et al. 2008). Pericolic inflammatory stranding is a frequent finding. Detection of complications such as pneumatosis, pneumoperitoneum, and pericolic fluid collections is

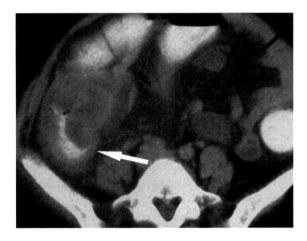

Fig. 10 A 37-year-old man who presented with acute pain in the right iliac fossa and fever. The patient was receiving chemotherapy for chronic lymphoid leukemia. MDCT shows marked thickening of the ascending colon and cecum (*arrow*). The findings are consistent with neutropenic enterocolitis (typhlitis)

important because they indicate a need for urgent surgical management (Frick et al. 1984; Shamberger et al. 1986). MDCT is helpful in assessing a favorable response to treatment and in identifying patients with intramural gas who need surgical resection (Wall and Jones 1992). Of interest, there have been cases of patients with neutropenic colitis and colonic pneumatosis who recovered after conservative therapy (Kirkpatrick and Greenberg 2003).

7.3 Differential Diagnosis

Distinction of typhlitis from other causes of colitis such as Crohn's disease or other infectious diseases may be difficult but the clinical history helps one make the correct diagnosis (Gayer et al. 2002; Da Ines et al. 2010). Clues to the diagnosis include the presence of marked thickening which is localized to the ascending colon in association with severe neutropenia (Fig. 10).

8 Radiation Colitis

8.1 Clinical Considerations

External radiation therapy can result in severe injury of the colon and rectum. Approximately, 50% of patients who receive more than 30 Gy of radiation therapy to the pelvis because of pelvic or genitourinary tract tumors will experience acute proctitis. Acute radiation injury to the rectum occurs within a few weeks of radiation exposure. Proctitis manifests itself as pain, self-limited diarrhea, tenesmus, and rectal bleeding (Otchy and Nelson 1993). This form of acute radiation injury is usually recognized clinically and treated symptomatically. It is self-limited and does not require imaging. Doses of 45–55 Gy induce chronic injury to the colon and rectum in 1–5% of patients, usually 6–24 months after completion of radiation therapy (Gilinsky et al. 1983; Kimose et al. 1989). Chronic injury is the result of radiation-induced endarteritis and damage to mesenchymal cells (Boudiaf et al. 2000).

8.2 MDCT Presentation

During the acute phase of radiation injury, MDCT shows nonspecific regular and symmetric wall thickening and inflammatory stranding adjacent to the affected region, which is typically the sigmoid colon and the rectum after pelvic radiation for prostate or cervical cancer. The MDCT appearance is nonspecific, but the clinical history helps suggest the correct diagnosis (Boudiaf et al. 2000).

A thickness of more than 10 mm of the presacral space in the anteroposterior plane and a thickening of the perirectal fascia are typical findings of chronic radiation-induced proctitis. They result in the so-called halo effect (Frommhold and Hubener 1981). Complications, such as fistulas, strictures, and abscesses, may also be demonstrated by MDCT. Once again, clinical history is the key to suggesting the diagnosis because the MDCT findings can be nonspecific.

8.3 Differential Diagnosis

MDCT findings in the active phase of radiation-induced injury of the colon are similar to those observed in graft-versus-host disease and in acute infectious proctitis. MDCT findings in the chronic phase of radiation-induced injury of the rectum raise the problem of tumor recurrence in the pelvis. In the other portions of the colon, MDCT findings such as strictures and fistulas may mimic chronic inflammatory diseases at a fibrous or chronic stage.

9 Graft-Versus-Host Disease

9.1 Clinical Considerations

Graft-versus-host disease is a severe complication of allogeneic bone marrow transplantation. This condition occurs when the donor T lymphocytes in the graft attack the transplant recipient's body. The gastrointestinal tract (predominantly the ileum and colon), skin, and liver are the primary organs affected. Graft-versus-host disease usually happens during the first 3 months after transplantation and affects approximately 15–50% of patients treated with allogeneic bone marrow transplantation (Kalantari et al. 2003). Clinically, this condition manifests itself as fever, diarrhea, vomiting, and sometimes gastrointestinal bleeding. Pathologically, there is a diffuse destruction and replacement of glandular structures by macrophages, lymphocytes, and plasmocytes. Glandular crypts of the colonic mucosa are involved by extensive lesions of necrosis.

9.2 MDCT Presentation

MDCT findings include colonic wall thickening, which may result in luminal narrowing. The terminal ileum can also demonstrates parietal thickening (Kalantari et al. 2003). Prolonged coating of the colon with contrast material has been reported in patients with severe mucosal disease. In these cases, the diluted barium can become trapped in the bowel wall because of mucosal healing from superficial ulcers (Ma et al. 1994). This intramural dissection of barium is not pathognomonic for graft-versus-host disease and has also been described in other conditions that cause severe mucosal ulceration, such as ischemic colitis. Other findings have been reported, such as a halo of decreased attenuation within the wall. The target sign can also be present when increased enhancement of the mucosa and submucosa is present (Kalantari et al. 2003). Inflammatory changes in the mesentery can be observed (Jones et al. 1986b). This latter finding is seen as increased attenuation of the mesentery with accompanying lymph nodes in some cases, similar to those observed in mesenteric panniculitis. In some cases, distension of the colon can be seen.

9.3 Differential Diagnosis

Colonic involvement in graft-versus-host disease is similar to that observed in radiation-induced colitis except for the length of involvement, which is usually less extensive in radiation-induced colitis. Although the colonic wall can be thickened, the thickening is less marked than in typhlitis and pseudomembranous colitis. In this regard, a colonic wall thickness of more than 7 mm excludes graft-versus-host disease (Kirkpatrick and Greenberg 2003). However, in ambiguous cases, the clinical history helps one make the specific diagnosis.

References

Adams GW, Rauch RF, Kelvin FM, Silverman PM, Korobkin M (1985) CT detection of typhlitis. J Comput Assist Tomogr 9:363–365

Balthazar EJ (1991) CT of the gastrointestinal tract: principles and interpretation. AJR Am J Roentgenol 156:23–32

Boudiaf M, Zidi SH, Soyer P, Lavergne-Slove A, Kardache M, Logeay O, Rymer R (1998) Tuberculous colitis mimicking Crohn's disease: utility of computed tomography in the differentiation. Eur Radiol 8:1221–1223

Boudiaf M, Soyer P, Pelage JP, Kardache M, Nemeth J, Dufresne AC, Rymer R (2000) CT of radiation-induced injury of the gastrointestinal tract: spectrum of findings with barium studies correlation. Eur Radiol 10:920–925

Bradley SJ, Weaver DW, Maxwell NP, Bouwman DL (1988) Surgical management of pseudomembranous colitis. Am Surg 54:329–332

Cao J, Liu WJ, Xu XY, Zou XP (2010) Endoscopic findings and clinicopathologic characteristics of colonic schistosomiasis: a report of 46 cases. World J Gastroenterol 16:723–727

Casola G, vanSonnenberg E, Neff CC, Saba RM, Withers C, Emarine CW et al (1987) Abscesses in Crohn disease: percutaneous drainage. Radiology 163:19–22

Choi D, Jin Lee S, Ah Cho Y et al (2003) Bowel wall thickening in patients with Crohn's disease: CT patterns and correlation with inflammatory activity. Clin Radiol 58: 68–74

Connor R, Jones B, Fishman EK, Siegelman SS (1984) Pneumatosis intestinalis: role of computed tomography in diagnosis and management. J Comput Assist Tomogr 8:269–275

Da Ines D, Petitcolin V, Lannareix W, Essamet W, Tournilhac O, Garcier JM (2010) CT imaging features of colitis in neutropenic patients. J Radiol 91:675–686

Fishman EK, Wolf EJ, Jones B, Bayless TM, Siegelman SS (1987) CT evaluation of Crohn's disease: effect on patient management. AJR Am J Roentgenol 148:537–540

Fishman EK, Kavuru M, Jones B (1991) Pseudomembranous colitis: CT evaluation of 26 cases. Radiology 180:57–60

Frager DH, Goldman M, Beneventano TC (1983) Computed tomography in Crohn disease. J Comput Assist Tomogr 7:819–824

Frager DH, Frager JD, Wolf EL, Rand LG, St Onge G, Mitsudo S, Bodner L, Brandt LJ, Beneventano TC (1986) Cytomegalovirus colitis in acquired immune deficiency syndrome: radiologic spectrum. Gastrointest Radiol 11:241–246

Frick MP, Maile CW, Crass JR, Goldberg ME, Delaney JP (1984) Computed tomography of neutropenic colitis. AJR Am J Roentgenol 143:763–765

Frommhold W, Hubener KH (1981) The role of computerized tomography in the after care of patients suffering from carcinoma of the rectum. J Comput Assist Tomogr 5:161–168

Funayama Y, Sasaki I, Naito H et al (1996) Psoas abscess complicating Crohn's disease: report of two cases. Surg Today 26:345–348

Furukawa A, Saotome T, Yamasaki M et al (2004) Cross-sectional imaging in Crohn disease. Radiographics 24: 689–702

Gayer G, Apter S, Zissin R (2002) Typhlitis as a rare cause of a psoas abscess. Abdom Imaging 27:600–602

Gilinsky NH, Burns DG, Barbezat GO, Levin W, Myers HS, Marks IN (1983) The natural history of radiation-induced proctosigmoiditis: an analysis of 88 patients. Q J Med 52:40–53

Gomez L, Martino R, Rolston KV (1998) Neutropenic enterocolitis: spectrum of the disease and comparison of definite and possible cases. Clin Infest Dis 27:695–699

Gore RM, Marn CS, Kirby DF, Vogelzang RL, Neiman HL (1984) CT findings in ulcerative, granulomatous, and indeterminate colitis. AJR Am J Roentgenol 143:279–284

Gore RM, Balthazar EJ, Ghahremani GG, Miller FH (1996) CT features of ulcerative colitis and Crohn's disease. AJR Am J Roentgenol 167:3–15

Gossios KJ, Tsianos EV (1997) Crohn disease: CT findings after treatment. Abdom Imaging 22:160–163

Herlinger H, Furth EE, Rubesin SE (1998) Fibrofatty proliferation of the mesentery in Crohn disease. Abdom Imaging 23:446–468

Hoeffel C, Crema MD, Belkacem A, Azizi L, Lewin M, Arrivé L, Tubiana JM (2006) Multi-detector row CT: spectrum of diseases involving the ileocecal area. Radiographics 26:1373–1790

Horton KM, Corl FM, Fishman EK (2000) CT evaluation of the colon: inflammatory disease. Radiographics 20:399–418

Imbriaco M, Balthazar EJ (2001) Toxic megacolon: role of CT in evaluation and detection of complications. Clin Imaging 25:349–354

Jafri SF, Marshall LB (1996) Ascites associated with antibiotic-associated pseudomembranous colitis. South Med J 89:1014–1017

Jobe BA, Grasley A, Deveney KE, Deveney CW, Sheppard BC (1995) Clostridium difficile colitis: an increasing hospital-acquired illness. Am J Surg 169:480–483

Jones B, Fishman EK, Hamilton SR et al (1986a) Submucosal accumulation of fat in inflammatory bowel disease: CT/pathologic correlation. J Comput Assist Tomogr 10: 759–763

Jones B, Fishman EK, Kramer SS (1986b) Computed tomography of gastrointestinal inflammation after bone marrow transplantation. AJR Am J Roentgenol 146:691–695

Kalantari BN, Mortelé KJ, Cantisani V (2003) CT features with pathologic correlation of acute gastrointestinal graft-versus-host disease after bone marrow transplantation in adults. AJR Am J Roentgenol 181:1621–1625

Kalra MK, Maher MM, Toth TL, Schmidt B, Westerman BL, Morgan HT et al (2004) Techniques and applications of automatic tube current modulation for CT. Radiology 233:649–657

Kawamoto S, Horton KM, Fishman EK (1999) Pseudomembranous colitis: can CT predict which patients will need surgical intervention? J Comput Assist Tomogr 23:79–85

Kelly CP, Pothoulakis C, LaMont JT (1994) Clostridium difficile colitis. N Engl J Med 330:257–262

Kimose HH, Fischer L, Spjeldmaes N, Wara P (1989) Late radiation injury of the colon and rectum: surgical management and outcome. Dis Colon Rectum 32:684–689

Kirkpatrick ID, Greenberg HM (2001) Evaluating the CT diagnosis of Clostridium difficile colitis: should CT guide therapy? AJR Am J Roentgenol 176:635–639

Kirkpatrick ID, Greenberg HM (2003) Gastrointestinal complications in the neutropenic patient: characterization and differentiation with abdominal CT. Radiology 226:668–674

Klingler PJ, Metzger PP, Seelig MH, Pettit PD, Knudsen JM, Alvarez SA (2000) Clostridium difficile infection: risk factors, medical and surgical management. Dig Dis 18:147–160

Kralovich KA, Sacksner J, Karmy-Jones RA, Eggenberger JC (1997) Pseudomembranous colitis with associated fulminant ileitis in the defunctionalized limb of a jejunalileal bypass: report of a case. Dis Colon Rectum 40:622–624

Kuehne SA, Cartman ST, Heap JT, Kelly ML, Cockayne A, Minton NP (2010) The role of toxin A and toxin B in Clostridium difficile infection. Nature 467:711–773

Latella G, Vernia P, Viscido A et al (2002) GI distension in severe ulcerative colitis. Am J Gastroenterol 97:1169–1175

Lee SS, Ha HK, Yang SK et al (2002) CT of prominent pericolic or perienteric vasculature in patients with Crohn's disease: correlation with clinical disease activity and findings on barium studies. AJR Am J Roentgenol 179:1029–1036

Lefèvre A, Soyer P, Vahedi K, Guerrache Y, Bellucci S, Gault V, Boudiaf M (2011) Multiple intra-abdominal venous thrombosis in ulcerative colitis: role of MDCT for detection. Clin Imaging 35:68–72

Ma LD, Jones B, Lazenby AJ, Douglas T, Bulte JW (1994) Persistent oral contrast agent lining the intestine in severe mucosal disease: elucidation of radiographic appearance. Radiology 191:747–749

Macari M, Balthazar EJ (2001) CT of bowel wall thickening: significance and pitfalls of interpretation. AJR Am J Roentgenol 176:1105–1116

Macari M, Balthazar EJ, Megibow AJ (1999) The accordion sign at CT: a nonspecific finding in patients with colonic edema. Radiology 211:743–746

Makanjuola D (1998) Is it Crohn's disease or intestinal tuberculosis? CT analysis. Eur J Radiol 28:55–61

McDonald JB, Middleton PJ (1976) Tuberculosis of the colon simulating carcinoma. Radiology 118:293–294

Merine D, Fishman EK, Jones B (1987a) Pseudomembranous colitis: CT evaluation. J Comput Assist Tomogr 11:1017–1020

Merine DS, Fishman EK, Jones B, Nussbaum AR, Simmons T (1987b) Right lower quadrant pain in the immunocompromised patient: CT findings in 10 cases. AJR Am J Roentgenol 149:1177–1179

Moir CR, Scudamore CH, Benny WB (1986) Typhlitis: selective surgical management. Am J Surg 151:563–566

Morris JB, Zollinger RM Jr, Stellato TA (1990) Role of surgery in antibiotic-induced pseudomembranous enterocolitis. Am J Surg 160:535–539

Otaibi AA, Barker C, Anderson R, Sigalet DL (2002) Neutropenic enterocolitis (typhlitis) after pediatric bone marrow transplant. J Pediatr Surg 37:770–772

Otchy DP, Nelson H (1993) Radiation injuries of the colon and rectum. Surg Clin North Am 73:1017–1035

Papa A, Scaldaferri F, Danese S, Guglielmo S, Roberto I, Bonizzi M, Mocci G, Felice C, Ricci C, Andrisani G, Fedeli G, Gasbarrini G, Gasbarrini A (2008) Vascular involvement in inflammatory bowel disease: pathogenesis and clinical aspects. Dig Dis 26:149–155

Philpotts LE, Heiken JP, Westcott MA, Gore RM (1994) Colitis: use of CT findings in differential diagnosis. Radiology 190:445–449

Ribeiro MB, Greenstein AJ, Yamazaki Y, Aufses AH Jr (1991) Intra-abdominal abscess in regional enteritis. Ann Surg 213:32–36

Ros PR, Buetow PC, Pantograg-Brown L, Forsmark CE, Sobin LH (1996) Pseudomembranous colitis. Radiology 198:1–9

Schindera ST, Nelson RC, DeLong DM, Jaffe TA, Merkle EM, Paulson EK, Thomas J (2007) Multi-detector row CT of the small bowel: peak enhancement temporal window—initial experience. Radiology 243:438–444

Schlatter M, Snyder K, Freyer D (2002) Successful nonoperative management of typhlitis in pediatric oncology patients. J Pediatr Surg 37:1151–1155

Shamberger RC, Weinstein HJ, Delorey MJ, Levey RH (1986) The medical and surgical management of typhlitis in children with acute nonlymphocytic (myelogenous) leukemia. Cancer 57:603–609

Soyer P, Martin-Grivaud S, Boudiaf M, Malzy P, Duchat F, Hamzi L, Pocard M, Vahedi K, Rymer R (2008) Linear or bubbly: a pictorial review of CT features of intestinal pneumatosis in adults. J Radiol 89:1907–1920

Talbot RW, Heppell J, Dozois RR, Beart RW Jr (1986) Vascular complications of inflammatory bowel disease. Mayo Clin Proc 61:140–145

Thoeni RF, Cello JP (2006) CT imaging of colitis. Radiology 240:623–638

Wagner ML, Rosenberg HS, Fernbach DJ, Singleton EB (1970) Typhlitis: a complication of leukemia in childhood. AJR Am J Roentgenol 109:341–350

Wall SD, Jones B (1992) Gastrointestinal tract in the immunocompromised host: opportunistic infections and other complications. Radiology 185:327–335

Wood BJ, Kumar PN, Cooper C, Silverman PM, Zeman RK (1995) Pneumatosis intestinalis in adults with AIDS: clinical significance and imaging findings. AJR Am J Roentgenol 165:1387–1390

Yamamoto K, Kiyohara T, Murayama Y et al (2005) Production of adiponectin, an anti-inflammatory protein, in mesenteric adipose tissue in Crohn's disease. Gut 54:789–796

Yilmaz T, Sever A, Gur S, Killi RM, Elmas N (2002) CT findings of abdominal tuberculosis in 12 patients. Comput Med Imaging Graph 26:321–325

Acute Gastritis and Enteritis

Denis Régent, Valerie Croisé-Laurent, Julien Mathias, Aurélia Fairise, Hélène Ropion-Michaux, and Clément Proust

Contents

1	**Acute Gastritis** 239
1.1	General Characteristics.. 240
1.2	The Main Aetiological Forms of Acute Gastritis 240
1.3	Diagnosis of Acute Gastritis by a CT Scan 242
2	**Acute Duodenitis and Enteritis**........................... 250
2.1	General Characteristics.. 250
2.2	Acute Infectious Conditions of the Duodenum and Small Intestine 252
2.3	Vascular Acute Inflammatory Conditions of the Duodenum and Small Intestine............................... 261
2.4	The Acute Appearance of Crohn's Disease in the Small Intestine 266
References.. 269

D. Régent (✉) · V. Croisé-Laurent · J. Mathias · A. Fairise · H. Ropion-Michaux · C. Proust
Service de Radiologie Adultes,
CHU Nancy-Brabois, Rue du Morvan,
54511 Vandoeuvre les Nancy Cedex, France
e-mail: d.regent@chu-nancy.fr

Abstract

In acute gastric or small bowel conditions, whether they are infectious, inflammatory, or ischemic, the CT scan objectifies submucosal oedema with parietal stratification, producing 'target' or 'double-halo' images that can be easily analysed in venous time. Precise analysis of proximal peritoneal reactions and of endoluminal content are the first steps of the diagnostic approach. In an acute clinical context, a number of hypotheses must be discussed (perforation, infection, arterial ischaemia, capillary hyperpermeability, congestion by portal venous stasis, etc.), some of which may be supported by abdominal/pelvic exploration, as a general rule complemented by thoracic exploration if there are no contraindications for the radiation risk (young subjects and women of childbearing potential). In all cases, the clinical context and laboratory tests are fundamental for orientating the diagnosis: a history of abdominal pain and diarrhoea, a state of acquired immunosuppression, a recent stay in a country where there are endemic parasites, a purpuric rash on the lower limbs, a marked inflammatory syndrome seen in laboratory tests, etc. are all signs providing pointers for the right direction which one needs to know how to find out by precise, directed questioning and clinical examination

1 Acute Gastritis

There are many different causes of acute gastritis. The most frequent complaints are due to limited histological lesions of the mucosa. They are diagnosed

P. Taourel (ed.), *CT of the Acute Abdomen*, Medical Radiology. Diagnostic Imaging,

exclusively by endoscopy and histology after biopsy. Only deep acute gastric lesions extending into the submucosa and the muscular layers can be seen during a CT examination performed because of a painful set of hyperalgesic epigastric symptoms with vomiting which may be haemorrhagic.

1.1 General Characteristics

The term 'acute gastritis' covers a very wide spectrum of inflammatory damage to the gastric mucosa, differentiated by distinct characteristics which depend on the depth of the parietal damage and the physiopathological mechanisms involved.

Two major groups can be differentiated:
1. Erosive gastritis, which includes the superficial forms, deep lesions and haemorrhagic forms.
2. Non-erosive gastritis, the main form of which is gastritis caused by *Helicobacter pylori*.

Most frequently, where involvement is limited to the mucosa, there is little or no correlation between the microscopic anatomopathological data and the clinical symptoms, which are often absent or non-specific (epigastric discomfort, nausea, vomiting). Diagnosis is essentially by endoscopy and biopsy, and there is no place here for any radiological method. There are many possible causes: alcohol, bile reflux, medicinal drugs, etc.

In severe erosive gastritis, in particular where there are deep ulcerations, and where the acute clinical picture reveals painful epigastric seizures associated with vomiting or haematemesis, a CT scan can be performed quite early and provides important semiotic data for a positive and differential diagnosis.

1.2 The Main Aetiological Forms of Acute Gastritis

1.2.1 Reactive Acute Gastritis or Reactive Gastropathy

There are many causes: non-steroidal anti-inflammatory drugs (NSAIDs), platelet aggregation inhibitors of the aspirin type whether they are administered orally or systemically, at therapeutic doses or in excessive doses, alcohol, stress, bile reflux and ischaemia. In NSAID gastritis, secondary to oral ingestion, the lesions are preferentially sited on the greater curvature owing to the effect of gravity (Table 1) (Levine 2008; Kim and Pickhardt 2007; Gelfand et al. 1999).

Table 1 Aetiology of acute gastritis and gastropathies

Drug-induced	Non-steroidal anti-inflammatory drugs and aspirin
	Cocaine
	Colchicine
	Antimitotic agents
Massive acute alcoholism with highly alcoholic drinks: whisky, vodka, gin	
Bacterial infections	*Helicobacter pylori*
	Helicobacter heilmanii
	Streptococci
	Staphylococci
	Enterobacteria of the genus *Proteus*
	Bacteria of the genus *Clostridium*
	Escherichia coli
	Tuberculosis
	Syphilis
Viral infections	Cytomegalovirus
Fungal infections	*Candida albicans*
	Histoplasmosis
Parasitic infections	Anisakiasis
Cardiogenic stress and shock	
Irradiation	
Allergies and food poisoning	
Biliary reflux	
Ischaemia	

1.2.2 Bacterial Gastritis

Phlegmonous gastritis is severe acute damage of bacterial origin, caused by various microorganisms such as *Escherichia coli*, *Pseudomonas aeruginosa*, *Clostridium perfringens*, *Enterobacter aerogenes*, *Proteus vulgaris*, *Staphylococcus aureus* or non-haemolytic streptococci; more rarely, its origin may be fungal (candidiasis, mucormycosis) (Jung et al. 2003; Asrani et al. 2007).

In general, it occurs in subjects in a poor general state of health. It is often secondary to massive ingestion of alcohol and coexists with respiratory infections. It is also found in AIDS patients (Fig. 1).

The infection affects the deep layers, the submucosa, muscularis propria and serous. It may have a gangrenous appearance and lead to peritonitis by

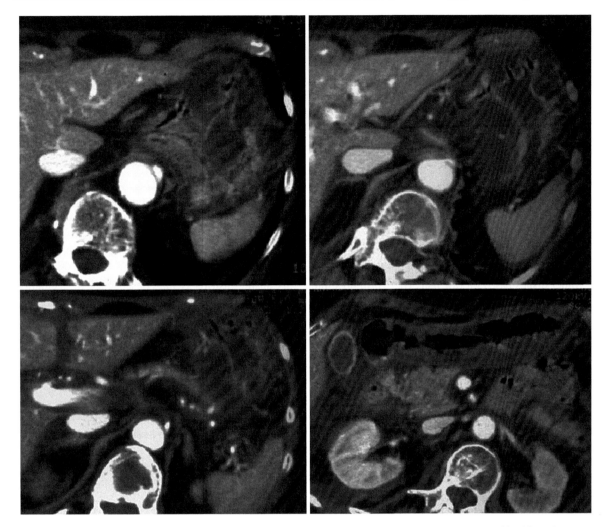

Fig. 1 Phlegmonous gastritis due to *Pseudomonas aeruginosa* (observed by C. Aubé, Angers). Very considerable oedematous thickening of the whole of the gastric body and fundus, in places exceeding 20 mm

perforation. The prognosis is very unfavourable, with a mortality rate of the order of 65%, even with treatment.

An intramural gastric abscess is a localised form of suppurative bacterial gastritis. It is a condition known since the time of Galen; diagnosis can be made with a CT scan when a liquid collection is seen within a gastric wall thickened by inflammation.

1.2.3 Other Infectious Causes of Severe Acute Gastritis

Other infectious causes of severe acute gastritis include:
- Viral infections, particularly cytomegalovirus (CMV) infections, generally seen in immuno-suppressed subjects, particularly in patients who have had transplants, those with cancer, and in AIDS. CMV gastritis may be haemorrhagic (Fig. 2). Acute gastritis caused by herpes simplex virus is exceptional.
- Acute fungal infections, in particular caused by *Candida albicans*, may be serious and even lethal. They occur above all in immunosuppressed subjects. This is also the case for the uncommon type of gastritis due to mucormycosis (predisposing factors are, above all, diabetes and also leukaemia, lymphoma, chronic renal impairment, solid organ transplant, septicaemia, severe burns, malnutrition, corticosteroid treatment and long-term antibiotic therapy). *Histoplasma capsulatum* can also be the cause of ulcerated gastritis, which can be erosive or with large rugae, but does not generally occur in an acute form.

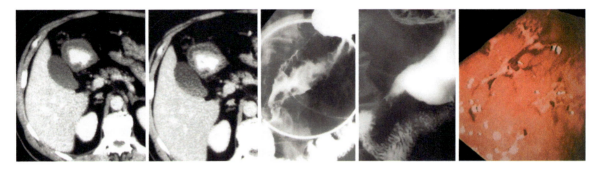

Fig. 2 Gastritis due to cytomegalovirus. Irregular thickening of the antral wall with submucosal hypodensity. Presence of eroded parietal nodules on the double contrast image. Endoscopy confirmed the presence of whitish ulcerations surrounded by hypervascularised folds of a nodular character

- Acute gastric parasitic infections, including anisakiasis caused by a nematode contaminating sushi or other dishes based on raw fish. The worm digs into the gastric mucosa along the greater curvature, leading to symptoms of acute pain that can persist for several days, linked to erosive and/or ulcerative lesions associated with large oedematous folds (Fig. 3).
- Gastric tuberculosis is generally a subacute condition most often found in the context of immunosuppression (AIDS) or disseminated tuberculosis.

Secondary syphilis has become a rare cause of gastritis that is generally subacute or chronic.

1.2.4 Haemorrhagic and Ulceronecrotic Acute Gastritis

As a general rule, haemorrhagic and ulceronecrotic acute gastritis are seen in patients who are critically ill, particularly with shock, severe infections, respiratory insufficiency or acute renal impairment, head injuries, extensive burns, etc. The mechanism is essentially ischaemia secondary to hypotension and hypovolaemic shock, to which are added the effects of the vasoconstrictor treatment administered, but the cause often remains unknown.

The lesions, essentially petechial or diffuse haemorrhages, are similar to those seen in acute drug-induced acute gastritis (aspirin, NSAID), except that their distribution is different, occurring in the fundus and body of the stomach.

1.2.5 Acute Gastritis Caused by Physical or Chemical Agents

Acute radiation gastritis is seen after exposure to more than 16 Gy and more frequently affects the antrum than the fundus; it can be complicated by pyloric stenosis.

Caustic gastritis is the consequence of accidental or voluntary ingestion of corrosive substances, usually acids (Fig. 4).

In both cases, a CT scan shows inflammatory parietal thickening and contributes to revealing early complications and associated lesions.

1.2.6 Idiopathic Inflammatory Gastritis May Quite Rarely Present in an Acute Clinical Picture

- Crohn's disease only affects the stomach in 2–7% of patients in whom the classic ileal and/or colic locations coexist.
- Eosinophilic gastritis is often seen in the context of eosinophilic gastroenteritis, but it may be encountered in association with many other conditions, such as food allergies (eggs, milk, soya proteins), collagenosis, digestive parasitosis, gastric cancer, lymphoma, Crohn's disease, vasculitis, drug allergies or *H. pylori* infection. The eosinophilic infiltrate can be limited to the mucosa or can extend to the whole intestinal wall.

1.3 Diagnosis of Acute Gastritis by a CT Scan

The semiotic data on which the positive diagnosis of acute gastritis and possibly the orientation of the aetiological diagnosis may be based need to be considered. Moreover, the direction taken by the differential diagnosis must take into consideration the other

Acute Gastritis and Enteritis

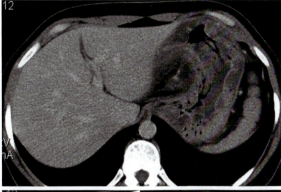
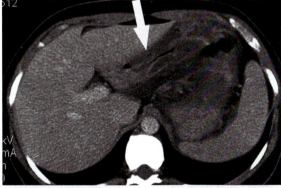
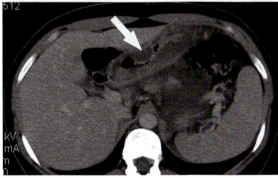

Fig. 3 Anisakiasis (observed by J.M. Hervochon, La Rochelle). Acute painful epigastric symptoms in a young woman. Very considerable diffuse oedematous thickening of the whole gastric body and antral region (*white arrow*) with oedematous infiltration of the lesser omentum. Aetiological questioning revealed recent ingestion of sushi and endoscopy confirmed anisakiasis

possible causes of 'acute' thickening of the gastric wall.

1.3.1 Positive Diagnostic Data for Acute Gastritis on a CT Scan

The main CT scan signs are seen in major transmural acute inflammatory conditions, in particular in bacterial phlegmonous gastritis, and include:

- Localised or diffuse thickening of the gastric wall with visible stratification indicating the oedema of the muco-submucosa complex; enhancement of the mucosal and muscle capillary networks, seen better in venous time with the 'target sign' appearance and best perceived if the stomach is distended with liquid (Jung et al. 2007). In other cases, a 'double halo' appears, defined as the juxtaposition of two concentric rings, the more internal, hypodense ring corresponding to the oedema of the submucosa, and the external, hyperdense ring corresponding to the thickening of the muscularis propria. This semiotic data are valuable for differentiating inflammatory parietal thickening from tumoral thickening (especially from an adenocarcinoma in which the collagen fibrous reaction stroma can be objectified by late enhancement in the postequilibrium phase).
- Oedematous hypertrophy of regular or nodular rugae is easier to analyse in a stomach distended with liquid.

Phlegmonous gastritis is a suppurative bacterial infection of the gastric wall. It can present in a diffuse or localised form, generally antral. Clinically, it appears in the form of acute abdomen combined with an infectious syndrome, epigastric pain, nausea, and vomiting—sometimes haemorrhagic in heavy drinkers—often following a serious respiratory infection. The different imaging techniques show the presence of localised or more diffuse parietal thickening, especially concerning the submucosa, that can be difficult to differentiate from a gastric adenocarcinoma on a CT scan (and by endoscopy!). The acute clinical context of the revelation, a septic and inflammatory picture in laboratory tests, an inflammatory reaction of the peritoneal serosa (thickened appearance with persistent enhancement, surrounding liquid reaction, etc.) and even, in certain cases, the appearance of a partially liquid parietal collection (gastric wall abscess) may orientate the diagnosis.

The presence of gas in a thickened gastric wall is a key sign that can be observed in various circumstances which must be clearly differentiated:

- Emphysematous gastritis is either a form of bacterial infectious gastritis caused by microorganisms producing large quantities of gas (by a mechanism similar to that incriminated in emphysematous cholecystitis) or phlegmonous gastritis of bacterial or fungal origin which can form an abscess

Fig. 4 Acute oesophagitis and gastritis after ingestion of bleach. The CT scan confirmed diffuse circumferential thickening of the lower oesophagus and all gastric walls with marked submucosal oedema

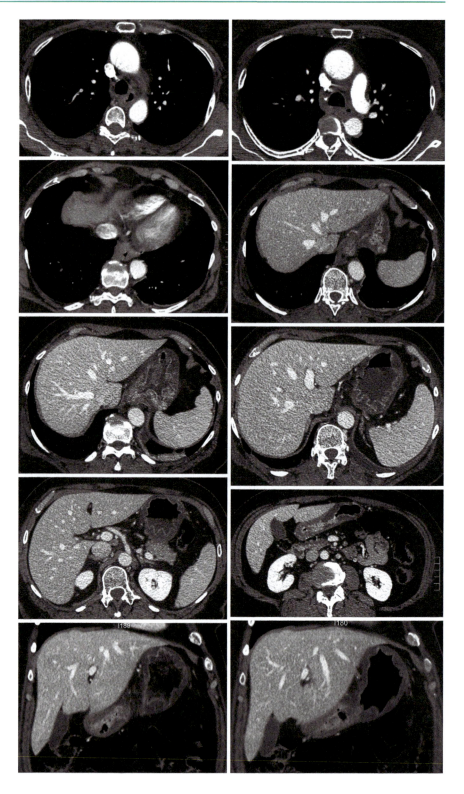

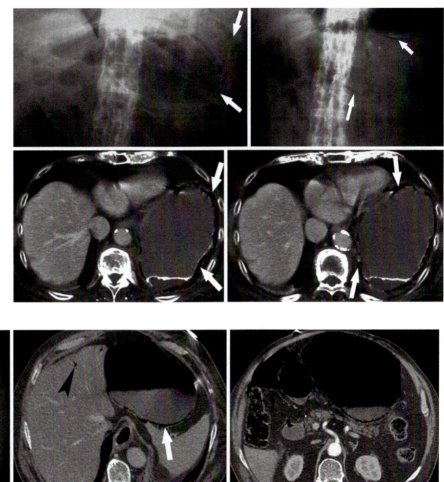

Fig. 5 Gastric emphysema in a patient with ankylosing spondylitis. The intraparietal gaseous images in a stomach distended with liquid are already clearly visible on the plain film pictures. The CT scan confirms the cystic gaseous dissection. The gastric emphysema occurred with gastroparesis. Clinical and radiological resolution after aspiration of the gastric contents

Fig. 6 Gastric emphysema in a 74-year-old patient with hepatic portal venous gas, of D3 after fitting of a total hip prosthesis. The abdominal plain film showed considerable gaseous distension of the stomach and, to a lesser degree, of the small intestine and colon, the whole picture corresponding to postoperative ileus. The CT scan confirmed the parietal gaseous dissection of the stomach (*white arrow*) and hepatic portal venous gas (*point of black arrow*). The condition evolved favourably after resumption of transit

(Jung et al. 2007; Loi et al. 2007). The appearance on the scan includes more or less extensive thickening of the gastric wall, generally in the fundus and the greater curvature with irregular bubbles of gas in spots or bunches; these gas bubbles remain in place whatever the subject's position or the degree of aspiration by the naso-gastric tube.

- Gastric emphysema is usually a regular linear infiltration of the gastric wall, which is not thickened or is little thickened, by gas from the gastric lumen, the surface of the peritoneal serosa or from the connections of the stomach with the oesophagus or duodenum. Gastric emphysema usually results from barotrauma without any infectious bacterial involvement; it is particularly seen in chronic liquid and or gas distension of the stomach whatever the mechanical (neoplastic antropyloric stenosis or stenosis of inflammatory origin by an ulcerative disease) or functional (gastroparesis) nature (Figs. 5, 6) (Buyt et al. 2003). This gastric emphysema is usually asymptomatic and is generally reabsorbed without treatment. A case has been reported in a 16-year-old adolescent boy, after he had ingested a large quantity of Coca Cola.

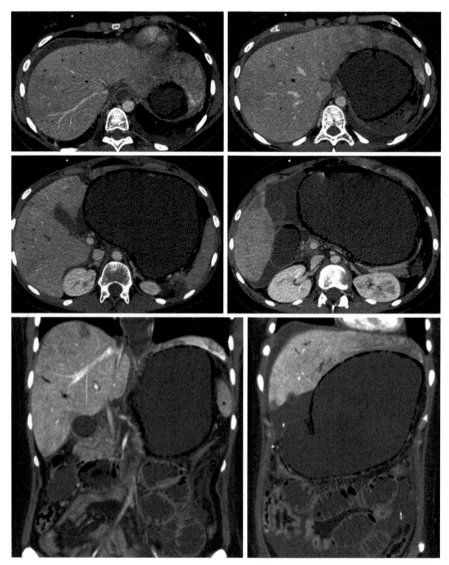

Fig. 7 Gastric necrosis. Transmural gastric necrosis in a 24-year-old patient with an antiphospholipid antibody syndrome and high-grade stenosis of the coeliac trunk by the arcuate ligament of the diaphragm. A CT scan was performed because of hyperalgesic painful epigastric symptoms. The CT scan confirmed the presence of massive gaseous dissection of the walls of the stomach, which were not enhanced after contrast medium injection. A large quantity of intraperitoneal fluid is present but the patient has a ventriculoperitoneal shunt for a cerebral expansive lesion. Hepatic portal venous gas is present. The surgical procedure confirmed transmural necrosis of the whole gastric wall

It was combined with hepatic portal venous gas and duodenal wall emphysema in a serious clinical condition which resolved with treatment (Hadas-Halpren et al. 1993).

The prognosis for these various conditions is therefore very different, and the presence of gas in the gastric wall must be carefully correlated with the clinical situation and probabilistic physiopathological hypotheses to correctly orientate therapeutic management.

1.3.2 Differential Diagnosis of Acute Gastritis on a CT Scan

CT interpretation in findings of gastritis must take into account clinical context and ancillary signs.

- Parietal pneumatosis of the stomach, seen in the context of painful acute abdomen and usually accompanied by intrahepatic portal venous gas, must be clearly differentiated from parietal emphysema. It is associated with the absence of parietal enhancement after injection of contrast medium and generally indicates transmural ischaemic necrosis of the stomach (Fig. 7). It can be observed after chemotherapy has been started in carcinomas (Fig. 8).
- Portal hypertensive gastropathy is a rare cause of digestive haemorrhage, and is generally not very severe in cirrhotic patients. Its probably multifactorial physiopathological mechanism remains open

Fig. 8 Tumoral necrosis in a 30-year-old patient with a very large anaplastic gastric adenocarcinoma. **a, b** Initial findings: massive thickening of the gastric wall with very voluminous hypodense adenopathies of the lesser omentum, coeliacs and splenic hilum. Presence of hepatic metastasis (*black arrow*). **c–f** One week after the start of chemotherapy: massive necrosis of the gastric wall tumour with lack of parietal enhancement and gaseous dissection. Massive metastatic and lymph node dissemination

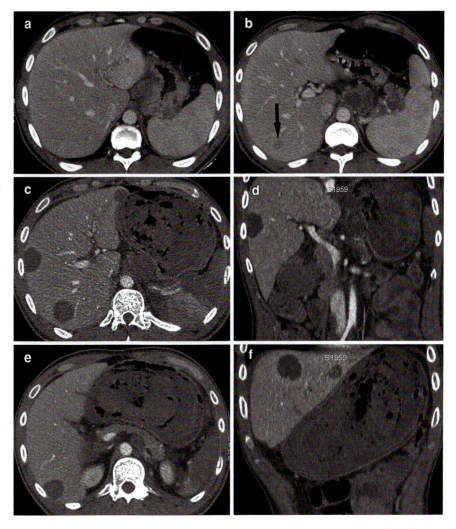

to discussion, involving raising of the pressure in the portal system, increasing splanchnic blood flow and local modifications to the regulation of microcirculation. The prevalence of portal hypertensive gastropathy varies from 7 to 98% in the series published, depending on the diagnostic criteria and the methods chosen for selecting patients. The circumferential thickening of the gastric wall with an image of parietal stratification by submucosal oedema, seen in severe portal hypertension with ascitic decompensation, may suggest the diagnosis (Figs. 9, 10) but it is known that there is no correlation between the portal pressure values measured, the severity of the cirrhosis, the degree of cellular dysfunction and the severity of the gastropathy when it is viewed endoscopically (Curvelo et al. 2000). Multiphase exploration objectifies defective segmental or subsegmental perfusion of the mucosa of the gastric body or fundus. This has been observed to disappear in the portal phase or during the postequilibrium phase in 75% of cases of endoscopically controlled portal hypertensive gastropathy but in only 11% of cirrhotic patients without endoscopically visible gastropathy. This method would therefore seem to provide useful, more specific information for diagnosis (Kim et al. 2008).

- Inflammatory reactions of the gastric wall during acute pancreatitis are frequent (one third of cases) and must be clearly identified. They have been known for a long time (Balthazar 1979) and predominate on the posterior wall, resulting in generally extensive oedematous muco-submucosal thickening in contact with anterior peripancreatic infiltrations and collections, whether recent or

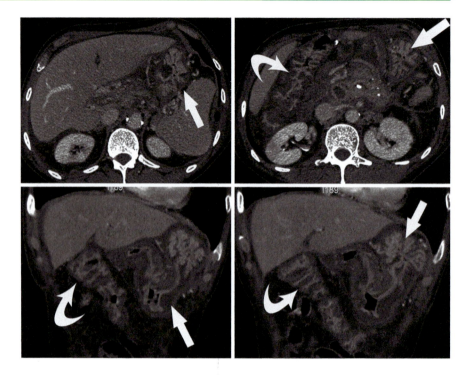

Fig. 9 Portal hypertensive gastritis. A 72-year-old cirrhotic patient with portal cavernoma and chronic calcifying pancreatitis. Very considerable submucosal oedema of the stomach wall (*straight white arrow*) and colon (*curved arrow*) in a context of extreme generalised oedema due to decompensated cirrhosis. The parietal submucosal thickening exceeds 15 mm in the body of the stomach

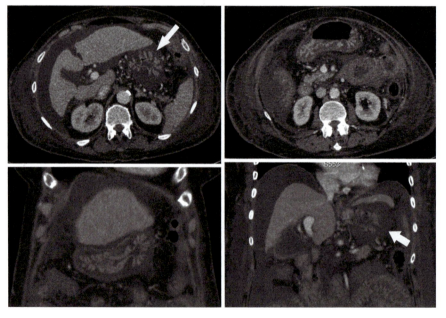

Fig. 10 Portal hypertensive gastritis in a patient with ascitic decompensated cirrhosis. Very considerable submucosal oedema of the whole stomach predominantly in the fundic region (*white arrow*)

organised (true pseudocysts) (Figs. 11, 12, 13). Analogous images can be seen on contact with infected collections (left-sided subphrenic abscesses) complicating ulcerous or surgical perforations (Chen et al. 2007; Brown et al. 1982).
- Persistent pseudotumoral hypertrophy of the gastric wall, in a context of epigastralgia which may be major, which is resistant to antiulcer treatment, in a young subject (in his 20s or 30s), with heterogeneous density and above all progressive enhancement increasing in the areas of tissue in the postequilibrium phase, indicating the significant presence of collagen, should bring to mind an inflammatory pseudotumour (Fig. 14). Only

Acute Gastritis and Enteritis

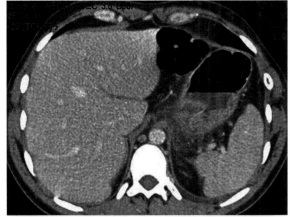

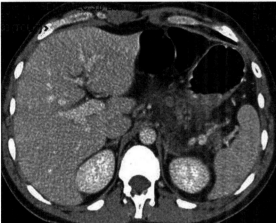

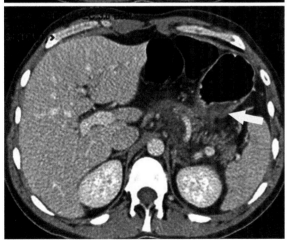

Fig. 11 Inflammatory reaction of the posterior wall of the fundus during acute caudal pancreatitis. The CT scan objectifies the parietal thickening limited to the floor and posterior wall of the fundus (*white arrow*) in direct relation to moderate inflammation of the caudal pancreas

surgical ablation can confirm the diagnosis as endoscopic biopsies cannot reach the significant areas.

- The presence of gastric trichophytobezoar, generally seen in trichotillomaniac girls, is associated with diffuse regular thickening, with intense, persistent enhancement of the gastric wall and no hypertrophy of the rugae (Fig. 15). The trichophytobezoar may extend a long way into the lumen of the duodenum and small intestine, producing Rapunzel's syndrome, named after the Grimm brothers' story with this name.
- Other possible causes of inflammatory thickening of the gastric wall which can be seen in the clinical context of acute abdomen include:
  - Lymphocytic varioliform gastritis, for which an immunoallergic origin is plausible. It appears as parietal thickening and large rugae with umbilicated nodules viewed by endoscopy, and an abundant liquid content in the stomach sometimes accompanied by gastric loss of proteins with oedema and hypoalbuminaemia. Associations with coeliac disease, collagenous colitis, lymphocytic colitis, Ménétrier's disease and *H. pylori* gastritis have been described.
  - Zollinger–Ellison syndrome with diffuse thickening of the gastric wall and rugae in the fundus with spontaneous liquid distension of the lumen by hypersecretion linked with hypergastrinaemia (Fig. 16). The endocrine lesion must be sought in the pancreaticoduodenal region; this may be small and hypervascularised (Fig. 17) or more voluminous and metastatic.
  - Ménétrier's disease, which can be revealed by pseudoulcerous pain. The parietal thickening is related to considerable hypertrophy of the muscularis propria and to cystic dilatation of mucosal glands, at the origin of a cerebriform hypertrophy of the fundic rugae (Fig. 18). The disease essentially affects middle-aged men, usually alcohol and tobacco users; it is accompanied by leakage of gastric protein, causing oedema and microcytic anaemia.
  - Submucosal fatty metaplasia or submucosal pseudolipomatosis, thickening of the submucosa

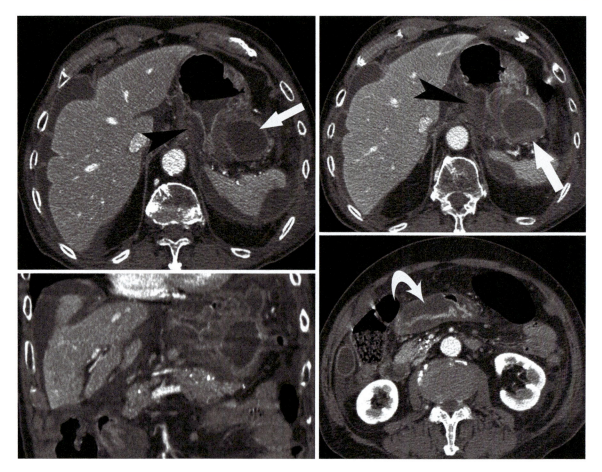

Fig. 12 Acute caudal pancreatitis with pseudocyst and peritoneal fluid effusion. The CT scan confirms massive gastric parietal thickening affecting the lesser curvature (*point of black arrow*), the fundus and the antral region (*curved white arrow*). The pseudocyst (*white arrow*) is the site of bleeding responsible for the hyperdensity of the lower part. Gastric parietal thickening is massive, exceeding 20 mm

with a regular homogeneous fatty density. Initially described in chronic inflammatory conditions of the small intestine and colon after corticosteroid therapy, then in patients treated by chemotherapy, in whom it can appear within a few weeks (Muldoney et al. 1995), it is, in fact, not unexceptional to see it in routine examinations, generally in overweight adults, more often men. It is easily identified because of its typical appearance (fat halo sign) (Fig. 19). It is much less frequent in the stomach than in the small intestine and colon, where it was observed in more than 20% of adult patients in a North American study. Obviously, it must not be confused with an acute inflammatory condition (Harisinghani et al. 2003).

2 Acute Duodenitis and Enteritis

2.1 General Characteristics

Acute inflammatory and infectious conditions of the small intestine may benefit from an emergency scan providing useful diagnostic data depending on the location and size of the anomalies objectified. Evidently, only severe infectious conditions that are

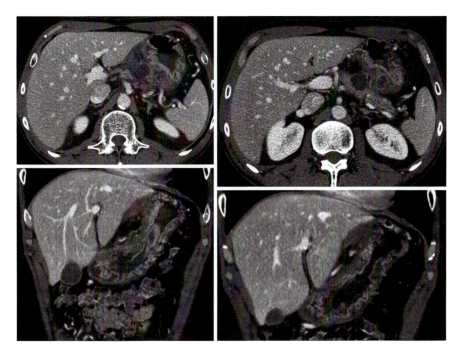

Fig. 13 Acute pancreatitis with small caudal pancreatic pseudocyst. Presence of a diffuse oedematous inflammatory reaction of the whole of the stomach wall

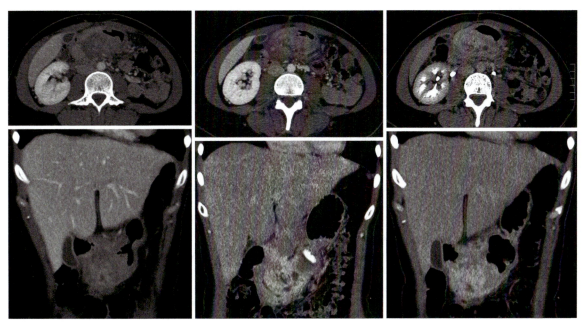

Fig. 14 Gastric inflammatory pseudotumour in a young (27-year-old) patient. Painful epigastric symptoms, ulcerous pain developing over the past 4 months resistant to proton pump inhibitors. Presence of parietal pseudotumoral thickening of the antral region with massive persistent enhancement accentuated on late images. Surgical procedures confirmed the diagnosis of an inflammatory pseudotumour complicating an intramural antral ectopic pancreas

resistant to treatment or which occur with major repercussions for the general condition of the patient necessitating hospitalisation will result in a scan being performed. In general, these are above all localised transmural lesions which can be identified better, with Crohn's disease and its complications in the lead

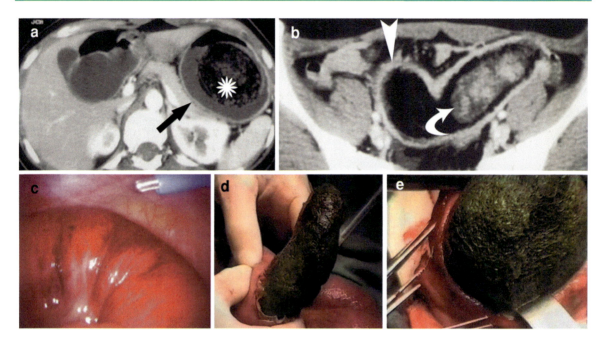

Fig. 15 Gastric and jejunal bezoar in a young (16-year-old) female trichotillomaniac patient. The heterogeneous spherical content of the gastric fundus (*white asterisk*) is accompanied by thickening of the gastric wall with significant persistent enhancement (**a**). Identical images are seen in the proximal jejunum (**b**), which confirmed a heterogeneous compact endoluminal foreign body (*curved white arrow*). Surgical exploration showed very considerable transparietal inflammatory reaction of the proximal jejunum affecting the serous side (**c**). The surgical procedure extracted the jejunal bezoar (**d**) and the gastric trichophytobezoar (**e**)

(Macari and Balthazar 2001; Thoeni and Cello 2006; D'Almeida et al. 2008; Macari et al. 2007).

In acute diffuse conditions, whether they are infectious or inflammatory, the scan objectifies submucosal oedema with parietal stratification of the loops, producing 'target' or 'double-halo' images that can be easily analysed in venous time (70 s after injection at 3 ml/s) (Gore et al. 2000). In the face of this, in an acute clinical context, a number of hypotheses must be discussed (arterial ischaemia, capillary hyperpermeability, congestion by portal venous stasis, etc.), some of which may be supported by abdominal/pelvic exploration, as a general rule complemented by thoracic exploration if there are no contraindications for the radiation risk (young subjects and women of childbearing potential).

In all cases, the clinical context and laboratory tests are fundamental for orientating the diagnosis: a history of abdominal pain and diarrhoea, a state of acquired immunosuppression, a recent stay in a country where there are endemic parasites, a purpuric rash on the lower limbs, a marked inflammatory syndrome seen in laboratory tests, etc. are all signs providing pointers for the right direction which one needs to know how to find out by precise, directed questioning and clinical examination (Figs. 20, 21).

2.2 Acute Infectious Conditions of the Duodenum and Small Intestine

The causes of acute infections of the small intestine are very different depending on whether they occur in an immunosuppressed context or not (Mazzie et al. 2007).

2.2.1 In immunocompetent subjects

Acute intestinal infections are rarely investigated by a CT scan (Macari et al. 2007). The possible causes include:
- *Giardia lamblia*, causing a parasitosis found throughout the world, the occurrence of which can be favoured by hypogammaglobulinaemia. This parasite attaches itself to the mucosa of the proximal small intestine (duodenum and jejunum) without invading it, resulting in a local inflammatory response with

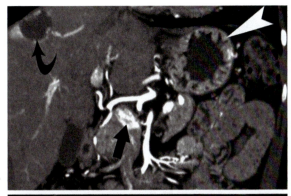

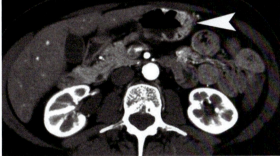

Fig. 16 Gastrinoma in a 50-year-old patient. The CT scan objectifies considerable hypertrophy of the gastric mucosal rugae with major enhancement (*point of white arrow*) and the presence of a hypervascularised lesion of the head of the pancreas corresponding to the gastrinoma (*black arrow*). There is a hepatic angioma (*curved black arrow*)

parietal thickening by submucosal oedema and problems of motility, more difficult to assess on cross-sectional images than on opacifications.

- *Ascaris lumbricoides* is responsible for one of the world's most frequent parisitoses. Its diagnosis is possible with a CT scan, which shows the worms surrounded by endoluminal liquid or distended by gas and thus appearing as linear clear areas (Hommeyer et al. 1995; Sherman and Weber 2005; Rodriguez et al. 2003). Occlusion by an endoluminal ascaris cluster is a classic way of detecting the parasite in countries where it is strongly endemic. It can be accompanied by perforation revealing the condition.
- Anisakiasis is an acute infection caused by the larva of *Anisakis*, a marine nematode ingested with preparations made from raw fish (sushi, raw anchovies) or undercooked fish. The larva causes an inflammatory reaction of the intestinal wall, which can be of major importance and can extend over a length of about 10 cm. Lesions of the small intestine may coexist with gastric and colic involvement and can be accompanied by allergic symptoms. Occlusive forms have been reported, often combined with ascites. Blood hypereosinophilia occurs frequently. From the point of view of a CT scan, the condition is very often situated in the terminal ileum and can extend into the adjacent colon. The pathological examination confirms the presence of an eosinophilic infiltration. An increase in specific IgE can support the diagnosis and must therefore be systematically assayed when one is faced with any histologically diagnosed 'eosinophilic gastroenteritis' (Fig. 20). Diagnostic certainty (endoscopic and/or laboratory tests) can avoid a surgical procedure since the condition develops favourably following drug-induced (or spontaneous) elimination of the parasite (Repiso et al. 2003; Ishida et al. 2007; Ortega-Deballon et al. 2005).
- *Strongyloides stercoralis* causes parasitosis which is particularly frequent in the tropics but which also occurs in temperate regions (e.g. the southeast of the USA). The larva of the parasite penetrates the organism through the skin, migrates into the respiratory system then is coughed up and swallowed and reaches the duodenum at the adult stage. The process can repeat itself, resulting in a cycle or endogenous reinfestation and visceral dissemination, particularly encephalic in immunosuppressed patients. The adult female infiltrates the lamina propria of the duodenum and jejunum, causing an inflammatory reaction there of variable intensity depending on the severity of the infestation. There is generally very marked hypereosinophilia. In severe forms, the dominant feature on a CT scan is major liquid distension of the digestive lumen, giving it the appearance of paralytic ileus or occlusion combined with more or less marked thickening of the wall. The colon can be simultaneously affected, with a scan appearance similar to that of ulcerative colitis (Kothary et al. 1999).
- Ileitis or enteritis due to *Salmonella* and *Shigella*, the most frequent acute infectious conditions found in countries with a high standard of living, is seen as regular circumferential thickening of the last 15 cm of the ileum wall readily extending to the adjacent

Fig. 17 Gastrinoma. Very considerable hypertrophy of the mucosal rugae over the whole stomach with major persistent enhancement. No sign of liquid hypersecretion. Presence of a small hypervascularised nodule at the isthmus of the pancreas corresponding to the gastrinoma

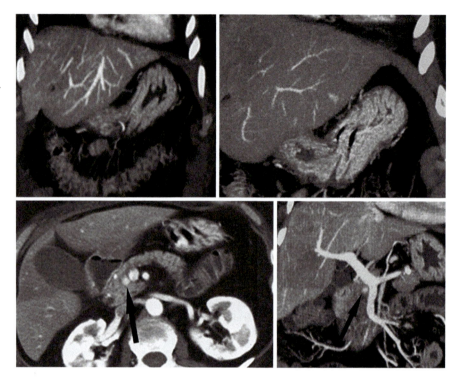

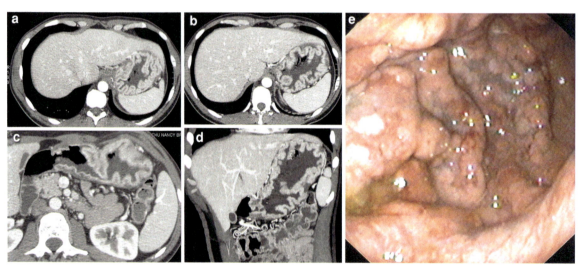

Fig. 18 Ménétrier's disease. The CT scan objectifies considerable hypertrophy with an encephaloid appearance of the rugae of the stomach, major enhancement of the mucosa and submucosal oedema (**a–c**). The stomach is hypersecretory (**c, d**) and endoscopy (**e**) confirms the encephaloid hypertrophy of the gastric rugae

colon to a lesser degree. The 'target sign' appearance of the acute lesions is found particularly in *Shigella* infections; satellite adenomegaly may be seen. The main sources of infection are poultry meat, eggs, milk products and undercooked meat. The severity of the symptoms is very variable and can be intense in immunosuppressed subjects. The 'cholera-like' very severe forms with watery diarrhoea and the dysenteric, sometimes haemorrhagic forms are combined with hyperallergic symptoms with fever and possible multiple organ failure (shigellosis) (Balthazar et al. 1966; Van Wolfswinkel et al. 2008).

Fig. 19 Gastric parietal pseudolipomatosis. Regular submucosal thickening of fatty density has occurred over the whole gastric wall (*white arrow*). This appearance coexists with deep android adiposity. The patient is asymptomatic

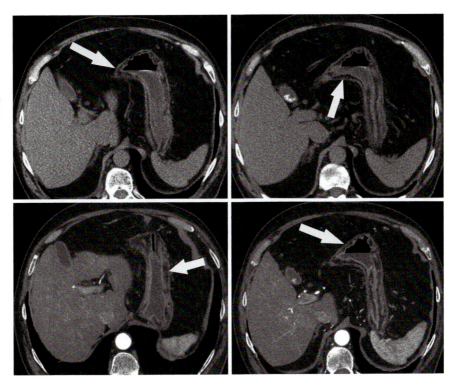

Fig. 20 Eosinophilic enteritis. Regular circumferential thickening of the walls of the duodenum and hypereosinophilic blood. Biopsies confirmed the diagnosis of eosinophilic enteritis without a parasitic cause being found

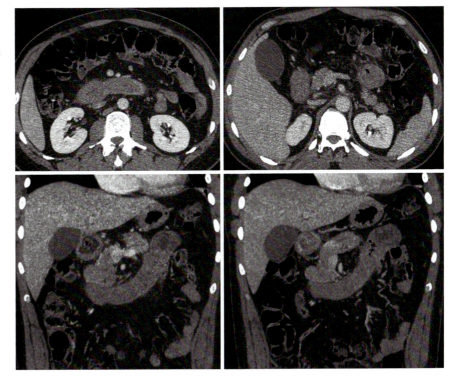

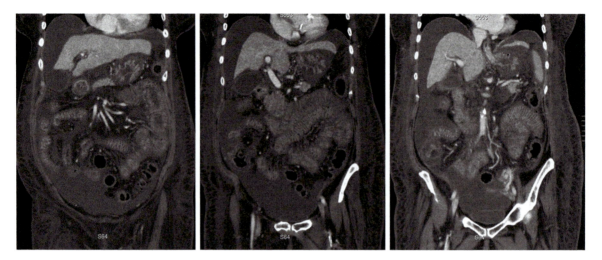

Fig. 21 Portal 'enteritis'. Ascitic oedematous decompensation of hepatic cirrhosis accompanied by diffuse submucosal oedema of the small intestine, colon and stomach. The multifactorial causes of this submucosal oedema include portal hypertension and hypoproteinaemia

- *Campylobacter jejuni* also affects the ileocaecal junction but it is generally a self-limiting disease. On the other hand, *Salmonella typhi* can lead to severe, sometimes haemorrhagic inflammation, essentially affecting the small intestine, causing hyperaemic and oedematous changes; the depth involved can result in perforation of the intestine.
- Yersiniosis is caused by *Yersinia enterocolitica* and *Yersinia pseudotuberculosis*. They affect the right ileocolic region, presenting clinically as a pseudo-appendicitis or as acute feverish diarrhoea with terminal ileitis combined with mesenteric lymph-adenitis. *Y. enterocolitica*, along with the bacteria in the genera *Salmonella* and *Campylobacter*, is the cause of most generally self-limiting bacterial cases of gastroenteritis. *Y. enterocolitica* above all affects young subjects. The disease is due to ingestion of contaminated food (pork meat, milk, water, tofu) or to blood transfusion. Faeces remain contaminated for 90 days after clinical resolution. Diagnosis of yersiniosis using imaging techniques is more the domain of echography than of CT scanning, considering the age of the subjects. The inflammatory circumferential thickening of the walls of the terminal ileum, the presence of regional mesenteric adenopathy and the absence of an image of appendicitis are all arguments in favour of this diagnosis. Severe septicaemia can be seen with the development of visceral abscesses specifically during treatment of iron overload with deferoxamine chelators (Abcarian and Demas 1991; Matsumoto et al. 1991; Antonopoulos et al. 2008).

2.2.2 In subjects seropositive for human immunodeficiency virus

Opportunistic acute infections of the small intestine are now much less frequent because of the efficacy of antiretroviral treatments which reduce the viral load and the frequency of all of these complications. It is thus in cases of resistance or escape from these treatments (highly active antiretroviral treatment) that a CT scan may be made of a patient with acute abdomen or a febrile diarrhoea syndrome in a seriously impaired general state of health. The degree of immunosuppression measured by the CD4 lymphocyte count is still the best guide for the radiologist when reading CT scan images. The imaging technique only supplies a guide to a range of probable causes; it only provides characteristic features in 12% of cases, and its essential role is to contribute to evaluation of the severity of the condition, and above all to screening for surgical complications (Wu et al. 1998; Koh et al. 2002).

- A CD4 lymphocyte count above 200/ml indicates relative immunocompetence and *Mycobacterium tuberculosis* is then the probable cause of the digestive disorders; with a lymphocyte count between 200/ml and 100/ml, there is some degree of

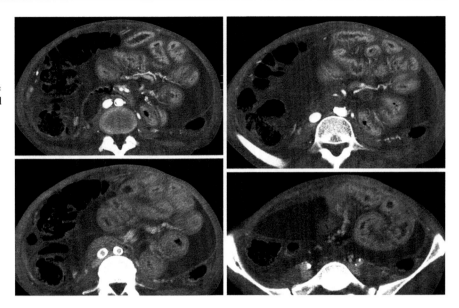

Fig. 22 Enteritis due to *Mycobacterium avium-intracellulare* (MAI) in an HIV-positive patient. Considerable submucosal thickening of the walls of the small intestine with thickened and enhanced mucosa and serosa, abundant ascites. Laboratory investigations confirmed infection by atypical mycobacteria

immunosuppression and many infectious agents may be involved, whereas below 100 CD4/ml CMV infections, infections by *Mycobacterium avium-intracellulare* and cryptosporidiosis must be envisaged in the first instance. The other significant elements which can be objectified and sought on CT scans include the presence of hepatic and/or splenic infectious focal lesions and light-centred adenopathies before and after injection of contrast medium, indicating tuberculosis, as well as the predominance of intestinal lesions on the terminal ileum and caecum.

- In contrast, in *M. avium-intracellulare* infection the area affected is frequently jejunal or diffuse and looks like Whipple's disease both radiologically and histologically (Figs. 22, 23). Visceral locations are rare, and the adenopathies are homogeneous because in these patients the very low CD4 lymphocyte count, generally below 100 and 50 CD4/ml, does not allow a caseous necrosis immune response to occur.
- Cryptosporidiosis is most often seen in deeply immunosuppressed states with CD4 lymphocyte levels below 50/ml but it can occur months later in the development of the disease with levels of more than 200/ml. The area affected is generally proximal, involving the duodenum/jejunum and upper ileum, but it can affect the whole digestive tract. It is not accompanied by adenopathy. The intestinal walls are moderately and regularly thickened and the loops are the site of liquid distension, which can be considerable (Fig. 24). Cryptosporidiosis, like CMV infection, can be accompanied by cholangiopathy, shown on the CT scan images as a generally moderate dilatation of the intrahepatic and extrahepatic bile ducts. The presence of a low stenosis of the main bile duct, in the papilla region, and the predisposition for developing alithiasic cholecystitis is the other characteristic describing biliary involvement.
- Gastrointestinal infections with *Isospora belli* cannot be distinguished clinically and radiologically from cryptosporidiosis; only microscopic examination of the faeces can provide an exact diagnosis.
- CMV intestinal infections preferentially concern the ascending caecum or the whole colon (pancolitis); the small intestine is rarely affected. The regular parietal thickening can be massive in severe forms, or even have a pseudotumoral polypoid appearance. It does not occur with adenopathy. The coexistence of biliary involvement is a diagnostic argument.
- Histoplasmosis can, in countries where it is endemic, give rise to digestive involvement when the CD4 count is below 100/ml. As with tuberculosis, it can be a primary infection or a reactivation. In the disseminated forms of histoplasmosis, the intestine is involved in 75% of cases. The aspects seen on a CT scan are identical to those encountered in tuberculosis: localisation on the terminal ileum and the ascending colon, generally regular concentric

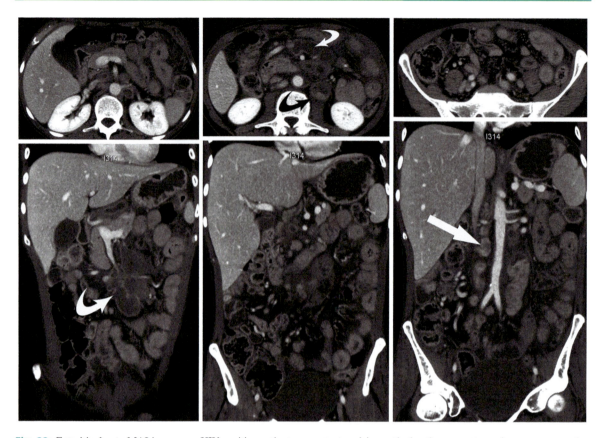

Fig. 23 Enteritis due to MAI in a young HIV-positive patient. Jejunoileal parietal abnormalities (thickening, hyperenhancement) accompanied by hypodense retroperitoneal mesenteric adenopathies were suggestive of tuberculosis, but the clinical context and in particular the very strong immunosuppression suggest more an MAI infection, which will be confirmed by laboratory investigations

parietal thickening, sometimes with pseudotumoral stenosis, infiltration of the adjacent peritoneum, hypodense regional adenopathy in the mesentery and retroperitoneum and possible hepatosplenic, adrenal glands and peritoneal nodular infectious focal lesions.

2.2.3 In neutropenic subjects

In particular during aplasia induced to treat malignant haemopathy by stem cell transplantation, cancer chemotherapy or after organ transplant, it is essential to have good knowledge of the factors orientating the diagnosis of acute gastrointestinal events after allogeneic haematopoietic stem cell transplantation, and in particular, the length of time since the patient became aplasic (Schmit et al. 2008; Kirkpatrick and Greenberg 2003; Beckett and Olliff 2005):

- Chemotherapy-related mucositis is the inevitable consequence of lesions of the mucosal barrier because of the toxicity of the aplastic drugs used. The initially inflammatory epithelial lesions ulcerate (approximately at day 15) then heal. On the CT scan, diffuse or segmental circumferential thickening of the wall of the digestive tube is seen with mucosal hyperaemia (alternation of hypoperfused and hyperperfused areas within the thickened walls). In general, there is little or no infiltration of the mesentery, nor is there adenopathy. The gastrointestinal tract is generally affected diffusely, and the clinical symptoms are moderate secretory diarrhoea and/or abdominal pain.
- Neutropenic enterocolitis most often involves the caecum (typhlitis or caecitis) but it is not unusual for the terminal ileum to be affected, which is a good argument in favour of the diagnosis and against the diagnosis of infectious colitis, in particular of pseudomembranous colitis due to *Clostridium difficile*. The affects are multifactorial,

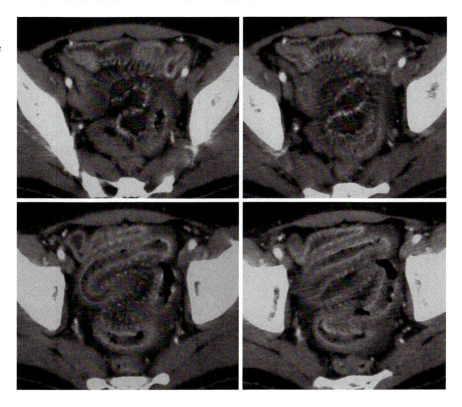

Fig. 24 Cryptosporidiosis and choleriform diarrhoea syndrome in an HIV-positive patient with a CD4 level below 50/ml. Diffuse submucosal thickening of all the ileal loops with increased mucosal contrast, hypervascularisation with the vasa recta showing a comb sign. Diagnosis of cryptosporidiosis was confirmed by laboratory tests

combining mucositis lesions, deep neutropenia, disturbances induced in the microbial flora and a haemorrhagic necrosis component of ischaemic origin. The CT scan shows circumferential thickening of the walls of the caecum (typhlitis), of the ascending colon and the terminal ileum, combined with moderate inflammatory infiltration of the adjacent peritoneum. In general, there is little ascites and no adenopathy. In severe cases, signs of ischaemia appear (parietal pneumatosis, lack of mucosal enhancement) or there are local complications: abscess, pneumoperiteum.

- The graft-versus-host reaction. After haematopoietic stem cell allotransplantation, the return to normal in immunological terms occurs in three phases:
  – During the first 10–30 days, the immune system is severely impaired by pancytopenia; local defences are weakened by mucitis.
  – Between 30 and 100 days after transplantation, the neutropenia corrects itself but with a delay for the lymphocytes, the cause of continued cellular and humoral immune deficiency. Infectious complications are thus frequent. An acute form of graft-versus-host reaction appearing as abdominal pain, and secretory diarrhoea can develop once the graft is functional. On the CT scan, abnormally intense enhancement of the mucosa of the digestive tract is seen very clearly predominating on the small intestine. This corresponds histologically to a destroyed mucosa, replaced by richly vascularised granulation tissue. The intestinal loops are generally distended with liquid with a circumferential submucosal oedema and a comb sign in the corresponding mesentery; on the other hand, there is only rarely infiltration of the mesentery. The alternation of healthy areas with pathological areas and the clinical context of haematopoietic stem cell transplantation are obviously major factors for making a diagnosis (Fig. 25).
  – After 100 days, a chronic form of graft-versus-host reaction can be seen which occurs mainly as a malabsorption syndrome without expression in imaging techniques.
- Acute fungal infections, in particular the disseminated invasive forms of aspergillosis, which may be the origin of necrotic ulcerative enteritis,

Fig. 25 Graft-versus-host reaction in a young patient who had received a transplant of haematopoietic stem cells. Diffuse thickening due to submucosal oedema with increased contrast in the mucosa of all the small intestine loops and the colon, in a graft-versus-host reaction

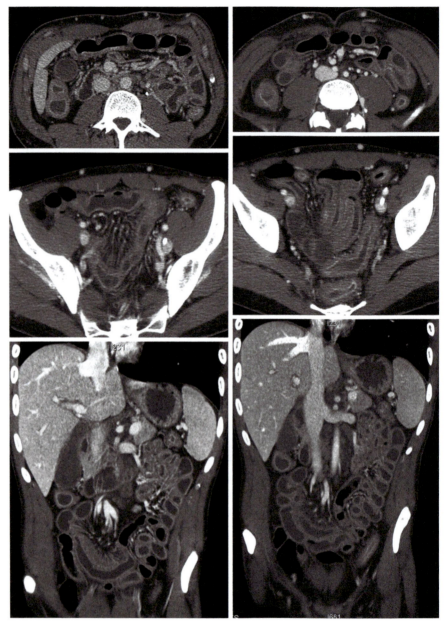

particularly concern the ileum, the walls of which are circumferentially thickened and the neighbouring mesentery is infiltrated. There is a very high risk of perforation and the symptoms are often not very specific, sometimes limited to a fever and abdominal pain without clear guarding. A CT scan is therefore of fundamental importance to confirm the parietal and peritoneal abnormalities of the ileocolic junction (Tresallet et al. 2004).

- Mucormycosis. This is seen in subjects treated for a malignant haemopathy, in immunosuppressed transplant patients, keto-acid diabetics, patients with cardiac and renal impairment and during chelator treatment for iron overload. Gastrointestinal involvement is uncommon, affecting the stomach more that the small intestine and colon. It is seen on a CT scan as a circumferential diffuse thickening of the walls of affected digestive

Fig. 26 Acute painful epigastric symptoms in a 29-year-old patient. The scan objectifies oedematous circumferential thickening of the proximal jejunal loops with discrete peritoneal fluid effusion accompanied by small mesenteric and peritoneal adenopathies. Purpura eruptions were seen on the lower limbs within hours of the examination, confirming the diagnosis of Henoch–Schönlein purpura

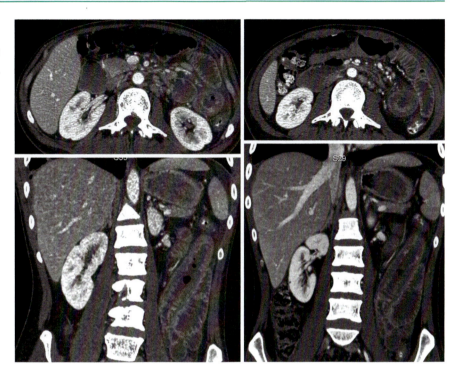

segments, which often coexist with hepatic focal localisations (Suh et al. 2000).

2.3 Vascular Acute Inflammatory Conditions of the Duodenum and Small Intestine

2.3.1 Acute Manifestations of Vasculitis on the Small Intestine

Most forms of vasculitis, in any case those concerning small and medium-sized vessels, may affect the small intestine. We should think of them each time we see images from a young patient suggesting ischaemic lesions in an unusual site, for instance in the stomach, above all the duodenum (ischaemia in the duodenum is practically always related to vasculitis), or the rectum, or when the small intestine and colon are simultaneously diffusely affected or when other viscera are affected, e.g. the uro-genital system (Ha et al. 2000; Ahn et al. 2009).

- Henoch–Schönlein purpura (sometimes called rheumatoid purpura) is vasculitis of small vessels characterised by the presence of serum IgA and the precipitation of immune complexes in the arterioles, capillaries and venules. It is most frequent in children, where it usually develops benignly, but a quarter of cases are seen in adults, more often in men (sex ratio 2:1), with a poorer prognosis because of more frequent and more severe renal involvement. The clinical triad of acute abdominal pain, arthralgia and palpable purpura must bring this diagnosis to mind. Abdominal pain occurs in 44% of cases of Henoch–Schönlein purpura in adults, preceding the skin lesions in 10–15% of patients. The CT scan shows an inflammatory thickening with double-halo signs of the digestive segments affected, loss of mesenteric fat transparency with vascular engorgement, and adenopathy; ascites is present in the severest forms (Figs. 26, 27). Complications due to perforation or occlusion by invagination are less frequent in children and the digestive lesions generally evolve favourably; the prognosis for the disease depends on the kidneys (Chung et al. 2006).
- Periarteritis nodosa (PAN) is a necrotising inflammatory vasculitis which affects the wall of small to medium-sized muscular arteries, leading to the formation of microaneurysms and stenoses. It particularly affects middle-aged men (in their 40s or 50 s; sex ratio 2:1–3:1) who, in 36% of cases, are carriers of the hepatitis B virus. Classical

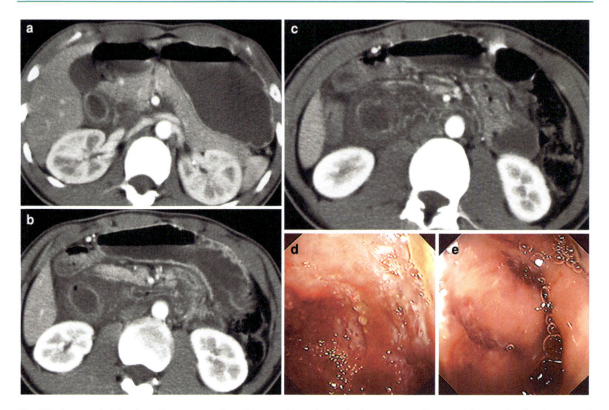

Fig. 27 Acute painful epigastric symptoms in a 21-year-old female patient. Considerable circumferential submucosal (**a–c**) oedema of the duodenum confirmed by endoscopy (**d**), which shows the hyperaemic (**d, e**) and haemorrhagic character of lesions due to Henoch–Schönlein purpura

antineutrophil cyloplasmic autoantibodies (cANCAs) are found in laboratory tests in many cases, but they are not specific (since they are also found in Wegener's granulomatosis, in Churg–Strauss syndrome and in microscopic polyangiitis). The digestive tract is affected in 50–70% of PAN cases, essentially the jejunum, which is the site of extensive submucosal oedema, which can be spontaneously hyperdense when it is haematic, with a double-halo image on biphasic acquisitions after contrast medium injection. Perforations and stenoses are complications of the vascular lesions. The scan, even with the spatial resolution of current machines, cannot objectify the microaneurysms that are easily shown by angiography (Rhodes et al. 2008; Jee et al. 2000).

- Microscopic polyangiitis (hypersensitivity vasculitis, leukocytoclastic vasculitis) is a condition identical to PAN which affects small-diameter vessels (arterioles, venules, capillaries). In most cases, cANCAs are present. Renal involvement is found in 90% of cases in the form of a necrotising glomerulonephritis. The effects on the digestive tract are identical to those seen in the other types of vasculitis: regular inflammatory thickening of the (generally ileal) walls, vascular engorgement, loss of mesenteric fat transparency and ascites.

- Wegener's granulomatosis histologically affects the intestinal tract in 24% of patients but is only expressed clinically in 10%. It affects the small intestine and colon. The appearance on a CT scan is identical to that seen in other forms of vasculitis. Acute forms are linked to intestinal perforations or extensive massive ischaemic necrosis (fulminating necrotising enterocolitis) (Pickhardt and Curran 2001).

- Churg–Strauss syndrome can exceptionally occur on intestinal-mesenteric structures (20% of cases), either in the form of ischaemic lesions secondary to vasculitis or by eosinophilic infiltration of the wall, which can be the cause of an occlusion or haemorrhagic diarrhoea (Rha et al. 2000).

- Acute-disseminated lupus erythematosus (ADLE) is a necrotising vasculitis of autoimmune origin which preferentially affects young female subjects.

The digestive effects are ischaemic, often haemorrhagic lesions consecutive to a real obliterating endarteritis. In physiopathological terms, the hypercoagulable state linked to the circulating antiphospholipid antibodies (anticardiolipin antibodies and lupus anticoagulant, which are encountered in 30–40% of patients with ADLE, as against 2% in the general population) appears to be of decisive importance in the occurrence of digestive symptoms. We speak of an antiphospholipid antibody syndrome when there are not enough diagnostic criteria for ADLE. Perforative and occlusive necrotic complications are classic. The whole digestive tract can be affected, but the predilection is for the territory of the superior mesenteric artery. In acute situations, the CT scan shows circumferential thickening of the walls of affected digestive segments, engorgement of mesenteric vessels, with a particular arrangement of the vasa recta of the ileum related to its shortening (comb sign), and adenopathy. Polyseritis is frequent (peritoneal, pleural, pericardial liquid effusions, etc.) and evokes the diagnosis. A high incidence of urogenital tract lesions has been reported (lupus glomerulonephritis, cystitis, hydronephrosis by fibrous changes to the ureterovesical junction or following vesicoureteral reflux secondary to a detrusor spasm). In everyday practice, these data are of very limited interest because of their rarity (Pagnoux et al. 2003; Kaushik et al. 2001).

- *Behçet's syndrome.* The gastrointestinal tract is affected in 10–50% of patients with Behçet's syndrome. The lesions affect the ileocaecal junction with a predilection for the terminal ileum and are the consequence of an inflammatory vasculitis preferentially affecting the venules. The deep ulcerations typical of the disease may be transmural, which explains the frequency of local complications such as haemorrhage, perforation, fistulae and localised or diffuse peritonitis, for the diagnosis of which the CT scan is particularly valuable. Parietal thickening can be massive, localised, asymmetric with a polypoid appearance, pseudotumoral or ulcerated in the centre (Chung et al. 2001).
- *Rheumatoid vasculitis.* In long-standing severe rheumatoid arthritis, with marked disorders in laboratory tests and in particular in male patients, acute intestinal inflammatory symptoms may be seen related to leukocytoclastic vasculitis of the

small venules. The diffuse thickening of walls of the small intestine and colon with double-halo enhancement, the possible infiltration of the mesentery and the peritoneal liquid reaction are identical to what is seen in the other forms of vasculitis.

2.3.2 Inflammatory Conditions with a Vascular Origin Excluding Forms of Vasculitis

- *Acute radiation enteritis of the small intestine* (Lyer et al. 2001). This is seen during the weeks immediately following pelvic irradiation, most often after doses higher than 45 Gy for uterine cervical cancers. It appears as an oedematous parietal thickening of the loops of the small intestine in the pelvis and lower abdomen. Limitation of the lesions to the field of irradiation with clear demarcation is highly evocative for this diagnosis (Fig. 28). The condition is usually resolved in a few weeks with symptomatic treatment. This acute effect, related to the direct action of ionising radiation on the lining epithelium, is different from chronic radiation enteritis, which is related to an obliterating endarteritis, the cause of fibrosing inflammation producing stenoses and fistulae, generally appearing several months to several years (2 months to 30 years) after irradiation.
- *Angio-oedema (or angioneurotic oedema) of the small intestine.* Angioneurotic oedema is a non-inflammatory condition characterised by acute episodes of capillary hyperpermeability with oedema of the skin of the face and of the respiratory and intestinal mucosae. The gastrointestinal condition is expressed as acute abdomen, generally resolving within 24–72 h, but there is a potential risk of death by hypovolaemic shock. The appearance of watery diarrhoea in the final phase of the attack is good diagnostic evidence. CT scan images show extensive inflammatory thickening of the walls of the digestive tract (stomach and small intestine) with liquid distension of the digestive lumens, congestion of mesenteric vessels and peritoneal fluid effusion. The cause of this disease is a hereditary or acquired lack of C1-esterase inhibitor, which should be determined by laboratory investigations. A personal or familial history of Quincke's oedema or minor forms (episodes of urticaria, transitory dyspnoea) should be sought but

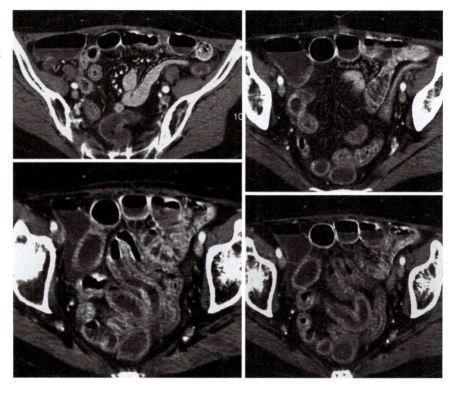

Fig. 28 Acute radiation enteritis. Regular moderate circumferential submucosal oedema of all the pelvic loops of the small intestine in a female patient irradiated during the previous 3 weeks for a neoplasia of the cervix of the uterus

the digestive events may precede cutaneous and respiratory symptoms by several years. There are paraneoplastic forms associated with lymphoproliferative syndromes, autoimmune diseases or cancers. Certain cases of this condition may be seen during treatment with conversion enzyme inhibitors (ACE inhibitors) (De Baker et al. 2001).

- *Buerger's disease (thromboangiitis obliterans)*. In young subjects who are usually heavy smokers this condition affects the vasa vasorum of arteries of intermediate size, leading to thrombosis and severe parietal inflammatory reactions. Digestive involvement is infrequent. Intestinal parietal symptoms are of the same type as those seen in vasculitis, but an angioscan shows the segmental thromboses of the medium-sized arteries. The context (young subject, heavy smoker) is fundamental to the diagnosis (Marder and Mellinghoff 2000).
- *Vasculitis linked to cocaine or heroine*. After just one inhalation of cocaine, the picture of acute abdomen can be seen on a CT scan, with images analogous to those seen in acute or subacute ischaemia of the digestive tract (Fig. 29). The colon is most often the site affected but the small intestine alone can be affected, essentially the ileum. The histological similarities between Buerger's disease and vasculitis due to cocaine have led some authors to suggest that there are close links between these two conditions (Herrine et al. 1998; Hagan and Burney 2007).

2.3.3 Drug-Induced Enterocolitis

Drug-induced enteropathies, are frequent but in general are not investigated using imaging techniques because of the usually minor character of their clinical symptoms (Chatelain et al. 2007).

- *Drug-induced Ileitis*
  – Ulcerated ileitis lesions can be seen after ingestion of NSAIDs, but are much less frequent than colic conditions. One of their particularities as they develop is the formation of diaphragm-like stenoses (Fig. 30).
  – Corticosteroids, tablets of iron salts or potassium chloride may lead to lesions similar to those caused by NSAIDs.
  – In all cases, the clinical picture can be acute with bloody diarrhoea, and peritonitis through perforation may be seen. The severity of the condition

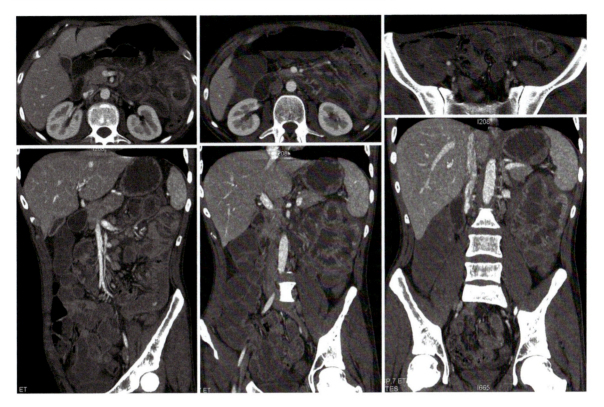

Fig. 29 Vasculitis in a heroine addict. The scan was performed for acute hyperalgesic pain and shows acute lesions predominantly on the proximal jejunum and characterised by considerable circumferential submucosal oedema with target sign enhancement, accompanied by small quantities of peritoneal fluid effusion

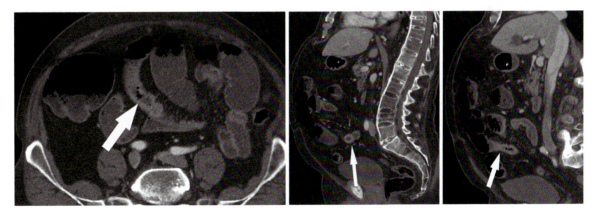

Fig. 30 Acute enteropathy due to non-steroidal anti-inflammatory drugs (NSAIDs). Moderately stenosing parietal circumferential thickening of the jejunum, with considerable lasting enhancement (*white arrow*). Double balloon enteroscopy confirmed the diagnosis of enteritis due to NSAIDs

is not related to how long treatment has been administered.
- *Enteropathy due to NSAIDs.* Diaphragm disease is a rare but specific complication of chronic prolonged use of NSAIDs. It is seen above all in middle-aged women taking NSAIDs over the long term for a rheumatic condition. It may be revealed clinically by an acute occlusive syndrome but usually attention is drawn to the condition by sub-occlusive episodes, chronic diarrhoea and weight

loss. Fine fibrous circular membranes, perforated in the centre, develop in the ileal lumen, opposite to valvules with which they interact. Histologically, the submucosa is the site of fibrous transformation, which would seem to correspond to the development of the ulcerous lesions caused by the NSAIDs (Zalev et al. 1996).

- *Necrotising ileocolitis due to treatment with Kayexalate and sorbitol.* An ulcerated condition of the distal ileum and the ascending colon, often accompanied by partial or transmural necrosis, which can then be complicated by perforation with peritonitis, may be seen in renally impaired subjects treated with Kayexalate for hyperkalaemia. In fact it is the sorbitol, a hypertonic solution administered to counteract the constipation induced by Kayexalate, which would seem to be the cause of the necrotising ileocolic lesions, through its direct toxic action on the mucosa and the local hypovolaemia that it induces due to its hypertonicity, and which causes a low local flow that can lead to parietal necrosis.
- *Ileal melanosis.* Like the much more frequent colic melanosis with which it can be associated, this is the consequence of long-term treatment for constipation by laxatives of the anthraquinone group. It is a feature of pathological anatomy which is not visible using imaging techniques.
- *Clofazimine enteropathy.* Clofazimine belongs to the phenazine group used in the treatment of leprosy, atypical mycobacterial infections and sometimes in graft-versus-host reactions, and after being used for several months can accumulate in the mucosa of the small intestine, the mesenteric ganglia and the greater omentum, giving them a brown-black or orangey coloration by which the condition can be identified in a pathological anatomy examination. The clinical picture is a combination of abdominal pain, vomiting and diarrhoea.

2.4 The Acute Appearance of Crohn's Disease in the Small Intestine

Crohn's disease can be revealed by an acute painful feverish episode with diarrhoea, or by an acute complication, such as an intestinal occlusion, deep abscess, fistula, perforation or digestive haemorrhage. In all these circumstances, a CT scan is often

performed quite quickly, and one must be able to identify the disease on the images produced, and its possible complications (Meyers et al. 1995; Lee et al. 2002; Madureira 2004; Gourtsoyianni et al. 2009).

It is obvious that, given an acute picture, even if questioning the patient or the clinical examination points towards Crohn's disease, the use of enteroclysis should be avoided and the examination should be performed usually without modifying the content of the loops or by performing enterography without a catheter, by ingestion of water or opacifying agent and in all cases taking care to minimise the dose of ionising radiation delivered to these patients, who are often young and who will be repeatedly subjected to CT scans as the condition develops.

Crohn's disease in the small intestine preferentially involves the terminal ileum, but, particularly in acutely revealed forms, it can affect almost the whole ileum or a shorter or longer segment of the jejunum and evidently the whole or part of the colon (Figs. 31, 32, 33).

Positive CT scan diagnosis of Crohn's disease in the small intestine is based on the criteria for transmural inflammation seen as:

- More than 3 mm parietal thickening
- Parietal stratification visible with double-halo finding in the active inflammatory forms
- The presence, above all, of the classic modifications of vascularisation on the mesenteric side of the loops affected: vascular jejunisation of the ileum (i.e. increase in the number of vasa recta per unit length, tortuosity and dilatation of these vessels) and a comb sign, which essentially reflect the shortening of the digestive segments involved and their mesentery which is, moreover, the site of fibrofatty infiltration (sclerolipomatosis).
- The presence of mesenteric adenopathies

The mesenteric vascular abnormalities indicate an active, developed, widespread condition seen in an acute clinical context. There is close correlation with the clinical Crohn's disease activity index.

In contrast, fibrostenotic lesions appear on the scan as:

- Regular uniform thickening, with no or little enhancement after injection of a contrast medium. However, it must be emphasised that the fibrosis can be enhanced, sometimes considerably, on delayed acquisitions. Delayed enhancement is therefore not a decisive predictive element for the efficacy of the medical treatment.

Acute Gastritis and Enteritis

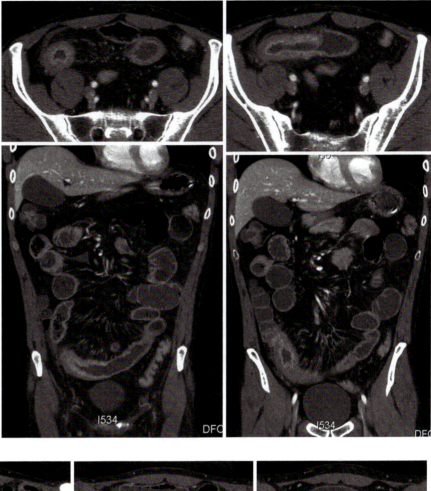

Fig. 31 Acute attack revealing Crohn's disease. Regular circumferential thickening of the final ileal loops with target sign image by enhancement of the mucosa and signs of transmural inflammation with comb sign appearance of the vasa recta

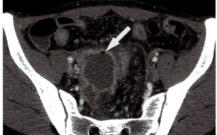
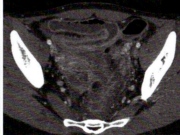
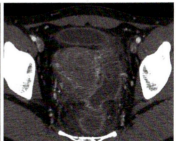

Fig. 32 Acute attack of Crohn's disease with pelvic peritonitis. Presence of acute inflammatory thickening of the ileal wall with signs of transmural inflammation. Multiple pelvic collections with one larger organised collection with a thick wall and gas bubbles (*white arrow*)

- Stenosis of the lumen and upstream distension with regular infundibuliform connection of the normal wall.

Target or double-halo enhancement images are also not themselves specific, even if this feature was initially described in Crohn's disease. Differential diagnosis should consider ischaemia, vasculitis, infectious enteritis, haematoma (Fig. 34), radiation enteritis and graft-versus-host reaction. Submucosal fatty metaplasia (or submucosal pseudolipomatosis) can lead to hesitation even more here than in the stomach. Its typical appearance of fatty density (the fat halo sign) and its existence in an overweight patient with excessive deep abdominal fat makes its easy to identify (Fig. 35).

Fig. 33 Phlegmon complicating an ileal Crohn's disease extending to the rectosigmoid junction. The CT scan shows the typical images of ileal Crohn's disease (*black arrow*). In the pelvis there is massive inflammatory infiltration of the adjacent mesenteric structures (*straight white arrow*) (**a–c**) with continuous extension at the rectosigmoid junction (*white curved arrow*) (**d**)

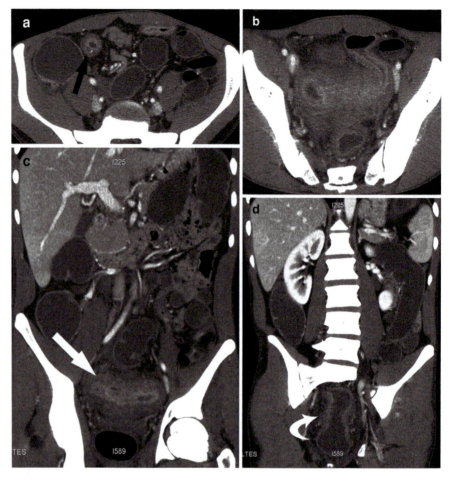

Fig. 34 Duodenojejunal parietal haematoma after ingestion of a large dose of Aspegic®. Presence of considerable circumferential thickening extending to the wall of the proximal jejunal loops. The patient had ingested relatively large quantities of Aspegic® during the days prior to the acute incident which revealed this

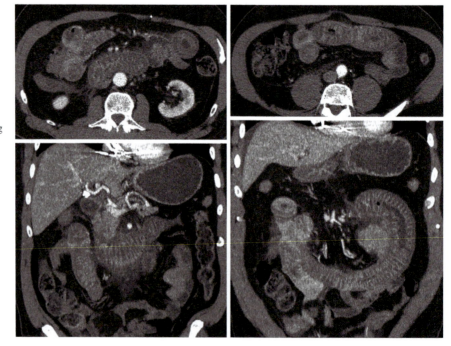

Fig. 35 Jejunal segmental submucosal metaplasia in an overweight patient. These images of parietal thickening with a fatty density seen in the context of painful abdominal symptoms led wrongly to the diagnosis of ischaemia of the small intestine and a misunderstanding of the real origin of the condition, which was biliary

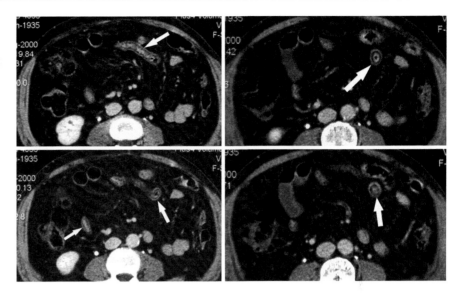

An emergency CT scan, even if it lacks precision and does not allow as fine an analysis as CT enteroclysis (Kohli and Maglinte 2009), does permit Crohn's disease to be diagnosed and shows the activity of the disease (Minordi et al. 2009). Obviously, it highlights local complications: inflammatory or fibrous stenosis, abscesses, fistulae, perforations and any possible remote lesions such as urinary calculi, venous and more rarely arterial thrombosis, spondyloarthropathy, sclerosing cholangitis, etc..

Meta-analyses have shown that there are no significant differences in diagnostic accuracy between CT and MRI (Horsthuis et al. 2008a, b). Given the necessity of limiting irradiation as much as possible, particularly in young patients, it therefore seems best to direct these patients wherever possible to MRI, all the more so as the additional information from diffusion sequences allows very effective assessment of the degree of activity of the disease, correlated perfectly with clinical/laboratory activity indices. Injected sequences can thus be avoided and T2-weighted sequences at the equilibrium state complemented with diffusion-weighted sequences allow one to effectively follow the spontaneous development of the disease and/or during treatment.

2.4.1 Summary

The appearance on a CT scan of localised or diffuse hypodense parietal thickening of the stomach and/or the small intestine, with visible stratification after injection in the context of acute abdomen should mean that several hypotheses need to be considered, for which exploration of the rest of the abdominal cavity may provide pros and cons of use for the aetiological diagnosis. It is usually, above all, the clinical history and carefully searching the patient's medical history which will guide this aetiological orientation. A radiologist is a clinician who must go well beyond the description of images if he wishes to provide the medical community with the services which this latter has the right to expect.

References

Abcarian PW, Demas BE (1991) Systemic *Yersinia enterocolitica* infection associated with iron overload and deferoxamine therapy. AJR Am J Roentgenol 157:773–775

Ahn E, Luk A, Chetty R, Buttany J (2009) Vasculitides of the gastrointestinal tract. Semin Diagn Pathol 26:77–88

Antonopoulos P, Constantinidis F, Charalampopoulos G, Dalamarinis K, Karanicas I, Kokkini G (2008) An emergency diagnostic dilemma; a case of *Yersinia enterocolitica* colitis mimicking acute appendicitis in a thalassenia major patient; the role of CT and literature review. Emerg Radiol 15:123–126

Asrani A, Avelline R, Abujudeh H, Lawrason J, Kaewlai R (2007) Intramural gastric abscess-preoperative diagnosis with CT. Emerg Radiol 14:253–256

Balthazar EJ (1979) Effects of acute and chronic pancreatitis on the stomach pattern of radiographic involvement. Am J Gastroenterol 72:568–580

Balthazar EJ, Charles HW, Megibow AJ (1966) Salmonella and shigella-induced ileitis: CT findings in four patients. J Comput Assist Tomogr 20:375–378

Beckett D, Olliff J (2005) Non infectious manifestations of stem cell transplantation. Br J Radiol 78:272–281

Brown BM, Federle MP, Jeffrey RB (1982) Gastric wall thickening and extragastric inflammatory process: a retrospective study. J Comput Assist Tomogr 6:782–785

Buyt L, Smeets P, Verstraete K (2003) Infectious emphysematous gastritis in multiple sclerosis. JBR-BTR 86:148–149

Chatelain D, Mokrani N, Flejou JF (2007) Entérocolites médicamenteuses. Ann Pathol 27:439–447

Chen TA, Lo GH, Lin CK, Lai KH, Wung HY, Yu HC, Hsu PI, Chen HH, Tsai WL, Chen WC (2007) Acute pancreatitis associated acute gastro-intestinal mucosal lesions: incidence, characteristic and clinical signification. J Clin Gastroenterol 41:830–834

Chung SY, Ha HK, Kim JH, Kim KW, Cho N, Cho KS, Lee YS, Chung DJ, Jung HY, Yang SK, Min YI (2001) Radiologic findings of Behcet syndrome involving the gastrointestinal tract. Radiographics 21:911–924

Chung DJ, Park YS, Huh KC, Kim JH (2006) Radiologic findings of gastrointestinal complications in an adult patient with Henoch Schönlein purpura. AJR Am J Roentgenol 187:w396–w398

Curvelo LA, Brabosa W, Rhohr R, Lanzoni V, Parise ER, Ferrari AP, Kondo M (2000) Underlying mechanism of portal hypertensive gastropathy in cirrhosis: a hemodynamic and morphological approach. J Gastroenterol Hepatol 24:1482–1483

D'Almeida A, Juse J, Onetto J, Restrepo R (2008) Bowel wall thickening in children: CT findings. Radiographics 28:727–746

De Baker AI, De Schepper AM, Vandevenne JE, Schoeters P, Michielsen P, Stevens WJ (2001) CT of angio-oedema of the small bowel. AJR Am J Roentgenol 176:649–652

Gelfand DW, Ott DJ, Chen MY (1999) Radiologic evaluation of gastritis and duodenitis. AJR Am J Roentgenol 173:357–361

Gore RM, Miller FH, Pereles FS, Yaghmai VY, Berlin JW (2000) Helical CT in the evaluation of acute abdomen. AJR Am J Roentgenol 174:901–913

Gourtsoyianni S, Zamboni GA, Romero JY, Raptopoulos VD (2009) Routine use of modified CT enterography in patients with acute abdominal pain. Eur J Radiol 69:388–392

Ha HK, Lee SH, Rha SE, Kim JH, Byum JY, Lim HK, Chung JW, Kim JG, Kim PN, Lee MG, Auh YH (2000) Radiologic features of vasculitis involving the gastrointestinal tract. Radiographics 20:779–795

Hadas-Halpren I, Hiller N, Guberman D (1993) Emphysematous gastritis secondary to ingestion of large amounts of Coca Cola. Am J Gastroenterol 88:127–129

Hagan IG, Burney K (2007) Radiology of recreational drug abuse. Radiographics 27:919–940

Harisinghani MG, Wittenberg J, Lee W, Chen S, Guttierez AL, Muller PR (2003) Bowel fat halo sign in patients without intestinal disease. AJR Am J Roentgenol 181:781–784

Herrine SK, Park PK, Wechsler RJ (1998) Acute mesenteric ischemia following intranasal cocaine use. Dig Dis Sci 43:586–589

Hommeyer SC, Hamill GS, Johnson JA (1995) CT diagnosis of intestinal ascaridiasis. Abdom Imaging 20:315–316

Horsthuis K, Stokkers PC, Stoker J (2008a) Detection of inflammatory bowel diseases: diagnostic performance of cross sectional imaging modalities. Abdom Imaging 33:407–416

Horsthuis K, Bipart S, Bennink RJ, Stoker J (2008b) Inflammatory bowel diseases diagnosed with US MR scintigraphy and CT: metaanalysis of prospective studies. Radiology 247:64–79

Ishida M, Harada A, Egawa S, Watabe S, Ebina N, Unno M (2007) Three successive cases of enteric anisakiasis. Dig Surg 24:228–231

Jee KN, Ha HK, Lee IJ, Kim JK, Sung KS, Cho KS, Kim PN, Lee MG, Lim HK, Choi CS, Auh YH (2000) Radiological findings of abdominal polyarteritis nodosa. AJR Am J Roentgenol 174:1675–1679

Jung C, Choi YW, Jeon SC, Chung WS (2003) Acute diffuse phlegmonous oesophagogastritis: radiologic diagnosis. AJR Am J Roentgenol 180:862–863

Jung JH, Choi HJ, Yoo J, Kang SJ, Lee KY (2007) Emphysematous gastritis associated with invasive gastric mucor mycosis: a case report. J Korean Med Sci 22:923–927

Kaushik S, Federle MP, Schur PH, Krishman M, Silverman SG, Ros PR (2001) Abdominal thrombotic and ischemic manifestations of the antiphospholipid antibody syndrome: CT findings in 42 patients. Radiology 218:768–771

Kim DH, Pickhardt PJ (2007) The stomach. In: Pickhardt PJ, Arluk GM (eds) Atlas of gastrointestinal imaging. Radiologic–endoscopic correlation. Saunders-Elsevier, Philadelphia, pp 61–112

Kim TU, Kim S, Woo SK, Lee JW, Lee TH, Jeong YJ, Heo J (2008) Dynamic CT of portal hypertensive gastropathy—significance of transient gastric perfusion defect sign. Clin Radiol 63:783–790

Kirkpatrick ID, Greenberg HM (2003) Gastrointestinal complication in the neutropenic patient: characterization and differentiation with abdominal CT. Radiology 226:668–674

Koh DM, Langroudi B, Padley SPG (2002) Abdominal CT in patients with AIDS. Imaging 14:24–34

Kohli MD, Maglinte DD (2009) CT enteroclysis in small bowel Crohn's disease. Eur J Radiol 83:398–403

Kothary NN, Muskie JM, Mathur SC (1999) Resident's teaching files. *Strongyloides stercoralis* hyperinfection. Radiographics 19:1077–1081

Lee SS, Ha HK, Yang SK, Kim AY, Kim TY, Kim PN, Lae MG, Myung SJ, Jung HH, Kim JH, Min YI (2002) CT of prominent pericolic or perienteric vasculature in patient with Crohn's disease: correlation with clinical disease activity and findings on barium studies. AJR Am J Roentgenol 179:1029–1036

Levine MS (2008) Inflammatory conditions of the stomach and duodenum. In: Gore RM, Levine MS (eds) Textbook of intestinal radiology, 3rd edn. Saunders-Elsevier, Philadelphia, pp 563–592

Loi TH, See JW, Diddapur RK, Issac JR (2007) Emphysematous gastritis: a case report and a review of the literature. Am Acad Med Singapore 36:72–73

Lyer RB, Jhingran A, Sawaf H, Libshitz HI (2001) Imaging findings after radiotherapy of the pelvis. AJR Am J Roentgenol 177:1083–1089

Macari M, Balthazar EJ (2001) CT of bowel thickening: significance and pitfalls of interpretation. Am J Roentgenol AJR 176:1105–1106

Macari M, Megibow AJ, Balthazar EJ (2007) A pattern approach to the abnormal small bowel; observation at

MDCT and CT enterography. AJR Am J Roentgenol 188:1344–1355

Madureira AJ (2004) The comb sign. Radiology 230:783–784

Marder VJ, Mellinghoff IK (2000) Cocaine and Buerger disease. Arch Intern Med 160:2057–2060

Matsumoto T, Ida M, Sakai T, Kimura Y, Fushima M (1991) Yersinia terminal ileites: sonographic findings in eight patients. AJR Am J Roentgenol 156:965–967

Mazzie JP, Wilson SR, Sadler MA, Khalili M, Javors BR, Weston SR, Katz DS (2007) Imaging of gastrointestinal tract infection. Semin Roentgenol 42:102–116

Meyers MA, McGuire PV (1995) Spiral CT demonstration of hypervascularity in Crohn disease 'vascular jejunization of the ileon' or the 'comb sign'. Abdom Imaging 20:327–332

Minordi LM, Vecchioli A, Buidi L, Poloni G, Fedeli G, Bonomo L (2009) CT findings and clinical activity in Crohn's disease. Clin Imaging 33:123–129

Muldoney SM, Balfe DM, Hammeman A, Wick MR (1995) 'Acute' fat deposition in bowel wall submucosa: CT appearance. J Comput Assist Tomogr 19:394–399

Ortega-Deballon P, Carabias-Hernandez A, Martin-Blasquez A, Garaulet P, Benoit L, Kretz B, Limones-Esteban M, Favre JP (2005) Anisakiase: une parasitose que le chirurgien doit connaître. Ann Chir 130:407–410

Pagnoux C, Mahr A, Guillevin L (2003) Manifestations abdominales et digestives des vascularites. Ann Med Interne (Paris) 154:457–487

Pickhardt PJ, Curran VW (2001) Fulminant enterocolitis in Wegener's granulomatosis. AJR Am J Roentgenol 177: 1335–1337

Repiso OA, Alcantara TM, Gonzalez de Frutos C, de Artaza VT, Rodriguez MR, Valle MJ, Martinez PJL (2003) Gastrointestinal anisakiasis. Study of a series of 25 patients. Gastroenterol Hepatol 26:341–346

Rha SE, Ha HK, Lee SH, Kim JH, Kim JK, Kim JH, Kim PN, Lee MG, Auh YH (2000) CT and MR imaging findings of bowel ischemia from various primary causes. Radiographics 20:29–42

Rhodes ES, Pekala JS, Gemery JM, Dickey KW (2008) Case 129: polyarteris nodosa. Radiology 246:322–326

Rodriguez EJ, Gama MA, Ornstein SM, Anderson WD (2003) Ascariasis causing small bowel volvulus. Radiographics 23:1291–1293

Schmit M, Bethge W, Beck R, Faul C, Claussen CD, Horger M (2008) CT of gastrointestinal complications associated with haematopoietic stem cell transplantation. AJR Am J Roentgenol 190:712–719

Sherman SC, Weber JM (2005) The CT diagnosis of ascariasis. J Emerg Med 28:471–472

Suh WS, Park CS, Lee MS, Lee JH, Chang MS, Woo JH, Lee IC, Ryu JS (2000) Hepatic and small bowel mucormycosis after chemotherapy in a patient with acute lymphocytic leukemia. J Korean Med Sci 15:351–354

Thoeni RF, Cello JP (2006) CT imaging of colitis. Radiology 240:623–638

Tresallet C, Nguyen-Thanh O, Aubriot-Lorton MH, Akakpo JP, Al Jijakli A, Cardot V, Chigot JP, Menegaux F (2004) Small bowel infarction from disseminated aspergillosis. Dis Colon Rectum 47:1515–1518

van Wolfswinkel ME, Lahri H, Wismans PJ, Petit PLC, van Genderen PJJ (2008) Early small bowel perforation and cochleovestibular impairment as rare complications of typhoid fever. Travel Med Infect Dis 7:265–268

Wu CM, Davis F, Fishman EK (1998) Radiologic evaluation of the acute abdomen in the patient with acquired immunodeficiency syndrome (AIDS): the role of CT scanning. Semin Ultrasound CT MR 19:190–199

Zalev AH, Gardiner JW, Warren RE (1996) NSAID injury to the small intestine. Abdom Imaging 23:40–44

Bowel Obstruction

Patrice Taourel, Denis Hoa and Jean-Michel Bruel

Contents

1	**Introduction**	273
2	**Gastroduodenal Obstruction**	274
3	**Small Bowel Obstruction**	277
3.1	Pathophysiology	277
3.2	Positive Diagnosis of SBO	278
3.3	Diagnosis of Site	281
3.4	Diagnosis of Obstruction Grade	282
3.5	Diagnosis of Causes	282
3.6	Diagnosis of Complications	291
4	**Large Bowel Obstruction**	296
4.1	Diagnosis of Mechanical Obstruction	296
4.2	Diagnosis of the Site of the Obstruction	297
4.3	Diagnosis of the Cause of the Obstruction	297
4.4	Diagnosis of Complications of the Obstruction	302
5	**Diagnostic Strategy**	305
References		306

Abstract

Bowel obstruction is a common clinical problem, and clinical signs and symptoms do not provide sufficient information for diagnosis or to guide management. CT is becoming a mainstay in diagnosing bowel obstruction and differentiating it from ileus, in locating the site of the obstruction, in identifying the transition point, in determining the cause of the obstruction, which may be intraluminal, intrinsic, or extrinsic, and finally in looking for a complication such as closed loop obstruction or ischemia. Multidetector row CT scanners permit high-quality reformatted series and particularly coronal reformatting useful in the identification of the transition point and in the analysis of the cause and of the mechanism of the obstruction. Because the management of obstruction has dramatically changed with a decrease in the proportion of patients who need surgery, of the time of surgery, which may be delayed, and of the type of surgery, with sometimes a coelioscopic procedure, a precise CT evaluation is now both the gold standard and the common approach in patients with suspected bowel obstruction.

1 Introduction

Acute intestinal obstruction is defined by the hindrance to the progression of the intestinal content due to a mechanical obstacle. It is responsible for approximately 25% of surgical admissions for acute abdominal conditions, with small bowel obstruction (SBO) accounting for about 65–75% of obstructions

P. Taourel (✉) · D. Hoa · J.-M. Bruel
Département d'Imagerie Médicale, Hôpital Lapeyronie,
371, avenue du Doyen Gaston Giraud,
34295 Montpellier Cedex 5, France
e-mail: p-taourel@chu-montpellier.fr

P. Taourel (ed.), *CT of the Acute Abdomen*, Medical Radiology. Diagnostic Imaging,
DOI: 10.1007/174_2010_85 © Springer-Verlag Berlin Heidelberg 2011

and large bowel obstruction (LBO) accounting for 25–35%, gastroduodenal obstruction being rarer and accounting for 1–2% of bowel obstructions. Bowel obstructions account for about 5–7% of all emergency department visits for abdominal pain, and reach 12% in patients older than 50 years (de Dombal 1994). The goals of imaging in a patient with suspected intestinal obstruction have been defined by Mondor et al. (1943) and summarized by Herlinger and Maglinte (1989) and are as follows:

- To confirm that it is a true obstruction and to differentiate it from an ileus
- To determine the level of obstruction
- To differentiate high-grade obstruction from incomplete obstruction
- To determine the cause of the obstruction
- To look for findings of strangulation
- To allow good management either medically or surgically by laparotomy or laparoscopy

This chapter deals with the findings, pitfalls, and accuracy of CT when answering these questions, discusses the impact of CT in the diagnosis and management of patients with suspected bowel obstruction, and recommends an approach for the diagnostic triage of such patients. The CT patterns, the causes, the potential severity, and the management of obstruction depend on the localization of the obstruction, and we will discuss separately gastroduodenal obstruction, SBO and LBO.

2 Gastroduodenal Obstruction

Gastroduodenal obstruction, also called gastric outlet obstruction, is clinically characterized by nausea and vomiting, which constitute the cardinal symptoms, whereas epigastric abdominal pain may lack and is usually related to the underlying cause.

Abdominal plain film often demonstrates the outline of the dilated gas-filled stomach with absence of gas distal to the duodenum. However, this pattern is not specific to gastroduodenal obstruction since it may be present in gastroparesis, also called delayed gastric emptying, a disorder in which the stomach takes too long to empty its contents. Gastroparesis occurs in numerous conditions, such as diabetes, postviral syndromes, surgery on the stomach or vagus nerve, use of medications, particularly anticholinergics and narcotics, smooth muscle disorders such as amyloidosis and scleroderma, nervous system diseases, and metabolic disorders. By showing a lesion at the junction between dilated bowel and collapsed bowel, CT differentiates gastroduodenal obstruction from gastroparesia.

The two main causes of gastroduodenal obstruction are malignant lesion and peptic ulcer disease. In the past, peptic ulcer disease accounted for most of the cases of obstruction. With the evolution of effective therapy for peptic ulcer disease, malignancy has emerged to be the most important cause of gastroduodenal obstruction.

Malignant obstruction of the gastric outlet is located mainly in the antropyloric region and is mostly due to advanced gastric neoplasia and is less commonly related to metastatic cancer or invasion of adjacent malignancies (bile duct cancer, gallbladder cancer) (Park et al. 2001). By contrast, malignant obstruction of the duodenum is mainly located at the level of the first part and the second part of the duodenum and is mostly due to invasion of the duodenum by a pancreatic cancer. Gastric neoplasia responsible for obstruction are adenocarcinoma and more rarely carcinoid tumors, whereas tumoral obstruction due to lymphomas (Buyn et al. 2003) or gastrointestinal stromal tumors seems to be exceptional (Sandrasegaran et al. 2005). Gastric adenocarcinomas which lead to obstruction are advanced cancer and may manifest themselves on CT as large, segmental, or diffuse wall thickening with irregular lobulation and often ulceration or as large, polypoid, fungating lesions (Ba-Salamah et al. 2003). Duodenal obstruction is encountered in an advanced stage of pancreatic cancer and is rarely present at the time of the diagnosis, for instance, in only three of 76 consecutive patients with pancreatic cancer (Valls et al. 2002), or in advanced peritoneal carcinomatosis (Fig. 1). Even if duodenal invasion is not itself a criterion for unresectability, it is often associated with criteria for unresectability, such as vascular invasion or liver metastasis well shown by CT. In metastatic disease, gastric and duodenal invasion may be associated. In a study describing imaging features of gastroduodenal obstruction in 438 consecutive women with ovarian cancer, the frequency of gastroduodenal obstruction was 2.5%, with five cases of predominant involvement of the gastric body and six of the gastric outlet and duodenum (Spencer et al. 2000).

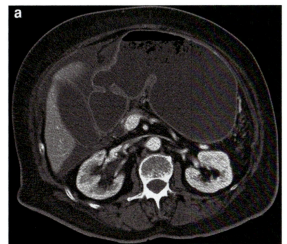
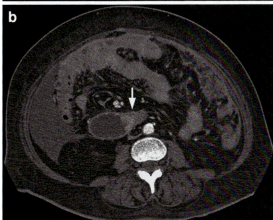
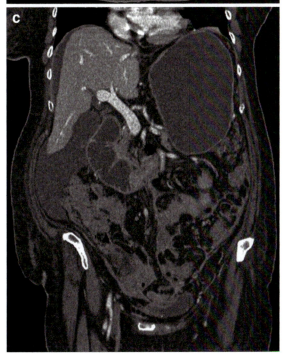

◀ **Fig. 1** Duodenal obstruction due to duodenal metastasis from an ovarian cancer. Axial slices (**a**, **b**) and coronal reformatting (**c**) show a dilatation of the stomach and of the first two parts of the duodenum. The tumoral mass is seen within the third part of the duodenum (*arrow*). Note also peritoneal carcinomatosis with involvement of the greater omentum

Gastroduodenal obstruction secondary to peptic ulcer disease remains prevalent and represents approximately 5–8% of ulcer-related complications (Behrman 2005). In 80% of cases, the obstruction is due to a duodenal ulcer, outlet obstruction due to gastric ulcer occurring less frequently. The stenosis is often short and may be difficult to identify by CT, making the differential diagnosis between obstruction related to peptic ulcer disease and gastroparesis difficult (Fig. 2).

Other causes of gastroduodenal obstruction mainly include gastritis and gastroenteritis, postsurgical strictures, adult congenital pyloric stenosis and volvulus for the stomach and pancreatitis, annular pancreas, superior mesenteric artery syndrome, Bouveret syndrome, bezoar, and intussusception for the duodenum.

Gastritis is a very common disease but is rarely responsible for gastric outlet obstruction. CT shows thickened gastric folds and wall thickening with soft-tissue attenuation. Eosinophilic gastroenteritis is a relatively classic cause of gastroduodenal obstruction with gastric and often duodenal esophageal involvement (Sheikh et al. 2009). Ingestion of corrosive substances may be responsible for severe gastritis, with fibrous scarring causing antral narrowing responsible for gastric outlet obstruction.

Adult idiopathic hypertrophic pyloric stenosis is a misleading anatomic and radioclinical entity of unknown cause. Only about 200 cases have been reported in the literature. It is a benign disease resulting from hypertrophy of the circular fibers of the pyloric canal. CT shows massive dilatation of the stomach, often without the identification of the wall pyloric thickening and upper gastrointestinal endoscopy which does not show any evidence of peptic ulcer disease or cancer allows both diagnosis and treatment by balloon dilatation of the pyloric sphincter (Franco and Dryden 2007).

Postoperative stenosis has become an increasing cause of gastric obstruction since the development of surgery for morbid obesity. Obstruction, with a reported incidence of up to 5%, may occur in several

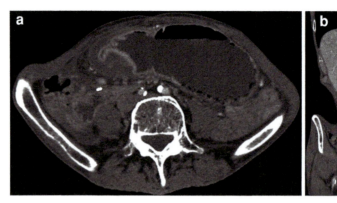

Fig. 2 Inflammatory stenosis of the antrum and of the first part of the duodenum shown on an axial slice (**a**) as well as on coronal reformatting (**b**). There is a thickening of the gastrointestinal wall responsible for a stenosis, with a dilatation of the gastric lumen. The stenosis was consecutive to an ulcer

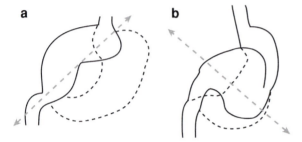

Fig. 3 Subtypes of gastric volvulus. Organoaxial volvulus (**a**) and mesenteroaxial volvulus (**b**)

locations and may result from several mechanisms. Potential sites include the gastrojejunostomy site, the jejunojejunostomy site, the mesocolic window, and behind the Roux limb (Peterson space). In the early postoperative setting, obstruction is often due to severe edema which will resolve spontaneously or can result from iatrogenic stenosis secondary to overzealous suturing. In the late postoperative setting, obstruction may result from fibrotic stenosis, internal hernias, or adhesions. Gastric outlet obstruction is generally the consequence of stricture located at the gastrojejunal anastomosis. The stenosis is better diagnosed by barium esophagography than by CT (Chandler et al. 2008).

The stomach is a relatively uncommon site of volvulus. Patients with acute gastric volvulus typically present with an acute clinical setting with sudden and intense epigastric pain, vomiting, and inability to pass a nasogastric tube in the stomach. CT allows one to differentiate the two forms of volvulus, i.e., organoaxial and mesenteroaxial forms (Fig. 3). The organoaxial form, which is the most common, occurs when the stomach rotates along its long axis and is generally associated with a paraesophageal hernia that follows the stomach along its long axis. This results in inversion of the greater curvature above the lesser curvature; the antrum is in the normal position. The mesenteroaxial form is much less common. It occurs when the stomach rotates along its short axis with consequent displacement of the antrum at the level of or above the gastroesophageal junction (Peterson et al. 2009) (Fig. 4).

Pancreatitis may lead to a gastroduodenal obstruction by two mechanisms: an inflammatory reaction of the gastroduodenal wall or a compression by pseudocysts. These two entities are well differentiated by CT.

Annular pancreas is an uncommon congenital abnormality responsible in adults for pancreatitis and duodenal obstruction and may be asymptomatic. Gastric outlet obstruction may be associated with incomplete or complete obstruction. The presence of pancreatic tissue posterolateral to the second part of the duodenum has both high sensitivity and high specificity for the diagnosis of annular pancreas; in the same way, a crocodile jaw appearance of pancreatic tissue anterior and posterior to the duodenum is highly suggestive of incomplete annular pancreas (Sandrasegaran et al. 2009).

Bouveret syndrome is a form of gallstone ileus with a stone impacted in the duodenum. Even if the stone is easily visible on CT, there are in some cases discrepancies between the diameter of the duodenum and the apparent size of the stone. Some findings such as the identification of air in dependent areas of the duodenal lumen, soft tissue surrounding the calcified part of the stone, or fat within the stone must be identified to better assess the size of the stone and to understand its involvement in the duodenal obstruction (Gan et al. 2008; Brennan et al. 2004).

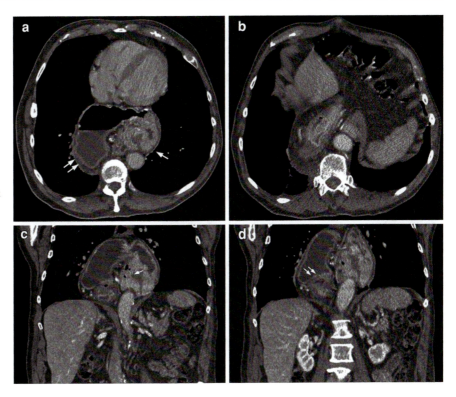

Fig. 4 Mesenteroaxial gastric volvulus. Axial slices (**a**, **b**) show the stomach within the thorax with the proximal part of the stomach (*arrow*) at the same craniocaudal level as the distal part (*double arrows*). On the coronal reconstructions (**c**, **d**), the gastroesophageal junction (*arrow*) and the gastroduodenal junction (*double arrows*) are almost at the same level

Superior mesenteric artery syndrome is characterized by the compression of the third part of the duodenum by the superior mesenteric artery. It is responsible for subacute or chronic forms of obstruction. CT shows a dilatation of the stomach and of the first and second parts of the duodenum, with a decrease of the superior mesenteric artery–aorta distance and angle (Unal et al. 2005).

Duodenoduodenal intussusception is rare, likely because mass in the duodenum is rare, and usually due to a tumoral lead point which is more often a benign tumor. CT easily demonstrates the collapsed intussusceptum lying within the opacified lumen of the distal intussuscipiens and one looks for a tumor at the leading point of the intussusceptum.

Duodenal bezoar is rarer in the duodenum than in the stomach or in the small bowel. However, bezoars located in the duodenum may be responsible for a gastric outlet obstruction. In a retrospective study of 34 cases of bezoar, only two involved the duodenum (Erzurumlu et al. 2005). Half of the patients had undergone gastric surgery. CT shows a nonenhanced intraluminal mass with gas bubbles and hypodense areas.

The outcome of a gastroduodenal obstruction depends more on the cause of the obstruction than on the dilatation of the stomach, with a high risk of gastric ischemia and perforation with peritonitis or mediastinitis in gastric volvulus if there is a delay between patient presentation and intervention. The identification of a gastric pneumatosis and or portal pneumatosis in the setting of a gastric dilatation is not specific to ischemia. Such findings may be present in gastroparesis due to the gastric dilatation and resolve when a nasogastric tube is passed into the stomach (Fig. 5).

3 Small Bowel Obstruction

3.1 Pathophysiology

Mechanical obstruction of the bowel lumen initially leads to an increase in intestinal contractions, which are intended to overcome the blockage. Peristaltis increases both above and below the obstructing lesion, so patients with obstruction may initially

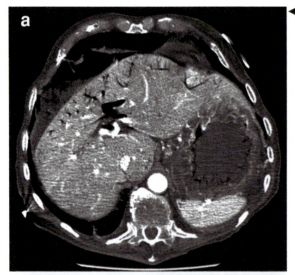
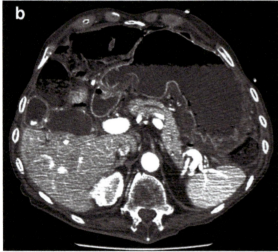
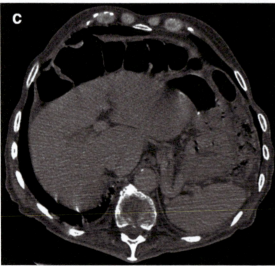

Fig. 5 Gastric pneumatosis consecutive to gastroparesy which spontaneously resolves. Axial slices (**a**, **b**) show a dilatation of the stomach, with parietal and portal pneumatosis. Intramural air spontaneously disappeared with the regression of the stomach dilatation, as seen on CT performed 1 week later (**c**)

present with the seemingly paradoxical finding of diarrhea. With the onset of muscle fatigue, peristaltic activity diminishes then ceases and the bowel dilates. Increased intraluminal pressures stimulate and increase the normal secretion of water and electrolytes into the bowel lumen and inhibit fluid resorption. Consequently, fluid accumulates in the bowel lumen, leading to further dilatation and increasing intraluminal pressure. Within certain limits, the bowel wall remains able to maintain an adequate blood supply through the process of stretching of its muscular layer with thinning of the wall and dilatation of blood vessels. Then, intraluminal pressures exceed capillary and venous pressures, mucosal perfusion diminishes, and bowel ischemia may result.

According to the process and the mechanism responsible for the obstruction, different pathophysiological responses may occur. In simple obstruction, considered when the bowel is occluded at one or several points along its course, the proximal part of the bowel is variably distended, depending on the severity (high grade vs. low grade) and duration of the process. In closed loop obstruction, considered when a bowel loop of variable length is occluded at both ends at two adjacent points, greater intraluminal pressures are generated and there is a risk of the distended closed bowel loops rotating around the axis of the mesenteric vessels, producing volvulus and arterial ischemia.

3.2 Positive Diagnosis of SBO

3.2.1 Clinical Considerations

The clinical diagnosis of SBO classically depends on four cardinal findings: abdominal pain, vomiting, constipation, and abdominal distension. However, the clinical findings differ with the degree and level of bowel obstruction and with the vascular status of the obstructed segment. In typical mechanical obstruction, abdominal pain is crampy and gradually increases in intensity, only to abate and recur. With time, increasing bowel distention inhibits motility and

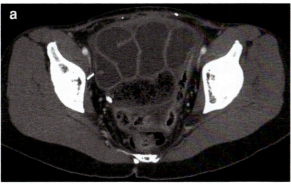 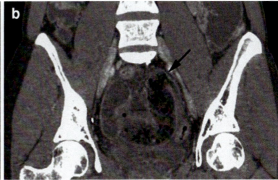

Fig. 6 Feces finding in a small bowel obstruction (SBO). Feces material within a small bowel loop well seen on the axial slice (**a**) as well as on coronal reformatting (**b**). The transition zone (*arrow*) just below the feces finding is better seen on the coronal view

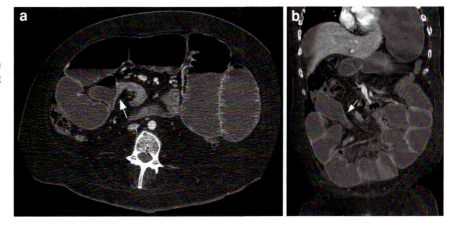

Fig. 7 SBO due to a unique adhesive band. The transition point is perfectly seen on the axial view (**a**) as well as on coronal reformatting (**b**). Note the presence of a beak finding at the transition zone

the pain tends to subside (Herlinger and Rubesin 1994). On the other hand, crampy abdominal pain may be present in other causes of acute abdomen such as renal colic. In the same way, vomiting or constipation is obviously not specific to acute abdomen.

3.2.2 CT Findings

The CT diagnosis of bowel obstruction is based on the presence of dilated bowel proximal to a transition zone and a collapsed distal bowel. The small bowel is considered dilated when its diameter is greater than 2.5 cm. The amount of intraluminal air versus fluid and the degree of dilatation of the small bowel are not reliable criteria to differentiate mechanical obstruction from ileus. Fluid-filled loops as large as 5 cm in diameter can be present in a nonobstructive ileus. In patients with dilated small bowel loops, the presence of a small bowel feces sign is a good ancillary finding of SBO. The small bowel feces sign is defined when intraluminal particulate material is identified in the dilated small bowel responsible for a mottled "feculent" appearance. Although not sensitive and seen in about 20% of cases of SBO, it is relatively specific to an SBO and facilitates the identification of the transition point since it occurs near the transition zone (Fig. 6) (Lazarus et al. 2004).

The identification of the transition point is the most accurate finding of an SBO. The transition point is determined by identifying a caliber change between the dilated proximal and collapsed distal small bowel loops (Fig. 7). The course of the small bowel needs to be tracked, and for that the use of a cine mode on a workstation or a picture archiving and communication system is more efficient than simply relying on static

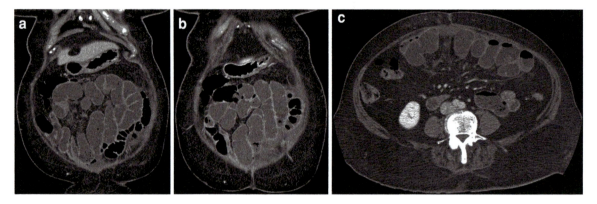

Fig. 8 SBO due to multiple matted adhesions. Coronal reformatting (**a**, **b**) show multiple transition zones. Note the anterior site of the bowel loops against the anterior abdominal wall shown on the axial slice (**c**)

images. Scrolling is generally performed in a retrograde fashion by starting at the rectum and proceeding proximally toward the cecum, ileum, and jejunum. If the transition point is located proximally (jejunum or duodenum), the position should be confirmed by using an anterograde approach, starting at the stomach (Silva et al. 2009; Khurana et al. 2002).

3.2.3 CT Pitfalls

The dilatation of small bowel loops, although not specific, is highly sensitive for the diagnosis of SBO. However, in some cases of SBO with rapidly developing strangulation, dilatation may be limited to one or two small bowel loops.

Although suggestive, the presence of a small bowel feces sign is not specific. By definition, for the small bowel feces sign to be present, particulate material must be within segments measuring greater than 2.5 cm in diameter, since feculent-appearing material may be seen within normal-caliber bowel loops in patients with cystic fibrosis, and in metabolic or infectious enteropathies. Furthermore, particulate material may also be present in the distal ileum owing to reflux through an incompetent ileocecal valve. Finally, small bowel feces must not be confused with bezoar characterized by a well-defined mass mottled with gas bubbles with an encapsulated wall and some fat-density debris floating in bowel lumen proximal to obstructive bezoar.

The transition point may be difficult to identify when SBO is due to matted adhesions defined as dense, multiple, short, and thick adhesive structures (Delabrousse et al. 2009). Furthermore, even if classically there is one transition point in simple bowel obstruction and there are two transition points in closed loop obstruction, more transition points may be present in simple as well as in closed loop obstruction (Fig. 8) (Sandhu et al. 2007).

3.2.4 CT Accuracy

The CT accuracy for the diagnosis of SBO is better than 90% in high-grade SBO and between 70 and 85% for low-grade SBO. Although intravenous injection is the standard in the evaluation of patients with suspected bowel obstruction, a recent study has shown that nonenhanced multidetector CT has comparable accuracy to enhanced multidetector CT in determining the presence or the absence of SBO and determination of the transition point (Atri et al. 2009). Multidetector CT allows one to scan the entire abdomen and pelvis at a nearly isotropic resolution, which gives good reformations. Coronal reformatting allows a better representation of the site of the dilated and nondilated bowel loops (Fig. 9). Several studies have shown that coronal reformations increase both agreement and confidence levels in the diagnosis of SBO. A recent French study has proved that the use of multiplanar evaluation improved the detection of the transition point from 85% with only axial slices to more than 90% (Hodel et al. 2009). This is a crucial finding for the management of patients with SBO.

3.2.5 CT Impact

The distinction between bowel obstruction and ileus is classically based upon clinical examination and abdominal plain film. In complete obstruction, distended loops of small bowel containing gas and fluid

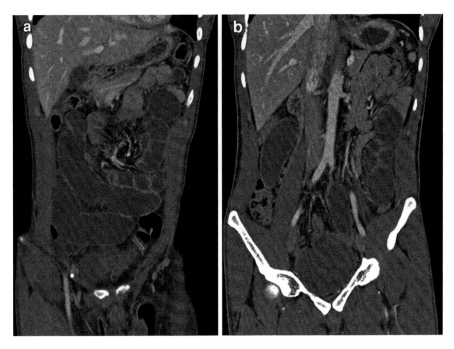

Fig. 9 Repartition of the nondilated bowel loops in an SBO. Coronal reformatting on an anterior (a) and posterior (b) plane show dilated and nondilated small bowel loops. The nondilated loops correspond to the proximal jejunal loops far from the site of the obstruction and distal pelvic ileal loops below the site of the obstruction

are usually present within 3–5 h of the onset. The interface between gas and fluid forms a straight horizontal margin in the upright or lateral decubitus view. Although gas–fluid levels are occasionally present normally, more than two gas–fluid levels in the small bowel are generally considered to be abnormal; however, gas–fluid levels are also very common in ileus. The presence of gas–fluid levels at different heights in the same loop has traditionally been considered strong evidence for mechanical obstruction; however, this pattern is insensitive and can also be demonstrated in some patients with adynamic ileus (Harlow et al. 1993). Furthermore, in severe complete obstruction, the bowel proximal to an obstruction may contain no gas and may be completely filled with fluid, producing sausage-shaped water-density shadows that can be difficult to diagnose. In one study, obstruction was not supported by abdominal radiographs read by an experienced gastrointestinal radiologist in 34% of surgically proven cases of SBO (Shrake et al. 1991). Consequently, CT plays a central role in the evaluation of patients with suspected SBO. For the diagnosis of SBO, it is particularly helpful in the following cases (Fig. 10):

- Clinical findings of obstruction with abdominal plain film showing no gas, likely meaning that bowel loops are completely filled with fluid
- Gas within one or two dilated loops
- Doubt between ileus and SBO

3.3 Diagnosis of Site

3.3.1 Clinical Considerations

The diagnosis of the site of a mechanical obstruction is not easily performed with only clinical data, even if vomiting is more pronounced in proximal SBO and abdominal distension is more pronounced in distal SBO.

The accurate determination of the site of the obstruction is becoming a major point when considering the management of patients with SBO, by permitting a safe laparoscopic division of adhesions that may be a suitable form of treatment of adhesive bands. Moreover, it may represent a valuable predictive factor in the management of adhesive SBO, since it has been shown that most patients with proximal SBO healed with conservative management, whereas distal SBO more frequently required surgery.

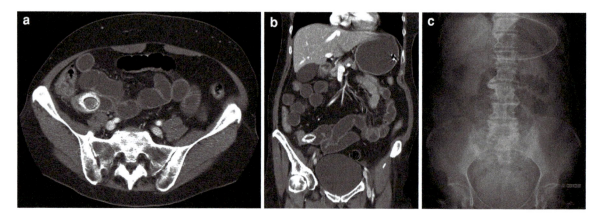

Fig. 10 SBO due to gallstone ileus. The axial slice (**a**) and coronal reformatting (**b**) clearly show the stone responsible for the SBO. Note that the stone is not seen on the abdominal plain film (**c**) and that most of the bowel loops do not contain air

3.3.2 CT Findings

CT determines the site of SBO by detecting the site of the transition zone and by surveying all the abdominal axial images and comparing the relative lengths of the prestenotic versus collapsed intestine. Attempting to determine the level of SBO solely on the basis of the site of transition in terms of the quadrant can result in misleading interpretations. Jejunal loops can be located in the pelvis, and ileal loops can be obstructed in the upper abdomen. When present, the small bowel feces finding is helpful to locate the transition zone in patients with SBO.

3.4 Diagnosis of Obstruction Grade

3.4.1 Clinical Considerations

Differentiating complete from partial grade obstruction is controversial. A low-grade obstruction is more likely than a high-grade obstruction to resolve spontaneously, and this could have an impact on the management of patients with bowel obstruction. In a study including patients with SBO due to adhesions (Hwang et al. 2009), all the 42 patients with incomplete low-grade obstruction were successfully managed without surgery, most of the patients with incomplete high-grade obstruction (43 of 58) were not operated on, whereas most of the patients with complete high-grade obstruction (22 of 28) were operated on. However, low-grade obstruction may theoretically be complicated by strangulation.

3.4.2 CT Findings

The diagnosis of the severity of the obstruction theoretically needs use of oral contrast material, with passage through the transition zone to the collapsed distal bowel loops indicating incomplete obstruction, which may be separated into high grade and low grade according to the amount and delay in the passage of contrast material. However, in clinical practice, oral contrast material is generally not given. Therefore, the severity of the obstruction is determined by the degree of collapse and the amount of residual contents in the portion of the bowel distal to the obstructed site.

3.5 Diagnosis of Causes

3.5.1 Clinical Considerations

The pattern of major causes of SBO has changed over the past five decades. The most common cause was originally external hernia. Now, adhesions compose 60–80% of the total number of SBOs in industrialized countries. The great majority (85%) of adhesions occur after surgery, the second cause is peritonitis, whereas the remaining causes are either congenital or uncertain causes. In patients who have undergone surgery, appendicectomy and gynecologic procedures are more prevalent as a cause of adhesive bands, whereas in patients who have not undergone surgery, inflammatory entities such as adnexitis and appendicitis are common precursors of adhesions. Among adhesive structures, adhesive bands, which are unique, long (more than 1 cm), and thin (less than

1 cm diameter), must be differentiated from matted adhesions, which are multiple, dense, short (less than 1 cm in diameter), and thick (more than 1 cm in diameter).

The second most common causes of SBO are neoplasm, hernias, and Crohn disease, each accounting for about 10%. A fourth miscellaneous group of causes includes inflammatory processes, intussusception, volvulus, endometriosis, ischemia, hematoma, congenital lesions, gallstones, foreign bodies, and bezoar (Fig. 10).

The prevalence of the different causes of SBO varies according to the clinical context.

In patients without a history of surgery, the diagnosis of a congenital adhesive band is still possible, since 5% of adhesive bands are encountered in such patients. Even if it is very rare, small bowel volvulus may occur in patients without adhesions or a predisposing abnormality such as malrotation or hernia, and the differential diagnosis between primary small bowel volvulus and volvulus complicating congenital band is impossible before surgery.

In patients with a previously treated cancer, obstruction is very common (Ha et al. 1998). It occurs in up to 30% of patients with a history of colorectal cancer and in as many as 40% of patients with ovarian cancer (Tang et al. 1995). Determining the cause of obstruction becomes a vexing problem since it may be benign postoperative adhesions, a focal malignant deposit, peritoneal carcinomatosis, ischemic stenosis due to radiation enteritis, or incisional entrapment. Malignant lesions represent the most common cause of obstructions; however, the percentage of benign causes of obstruction ranges from 18 to 38% on the basis of the distribution of the primary cancer. Benign obstruction is more likely if pelvic irradiation was used in the management of the primary tumor, whereas the risk of malignant obstruction is increased if the patient has a known metastatic cancer or if the primary cancer was in an advanced stage or of gynecologic origin. In patients with SBO due to advanced intra-abdominal malignancy, occult synchronous colonic obstruction is present in nearly half of patients. This must be kept in mind before bypass surgery.

In patients with occlusion and fever, the three most classic causes are mesocoeliac appendicitis, sigmoid diverticulitis, and biliary ileus. However, other causes may be responsible for this clinical setting (Table 1).

Table 1 Causes of small bowel obstruction (*SBO*) with fever

Mesocoeliac appendicitis

Sigmoid diverticulitis

Biliary ileus

Pelvic peritonitis from salpingitis origin

Meckel diverticulitis

Inflammatory stenosis (Crohn disease)

Complicated SBO with strangulation

Furthermore, fever may be a sign of complicated obstruction with strangulation and ischemia.

In patients with Crohn disease, SBO may result from three different causes: it may be due to the acute presentation of the disease with a transmural acute inflammatory process; it can result from a long-standing process with cicatricial stenosis; or it may be due to inflammatory or postoperative adhesions or to incisional hernias.

Hernias are classified according to the anatomic location of the orifice through which the bowel protrudes. They are differentiated as external and internal hernias. External hernias result from a defect in the abdominal and pelvic wall at sites of congenital weakness or previous surgery. Internal hernias, which are less common, occur when there is protrusion of the viscera through the peritoneum or mesentery and into a compartment within the abdominal cavity (Armstrong et al. 2007). Both external and internal hernias may be congenital or acquired. The diagnostic hypothesis for the cause of an SBO must take into account these probability data and the clinical context (Table 2). Furthermore, systematic evaluation of imaging data must also be performed by looking for one of the three major categories of SBO, as stated by Herlinger and Rubesin (1994): intraluminal, intrinsic, and extrinsic (Table 3). Most extrinsic causes produce obstruction by flattening, twisting, or kinking the small bowel. Intrinsic lesions constrict the lumen by thickening of the bowel wall, and intraluminal causes obturate the bowel lumen.

3.5.2 CT Findings

Intraluminal causes of obstruction include gallstones (mostly in elderly women) which may be visible on CT but not on plain radiography (Fig. 10), fecal impaction in patients with cystic fibrosis, related to inadequately controlled intestinal absorption

Table 2 Causes of SBO according to the clinical context

History of abdominal surgery	Malignancy context	Crohn disease	AIDS context	Septic context
Adhesions	Adhesions (if history of surgery)	Inflammatory transmural stenosis	Frequency of intussusceptions due to infectious enteritis, lymphoid hyperplasia, mesenteric adenopathy, Kaposi sarcoma, and non-Hodgkin lymphoma	Appendicitis
External hernias	Peritoneal carcinomatosis	Chronic stricture		Sigmoid diverticulitis
Incisional hernias	Focal malignant deposit	Postsurgical or inflammatory adhesions		Meckel diverticulitis
Laparoscopic port site hernias	Intussusception due to metastasis (melanoma)			Salpingitis
Parastomial hernias	External hernias			
Internal hernias	Incisional hernias			
Transmesenteric hernias	Laparoscopic port site hernias			
	Paratonial hernias			

secondary to pancreatic insufficiency, ingested foreign bodies occurring in mentally disturbed or retarded or elderly patients, and bezoars, which are most frequent in patients who have undergone gastric outlet resection or who have small bowel diverticula. The detection of a small bowel foreign body or bezoars requires one to look for an underlying obstructive lesion.

CT findings of gallstone ileus are pathognomonic of pneumobilia, ectopic gallstone, and SBO. Fecal impactions are generally distal in the small bowel with feculent filling defect. Among foreign bodies usually occurring in children or disturbed patients, a particular epidemiological context must be known: the retention of endoscopic capsules used to evaluate inaccessible portions of the bowel when there is an associated bowel lumen narrowing. CT shows the SBO with evidence of a foreign body at the transition zone. The diagnosis of bezoar is performed by the identification of a well-defined mass mottled with gas bubbles associated with an encapsulating wall and fat-density debris within the bowel lumen (Delabrousse et al. 2008).

Intussusception may be considered as an intraluminal cause of SBO, since it obturates the lumen by pushing a proximal small bowel loop and part of its mesentery into the lumen of the small bowel distal to it, even if various extrinsic or intrinsic processes may result in intussusception. The typical imaging features of enteroenteric intussusception are as follows (Gayer et al. 1998): a distended loop of bowel (the intussuspiens) with a thickened wall; an eccentrically positioned intraluminal intussuseptum; and a crescentic area of fat-density mass representing invaginated fat from the mesentery of the intussusceptum (Fig. 11). CT can also demonstrate the cause of the intussusception by showing the leading point and can suggest its nature by its density: lipoma, cystic mass from a mucocele, or solid mass (Warshauer and Lee 1999). In some cases, CT may show multiple polypoid tumors, which suggest a diagnosis of metastases, especially from malignant melanoma, or Peutz–Jeghers syndrome. The great majority of intussusceptions responsible for an SBO are related to a tumoral cause, but intussusception is almost never the presenting sign of undiagnosed malignancy (Wang et al. 2009; Marinis et al. 2009). By contrast, numerous intussusceptions are asymptomatic without any finding of obstruction, fortuitously discovered by CT, often transient, and without a leading point (Huang and Warshauer 2003; Horton and Fishman

Table 3 Causes of SBO in adults

Extrinsic lesions	Intrinsic lesions	Intraluminal causes
Adhesions	Tumors infiltrating the wall of the small bowel	Obstruction
Hernia	Adenocarcinoma	Gallstone
External	Carcinoid tumor	Bezoar
Inguinal	Lymphoma (rare)	Foreign body
Femoral	Leiomyosarcoma (rare)	Ascaris
Obturator	Inflammatory conditions	Meconium
Sciatic	Crohn disease	Intussusception
Perineal	Tuberculosis	Adhesions
Supravesical	Potassium chloride stricture	Tumor
Spigelian	Eosinophilic gastroenteritis	Duplication
Lumbar	Vascular	Inverted Meckel diverticulum
Incisional	Radiation enteropathy	
Umbilical	Ischemia	
Internal	Hematoma	
Paraduodenal	Posttraumatic	
Epiploic foramen	Thrombocytopenia	
Diaphragmatic (traumatic)	Anticoagulants	
Transomental	Henoch–Schönlein purpura	
Transmesenteric		
Iliac fossa		
Masses		
Extrinsic tumors in mesentery		
Lymphoma		
Peritoneal metastasis		
Carcinoid		
Desmoid		
Abscesses		
Diverticulitis		
Pelvic inflammatory disease		
Crohn disease		
Appendicitis		
Aneurysm		
Hematoma		
Endometriosis		

2008). Intussusception constitutes a relatively common cause of SBO in AIDS patients, and it may be related to numerous causes: infectious enteritis, lymphoid hyperplasia, mesenteric adenopathy, Kaposi sarcoma, and non-Hodgkin lymphoma (Rabeneck 1995).

Intrinsic causes include tumor, inflammatory disease, ischemia, and hematoma. Tumors that are responsible for SBO by infiltration of the bowel wall are mainly adenocarcinoma, primary carcinoid, and metastases. Adenocarcinomas appear as an annular infiltrating lesion located in the duodenum or in the proximal jejunum, although more distal sites are possible (Fig. 12). Conversely, bowel metastases (e.g., from melanoma) usually involve the distal small

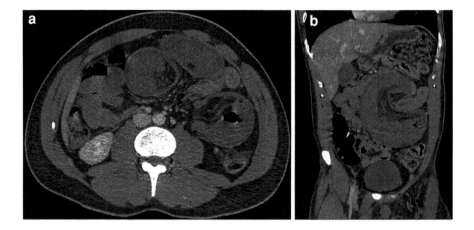

Fig. 11 Small bowel intussusception seen on the axial slice (**a**) and coronal reformatting (**b**)

bowel, making an annular infiltrative lesion in the distal ileum more likely to be a metastasis, especially in the setting of a known primary malignancy. Primary carcinoids obstruct the bowel more by desmoplastic changes (extrinsic process) than the tumor itself, which may be difficult to visualize. The SBO consecutive to inflammatory disease is more often due to Crohn disease and bowel obstruction may be the first manifestation of the disease. Ultrasonography and CT show circumferential inflammatory thickening of the bowel wall, fibrofatty changes (Fig. 13), and abscess in some cases. Other primary inflammatory causes of SBO include tuberculosis and manifestations of Behçet syndrome, both invading the terminal ileum, and ulcerative jejunoileitis complicating celiac disease and occurring in the proximal jejunum. Chronic mesenteric ischemia is responsible for a thickening of the bowel wall, which may be responsible for an SBO. Radiation enteropathy is a form of ischemia since radiation-induced small-vessel occlusions may produce chronic ischemia anywhere in the alimentary tract. CT shows bowel wall thickening with occasional visualization of the target sign. An important clue for diagnosis is that bowel changes are confined to the radiation port (Furukama et al. 2001). Spontaneous intramural hematoma is most commonly caused by excessive anticoagulation. Other causes include coagulopathy, collagen vascular disease, and Henoch–Schönlein purpura. CT shows thickening of the bowel wall occurring mainly in the duodenum and in the proximal jejunum with a characteristic ring pattern of high attenuation on nonenhanced slices (Fig. 14).

Extrinsic causes are the most common causes of SBO. Most extrinsic lesions are adhesions, which are the causes of SBO in approximately 70% of cases. The CT diagnosis of adhesion was classically considered as difficult because it was based on negative findings. The diagnosis is evoked from the presence of an abrupt change in bowel caliber without evidence of another cause of obstruction, the adhesive band itself being unidentifiable by CT. However, thin slices and multiplanar reformation have improved the diagnosis of adhesions. They allow the transition point to be viewed with more confidence and permit one to better individualize two CT signs of adhesive bands (Fig. 15): the beak sign, which is a beaklike narrowing without any mass at the transition zone, described more than 15 years ago (Balthazar et al. 1992; Balthazar and George 1994; Ha et al. 1993), and the fat notch sign, which corresponds to the extraluminal compression made by a band on the bowel at the transition zone (Petrovic et al. 2006). These findings are seen in adhesive bands in more than 60% of cases, whereas they are rarely encountered in matted adhesions (Delabrousse et al. 2009).

Although most small bowel volvulus are complications of bowel obstruction due to adhesions, midgut volvulus constitutes a primary cause of small bowel volvulus. The major predisposing factor for midgut volvulus is malrotation of the small bowel. In a malrotation, there is abnormal fixation of the small bowel mesentery, which results in an abnormally short mesentery root. This favors the twisting of the small bowel around its mesentery. With CT, one will look for a swirling of vessels in the mesentery root (Fig. 16), an abnormal relationship between the superior mesenteric artery and

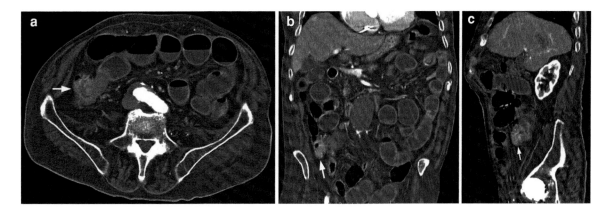

Fig. 12 SBO due to an adenocarcinoma of the terminal ileum. The axial slice (**a**) as well as coronal (**b**) and sagittal (**c**) reformatting show a dilatation of the entire small bowel. Note an enhanced, important and short thickening of the terminal ileum wall suggesting a malignant tumor of the terminal ileum (*arrow*). Surgery confirmed an adenocarcinoma

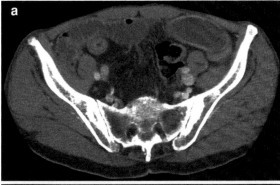

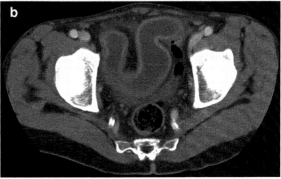

Fig. 13 SBO due to Crohn disease. Axial slices (**a**, **b**) show a thickening of the distal ileum which involved a long segment of intestine. The involved ileum has an enhanced wall with a target finding. Note also a sclerolipomatosis suggestive of Crohn disease

vein, and abnormal position of the angle of Treitz positioned below and to the right of the left L1 pedicle (Silva et al. 2009).

Hernias are the second most common cause of SBO. Approximately 95% of obstructions caused by hernias are external. External hernias, which include inguinal, femoral, umbilical, spigelian, and incisional hernias, consist of a peritoneal sac that protrudes through a weakness or defect in the muscular layers of the abdomen. Diagnosis of external hernias is based on clinical examination, and generally external hernias are treated before occlusive complications. However, in obese patients, the clinical diagnosis may be difficult and patient imaging is required. Indirect inguinal hernias are by far the most common cause of hernias This type of hernia is localized laterally to the inferior epigastric vessels and anteromedially to the spermatic cords and may reach the scrotum. Femoral hernias are far less frequent than inguinal hernias, are encountered in women, and generally reach the superior part of the thigh, at the level of the Scarpa triangle, and when they are small, they may be difficult to distinguish from inguinal hernias. CT is very helpful in differentiating direct inguinal hernia, indirect inguinal hernia, and femoral hernia by using the pubic tubercle as a reference point (Delabrousse et al. 2005) (Figs. 17, 18). Umbilical and subumbilical hernias are the second most common cause of external hernias and are easily diagnosed by CT. Postoperative external hernias are common and include incisional hernia, most frequently occurring in midline or paramidline incision, laparoscopic port site hernias, and parastomial hernias. Obturator hernias and spigelian hernias constitute rarer forms of external hernia, for which CT has a great contribution to the diagnosis (Stabile Ianora et al. 2000). Richter hernia is a special type of external hernia in which a portion of the bowel wall circumference, rather than a

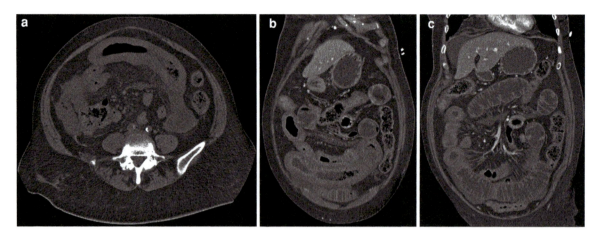

Fig. 14 SBO due to spontaneous hematoma of the small bowel. The axial slice before contrast material administration (**a**) shows a huge, symmetric, and spontaneously hyperdense thickening of bowel wall. Coronal reformatting (**b**, **c**) shows that the thickening is extensive and leads to a small bowel dilatation

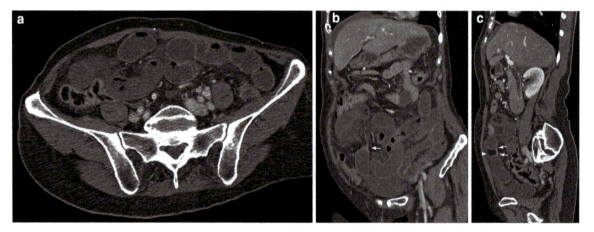

Fig. 15 SBO due to a unique adhesive band with a beak finding and a fat notch finding. The axial slice (**a**) shows a dilatation of the small bowel with a collapsed colon. The transition zone is not well seen, whereas it is clearly seen on coronal (**b**) and sagittal (**c**) reformatting with two beak findings (*arrows*) and a fat notch finding (*arrowhead*). Surgery confirmed the unique anterior adhesive band

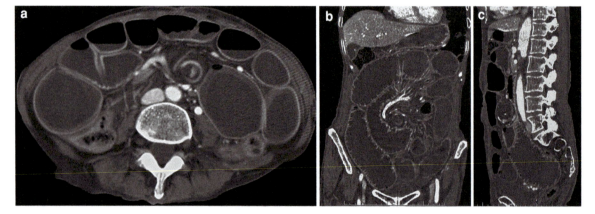

Fig. 16 Whirl sign in primary volvulus of the small bowel. The axial slice (**a**) and coronal (**b**) and sagittal (**c**) reformatting clearly show a whirl finding with swirling of the mesenteric vessels around the mesentery

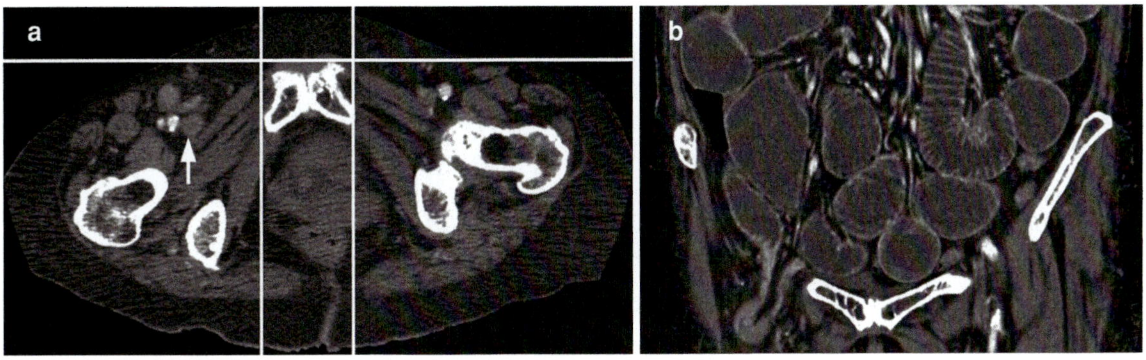

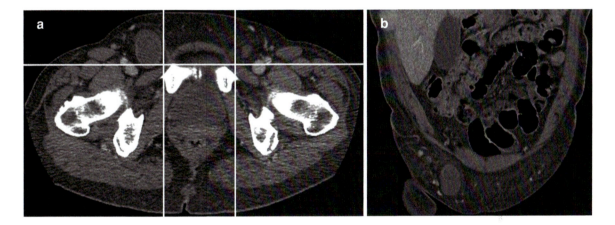

Fig. 17 Right femoral hernia. Construction of orthogonal lines on the axial slice (**a**) focused on the pubic tubercles allows one to differentiate femoral hernia (*arrow*) located dorsal to the axial axis from inguinal hernias located ventral to the axial axis. The coronal view (**b**) clearly shows the herniated small bowel

Fig. 18 Right-sided direct inguinal hernia. Construction of orthogonal lines on the axial slice (**a**) focused on the pubic tubercles allows one to differentiate inguinal hernia located ventral to the axial axis from femoral hernias located dorsal to the axial axis, and to differentiate direct inguinal hernia lateral to the sagittal axis from indirect hernia crossing medially the sagittal axis. The coronal view (**b**) clearly shows the herniated small bowel

whole loop, becomes entrapped in a tightly constricting hernia orifice. Richter hernias more rapidly progress to bowel wall necrosis than other strangulated hernias and present with symptoms of ischemia rather than obstruction because the lumen remains open.

In comparison with external hernias, internal hernias are uncommon and remain a vexing problem for CT (Blachar et al. 2001; Takeyama et al. 2005). The two most common internal hernias are paraduodenal hernias and transmesenteric or transmesocolic hernias. Paraduodenal hernias account for approximately 50% of all internal hernias. The small bowel is entrapped between the posterior and the mesocolon in a hernia sac. CT shows that the anterior wall of the sac contains the inferior mesenteric vein and left colic artery in left-sided paraduodenal hernia and the superior mesenteric vein and the right colic artery in right-sided paraduodenal hernia, and these vessels constitute a landmark above the encapsulated bowel loops (Warshauer and Mauro 1992). Transmesenteric and transmesocolic hernias are becoming more common because of transplants and bariatric surgery in which surgical defects in the mesocolon are created to accommodate a Roux loop. CT shows small bowel located laterally to the colon (Fig. 19) and overall directly adjacent to the abdominal wall, and mesenteric vessels stretched and following the course of the herniated bowel (Martin et al. 2006). Other internal hernias include herniation through the foramen of Winslow (Fig. 20), pericecal, intersigmoid, supravesical, and pelvic hernias, including hernias through

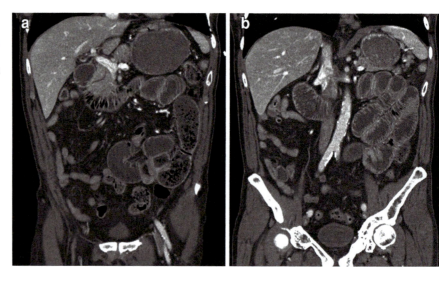

Fig. 19 Transmesenteric hernia shown on coronal views (**a**, **b**). Note the lateral position of the small bowel loops which are dilated with a feces content. The bowel loops are encapsulated. The diagnosis of internal hernia was not performed preoperatively

the broad ligament. Table 4 summarizes CT findings in these different hernias.

Extrinsic causes of SBO other than adhesions and hernias include a wide variety of neoplastic, inflammatory, and vascular processes. Extrinsic masses cause obstruction by two main mechanisms: compression of the lumen by the mass and distortion of the lumen by a desmoplastic process. The most common cause of extrinsic masses is carcinomatosis, most often from ovarian carcinoma. However, any peritoneal process, such as carcinoid desmoplastic reaction which often results in retraction of surrounding loops of small bowel, tuberculous peritonitis, desmoid tumors, severe radiation changes, or peritoneal endometriosis from the small bowel serosa, may mimic peritoneal metastases. In the same way, an inflammatory process may agglutinate the bowel loops responsible for an SBO (Fig. 21)

Abdominal cocoon, also referred to as sclerosing encapsulating peritonitis, is a rare extrinsic cause of SBO. It is characterized by forming a fibrous membranelike sac, which encases the loops of small bowel and causes subacute and recurrent episodes of bowel obstruction. CT shows totally or partially obstructed loops of small bowel concentrated to the center of the abdomen and a thickening of the peritoneal membrane (Tombak et al. 2010).

3.5.3 CT Pitfalls

As previously said, the lack of identification of a lesion in adhesion was classically a cause of lack of confidence. However, the identification of a beak sign or a fat notch sign at the transition zone dramatically increases the radiologist's ability to affirm an adhesive band. In some cases, at the level of the beak finding, there is some thickening of the bowel wall which may evoke an intrinsic bowel lesion. By contrast with adhesive band, the diagnosis of matted obstruction, for which the beak sign and the fat notch sign are generally missing, remains difficult.

The diagnosis of internal hernias remains very challenging, and even though numerous case reports of CT diagnosis of internal hernia have been published, mostly the pictures are correctly interpreted only after the surgical procedure. The diagnostic criteria making diagnostic possible include abnormal location of bowel, encapsulation, and crowding of bowel loops, but these findings are not pathognomonic and key points such as an abnormal location of a vessel, an abnormal distance between the portal vein and the inferior vena cava, or a surgical context consistent with a mesocolic defect must be looked for. In clinical practice, paraduodenal hernias are more often diagnosed preoperatively because of their relative frequency (Fig. 22)

Endometriosis is a common disease, but is rarely revealed by an SBO, and findings such as a solid nodule penetrating the bowel wall or a transition point which appears as a short circumferential mural thickening and on surgery a stricture due to fibrosis secondary to endometriotic implants looking like an adhesive band are often difficult to identify (Silva et al. 2009).

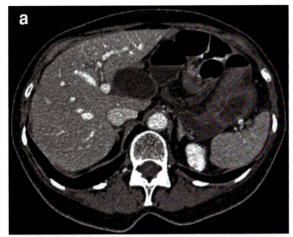

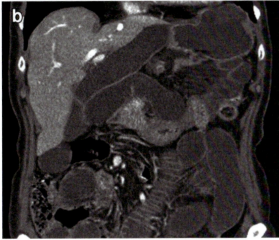

Fig. 20 Foramen of Winslow hernia. The dilated small bowel loops are encapsulated and localized in the lesser sac. The axial slice (**a**) show the loops within the lesser sac, whereas the coronal view (**b**) show bowel loops passing through the foramen of Winslow

The CT diagnosis of intussusception is easy with a pathognomonic finding, but a leading mass as the cause of the intussusception may be difficult to differentiate from the soft-tissue pseudotumor that represents the intussusception itself (Aufort et al. 2005; Tresoldi et al. 2008).

3.5.4 CT Impact

The practical value of knowing the cause of SBO before surgery has dramatically improved treatment in the last decade. The philosophy of never letting the sun set or rise on SBO has been followed by management according to the cause and the severity of the obstruction. Most modern surgeons actually recommend an emergent operative management in hernias, a more delayed surgical management in malignant focal tumor, a medical management in most cases of peritoneal carcinomatosis, radiation enteritis, or jejunal hematoma, a conservative management in Crohn disease when an acute flare is causing bowel obstruction whereas obstruction caused by a chronic fibrotic structure may in some cases necessitate surgical resection, and treatment of adhesions, balancing between medical treatment and surgical exploration according to the patient's status, the location of the adhesions, and above all the suspicion of strangulation. The distinction between adhesive bands and matted obstruction is of importance because the risk of closed loop obstruction and strangulation is dramatically higher in adhesive bands, whereas a higher rate of surgical accidental bowel perforation seems to be associated with matted adhesions. In clinical practice, fewer than 50% of patients with a CT diagnosis of adhesion are operated.

3.6 Diagnosis of Complications

3.6.1 Clinical Considerations

Strangulation occurs in about 10% of SBO cases. It represents the main factor of morbidity and mortality, with a mortality above 10%, increasing with the diagnostic delay. It is characterized by an impaired vascular circulation to the obstructed intestine. Balthazar and George (1994) have very clearly summarized the mechanisms which lead to a strangulation:

1. The first event is a closed loop or incarcerated intestinal obstruction due to adhesions or hernias, in which a loop of bowel is occluded at two or more adjacent points along its course. There is a mechanical obstruction proximal to the involved bowel segment. The length of the closed loop is variable, from a single loop to several loops of bowel. If the length of the closed loop is sufficient, the loop may twist and produce a volvulus. It the length of the closed loop is short (e.g., in some external hernias), the bowel proximal to the obstacle may twist. Volvulus is a common but not invariable complication of an incarcerated loop. It tends to occur in patents with high degrees of obstruction, but once developed, it further

Table 4 CT patterns in internal hernias

	Relative incidence	Mechanism	CT position of the loops	Key points
Left-sided paraduodenal hernia	+++	Congenital	Encapsulated loops between the stomach and pancreas or behind the pancreas or between the transverse colon and the left adrenal gland	Inferior mesenteric vein displaced anteriorly
Right-sided paraduodenal hernia	++	Congenital	Encapsulated loops lateral and inferior to the descending duodenum	Superior mesenteric artery displaced anteriorly (located in the anteromedial border of the sac)
Pericecal hernia	++	Congenital or acquired	Clustered loops posterior and lateral to the ascending colon	
Foramen of Winslow hernia	+	Congenital	Small bowel loops and sometimes ascending colon in the lesser sac	Mesentery between the abnormally distant portal vein and the inferior vena cava
Transmesenteric and transmesocolic hernias	+++	Acquired (in adults)	Small bowel loops lateral to the colon	Displaced omental fat with small bowel directly abutting abdominal wall. Epidemiological data: history of Roux-en-Y surgery (liver transplant, bariatric surgery)
Intersigmoid hernias	+	Congenital or acquired	Clustered small bowel loops posterior and lateral to the sigmoid colon	
Hernias through the broad ligament	+	Congenital or acquired	Clustered bowel loops compressing the rectosigmoid dorsolaterally and the uterus ventrally	Mesenteric fat tissue and vessels penetrating the broad ligament

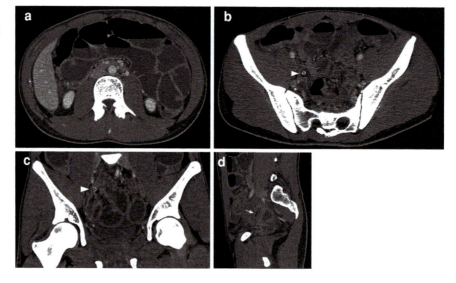

Fig. 21 SBO due to appendicitis. The upper axial slice (**a**) show a dilatation of the small bowel with a collapsed descending colon. The pelvic slice (**b**) and coronal (**c**), and sagittal (**d**) reconstructions show agglutination of the small bowel loops on an appendicitis (*arrow*) with an appendicolith (*arrowhead*)

aggravates the mechanical obstructive process and contributes to the development of mesenteric ischemia.
2. The second event is strangulation, which is defined as a closed loop obstruction associated with intestinal ischemia. The severity and duration of the intestinal and mesenteric obstructive process determines the severity of the ischemia. Initially, the venous return of blood from the involved bowel segment is compromised because intraluminal pressure exceeds venous pressure, with congestive changes affecting the bowel wall and the mesentery, while the influx of arterial blood continues. Ischemia may resolve with an emergent surgical

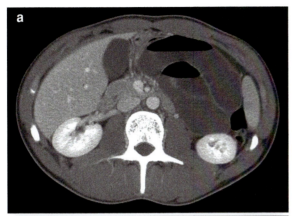

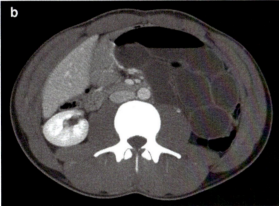

Fig. 22 Left-sided paraduodenal hernia shown on two axial slices (**a**, **b**)

treatment of the cause. Increasing distension also predisposes the closed loop to rotation about its mesentery. Then arterial insufficiency follows, aggravating the anoxia and further contributing to the rapid development of gangrene and perforation.

The clinical diagnosis of strangulation is difficult. Intestinal strangulation is suspected when the intermittent crampy pain becomes continuous and increases in severity, and in patients with tachycardia, fever, peritoneal irritation, and leukocytosis. However, these findings cannot reliably differentiate simple from strangulated obstruction, which means that before the development of CT, strangulation was not diagnosed preoperatively in about 75% of patients with surgically proved strangulation.

3.6.2 CT Findings

In strangulating SBO, the CT findings can be divided into two categories: findings indicative of closed loop obstruction and findings indicative of strangulation.

Closed loop obstruction. In closed loop obstruction, CT shows incarcerated small bowel with a radial distribution and stretched mesenteric vessels converging toward torsion (Fig. 23) and a U- or C-shaped dilated bowel loop and at the site of torsion, the presence of two adjacent collapsed, round, oval, or triangular loops, the beak sign appearing as a fusiform tapering when the bowel is imaged in longitudinal section. The whirl sign is a classic sign of closed loop obstruction. It appears as a twist of bowel wrapping around a single constrictive focus of mesentery with a spiral arrangement of mesenteric vessels (Khurana 2003).

Strangulation. CT shows bowel wall and mesentery abnormalities (Balthazar et al. 1997; Catel et al. 2003) (Table 5). Bowel wall findings are a circumferential thickening wall, increased attenuation, a target or a halo sign, or, on the contrary, a bowel wall thinning that corresponds to late mucosal desquamation, a pneumatosis, or a lack of enhancement of the wall of the incarcerated bowel after intravenous administration of contrast material (Figs. 23, 24). This last finding is the most specific finding of strangulation. The nonenhanced bowel wall is responsible for the disappearing loop sign, which refers to isodense bowel wall indistinguishable from adjacent mesenteric fluid. Before intravenous administration of contrast material, bowel wall hemorrhage with a spontaneously hyperdense wall (Fig. 25) is a good finding of ischemia, and needs a narrow window to be identified. Mesentery abnormalities include congestion, blurring, haziness, and obliteration of the mesenteric vessels and fluid or hemorrhage in the mesentery.

Theoretically, the CT appearance in strangulating obstruction depends on the stage of the strangulation. When the blood inflow is higher than venous outflow, the appearance of the bowel loop is that of a loop with impaired mesenteric venous drainage: bowel wall thickening with mesenteric engorgement and mesenteric edema, abnormal enhancement of the bowel wall is usually present with increased attenuation, a halo sign, or a target sign. At a more advanced stage of the disease, the arterial supply and the bowel wall may be thin and nonenhanced.

3.6.3 CT Pitfalls

The whirl sign, which indicates a rotation of the mesentery, is suggestive of a closed loop obstruction. However, this sign is not specific and may be present in patients with altered mesenteric anatomy due to

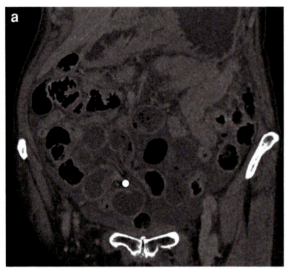
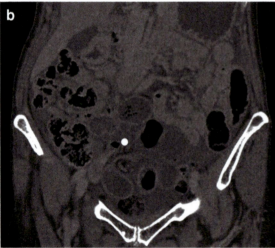
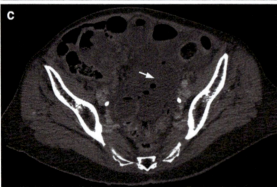

Fig. 23 Closed loop obstruction with several converging beak findings. Coronal views (**a**, **b**) show dilated bowel loops with several beak findings converging toward the same point (*right dot*). This is very suggestive of a closed loop obstruction. Note also the lack of enhancement of the bowel wall on the axial slice (**c**), suggestive of strangulation (*arrows*)

Table 5 CT features of ischemia in SBO

Bowel wall findings
  Without injection phase
    Increased attenuation
  Arterial phase
    Decreased or delayed wall enhancement
    Pneumatosis
    Wall thinning
  Venous phase
    Circumferential thickening
    Target or halo sign
Mesentery
  Blurring of mesenteric fat
  Interloop fluid
  Congestion of mesenteric vessels
Combined
  Disappearing loop sign

prior bowel surgery. In a large retrospective study at Memorial Sloan-Kettering, most CT scans in patients with small bowel volvulus had a whirl sign, but most whirl signs were not due to volvulus (Gollub et al. 2006). However, it must be known that in patients with bowel obstruction, the presence of a whirl sign has great value in predicting the need for surgery (Duda et al. 2008).

Among classic findings of bowel strangulation, it is well known that a thickening of the bowel wall, a target finding or a halo finding is not specific and may be present in infectious or inflammatory bowel disease. It has more recently been shown that a pneumatosis might be the consequence of the bowel distension in the lack of ischemia. The only finding specific to ischemia is the lack of enhancement of the bowel wall. It may be difficult to affirm if the bowel wall is thin, and above all if there is no fluid around the bowel wall permitting one to identify the disappearing loop sign. Contrary to common opinion, the arterial phase is not useful to evaluate the bowel wall enhancement, the portal phase is preferable, and in some cases, some residual enhancement of the bowel wall may be shown only on the delayed phase, but delayed enhancement of the bowel wall may be considered as a finding of ischemia, as may be a lack of enhancement.

Bowel Obstruction

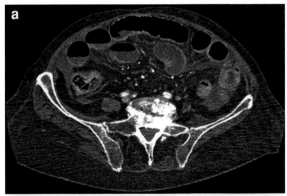
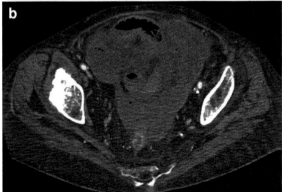
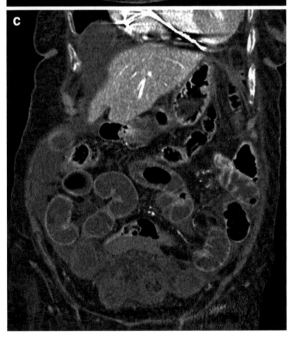

Fig. 24 Strangulating obstruction. The upper axial pelvic slice (**a**) shows dilated small bowel loops with normal wall enhancement. At a lower level (**b**), the wall of the dilated bowel loops is not identified because it is not enhanced and with the same density as the bowel content. Coronal reformatting (**c**) shows the upper enhanced and lower nonenhanced small bowel loops

3.6.4 CT Accuracy

Several studies have investigated the accuracy of CT for the diagnosis of bowel ischemia among patients with SBO. The reported accuracies of CT in these retrospective studies are good, with sensitivities reported from 76 to 100% and specificities ranging between 76 and 100% (Balthazar et al. 1997; Zalcman et al. 2000; Kim et al. 2004; Mallo et al. 2005). By contrast, a review of prospective interpretation in patients with suspected SBO found very poor performance for detecting ischemia, with only 14.8% sensitivity but a specificity of 94% (Sheedy et al. 2006). In our experience, discrepancies between CT and surgical findings are more due to CT false positives, with findings of ischemia not confirmed at surgery. We also found a lack of enhancement or a delayed enhancement of the bowel wall as a highly specific finding of bowel ischemia. However, the sensitivity ranges from 33 to 50% in the published experiences (Sheedy et al. 2006; Catel et al. 2003).

There is a main difficulty in the evaluation of CT in strangulating obstruction: the delay between CT and surgery, which hinders correlation between CT and surgical findings. Ischemia may have worsened between CT and surgery or, on the contrary, ischemic bowel wall may have been reperfused during this time. Furthermore, surgery is not an absolute gold standard since we have encountered patients with CT findings of strangulation, not confirmed by a first surgical investigation and recognized during a second surgical investigation, this latter investigation being performed because no improvement of the clinical status of the patient.

3.6.5 CT Impact

Despite these limitations, CT has a great impact on the diagnosis of strangulation. Clinical findings of strangulation are lacking in about 75% of cases in patients with strangulation, and a conservative attitude in patients with SBO is more and more recommended since in patients with adhesions unnecessary additional abdominal interventions represent a source for future occlusive episodes. Consequently, information regarding ischemic complications in patients with SBO is important for the surgeon in order to plan the correct time for a surgical therapy. Regression analysis of multiple clinical biological and CT preoperative criteria has demonstrated that

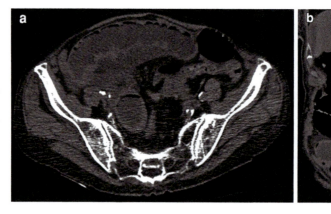

Fig. 25 Strangulating obstruction CT performed without intravenous administration of contrast material. On axial (a) as well as on coronal (b) reformatting the wall of a low and anterior bowel loop is spontaneously hyperdense. This is suggestive of strangulation

reduced wall enhancement on CT was the most significant factor of strangulation (Jancelewicz et al. 2009)

4 Large Bowel Obstruction

4.1 Diagnosis of Mechanical Obstruction

4.1.1 Clinical Considerations

The clinical diagnosis of LBO classically depends on four cardinal findings: abdominal pain, constipation or obstipation, abdominal distention, and vomiting if the ileocecal valve is incompetent. However, diagnosis can be difficult because clinical findings differ with the degree and level of bowel obstruction and with the vascular status of the obstructed segment. In typical mechanical obstruction, abdominal pain is crampy and gradually increases in intensity, only to abate and recur. With time, increasing bowel distention inhibits motility and the pain tends to subside. Furthermore, because most colonic obstructions are due to cancer, patients are often elderly and have symptoms related to the tumor location, with fewer acute symptoms than with SBO. However, crampy abdominal pain can occur with other causes of acute abdomen, such as renal colic. In the same way, vomiting or constipation is not specific to mechanical obstruction. As its name indicates, colonic pseudoobstruction is the main differential diagnosis of LBO. Colonic pseudoobstruction is a syndrome in which the clinical features resemble those of mechanical obstruction, that is, failure of motility associated with pain and abdominal distention, but there is no mechanical obstruction (De Giorgio and Knowles 2009). Abdominal plain film is the classic imaging modality used to confirm the diagnosis of LBO. However, in about one third of patients supposed to have mechanical obstruction on clinical examination, abdominal plain film shows no obstruction. Conversely, about 20% of patients suspected of having colonic pseudoobstruction have mechanical LBO.

4.1.2 CT Findings

The CT diagnosis of LBO is based on the presence of a dilated colon proximal to a transition zone and a collapsed distal colon. The large bowel is considered dilated when its diameter is more than 8 cm. However, a colon diameter larger than 10 cm may be present in colonic pseudoobstruction. Conversely, proximal colonic dilatation with gas, feces, or fluid, with an abrupt transition zone and a collapsed distal colon, is a reliable and convincing finding of LBO.

4.1.3 Pitfalls and Limitations

CT has limitations in the diagnosis of colonic obstruction, with false-negative and false-positive results.

False-negative CT diagnosis in LBO may be encountered in patients with partly obstructing carcinoma of the colon, with no significant proximal dilatation. CT interpretation in these cases requires proper colon cleaning and the use of air insufflation. An obstructive process at the ileocecal valve or the colonic flexure with residual fecal content in the distal colon may also lead to an erroneous diagnosis of ileus. Furthermore, despite an obstruction leading to LBO, distal colonic segments may be filled with gas.

False-positive diagnosis may be due to some pattern of ileus with dilatation of the small bowel and the ascending colon and a distal totally collapsed colon that should not lead to a diagnosis of colonic obstruction unless a colonic lesion is visualized at the transition zone. In fact, there is often a dilatation limited to the ascending and transverse colon in colonic pseudoobstruction. In a retrospective study including eight cases of colonic pseudoobstruction, the transition zone was located in six patients at the splenic flexure and in the other two patients in the midportion of the transverse and descending colon (Choi et al. 2008).

4.1.4 Accuracy

In contrast to SBO, which has been studied extensively, the value of CT in the diagnosis of LBO has been established in only two studies (Frager et al. 1998; Beattie et al. 2007): one study reported a sensitivity of 96% and a specificity of 93% and the other study reported a sensitivity and a specificity of 91%.

4.1.5 CT Impact

In all situations of suspected LBO, no matter how clear the diagnosis appears on plain radiography, another imaging test must be performed to differentiate mechanical obstruction from pseudoobstruction. Although contrast enema and CT are still the tests recommended, both tests having good sensitivity and specificity, CT has at least five advantages (Taourel et al. 2003): it is easier to perform; it is always diagnostic, in opposition to contrast enema, for which the patient may not retain the contrast material or may not tolerate insertion of the rectal tube; it is better for investigating the cause of the obstacle; it allows more accurate measurement of bowel diameter; and it is better for analyzing the viability of the colonic wall.

4.2 Diagnosis of the Site of the Obstruction

4.2.1 Clinical Considerations

The diagnosis of an LBO site is not done easily with only clinical data. Lesions at the ileocecal valve or ileocolic intussusception cause acute symptoms with vomiting, but lesions in the ascending colon cause more insidious manifestations because the lumen is wide and the contents are semiliquid. Left-sided lesions cause major abdominal distention with progressive constipation and ultimately obstipation. The determination of the LBO site due to cancer is important for the surgical procedure, particularly when laparoscopic surgery is scheduled.

4.2.2 CT Findings

It is generally easier to follow the course of the large bowel than that of the small bowel on CT slices, and CT is accurate in establishing the exact point of transition between the dilated and collapsed colon. Misinterpretations may be encountered between an obstructing terminal ileal lesion and a cecal lesion.

4.3 Diagnosis of the Cause of the Obstruction

4.3.1 Clinical Considerations

The main cause of LBO is constituted by malignant lesions (Fig. 26). In a study including 234 consecutive patients who underwent emergency surgery for colonic obstruction, colorectal cancer accounted for 82% of obstructions (Biondo et al. 2004). The second most common causes were extracolonic cancer and volvulus, each representing in the same study about 5% of causes. Rarer causes included diverticular disease, hernias, ischemic colitis, inflammatory mass, colonic tuberculosis, and colonic invagination.

The sigmoid colon constitutes the most common site of obstructive colon cancer because of its relatively narrow diameter and solid fecal contents. In the same way, nearly 20% of sigmoid cancers are complicated by some degree of obstruction.

Volvulus represents the second most common cause of LBO. Colonic volvulus requires a segment of redundant mobile colon and relatively fixed points around which the volvulus can occur. As a consequence, the sigmoid colon (70%), the cecum (25%), and the transverse colon (5%) are the most common sites of volvulus. Other contributing factors are distention of the colon by feces or gas, increased muscular activity, and changes in the intraperitoneal relationship as seen in pregnancy (sigmoid volvulus is the first cause of obstruction in pregnant woman) or parturition, previous abdominal surgery resulting in adhesions, congenital abnormalities such as malrotation, and acquired obstructive lesions in the distal colon. The diagnosis of colon volvulus is often

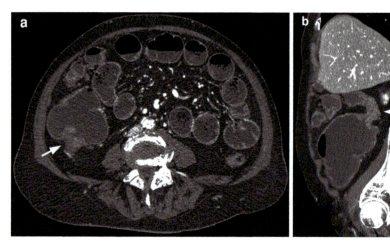

Fig. 26 Large bowel obstruction (LBO) due to ascending colon cancer. The axial slice (**a**) shows dilated small bowel loops and cecum with a short thickening of the wall of the ascending colon (*arrow*). Sagittal reformatting (**b**) shows clearly the relationship between the proximal dilated colon, the tumor (*arrow*), and the distal collapsed colon

evident on abdominal plain film. This shows a greatly distended paralyzed loop with fluid–fluid levels, mainly on the left side, extending toward the diaphragm with a "northern exposure sign", meaning that the sigmoid colon extends cranially beyond the level of the transverse colon, and a "coffee bean sign", referring to the coffee-bean-like shape that the dilated sigmoid colon may assume in a sigmoid volvulus. In the cecum volvulus, a distended cecum is typically positioned in the left upper quadrant; however, in nearly half of cases of cecal volvulus, the cecum twists in the axial plane, rotating around its long axis and appears in the right lower quadrant.

Diverticulitis is a classic but relatively rare cause of LBO. Several mechanisms may lead to an obstruction in patients with diverticulitis: adherence of small bowel loops to an inflammatory focus, a pelvic colon angulated by adhesions, pericolic fibrosis, or compression by intramural or extramural abscesses. In our experience, bowel obstruction consecutive to diverticulitis is more often SBO by agglutination of the bowel loops (Kim et al. 1998), and LBO due to colitis is mainly due to ischemic colitis.

4.3.2 CT Findings

CT may diagnose intraluminal, intrinsic, and extrinsic causes of bowel obstruction.

Intraluminal causes of colonic obstruction are often in the sigmoid colon, which is the narrowest portion of the colon. The most frequent cause is fecal impaction, which is a rather common cause of LBO in elderly and inactive patients. Other intraluminal objects that may cause LBO include gallstones (mostly in elderly women), foreign bodies in mentally ill or disturbed patients, medications such as antacid containing nonabsorbable aluminum hydroxide antacid gel given to prevent hyperphosphatemia, and bezoars, which usually do not affect the colon unless there is a stricture. Intussusception may be considered as an intraluminal cause of LBO because it occludes the lumen of the colon by pushing an ileal loop or the proximal colon and part of its mesentery into the lumen of the colon distal to it, even if various extrinsic or intrinsic processes may result in intussusception. The typical CT features of ileocolic or colocolic intussusception include a distended bowel loop (the intussuscipiens) with a thickened wall, an eccentrically positioned intraluminal intussusceptum, and a crescentic area of fat density representing invaginated fat from the mesentery of the intussusceptum. CT can also demonstrate the cause of intussusception by showing the leading mass and suggesting its nature by its density: fat-containing lipoma, cystic mass from a mucocele, or solid tumor. In contrast to ileoileal intussusception, colocolic intussusceptions are more usually due to large bowel tumor (Wang et al. 2009) (Fig. 27).

Intrinsic causes include tumor, diverticulitis, inflammatory disease, and ischemic colitis. In colon cancer, CT shows an asymmetric and short thickening of the colon wall (Fig. 28) or an enhanced soft tissue mass. The dilatation of the colon proximal to the tumor makes the identification and the analysis of the

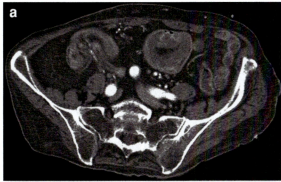
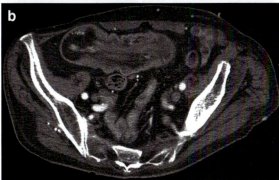
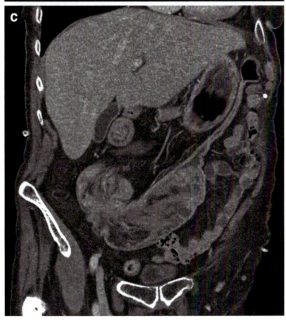

Fig. 27 Colocolic intussusception due to colon cancer. Axial slices (**a**, **b**) and coronal reformatting (**c**) show the intussuscipiens and the intracolic intussusception. Note the presence of several enhanced vessels in the mesentery which are adjacent to the intussuscepted colon. The tumoral lead point is difficult to distinguish from the intussuscepted bowel

tumor easier. Three-dimensional reconstruction images can demonstrate the transition point between the dilated and collapsed colon in problem cases (Filippone et al. 2007). In diverticulitis, thickening of the bowel wall is symmetric, more moderate, and extended on a longer segment. Moreover, pericolic changes are more important with fat stranding and, in some cases, phlegmon or intramural or extramural abscesses. In typhilitis, which occurs in neutropenic patients undergoing chemotherapy for acute leukemia, CT demonstrates cecal distention and circumferential thickening of the cecal wall. Crohn disease and ulcerative colitis are rarely the cause of LBO. The location of the involved segment and the extent and appearance of wall thickening may help distinguish these entities. In ischemic colitis, CT typically demonstrates circumferential, symmetric wall thickening (Fig. 29), often with a double-halo sign or a target sign. Pericolic fat stranding is present in 60% of patients with ischemic colitis (Balthazar et al. 1999). CT is helpful in distinguishing tumoral from ischemic segments in patients with ischemic colitis proximal to colonic carcinoma. The tumoral segment has an irregular thickening and heterogeneous enhancement by contrast material, with the ischemic segment generally smoothly thickened and homogeneously enhanced. Radiation colitis is a form of ischemic colitis, and the stricture is generally responsible for the obstruction. The sigmoid colon and the rectum are affected most frequently because radiation therapy is used for pelvic disease.

Extrinsic causes include volvulus, hernias, adhesions, and compression by diseases from adjacent organs.

Cecal volvulus results from an abnormal mobility of the cecum because of congenital improper fusion of the cecal mesentery with the posterior parietal peritoneum. The CT appearance depends on the pathophysiological mechanism of the volvulus (Delabrousse et al. 2007). Three types of cecal volvulus are defined: the axial torsion type, the loop type, and the bascule type (Fig. 30).

1. In the axial torsion type (Fig. 31), the cecum rotates along its long axis and twists in the axial plane. The distended cecum is located in the right side of the lower abdomen. The whirl sign composed of

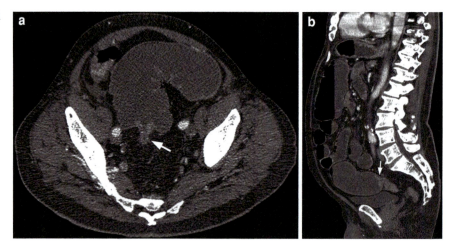

Fig. 28 LBO due to sigmoid colon cancer. The axial slice (a) and sagittal reformatting (b) show the sigmoid carcinoma (*arrow*) responsible for LBO

spiraled vessels and loops of collapsed cecum is well seen and distal ileum is present in a clockwise appearance.
2. In the loop type, the distended cecum both twists and inverts. The distended cecum is located in the left upper quadrant. The whirl sign is well seen. A counterclockwise appearance is present.
3. In the bascule type, the distended cecum folds anteriorly without any torsion. The distended cecum is located in the central abdomen and the whirl sign is absent.

Three-dimensional imaging may allow selection of the optimal plane for viewing the volvulus and localizing the precise source of torsion (Moore et al. 2001).

The transverse colon is the rarest site of colonic volvulus, but it is associated with the highest mortality. Transverse colon volvulus occurs in the setting of abnormal fixation of a long transverse colon. CT shows a beaklike narrowing of the transverse colon at the volvulus site and an adjacent whirl sign.

The sigmoid colon is the most common site of colonic volvulus. CT shows a whirl pattern of the collapsed colon, twisted mesentery, and enhanced engorged vessels, with a bird beak aspect of the afferent and efferent segments (Catalano 1996), constituting a closed loop obstruction. This represents the classic form of sigmoid volvulus (Figs. 32, 33). A new form of sigmoid volvulus has been described recently (Levsky et al. 2010): the organoaxial volvulus, for which the sigmoid colon rotates along its long axis with only one point of beak finding, the proximal colon running at a distance from the site of volvulus.

LBO secondary to hernias or adhesions is much less common than SBO because of the relatively fixed nature of the colon and its larger caliber. Extrinsic compression may be caused by endometriosis, which involves the rectum and the distal sigmoid colon, with thickening that may simulate a colon cancer on CT; actinomycosis, which must be considered in a woman with prolonged use of an intrauterine device (Yeguez et al. 2000); pancreatitis, or more often, involvement due to extracolonic neoplasm either directly or by serosal metastasis. The rectum or the sigmoid may be obstructed by direct invasion from gynecologic and prostatic neoplasms and by drop metastases to the pouch of Douglas. Pelvic lipomatosis, benign pelvic masses, retroperitoneal fibrosis, and pregnancy can compress the colon but rarely lead to LBO.

4.3.3 Pitfalls and Limitations

False-positive pictures of narrowing in the colon may be encountered when the colon is collapsed. In these cases, supplementary scanning in the left-side-up position if the descending colon is suspicious, or in the right-side-up position if the ascending colon is suspicious, shifts colonic air and opens up the suspicious segment, ruling out true obstruction (Beattie et al. 2007).

False-positive diagnosis of rectal lesion may be encountered in patients with circumferential thickening of the rectal wall. In these cases, air insufflation

Bowel Obstruction

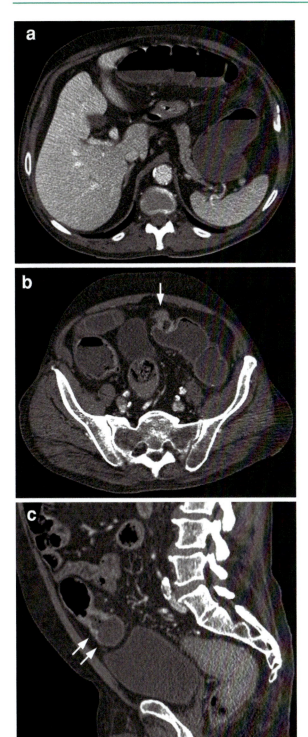

Fig. 29 LBO due to ischemic colitis. Axial slices (**a**, **b**) show a colonic dilatation due to a short stenosis with a symmetric thickening of the sigmoid wall (*arrow*). Sagittal reformatting (**c**) shows distal colon which is not entirely collapsed (*double arrows*). The CT diagnosis was LBO due to cancer with the diagnosis of ischemic colitis revealed by surgery and pathologic analysis

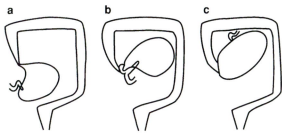

Fig. 30 Subtypes of cecal volvulus: organoaxial volvulus (**a**), loop type volvulus (**b**), and cecal bascule type (**c**)

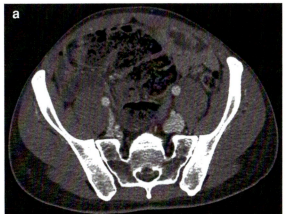

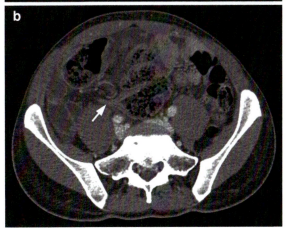

Fig. 31 Cecal volvulus of the axial torsion type. Axial slices (**a**, **b**) show a distended cecum medially located with a beak finding well seen in **b** (*arrow*). Note also the whirl sign shown in **b**. The cecum has not moved in the left upper quadrant but is medially located because of the lack of posterior mesocecum, which favors motility

with rectal distention can make the thickening disappear.

False-negative diagnoses may be encountered in partial colonic obstruction, where there is no proximal dilatation to delineate the obstructing lesion and

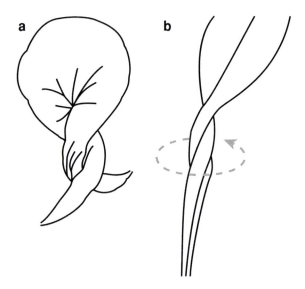

Fig. 32 Subtypes of sigmoid volvulus. Classic form of volvulus with two loops obstruction (**a**) and organoaxial volvulus (**b**)

particularly when the lesion is located at the splenic flexure; in these cases, CT images are much more difficult to interpret without proper colon cleaning and air insufflation.

Colon volvulus may be difficult to diagnose on CT. Visualization of the beak sign requires thin slices and should be in the axial plane. This underlines the potential usefulness of three-dimensional imaging.

Some causes of colonic obstruction may be difficult to characterize, such as radiation colitis and endometriosis. For this latter cause, the diagnosis must be considered in a woman of childbearing age who has a rectal or sigmoid obstructing tumor and normal endoscopy findings (Thomassin et al. 2004) (Fig. 34).

The appearance of colon cancer may mimic diverticulitis, especially if tumor involvement of the wall has resulted in infiltration of the pericolic fat. As demonstrated by Padidar et al. (1994), fluid in the root of the sigmoid mesentery and engorgement of the adjacent sigmoid mesenteric vasculature favor the diagnosis of diverticulitis. However, pericolic lymph nodes in patients with suspected diverticulitis should raise the suspicion of colon cancer (Chintapalli et al. 1999). In some cases, it may be impossible to distinguish diverticulitis from perforated carcinoma. Otherwise, differential diagnosis between ischemic colitis and colon cancer may be problematic.

Classically, ischemic involvement is greater with concentrically and smoothly thickened wall. However, ischemic thickening responsible for obstruction may be short and important.

Different causes of colonic obstruction may be associated, for instance, fecal impaction in the rectum or an obstructing tumor may lead to a colonic ischemia that can worsen the obstruction. Distinguishing tumoral from ischemic segments in patients who have ischemic colitis proximal to colonic carcinoma is important to obtain a true evaluation of the length of the tumoral segment and to adapt the surgical procedure. Before identifying a foreign body as the cause of a LBO, one must carefully look for a tumor responsible for the blockage of the foreign body (Fig. 35).

4.3.4 Accuracy

In the only two studies (Frager et al. 1998; Beattie et al. 2007) focused on CT findings of LBO, a correct preoperative pathologic diagnosis was established by CT in, respectively, 89% of patients (40 of 45) and 70% of patients (14 of 20) in whom obstruction was diagnosed by CT.

4.3.5 CT Impact

One of the advantages of CT in comparison with contrast enema classically considered as the gold standard imaging method in LBO is it can better analyze the characteristic of the thickening bowel wall responsible for a stenosis and differentiate tumor from other intrinsic stenoses. Furthermore right-sided colonic obstructions are difficult to characterize and in cases of cecal volvulus of the axial torsion type because the cecum is normally located, abdominal plain film and contrast enema may fail to identify the cause of the obstruction.

Consequently, CT is becoming the reference examination in the assessment of LBO.

4.4 Diagnosis of Complications of the Obstruction

4.4.1 Clinical Considerations

Traditionally, the diagnosis of bowel obstruction has been performed by clinical examination and abdominal plain film, the key point being to differentiate mechanical obstruction from ileus. Bowel obstruction was treated emergently by surgery, whereas ileus was

Bowel Obstruction

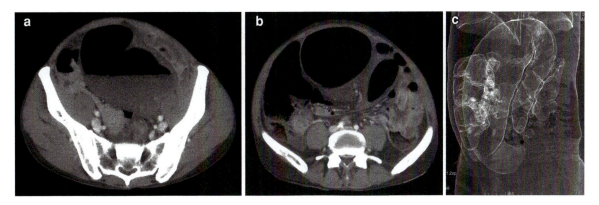

Fig. 33 Sigmoid volvulus with two loops obstruction. Axial slices (**a**, **b**) show the two distended loops with an inverted-U pattern. Three-dimensional volume rendering (**c**) shows clearly the mechanism of the volvulus with the two distended loops converging toward the same point (*star*)

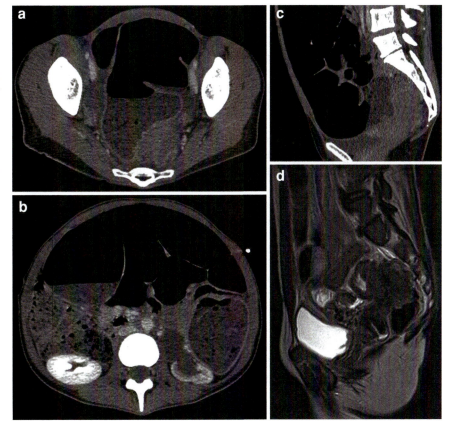

Fig. 34 LBO due to pericolic endometriosis in a woman of childbearing age. Axial slices (**a**, **b**) show an enhanced mass located at the junction between the sigmoid and the rectum responsible for an LBO. On sagittal CT reformatting (**c**) and the sagittal T2-weighted MRI slice (**d**), the relationship between the mass, in hyposignal T2, and the colon is clearly seen. A colostomy was performed in an emergency and revealed that the colon was compressed by the mass, with pathologic analysis of the mass diagnosing endometriosis

managed medically. However, in patients with bowel obstruction, management should depend on the site, cause, and viability of the bowel. The main complication of an LBO is peritonitis due to perforation. Indeed, progression of LBO, particularly in the presence of a competent ileocecal valve, may result in cecal perforation with fecal peritonitis. Some rules are generally followed for the treatment of patients with LBO:

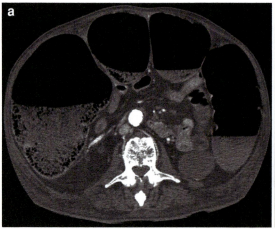
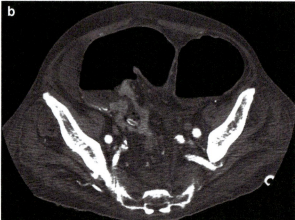

Fig. 35 LBO due to sigmoid cancer with an intraluminal foreign body. The upper axial slice (**a**) shows a distended colon and the lower slice (**b**) shows an irregular thickening of the sigmoid wall suggestive of colon cancer. Note the presence of a foreign body at the site of the obstruction

- Bowel obstruction with perforation or ischemia requires emergent surgery.
- Sigmoid volvulus is treated initially by endoscopic detorsion unless it is complicated by peritonitis, which requires surgery.
- Ideally obstruction due to colon cancer is first medically managed to prepare the colon for surgery, with resection of the tumor and anastomisis in one stage.

These rules underscore the importance of diagnosing the potential complications of LBO.

4.4.2 CT Findings

In LBO due to cancer, pneumatosis affecting the proximal colon wall suggests an infarction. In the same way, dilatation of the cecum, proximal to an obstructing colon cancer, to 12-cm diameter is a risk factor for diastatic perforation. The perforation may arise from the tumor itself or from the distended cecum above the tumor. In the former instance, free pneumoperitoneum is rare; more often, small air bubbles with fluid and mesenteric stranding are detected in the pericolic fat. In the case of perforation from the distended cecum above the tumor, pneumoperitoneum is abundant (Fig. 36).

In colonic volvulus, CT findings of ischemia are sought in the colonic wall and the mesocolon. Bowel wall abnormalities include circumferential thickening, increased attenuation, target or halo sign, and extreme lack of mural enhancement of the incarcerated bowel after intravenous administration of contrast material. Mesocolonic abnormalities include congestion, blurring, haziness, obliteration of the mesocolic vessels, and fluid or hemorrhage in the mesocolon. This may be crucial for the therapeutic choice between sigmoidoscopic decompression with insertion of a rectal tube in patients without findings of infarct or perforation and emergent sigmoid resection for other patients. However, the usefulness of CT in differentiating between sigmoid volvulus with and without infarction has not been evaluated.

4.4.3 CT Pitfalls

Although being a classic sign of ischemia, cecal pneumatosis in dilated cecum proximal to bowel cancer may be the consequence of the dilatation without any finding of ischemia (Taourel et al. 2004). Otherwise, the assessment of the wall enhancement of the sigmoid colon is very difficult because of the spontaneous contrast between colonic wall and air which fills the colonic lumen. Therefore, in clinical practice the therapeutic choice in sigmoid volvulus between endoscopic aspiration and surgery relies on clinical data.

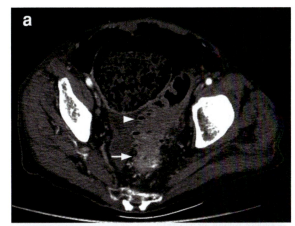
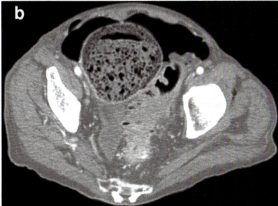
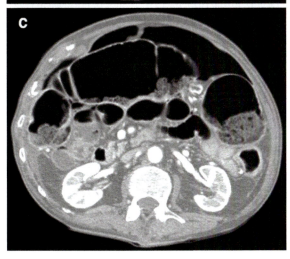

Fig. 36 Diastatic cecal perforation consecutive to LBO due to sigmoid cancer in a patient with diverticulosis. The axial slice (**a**) shows a thickening of the sigmoid wall more pronounced and more enhanced in its lower part; the lower thickened wall corresponded to cancer (*arrow*), whereas the upper wall corresponded to diverticulosis (*arrowhead*). On the slices with lung window (**b**, **c**), a pneumoperitoneum and a huge amount of stool outside the colon (**b**) are clearly seen, consequences of bowel perforation

5 Diagnostic Strategy

In patients with suspected intestinal obstruction, the primary diagnostic triage is based on clinical, laboratory, and abdominal plain film findings, which allow the schematic individualization in the following four situations:

1. There is a strong suspicion of paralytic ileus. The cause must be investigated by clinical and laboratory examinations and in some cases by ultrasonography or CT.
2. There is a strong suspicion of SBO. If there are findings of strangulation or the cause of the SBO is obvious and needs emergent surgical management, surgery must be performed without other investigations. In other patients with acute symptoms, CT helps in the search for the mechanism and cause. In patients with nonacute symptoms (suspicion of low-grade obstruction), CT with enteroclysis is a good alternative to CT.
3. There is a strong suspicion of LBO. If abdominal plain film shows signs of volvulus, which is more common in the sigmoid colon than in the cecum, treatment of the volvulus must be performed (colonoscopic or surgical detorsion in sigmoid volvulus and surgery in cecal volvulus). The benefit of CT for therapeutic choice in sigmoid volvulus remains to be evaluated. If there is no finding of volvulus, stenosis is the presumed cause of LBO. In complicated diverticulitis, CT is considered the method of choice in its diagnosis and for staging complications. Contrast enema traditionally is the recommended radiologic examination for evaluating patients with suspected obstructing colonic carcinoma. However, the findings may be incomplete because the patient cannot retain the contrast material or tolerate the rectal tube and may be inconclusive in right-sided colonic obstruction. In addition, it is associated with an increased risk of barium inspissation and may necessitate a delay before surgery to adequately clean the colon. CT examination is widely accepted as faster and simpler to perform and interpret and gentler on the patient. CT has the advantages of diagnosing the tumor, evaluating its local and metastatic spread, and searching for synchronous cancer of the colon, which is found in nearly 10% of patients

References

Armstrong O, Hamel A, Grignon B et al (2007) Internal hernias: anatomical basis and clinical relevance. Surg Radiol Anat 29:333–337

Atri M, McGregor C, McInnes M et al (2009) Multidetector helical CT in the evaluation of acute small bowel obstruction: comparison of non-enhanced (no oral, rectal or IV contrast) and IV enhanced CT. Eur J Radiol 71:135–140

Aufort S, Charra L, Lesnik A, Bruel JM, Taourel P (2005) Multidetector CT of bowel obstruction: value of post-processing. Eur Radiol 15:2323–2329

Balthazar EJ, George W (1994) Holmes lecture CT of small-bowell obstruction. AJR Am J Roentgenol 162:255–261

Balthazar EJ, Birnbaum BA, Megibow AJ et al (1992) Closed-loop and strangulating intestinal obstruction: CT signs. Radiology 185:769–775

Balthazar EJ, Liebeskind ME, Macari M (1997) Intestinal ischemia in patients in whom small bowel obstruction is suspected: evaluation of accuracy limitations, and clinical implications of CT in diagnosis. Radiology 205:519–522

Balthazar EJ, Yen BC, Gordon RB (1999) Ischemic colitis: CT evaluation of 54 cases. Radiology 211:381–388

Ba-Salamah A, Prokop M, Uffmann M et al (2003) Dedicated multidetector CT of the stomach: spectrum of diseases. Radiographics 23:625–644

Beattie GC, Peters RT, Guy S, Mendelson RM (2007) Computed tomography in the assessment of suspected large bowel obstruction. ANZ J Surg 77:160–165

Behrman SW (2005) Management of complicated peptic ulcer disease. Arch Surg 140:201–208

Biondo S, Pares D, Frago R et al (2004) Large bowel obstruction: predictive factors for post-operative mortality. Dis Colon Rectum 47:1889–1897

Blachar A, Federle MP, Dodson SF (2001) Internal hernia: clinical and imaging findings in 17 patients with emphasis on CT criteria. Radiology 218:68–74

Brennan GB, Rosenberg RD, Arora S (2004) Bouveret syndrome. Radiographics 24:1171–1175

Buyn JH, Ha HK, Kim AY et al (2003) CT findings in peripheral T-cell lymphoma involving the gastrointestinal tract. Radiology 227:59–67

Catalano O (1996) Computed tomographic appearance of sigmoid volvulus. Abdom Imaging 21:314–317

Catel L, Lefèvre F, Lauren V et al (2003) Small bowel obstruction from adhesions: which CT severity criteria to research? J Radiol 84:27–31

Chandler RC, Srinivas G, Chintapalli KN, Schwesinger WH, Prasad SR (2008) Imaging in bariatric surgery: a guide to postsurgical anatomy and common complications. AJR Am J Roentgenol 190:122–135

Chintapalli KN, Chopra S, Ghiatas AA et al (1999) Diverticulitis versus colon cancer: differentiation with helical CT findings. Radiology 210:429–435

Choi JS, Lim JS, Kim H et al (2008) Colonic pseudoobstruction: CT findings. AJR Am J Roentgenol 190:1521–1526

de Dombal FT (1994) Acute abdominal pain in the elderly. J Clin Gastroenterol 19:331–335

De Giorgio R, Knowles CH (2009) Acute colonic pseudo-obstruction. Br J Surg 96:229–239

Delabrousse E, Michalakis D, Sarliève P et al (2005) Value of the public tubercle as a CT reference point in groin hernias. J Radiol 86:651–654

Delabrousse E, Sarliève P, Sailley N et al (2007) Cecal volvulus: CT findings and correlation with pathophysiology. Emerg Radiol 14:411–415

Delabrousse E, Lubrano J, Sailley N et al (2008) Small-bowel bezoar versus small-bowel feces: CT evaluation. AJR Am J Roentgenol 191:1465–1468

Delabrousse E, Lubrano J, Jehl J et al (2009) Small-bowel obstruction from adhesive bands and matted adhesions: CT differentiation. AJR Am J Roentgenol 192:693–697

Duda JB, Bhatt S, Dogra VS (2008) Utility of CT whirl sign in guiding management of small-bowel obstruction. AJR Am J Roentgenol 191:743–747

Erzurumlu K, Malazgirt Z, Bektas A et al (2005) Gastrointestinal bezoars: a retrospective analysis of 34 cases. World J Gastroenterol 11:1813–1817

Filippone A, Cianci R, Storto ML (2007) Bowel obstruction: comparison between multidetector-row CT axial and coronal planes. Abdom Imaging 32:310–316

Frager D, Rovno HDS, Baer JW, Bashist B, Friedman M (1998) Prospective evaluation of colonic obstruction with computed tomography. Abdom Imaging 23:141–146

Franco LM, Dryden NJ (2007) Gastric-outlet obstruction. N Engl J Med 356:942

Furukama A, Yamasaky M, Furuichi K et al (2001) Helical CT in the diagnosis of small bowel obstruction. Radiographics 21:341–355

Gan S, Roy-Choudhury S, Agrawal S et al (2008) More than meets the eye: subtle but important CT findings in Bouveret's syndrome. AJR Am J Roentgenol 191:182–185

Gayer G, Apter S, Hofmann C et al (1998) Intussusception in adults: CT diagnosis. Clin Radiol 53:53–57

Gollub M, Yoon S, Smith L, Moskowitz C (2006) Does the CT whirl sign really predict small bowel volvulus?: experience in an oncologic population. J Comput Assist Tomogr 30:25–32

Ha HK, Park CH, Kim SK et al (1993) CT analysis of intestinal obstruction due to adhesions: early detection of strangulation. J Comput Assist Tomogr 17:386–389

Ha KH, Shin BS, Lee SI et al (1998) Usefulness of CT in patients with intestinal obstruction who have undergone abdominal surgery for malignancy. AJR Am J Roentgenol 171:1587–1593

Harlow CL, Stears RL, Zeligman BE, Archer PG (1993) Diagnosis of bowel obstruction on plain abdominal radiographs: significance of air-fluid levels at different heights in the same loop of bowel. AJR Am J Roentgenol 161:291–295

Herlinger H, Maglinte DDT (1989) Small bowel obstruction. In: Herlinger H, Maglinte DDT (eds) Clinical radiology of the small bowel. Saunders, Philadelphia, pp 479–509

Herlinger H, Rubesin SE (1994) Obstruction. In: Gore RM, Levine MS, Laufer I (eds) Textbook of gastrointestinal radiology. Saunders, Philadelphia, pp 931–966

Hodel J, Zins M, Desmottes L et al (2009) Location of the transition zone in CT of small-bowel obstruction: added value of multiplanar reformations. Abdom Imaging 34:35–41

Horton KM, Fishman EK (2008) MDCT and 3D imaging in transient enteroenteric intussusception: clinical observations and review of the literature. AJR Am J Roentgenol 191:736–742

Huang BY, Warshauer DM (2003) Adult intussusception: diagnosis and clinical relevance. Radiol Clin North Am 41:1137–1151

Hwang JY, Lee JK, Lee JE et al (2009) Value of multidetector CT in decision making regarding surgery in patients with small-bowel obstruction due to adhesion. Eur Radiol 19:2425–2431

Jancelewicz T, Vu LT, Shawo AE (2009) Predicting strangulated small bowel obstruction: an old problem revisited. J Gastrointest Surg 13:93–99

Khurana B (2003) The whirl sign. Radiology 226:69–70

Khurana B, Ledbetter S, McTavish J, Wiesner W, Ros PR (2002) Bowel obstruction revealed by multidetector CT. AJR Am J Roentgenol 178:1139–1144

Kim AY, Bennet GL, Bashist B, Perlman B, Megibow AJ (1998) Small-bowel obstruction associated with sigmoid diverticulitis: CT evaluation in 16 patients. AJR Am J Roentgenol 170:1311–1313

Kim JH, Ha HK, Kim JK et al (2004) Usefulness of known computed tomography and clinical criteria for diagnosing strangulation in small-bowel obstruction: analysis of true and false interpretation groups in computed tomography. World J Surg 28:63–68

Lazarus DE, Slywotsky C, Bennett GL, Megibow AJ, Macari M (2004) Frequency and relevance of the "small-bowel feces" signs on CT in patients with small-bowel obstruction. AJR Am J Roentgenol 183:1361–1366

Levsky JM, Den EI, DuBrow RA, Wolf EL, Rozenblit AM (2010) CT findings of sigmoid volvulus. Am J Roentgenol 194:136–143

Mallo RD, Salem L, Lalani T et al (2005) Computed tomography diagnosis of ischemia and complete obstruction in small bowel obstruction: a systematic review. J Gastrointest Surg 9:690–694

Marinis A, Yiallourou A, Samanides L et al (2009) Intussusception of the bowel in adults: a review. World J Gastroenterol 28(15):407–411

Martin LC, Merkle EM, Thompson WM (2006) Review of internal hernias: radiographic and clinical findings. AJR Am J Roentgenol 186:703–717

Mondor H, Porcher P, Olivier C (1943) Radiodiagnostics urgents: abdomen. Masson, Paris, p 340

Moore CJ, Corl FM, Fishman EK (2001) CT of cecal volvulus: unraveling the image. AJR Am J Roentgenol 177:95–98

Padidar AM, Jeffrey RB Jr, Mindelzun RE, Dolph JF (1994) Differentiating sigmoid diverticulitis from carcinoma on CT scans: mesenteric inflammation suggests diverticulitis. AJR Am J Roentgenol 163:81–83

Park KB, Do YS, Kang WK et al (2001) Malignant obstruction of gastric outlet and duodenum: palliation with flexible covered metallic stents. Radiology 219:679–683

Peterson CM, Anderson JS, Hara AK et al (2009) Volvulus of the gastrointestinal tract: appearances at multimodality imaging. Radiographics 29:1281–1293

Petrovic B, Nikalaidis P, Hammond NA, Grant TH, Miller F (2006) Identification of adhesions on CT in small bowel obstruction. Emerg Radiol 12:88–93

Rabeneck L (1995) AIDS associated intussusception in young adults. J Clin Gastroenterol 21:158–162

Sandhu PS, Joe BN, Coakley FV et al (2007) Bowel transition points: multiplicity and posterior location at CT are associated with small-bowel volvulus. Radiology 245:160–167

Sandrasegaran K, Rajesh A, Rushing DA et al (2005) Gastrointestinal stromal tumors: CT and MRI findings. Eur Radiol 15:1407–1414

Sandrasegaran K, Patel A, Fogel EL, Zyromski NJ, Pitt HA (2009) Annular pancreas in adults. AJR Am J Roentgenol 193:455–460

Sheedy SP, Earnest F 4th, Fletcher JG et al (2006) CT of small-bowel ischemia associated with obstruction in emergency department patients: diagnostic performance evaluation. Radiology 241:729–736

Sheikh RA, Prindiville TP, Pecha RE, Ruebner BH (2009) Unusual presentations of eosinophilic gastroenteritis: case series and review of literature. World J Gastroenterol 15:2156–2161

Shrake PD, Res DK, Lappas JC et al (1991) Radiographic evaluation of suspected small-bowel obstruction. Am J Gastroenterol 86:175–178

Silva AC, Pimenta M, Guimarães LS (2009) Small bowel obstruction: what to look for. Radiographics 29:423–439

Spencer JA, Crosse BA, Mannion RA et al (2000) Gastroduodenal obstruction from ovarian cancer: imaging features and clinical outcome. Clin Radiol 55:264–272

Stabile Ianora AA, Midiri M, Vinci R, Rotondo A, Angelelli G (2000) Abdominal wall hernias: imaging with spiral CT. Eur Radiol 10:914–919

Takeyama N, Gokan T, Ohgiya Y et al (2005) CT of internal hernias. Radiographics 25:997–1015

Tang E, Davis J, Silberman H (1995) Bowel obstruction in cancer patients. Arch Surg 130:832–837

Taourel P, Kessler N, Lesnik A et al (2003) Helical CT of large bowel obstruction. Abdom Imaging 28:267–275

Taourel P, Garibaldi F, Arrigoni J et al (2004) Cecal pneumatosis in patients with obstructive colon cancer: correlation of CT findings with bowel viability. AJR Am J Roentgenol 183:1667–1671

Thomassin I, Bazot M, Detchev R et al (2004) Symptoms before and after surgical removal of colorectal endometriosis that are assessed by magnetic resonance imaging and rectal endoscopic sonography. Am J Obstet Gynecol 190:1264–1271

Tombak MC, Apaydin FD, Colak T et al (2010) An unusual cause of intestinal obstruction: abdominal cocoon. AJR Am J Roentgenol 194:176–178

Tresoldi S, Kim YH, Blake M et al (2008) Adult intestinal intussusception: can abdominal MDCT distinguish an intussusception caused by a lead point? Abdom Imaging 33:582–588

Unal B, Aktaş A, Kemal G et al (2005) Superior mesenteric artery syndrome: CT and ultrasonography findings. Diagn Interv Radiol 11:90–95

Valls C, Andia E, Sanchez A et al (2002) Dual-phase helical CT of pancréatic adenocarcinoma: assessment of resectability before surgery. AJR Am J Roentgenol 178:821–826

Wang N, Cui XY, Liu Y et al (2009) Adult intussusception: a retrospective review of 41 cases. World J Gastroenterol 15:3303–3308

Warshauer DM, Lee JK (1999) Adult intussusception detected at CT or MR imaging: clinical-imaging correlation. Radiology 212:853–860

Warshauer DM, Mauro MA (1992) CT diagnosis of paraduodenal hernia. Gastrointest Radiol 17:13–15

Yeguez JF, Martinez SA, Sands LR, Hellinger MD (2000) Pelvic actino-mycosis presenting as malignant large bowel obstruction: a case report and a review of the literature. Am Surg 66:85–90

Zalcman M, Sy M, Donckier V, Closset J, Van Gansbeke D (2000) Helical CT signs in the diagnosis of intestinal ischemia in small-bowel obstruction. AJR Am J Roentgenol 175:1601–1607

Bowel Perforations

Patrice Taourel, Joseph Pujol, and Emma Pages-Bouic

Contents

1	**Introduction**	309
2	**Pathology**	310
2.1	Definition of a Bowel Perforation	310
2.2	Causes of GI Tract Perforations	310
3	**Clinical Findings**	314
3.1	Peritoneal Syndrome	314
3.2	Clinical Presentation According to the Cause	315
4	**CT Findings**	315
4.1	Direct Findings	315
4.2	Indirect Findings	315
4.3	CT Findings According to the Cause	316
5	**CT Pitfalls**	319
6	**CT Accuracy**	320
7	**CT Impact**	323
8	**Diagnosis Strategy**	325
8.1	No Orientation Element in the Anamnesis	325
8.2	Diagnosis Oriented by Anamnestic Context	325
8.3	Postoperative or Postendoscopy Situations	325
References		326

P. Taourel (✉) · J. Pujol · E. Pages-Bouic
Département of Imaging, Hôpital Lapeyronie,
371, avenue du Doyen Gaston Giraud,
34295 Montpellier Cedex 5, France
e-mail: p-taourel@chu-montpellier.fr

Abstract

Gastrointestinal tract perforation is an emergent condition that requires prompt surgery. Diagnosis largely depends on imaging examinations, and correct diagnosis of the presence, level, and cause of perforation is essential for appropriate management and surgical planning. Although plain radiography classically remains the first imaging modality, the high clinical efficacy of computed tomographic examination in this field has been well recognized. CT semiology is based on direct findings, including the identification of the bowel wall interruption, and indirect findings, including a pneumoperitoneum, a peridigestive infiltration, and a bowel wall thickening. These findings have different patterns according to the cause and the site of the bowel perforation. This chapter deals with the CT findings, CT pitfalls, and CT impact in the diagnosis and management of bowel perforation.

1 Introduction

Gastrointestinal (GI) tract perforations are a common cause of acute abdominal pain syndrome. They account for 1–3% of cases acute abdomen syndrome. Diagnosing intestinal perforation is a surgical emergency.

As for suspicion of obstruction and colic pain, suspected perforation remains one of the indications for abdominal plain film (APF). Nevertheless, the development of computed tomography (CT) in clinical management of acute abdominal pain along with the setting up of an accurate and efficient semiology allowed improved diagnosis of GI tract perforations with respect to the presence, localization site, and cause.

Early diagnosis of GI tract perforation together with identification of the site and cause improves the prognosis of GI tract perforation and has a great impact on the therapeutic choice, including the type of surgery and the means of access.

2   Pathology

2.1   Definition of a Bowel Perforation

GI perforations are discontinuities of the GI wall which allow intestine lumen and peritoneal cavity or subperitoneal or retroperitoneal spaces to communicate.

The peritoneal irritation may be caused by a purulent fluid, as well as by an aseptic fluid (at least at the beginning of the evolution), in particular in the case of perforation of a gastroduodenal ulcer. Peritonitis may be generalized or localized. When the fluid bathes the entire peritoneal cavity, it is a generalized peritonitis. When only part of the abdominal cavity is involved, it is a localized peritonitis. Some localized peritonitis clinically manifest themselves as plastic peritonitis, also called plastron, due to an inflammatory reaction of the surroundings organs (epiploic fat in particular). On palpation, the plastron makes up a resisting mass, a "boardlike" abdominal wall.

2.2   Causes of GI Tract Perforations

GI tract perforations can affect any segment of the digestive tract, and complicate every digestive disease, whether tumoral, inflammatory, ischemic, postradiation, or ulcerous. Nevertheless, in order of frequency, perforations are most often the complication of a gastroduodenal ulcer or a sigmoid diverticulitis.

2.2.1   Esophageal Perforation

Spontaneous perforations—not caused by a trauma (mostly from iatrogenic or endoscopic causes)—of the esophagus are commonly known as Boerhaave

syndrome. It differs from Mallory–Weiss syndrome, in which lesions, often linear, occur within the mucosa and the submucosa, and are characterized by an upper hemorrhage (Rubesin and Levine 2003). Similarly to Mallory–Weiss syndrome, it is postulated to result from a sudden rise in intraluminal esophageal pressure, commonly associated with vomiting (typically with alcoholism), which can induce a dilatation of the lower esophagus, up to 5 times its normal diameter. Perforation typically occurs at the weakest point in the esophagus, at the left posterolateral wall of the lower third of the esophagus (Korn et al. 2007). Mediatinitis frequently is seen late in the course of illness. The contiguous pleura is often ruptured.

2.2.2   Gastroduodenal Perforation

Perforations of a gastroduodenal ulcer represent the leading cause of GI tract perforations. As an example, in the largest series assessing multidetector CT in GI perforations, more than half of the perforations were related to a gastroduodenal ulcer (Imuta et al. 2007). On the anatomopathologic plan, chronic ulcer is a round or oval-shaped loss of deep substance, with sharp margins, covered with a fake yellowish membrane, amputating the muscularis, which becomes sclerous. Depending on the depth of the parietal lesion, true ulcer must be distinguished from abrasion, erosion, and ulceration. Perforations complicate 2–10% of peptic ulcers (Ramakrishinan and Salinas 2007; Behrman 2005). They more frequently affect the first part of the duodenum and its anterior face, and more rarely the gastric antrum and the lesser curvature. The prevalence of perforations is the same for both gastric and duodenal ulcers. However, duodenal ulcers are 3 times more frequent than gastric ulcers. The causes of perforations are dependent on multiple factors, and are commonly associated with *Helicobacter pylori* infections. Intake of nonsteroidal anti-inflammatory drugs is found in about half of cases of perforated ulcers. Cocaine was shown as an important causative factor in perforated juxtapyloric ulcers in a series of patients from an urban hospital (Feliciano et al. 1999). Other rarer causes are associated with an increased prevalence of digestive ulcer, such as Zollinger–Ellison syndrome, in which ulcers are more likely jejunum ulcers, and Crohn disease.

Gastric tumor perforations are rarer than ulcer perforations and can be associated with adenocarcinoma, leiomyosarcoma, or lymphoma. The perforation is

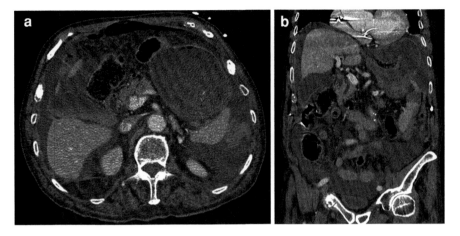

Fig. 1 Gastric volvulus. Axial (a) and coronal (b) views show a distended stomach with a hyperdense content, a thickened gastric wall, and a pneumoperitoneum

seldom the reason for the discovery of the gastric tumor. Gastric penetrations associated with a lymphoma are often due to a lymphoma of the mucosa-associated lymphoid tissue type. The perforation may either be related to the evolution of the disease itself or secondary to chemotherapy.

Gastric perforation may complicate gastric volvulus (Fig. 1), which is a disease with a high rate of perforation.

At the duodenal level, except from ulcer and tumor perforations, duodenal diverticulum is a typical but rare cause of digestive perforation. The most frequent duodenal diverticula are juxtapapillary diverticula created by herniation of the mucosa or submucosa through the muscularis mucosae at a weak spot known as the duodenal window. Perforation of those diverticula is a rare complication, and is most commonly of a retroperitoneal site.

2.2.3 Small Bowel Perforations

Perforations of the small bowel are rare, besides those related to ischemic causes. Perforations of ischemic origin occur either in a context of mechanical obstruction as a complication of ischemic digestive strangulation or in a context of primary ischemia as a severity factor, most frequently associated with arterial ischemia or low-debit ischemia, rather than venous ischemia. Other causes are rare and account for one case per year and for every 350,000 inhabitants (Kimchi et al. 2002). They include Crohn disease, tumor, infection (tuberculosis, opportunist infection), and jejunal or Meckel diverticulitis. The pathophysiological changes, the frequency, and the site of the perforation differ according to the cause.

Small bowel perforation complicating mechanical occlusion Obstruction is due to a band or internal or external hernia. Strangulation complicates a mechanism of incarceration with a severe proximal distension which induces a venous stasis, followed by an arterial stasis, with pneumatosis and/or perforation.

Small bowel perforation complicating primary small bowel ischemia This is a major complication of digestive ischemia.

Crohn disease Besides ischemia, this is a leading cause of small bowel perforation. Nevertheless, perforations represent a rare complication of Crohn disease, with an incidence of 1%. Other Crohn disease perforating complications exist, such as loop–loop bowel fistula and vesicular fistula.

Tuberculosis Abdominal tuberculosis can affect any organ, although it is often secondary to pulmonary tuberculosis. The ileocecal region is the most frequently affected area in digestive tuberculosis (Ha et al. 1999). Perforations observed in digestive tuberculosis are rare, accounting for 1–10% of all cases.

Lymphoma Roughly all lymphomas affecting the digestive wall are non-Hodgkin lymphomas, mostly of B type. The small bowel is, besides the stomach, the mots common lymphoma digestive affection. Lymphoma represents the most frequent cause of small bowel tumor perforation. Such perforations are more frequent in digestive affections associated with a B-type lymphoma and can be chemotherapy-induced (Ghai et al. 2007). Lymphomatous affections can be either secondary, with digestive localizations associated with splenic or hepatic lymph nodes, or primary,

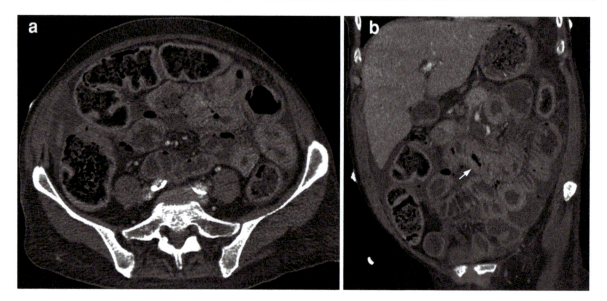

Fig. 2 Small bowel tumor perforation under chemotherapy. Axial (**a**) and coronal (**b**) views show a thickening of the bowel wall involving a large part of the small bowel because of peritonitis but which is more pronounced at the site of the tumor (*arrow*). Close to the tumor there is nonluminal fluid and air, which show the site of the perforation. A malignant tumor of the small bowel treated by chemotherapy was known in this patient

with digestive tract localization only. Other malignant small bowel tumors may be perforated and so may be revealed by acute abdomen. Otherwise, in a patient with a known small bowel tumor, chemotherapy may favor perforation (Fig. 2).

Small bowel diverticulitis The small bowel diverticulum can be either of a jejunal site, typically localized on the mesenteric border of the intestine, or of an ileal site, associated with a congenital Meckel diverticulum. Jejunal diverticula are acquired, mostly occurring between the sixth and the seventh decade of life. They do not have muscular lining. Up to 10% of patients presenting with jejunal diverticulitis will have a small bowel perforation (Park et al. 2005) and hemorrhage; perforations being the most frequent complications. Complications secondary to Meckel diverticulitis are rare, occurring in 2% of patients presenting with Meckel diverticulum (Park et al. 2005) (Fig. 3). Meckel diverticulum is a congenital abnormality, occurring in 1–3% of the population.

Jejunal ulcer Jejunal ulcers can complicate Zollinger–Ellison syndrome. Zollinger–Ellison syndrome is characterized by hypersecretion of gastrin produced by either pancreatic or duodenal endocrine tumors. It is associated with ulcerations and jejunal ulcers which can be perforated.

Vasculitis (aka angiitis) Numerous vasculitides can lead to intestinal perforation, which typically occur during attacks of the disease, and exceptionally are the only manifestations. An anatomoclinical mismatch often exists, and lack of abdominal contracture is sometimes seen, especially in corticoid-treated patients. Small bowel involvement predominates at the ileal level, and perforations are often multiple. Vasculitides are defined by an inflammation associated with necrosis of the vascular wall. They are classified by anatomical and histological criteria, as well as by the caliber of the affected blood vessels, and the presence or absence of vascular granuloma and parietal necrosis (Pagnoux et al. 2003). Vasculitides mainly leading to intestinal perforation include polyarteritis nodulosa, Wegener syndrome, Churg–Strauss syndrome, Behçet syndrome, and rheumatoid-arthritis-associated vasculitides, with polyarteritis nodulosa and Behçet syndrome being the most frequent. In Behçet syndrome, digestive involvement occurs in 10–50% of patients with relatively ubiquitous localization, predominating in the terminal ileus and cecum. Predominant lesions are generally large

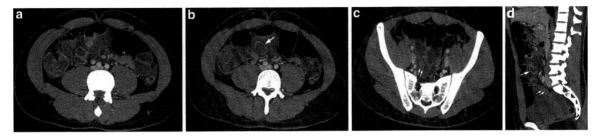

Fig. 3 Perforated Meckel diverticulum. The axial slice (**a**) shows extraluminal fluid and air within the mesentery suggestive of a small bowel perforation. On a slightly lower slice (**b**), distended Meckel diverticula with a very enhanced wall are individualized (*arrow*). On a pelvic slice (**c**), the appendix is well seen (*double arrows*) with abnormally enhanced wall because of reaction to peritonitis. Sagittal reformatting (**d**) shows both the Meckel diverticula (*arrow*) and the appendix (*double arrows*), both having abnormally enhanced walls. Surgery confirmed the perforation of a Meckel diverticulum

and deep ulcers. Ulcers mostly affect the ileocecal region, being more diffuse and less deep at the colic level (Chung et al. 2001).

Foreign body The most frequent sites of intestinal perforation due to a foreign body are the esophagus and the ileal, ileocecal, and rectosigmoid regions. As little as 1% of ingested foreign bodies is responsible for an intestinal perforation, even though this complication is systematically looked for. Fish bones are the leading cause of intestinal perforation due to a foreign body.

2.2.4 Appendiceal Perforation

Appendiceal perforations complicate about 25% of cases of acute appendicitis and represent the natural evolution pattern of ulcerated appendicitis.

2.2.5 Colic Perforation

Sigmoid diverticulitis Colic diverticulosis is a condition commonly occurring in developed countries. It affects up to two thirds of the population beyond 65 years, and can lead to clinical symptoms in about a quarter of patients. Nevertheless, among affected patients, only a few will develop a diverticular perforation. It is considered that as few as 10% of patients hospitalized for a sigmoid diverticulitis will require surgery due to a generalized peritonitis by perforation. Peritonitis in the context of acute diverticulitis is mostly localized peritonitis which corresponds to a poorly limited pelvic abscess, with a risk of secondary rupture leading to a two-step generalized peritonitis. Generalized peritonitis is most often the consequence of a ruptured diverticular abscess in the peritoneum. Depending on whether or not there is a communication between the initial abscess and the colic lumen, peritonitis will be stercoral or purulent (Loiseau et al. 2005).

More rarely, diverticular peritonitis can occur without a preliminary abscess, during perforation of the colic wall from vascular origin (Tagliacozzo and Tocchi 1997).

Lastly, a pseudotumoral sigmoiditis can lead to a mechanical obstruction of the colon complicated with a diastatic perforation of the cecum. This phenomenon more often complicates colon obstructions from neoplasic origin.

Tumoral colic perforation Colic tumors can cause perforations following two mechanisms:
1. By a direct perforation from tumoral origin
2. By a diastatic perforation of the cecum, upstream from a tumor, most often sigmoid, complicated with a mechanical obstruction

In a retrospective study including 1,650 patients with a colorectal adenocarcinoma, a 3% prevalence of perforations was shown (Chen and Sheen-Chen 2000). An association with a colic mechanical obstruction was shown in all 48 cases of perforation. In 35 of the cases, the perforation was located at the tumor site, whereas it was proximal in the remaining 13 cases. As a comparison, a mechanical obstruction existed in 10% of patients. According to other authors, the incidence of colic perforations would be higher in colon cancer patients treated with an antiangiogenic such as Avastin® (Saif et al. 2007;

Heinzerling and Huerta 2006). Such antiangiogenic treatment could even explain the rise of colic perforation complicating a neoplasia with no mechanical obstruction.

Other causes of colic perforation Many inflammatory colitises (often of right development) or ischemic colitises can cause a colic perforation. The cecum is predisposed to perforation as the intraluminal pressure increases, such as in colic mechanical obstruction as discussed above, or in idiopathic cecal distension. Stercoral colitis can lead to highly serious stercoral peritonitis. Stercoral peritonitis mostly affects elderly as well as laid-up patients. The perforation is typically located on the antimesenteric border of the intestine, which is less vascularized than the mesenteric border and more sensitive to mechanical constraint (Facy et al. 2007). Stercoral peritonitis is typically located in the sigmoid colon or upper rectum as a fecaloma more frequently develops in the distal colon. The diagnosis is made upon the presence of colic distension by fecal material and the presence of intraperitoneal material. The prognosis of stercoral peritonitis is very severe.

2.2.6 Rectal Perforation

Rectal perforations are mostly related to a foreign body, or from iatrogenic origin complicating a surgical or endoscopic gesture. They can also occur following a cleansing enema or maneuver to extract fecaloma with the constitution of a stercoral peritonitis (Fig. 4).

3 Clinical Findings

3.1 Peritoneal Syndrome

The onset is most often characterized by a syndrome of acute abdominal pain, sometimes "stab"-like. Pain, initially localized, quickly becomes generalized and increased during early and abundant vomiting episodes. Transit modifications (subocclusion) occur later.

General signs depend on the cause of the perforation and time elapsed from the perforation. They are typically dependent on the time of onset, and include fever, tachycardia, dyspnea, and oliguria. Septic

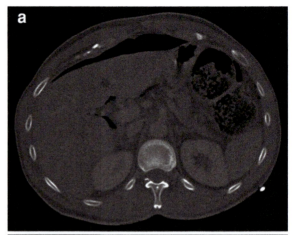
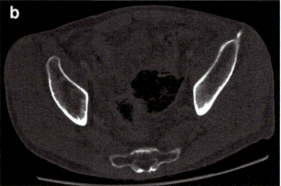

Fig. 4 Iatrogenic perforation located at the junction between the sigmoid colon and the rectum. The upper axial slice (**a**) shows a free pneumoperitoneum, and the lower axial slice (**b**) shows stool outside the colic tract. At surgery, the perforation complicating a cleansing enema was located at the junction between the sigmoid colon and the rectum

shock with multiple organ failure can occur, especially with elderly and immunosuppressed patients. Patients may present with a grayish complexion, and hollow eyes (peritoneal face).

On examination, the pathognomonic sign is the contracture of the abdominal wall. In a lean and fit patient, muscles are visible, and the abdomen stops moving with respiration. The contracture is spontaneous, permanent, painful, and invincible. It is typically generalized to the entire abdomen, sometimes predominant at the site of the causative lesion. It must be appreciated on the basis of the musculature and the age of the subject. It can therefore be very discrete, even absent in elderly patients. It can be masked by analgesic treatment such as morphine. Pelvic touch is very painful, because of the peritoneal irritation.

3.2 Clinical Presentation According to the Cause

Several clinical and anamnestic signs can indicate the site of intestinal perforation. Ulcerous perforations affect men more than women, with the same incidence with regard to age, whereas small bowel perforation, appendiceal perforation, and colic perforations mostly affect the elderly.

In esophageal perforations, pain is localized to the thorax base or the epigastrium. Vomiting, cervical subcutaneous emphysema, and respiratory distress are late presentations. Two signs with a strong orientation value are the rise of pain in a context of violent vomiting and the patient's background, including ulcer history, neurologic history, and alcohol intake.

In gastroduodenal ulcer perforations, the site of pain—epigastric at first, which can radiate to the iliac fossa or to the shoulders—the epidemiologic context—intake of drugs with gastric wall toxicity, such as anti-inflammatory drugs, which are responsible for about half of ulcer perforations (Ramakrishinan and Salinas 2007), a great stress (recent surgery), and a young age orientate one toward diagnosis. In the case of frequent ulcerous attacks, adherences with neighboring organs can form around the first duodenum (liver, gallbladder, and colon). In this case, the perforation does not manifest itself with acute-generalized peritonitis symptoms but rather as acute pain localized in the right upper quadrant.

In small bowel perforations, the peritoneal syndrome is in general less obvious, the rise of the pain is less sudden, a fever is found in half of cases, and symptoms of obstruction can lead to a mechanical obstruction of the small bowel, in a context of infection.

Appendiceal perforations complicate from 18 to 35% of cases of appendicitis, appendicitis being the most frequent cause of abdominal emergency in a surgery department. Differentiating between appendicitis and complicated appendicitis with perforation is challenging when the clinical features are compatible with appendicitis. Flamant's criteria (Flamant 1995), used to postpone an eventual hospitalization (namely, lack of defense, lack of fever beyond 38°C, and lack of hyperleucocytosis), typically allow a perforated appendicitis to be excluded.

Colic perforations are in general complications of diverticular sigmoiditis and colic tumors. They thus occur in the elderly, with less sudden clinical presentation and symptoms of abdominal infection in case of a diverticulitis, or episodes of subocclusion with altered general state in case of a colon cancer.

4 CT Findings

4.1 Direct Findings

Direct visualization of a localized rupture of the digestive tract wall and of a communication between the intestinal content (air or liquid) and the peri-intestinal atmosphere is pathognomonic of the site of intestinal perforation (Fig. 5). It is a CT finding whose visualization can be favored by using fine sections and multiplanar reconstructions.

4.2 Indirect Findings

4.2.1 Pneumoperitoneum

A pneumoperitoneum is the cardinal sign of digestive perforation (Cho and Baker 1994). On CT, the pneumoperitoneum is easily visible as large windows and fine slices are used (Rubesin and Levine 2003; Grassi et al. 2004). The presence and the amount of free air in the peritoneum depend on the anatomical site and extension of the perforation, on preexisting intestinal distension, and moreover, on the time elapsed from the perforation to the scan. The site of a pneumoperitoneum, whether localized or not localized, points toward a perforation of the adjacent bowel, particularly when extraluminal free air is in little abundance (Kim et al. 2009).

4.2.2 Fatty Infiltration

A localized fatty infiltration adjacent to an intestinal segment points, with a less valuable diagnostic value than for the pneumoperitoneum, toward the perforation of this particular intestinal segment.

4.2.3 Intestinal Wall Thickening

A localized thickening of the intestinal wall in acute abdomen syndrome with a pneumoperitoneum orientates one toward the cause (by analyzing the thickening features) and the site of the perforation. Inversely, an extended thickening of the intestinal

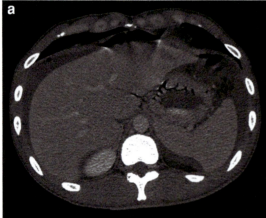
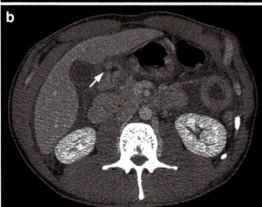
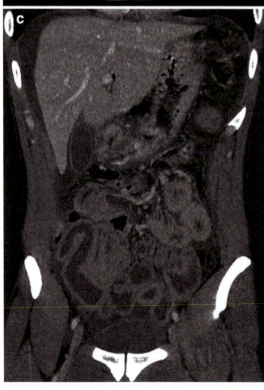

◄ **Fig. 5** Small bowel thickening consecutive to a gastroduodenal ulcer perforation. The upper axial slice (**a**) shows a free pneumoperitoneum and peritoneal fluid, whereas the duodenal discontinuity (*arrow*) is well seen on the slice in (**b**). Note the thickening of the small bowel wall seen on the axial view (**b**) and coronal reformatting (**c**)

wall has a poor diagnostic value and can simply be the consequence of peritonitis (Fig. 5).

4.3 CT Findings According to the Cause

4.3.1 Esophageal Perforation

CT is used to look for indirect signs: a mediastinal posterior collection of liquid revealing a mediastinitis, a posterior pneumomediastin that can diffuse to the retroperitoneum, parietal signs as a localized thickening of the esophageal wall. Exceptionally, it will identify parietal wall discontinuity, as a direct sign of the perforation.

4.3.2 Gastroduodenal Perforation

Identification of a rupture in the intestinal wall, most commonly in the duodenal bulb or prepyloric region, is a direct sign of a perforated gastroduodenal ulcer (Fig. 6).

Indirect CT findings of an ulcer perforation typically are the presence of an abundant pneumoperitoneum, free air around the falciform ligament, perigastroduodenal fatty infiltration, interduodenopancreatic fluid, and gastroduodenal thickening (Chen et al. 2001; Ongolo-Zogo et al. 1999).

Considering the predominant bulbar localization of duodenal ulcer, the perforation is intraperitoneal. A retroperitoneal localization, which is visualized by imaging as leaking of extraintestinal gas, in the right anterior pararenal space indicates a duodenal perforation beyond the bulbar segment, often related to a duodenal diverticulum or a perforation from GI endoscopy (Yagan et al. 2009).

The perforation is not always related to an ulcer. It can originate from a tumor. Such a diagnosis must be suspected in patients with an important irregular thickening of the gastric wall.

The perforation can be limited to the gastric wall, but can be extended to the colic wall with formation of a gastrocolic fistula. This event is rare. It can be found in tumoral gastric perforations, in Crohn diseases with gastric and colic involvement, and

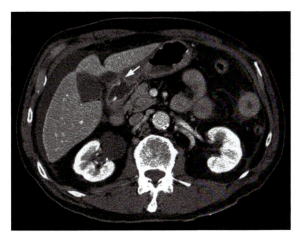

Fig. 6 Perforation due to an antropyloric ulcer. The discontinuity of the anterior wall of the gastric wall is well identified (*arrow*) on these 3-mm axial reconstructions

exceptionally in certain ulcers affecting patients treated with nonsteroidal anti-inflammatory drugs (Ramakrishinan and Salinas 2007).

As described above, perforations of a duodenal diverticulum are mostly retroperitoneal. In a small series including eight cases, both a retroperitoneum and retroperitoneal fatty infiltration were found in all cases, with an associated pneumoperitoneum in three of the cases (Fig. 7). A second or third duodenum localized diverticulum was identified in seven of the cases (Ames et al. 2009).

4.3.3 Small Bowel Perforation

CT findings of small bowel perforation are findings of air bubbles within the mesentery fluid collection with a pneumoperitoneum (Kimchi et al. 2002), localized fatty infiltration in the mesentery, or a localized. Thickening of the small bowel wall often exists, with little prognostic value with respect to the site, as the thickening could result from peritonitis, hence indicating either a colic or a gastroduodenal perforation.

Small bowel perforation complicating a bowel obstruction CT (Catel et al. 2003) will show signs of mechanical obstruction, signs of incarceration and strangulation with a localized edema, a venous congestion, or and mostly, an intestinal wall thinning or an intestinal pneumatosis revealing an infarcted intestine.

Acute ischemia of the mesentery CT will show parietal findings with a localized or not localized defect enhancement of the intestine wall revealing parietal distress, and vascular signs, thrombus, most often proximal, in the superior mesenteric artery, or embolus sited on arterial bifurcation.

Crohn disease CT shows a thickening of the intestinal wall, a marked fatty infiltration (sclerolipomatosis), and an increased parietal vascularization. Perforation in a Crohn disease setting complicates an evolved Crohn disease, with common fistula and abscess formation (Furukawa et al. 2004) (Fig. 8).

Digestive lymphoma In addition to a small bowel parietal thickening, criteria favoring a lymphoma are findings of an ectatic digestive lumen, of adenomegaly, or the extent of thickening. However, in type T lymphoma, moderate thickening and missing lymph nodes can make a differential diagnosis with inflammatory involvement difficult (Byun et al. 2003).

Small bowel diverticulitis CT will show signs of complicated jejunal diverticulitis, or signs of Meckel diverticulitis, by individualizing thickened diverticula with peridiverticular fatty infiltration, and the presence of small pneumoperitoneum bubbles more often localized around the diverticulum than free, and close to the anterior parietal peritoneum (Hibben et al. 1995). A Meckel diverticulum containing air, liquid, or fecal material is sometimes visualized. The diverticulum wall can be thickened (Fig. 3) or with no enhancement, and even interrupted, revealing a perforated diverticulum.

Digestive tuberculosis Tuberculous perforations affect the terminal ileus, with a thickened ileocecal valvule and a thickened ileal and cecal wall. A small bowel obstruction is often associated, as a consequence of the stenosis of the terminal ileus. Enlarged lymph nodes with a hypodense center may be seen. The main differential diagnoses are Crohn disease and ileocecal lymphoma.

Jejunal ulcer In jejunal ulcer perforations occurring in the setting of Zollinger–Elisson syndrome, scan findings include a localized defect of the digestive wall, sited at a proximal jejunal loop, with associated extraluminal air bubbles, and with a localized infiltration of fat close to the pathologic loop, as seen in gastroduodenal ulcer perforations.

Foreign body In addition to indirect signs of perforation, such as localized extradigestive collection,

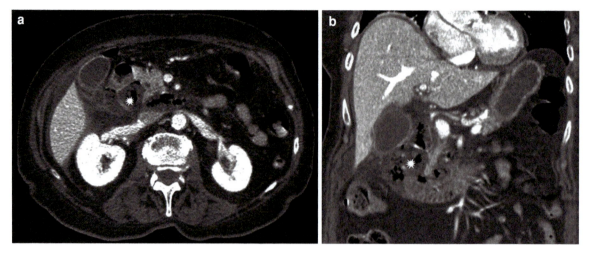

Fig. 7 Perforation of a duodenal diverticulum. Axial (**a**) and coronal (**b**) views show the diverticulum (*star*) adjacent and posterior to the second part of the duodenum on the axial slice. There is a rounded collection with air and fluid along the lateral surface of the diverticulum. Note also the presence of both a retropneumoperitoneum and a pneumoperitoneum

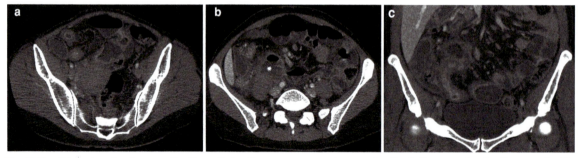

Fig. 8 Small bowel perforation complicating a Crohn disease. The lower axial slice (**a**) and the coronal view (**c**) show Crohn disease findings with wall thickening of the terminal ileum, target sign on the distal ileum, and sclerolipomatosis. The upper axial slice (**b**) shows an abscess (*star*) located in front of the right psoas muscle

fatty infiltration, and thickening of the involved digestive wall, direct visualization of a foreign body, either calcified or metallic, through the digestive wall allows a diagnosis to be made with certainty (Goh et al. 2006) (Fig. 9).

Vascularitis In polyarteritis nodulosa, the scan will show digestive wall thickening related to ischemia, imaging of thrombosis of the portal venous system, and signs of hepatic, splenic, or renal infarction. It will also detect signs of pancreatitis, or cholecystis. In Behcet syndrome, ulcers are reliably displayed by digestive opacification. On CT, digestive wall thickening is important, sometimes being circumferential and mass-shaped, and sometimes being voluminous, which can be mistaken for digestive tumors (Pagnoux et al. 2003). As compared with Crohn disease, ulcerations are wider and deeper, and peridigestive inflammatory infiltration is less important, with little or no sclerolipomatosis.

4.3.4 Appendiceal Perforation

Semiology, which allows complicated and uncomplicated appendicitis to be distinguished, is based on the presence of abscesses, phlegmon, extraluminal air, extraappendiceal stercolith, and a defect in enhancement of the appendiceal wall and ileus. All such signs are in favor of a perforated appendicitis. A free pneumoperitoneum is very rare in appendiceal perforations (Fig. 10).

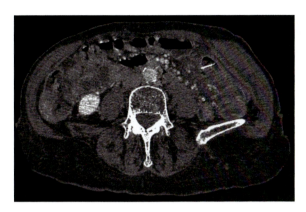

Fig. 9 Foreign body going through the small bowel wall. The foreign body is clearly seen and was related to a rabbit bone

4.3.5 Colic Perforation

CT is now the reference standard for evaluating complications of colic diverticular disease (Loiseau et al. 2005; Zins et al. 2007). It individualizes signs of diverticulitis, with thickening of the colic wall commonly involving the sigmoid, perisigmoid fatty infiltration, and diverticula. It shows signs of perforation, such as extraluminal air, localized in the mesosigmoid region, or at a distance in the pelvis, or as a free subdiapharagmatic pneumoperitoneum which may be very limited (Fig. 11) because the perforation is closed by the adjacent inflamed mesosigmoid. It shows pericolic or pelvic abscesses, further evaluating their size, as well as extradigestive materials, revealing a stercoral peritonitis.

CT findings (Lorhmann et al. 2005) correlate well with surgical findings; hence, complications can be graded according to the Hinchey grading system (Hinchey et al. 1978).
- Stage I, in which there is a phlegmon or a pericolic abcess
- Stage II, in which either the phlegmon or the pericolic abscess is voluminous, or there are pelvic or retroperitoneal or abdominal abscesses at a distance
- Stage III, with a purulent generalized peritonitis
- Stage IV, with a stercoral peritonitis

The diagnosis of tumoral colic perforation has to be proposed when extraluminal air is adjacent to the thickened colic wall, revealing a tumor. Common findings are major peritumoral fatty infiltration and small amounts of extraluminal air. In contrast, in cecal diastatic perforations, with accompanying CT signs of large bowel obstruction and a distended colon, the pneumoperitoneum is often highly abundant. A cecal parietal pneumatosis is sometimes associated with such an abundant pneumoperitoneum, pointing toward the site and mechanism of perforation, although not specific to cecal transmural distress in the setting of colic mechanical obstruction (Taourel et al. 2004).

In stercoral perforations, diagnosis is made upon a coexisting free peritoneum and a very important colic distension by materials. The colon wall is distended and sometimes thickened, and pericolic fat is infiltrated (Heffernan et al. 2005).

In perforation complicating an ischemic colitis, CT frequently shows a lack of enhancement of the bowel wall (Fig. 12)

4.3.6 Rectal Perforation

On CT, extraluminal air in the perirectal fat is the most frequent finding. Additional findings include presacral fluid, extraluminal feces, and rectal wall thickening (Zissin et al. 2008).

5 CT Pitfalls

The main potential error in diagnosing a pneumoperitoneum by CT is confusion between intraluminal and extraluminal air, and more particularly, doubt between intraperitoneal and preperitoneal air in the case of a small anterior pneumoperitoneum, the latter diagnosing issue especially arising in abdomen trauma.

Even when optimum imaging examination (CT with fine sections and a wide window) is used, a pneumoperitoneum may not be present in a true digestive perforation (false negative) (Grassi et al. 2004). In contrast, a pneumoperitoneum may be present in the absence of a digestive perforation (false positive).

A false negative can be related to digestive perforation without pneumoperitoneum formation. This has been well demonstrated in a study (Grassi et al. 2004) using a series of gastroduodenal perforations. A pneumoperitoneum could not be found by CT in some cases, but was detected in a few of the cases by delayed scans (beyond 6 h). Nevertheless, a free pneumoperitoneum can be delayed as well. A localized pneumoperitoneum adjacent to the perforation is found in roughly all nontraumatic perforations of

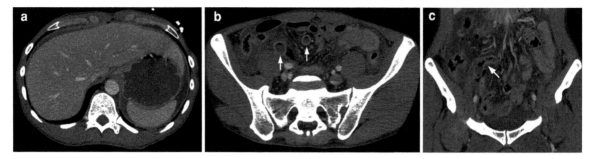

Fig. 10 Peritonitis consecutive to an appendiceal perforation. The upper axial slice (**a**) shows a free pneumoperitoneum. The lower axial slice (**b**) shows a collection in the right lower quadrant with dilatation of the appendix (*arrow*) and important enhancement of the appendix wall, which is thickened. The coronal view (**c**) shows the appendicitis in its length

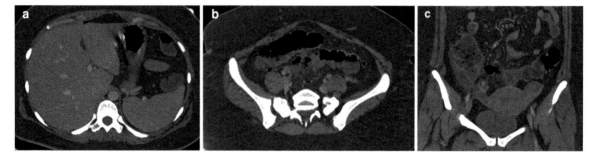

Fig. 11 Perforation of sigmoid diverticulitis. The upper axial slice (**a**) shows a free pneumoperitoneum, whereas the lower slice (**b**) and coronal reformatting (**c**) show a thickening of the sigmoid wall with fat stranding. Note also the presence of air bubbles outside the bowel

nonappendiceal origin (Imuta et al. 2007) involving intraperitoneal segments of bowel.

Excluding a pseudopneumoperitoneum notably related to preperitoneal air, with air confined to the inner layer of the abdominal wall and external to the parietal peritoneum, a false positive correspond to the presence of a documented pneumoperitoneum, with no digestive perforation. A false positive can originate from the thorax, digestive organs, or gynecologic organs (Table 1) (Catel et al. 2003). Finally, a retropneumoperitoneum can be related to a diffuse pneumomediastinum.

For the diagnosis of the perforation's cause, in a patient with a pneumoperitoneum, the identification of a thickening of the bowel wall pointing toward the site of the perforation may be misleading: a thickening of the bowel may be the consequence of the peritonitis due to the perforation of another part of the GI tract. This specifically involves the small bowel with thickening of the small bowel wall, which may make differential diagnosis between small and large bowel perforation difficult (Fig. 13). In the same way, the site of the pneumoperitoneum does not point toward the site of the perforation when the pneumoperitoneum is abundant, and this may correspond to a gastroduodenal or a colic perforation (Fig. 14).

6 CT Accuracy

CT is very accurate for pneumoperitoneum identification, even if it is poorly abundant or localized. Reading requires the use of wide windows. A 1-mm section can be useful for identification of a small pneumoperitoneum. CT is likely to very accurately diagnose a pneumoperitoneum, as long as it exists.

Classic indirect CT signs pointing toward an ulcer perforation are the presence of an abundant pneumoperitoneum, air located around the round ligament, outlining of the falciform ligament, infiltration of perigastroduodenal fat, and the finding of a gastroduodenal thickening. In a retrospective study

Bowel Perforations

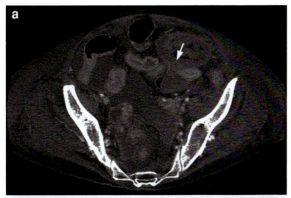

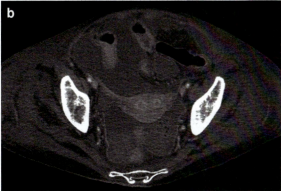

Fig. 12 Ischemic colitis complicated by perforation. The upper axial slice (**a**) shows a collection in the peritoneum with the peritoneal membrane, which is enhanced. The descending colon is thickened without enhancement of its posterior wall (*arrow*). The lower axial slice (**b**) shows some air bubbles within the collection located in the Douglas pouch. Note also the enhanced peritoneum

Table 1 Causes of pneumoperitoneum without bowel perforation

Pseudopneumoperitoneum on abdominal plain film
  Lucency under the diaphragm
    Fatty area under the diaphragm (more common in obese patients or in patients with corticoid)
    Nonperitoneal gas
    Properitoneal gas
    Gas within lung trapped under a lung collapse
  Air within the bowel
    Chilaiditi syndrome
    Stomach closed to the diaphragm
    Emphysematous cholecystitis or pyelonephritis

True pneumoperitoneum
  Thoracic causes
    Diffusion of pneumothorax or pneumomediastinum
  Abdominal causes
    Abdominal surgery
    Perioneal dialysis
    Endoscopy: pneumoperitoneum is due to the diffusion of intraluminal air
    Gastroparesy
    Pneumatosis cystoides intestinalis
  Female genital tract causes
    Hysterectomy
    Sexual intercourse or cunnilingus
    Pelvic examination
    Athletic activities such as waterskiing

(Ghekiere et al. 2007a) including 81 digestive perforations, about half of which related to a gastroduodenal perforation, we demonstrated the lack of specificity of indirect signs. The presence of air around the ligamentum teres or visualization of the falciform ligament outlined by some air could be related to a perforation from any other origin when the pneumoperitoneum is abundant. A reactive gastroduodenal thickening could also indicate peritonitis from another cause. In our series, the best indirect sign of a gastroduodenal perforation was the presence of fluid localized between the duodenum and the head of the pancreas. This sign had a positive predictive value greater than 90% for diagnosing a perforated ulcer. In contrast, the presence of an abundant pneumoperitoneum or a pneumoperitoneum outlining the falciform ligament and also a pneumoperitoneum within the lesser sac had a positive predictive value ranging from 40 to 52% for the diagnosis of a gastroduodenal ulcer perforation. More recently, a Korean study has confirmed that evaluation of the site of the pneumoperitoneum, and more specifically the presence of periportal free air around the round or falciform ligament were only ancillary findings in the diagnosis of a gastroduodenal perforation (Choi et al. 2009). In contrast, a pneumoperitoneum only localized within the mesentery points toward a small bowel perforation, whereas a free pneumoperitoneum localized within the submesocolic space points toward a colic perforation.

Direct visualization of the site of perforation is a major advantage of multidetector CT, owing to thin sections (Fig. 15) and multiplanar reconstructions. In a study by Chen et al. (2001), analyzing ulcer

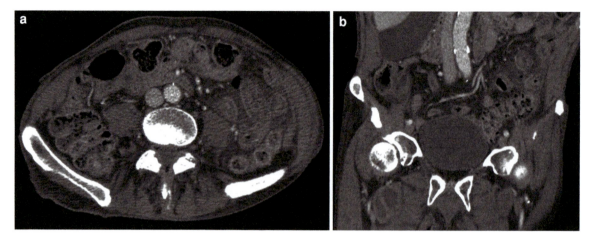

Fig. 13 Sigmoid perforation with reactive thickening of the small bowel. Axial slices (**a**) show thickening of the small bowel wall, peritoneal fluid, and some extraluminal air bubbles. On the coronal reformatting (**b**), sigmoid diverticula are well identified with some slight thickening of the sigmoid wall. Surgery showed perforated sigmoid diverticulitis

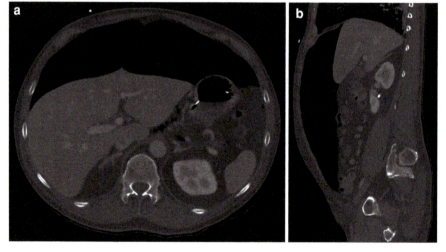

Fig. 14 Big pneumoperitoneum without any value for the perforation localization. The axial view (**a**) and sagittal reformatting (**b**) show a big pneumoperitoneum in a patient hospitalized in an intensive care unit. There is no argument for a gastric versus a colic perforation. At surgery, there was a tear in the lesser curvature of the stomach complicating cardiac massagea

perforations, discontinuity of the digestive wall was never visualized, as CT was performed using centimeter sections. In another study, performed using 3-mm sections, discontinuity of the digestive wall was visualized in 60% of patients with a perforated ulcer (Ongolo-Zogo et al. 1999). In a retrospective series of 15 perforated gastroduodenal ulcers, Cazejust et al. (2007) directly individualized the parietal rupture in eight cases by using a 16-detector CT scanner and millimeter sections.

In our experience (Ghekiere et al. 2007b), in a retrospective study including 40 patients with non-traumatic digestive perforations from various sites and causes, the utility of thin sections and reconstruction significantly allowed direct identification of the route of perforation. Identification was possible in 5–20% of the cases, depending on the readers, using 5-mm sections in the axial plane, in 28–48% of the cases using both 1- and 5-mm sections, and in 43–53% of the cases using both thin slices and sagittal coronal and axial planes. Coronal plane sections proved useful in detecting perforations of both the superior and the inferior wall of the antrum and the bulb or first part of the duodenum. In a study by Hainaux et al. (2006) including 85 patients with various causes of both trauma and nontrauma perforations, the route of perforation was visualized in 29 cases out of 85 (34.1%), using a four-detector CT

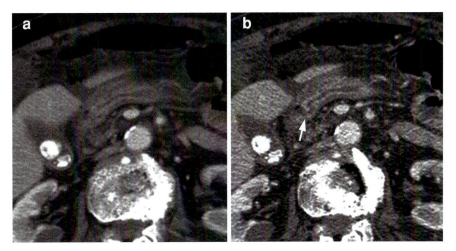

Fig. 15 Impact of slice thickness on the identification of a perforated gastrointestinal ulcer. The antral lumen and the defect in the antral wall are better seen on the 1-mm-thick slice (**b**) than on the 5-mm-thick slice (**a**)

scanner and 2.5-mm sections. These authors also illustrated the potential utility of multiplanar reformatting for identifying the parietal rupture.

CT semiology in diagnosing appendiceal perforation has been validated by three retrospective studies following the same method. The results are summarized in Table 2. All three studies found specific signs of appendicitis, although with a relatively low sensitivity, especially for one specific case of extra-appendiceal stercolith. A localized defect in enhanced appendiceal wall was reported as the most sensitive sign of appendicitis (Bixby et al. 2006). However, thin sections, which are more sensitive to artifacts related to surrounding bone structures or digestive peristaltic movement, could be responsible for a false positive, owing to visualization of a localized digestive wall defect, with no true perforation. Findings of peritoneal fluid, either free or localized, are not a specific sign of appendiceal perforation.

7 CT Impact

The advantages in identifying the site of perforation in patients presenting with digestive perforation deserve to be discussed, as it can be advocated that a peritonitis from digestive perforation may require, whatever its site, emergency surgery. Nevertheless, the type of surgery depends on the site and cause of perforation.

In patients with gastroduodenal ulcer perforation, laparoscopy is an interesting choice, as shown in a number of randomized studies comparing laparoscopic with laparotomic repair of perforated ulcer (Lau et al. 1996; Druart et al. 1997; Siu et al. 2002). A laparoscopic intervention is often recommended in gastroduodenal ulcer perforations of the anterior or lateral site, whereas perforations of the posterior face of the stomach or duodenum could be better managed by regular open abdomen surgery owing to difficult access to the posterior wall of the antropylorobulbar region in peritoneoscopy (Mabrut et al. 2007).

Unlike gastroduodenal ulcer perforations, small bowel perforations are best treated by laparotomy.

For colic perforation, perforations from tumor will be repaired by open abdomen surgery. In contrast, management of perforations from sigmoid diverticulitis depends on the evolution of the disease, as well as on the surgery team practice. The French Society of Gastroenterology and Surgery has given recommendations for management of diverticulitis based on the morphologic assessment of complications by means of a CT scan and Hinchey classification:

– Hinchey grading stage I (phlegmon or colic abscess): After medical treatment and/or CT-guided drainage, resection and anastomosis is the recommended surgical procedure, eventually associated with a protective colostomy. A laparoscopic procedure may be used.
– Hinchey grading stage II: CT-guided drainage and sampling for further microbiology analysis is recommended for abscesses greater than 5 cm. In the case of efficient drainage, primary resection followed by anastomosis is recommended. In the case of a failed drainage or if drainage is not possible, surgical treatment with anastomosis,

Table 2 Accuracy of computed tomography for the diagnosis of perforation in appendicitis		Horrow et al. (2003)	Bixby et al. (2006)	Tsuboi et al. (2008)
	Number of patients	94	244	102
	Appendiceal perforation (%)	41.4	25.4	39.2
	Slice thickness (mm)	5–10	3.2	2–3
	Ileus			
	Sensitivity (%)		53	
	Specificity (%)		93	
	Extraintestinal gas			
	Sensitivity (%)	36	35	22.5
	Specificity (%)	100	98	100
	Abscess			
	Sensitivity (%)	36	34	37.5
	Specificity (%)	100	99	100
	Localized defect of enhancement			
	Sensitivity (%)	64	64	95
	Specificity (%)	100	80	96.8
	Extraluminal appendicoloth			
	Sensitivity (%)	20		32.5
	Specificity (%)	100		100
	Phlegmon			
	Sensitivity (%)	46.5		40
	Specificity (%)	94		95

associated or not associated with protective colostomy is recommended.

- Hinchey grading stage III (generalized purulent peritonitis): A sigmoid resection is recommended. Depending on both the local and the general state of the patient, either resection and anastomosis (associated or not associated with protective ostomy) or the Hartmann procedure will be chosen.
- Hinchey grading stage IV (stercoral peritonitis): The Hartmann procedure is the reference intervention.

A dedicated CT assessment of a complicated diverticulitis not only allows for a modified emergency management, but is also required for later management, as a prophylactic surgery is recommended in the case of a diverticulitis attack with serious signs on the CT scan (namely, abscess or extraluminal leaking of air or contrast liquid).

Similarly, preoperative diagnosis of appendiceal perforation is valuable as it can affect the prognosis of appendicitis, as well as the therapeutic management. Preoperative findings of a localized appendiceal perforation with peritonitis is a reason for switching from an appendectomy by celioscopy to a laparotomic procedure (Liu et al. 2002). Furthermore, medical therapy with intravenous antibiotics combined or not combined with percutaneous drainage may not only limit the extent of surgery, but may also allow, at least, one-step surgery to be undertaken. Finally, medical treatment of uncomplicated appendicitis represents a therapeutic option likely to develop in the future. Indeed a recent analysis of the disconnect between the incidence of nonperforated and perforated appendicitis with a decrease of nonperforated appendicitis and an increase of perforated appendicitis has some implications for pathophysiology and potentially for management of an appendicitis. This may advocate individualization of two different conditions, a perforated appendicitis not necessarily evolving from an appendicitis that has not been surgically treated (Livingston et al. 2007).

8 Diagnosis Strategy

In a patient with a suspected digestive perforation, the diagnostic strategy relies on the wide use of CT, which is the reference examination in management of acute abdomen. APF is only valuable when it shows a pneumoperitoneum. However, a digestive perforation can definitively not be excluded upon normal APF radiography. In practice, three clinical situations can be individualized:

1. There is no orientation element in the anamnesis.
2. An anamnestic context exists, allowing the diagnosis to be orientated.
3. Acute abdomen symptoms arise either early after surgery or after a coloscopy.

8.1 No Orientation Element in the Anamnesis

This is the most frequent clinical situation. The patient has no particular history, or the history is either unknown or not reported at the time of examination. Before abdominal symptomatology highly evoking a digestive perforation, APF radiography will confirm a pneumoperitoneum. Nevertheless, in most cases, a CT scan will be performed to identify the site and cause of the digestive perforation.

8.2 Diagnosis Oriented by Anamnestic Context

An anamnestic context exists, which can be a known bowel or colon disease, or intake of GI-toxic drugs such as anti-inflammatory drugs (corticoids, acetyl-salicylic acid). When a gastroduodenal ulcer perforation is suspected because of an acute gastric pain combined with anti-inflammatory drug intake, APF detection of a pneunoperitoneum will suffice for further therapeutic management. In the case of a negative APF finding, endoscopy or a CT scan seeking a complicated digestive disease or differential diagnoses will be discussed.

Besides a clinical context of perforated ulcer, associated with an APF finding of a pneumoperitoneum, CT will be used to assess the known disease, for instance, Crohn disease, and its complications.

8.3 Postoperative or Postendoscopy Situations

In postoperative follow-up of abdominal surgery, abdominal pain may indicate a complication from surgery such as fistula formation. The presence of a pneumoperitoneum questions its origin: a residual postoperative pneumoperitoneum or a pneumoperitoneum revealing either an anastomotic fistula in the case of intestinal anastomosis or an iatrogenic perforation of the GI tract. The extent of the pneumoperitoneum and the presence or absence of localized inflammatory signs can orientate the diagnosis toward either a residual postoperative pneumoperitoneum or a GI tract perforation. Postoperative pneumoperitoneums are very frequent, with CT detection of a postoperative pneumoperitoneum reported in up to 44–87% of patients after abdominal surgery (Gayer et al. 2000; Earls et al. 1993). They are typically poorly abundant, less than 10 ml in most patients, with lean patients and men presenting with a more abundant pneumoperitoneum. However, they can be larger in case of surgical drainage (Gayer et al. 2000). The abundance of such a postoperative pneumoperitoneum decreases with time.

In clinical practice, if postoperative perforation is suspected for a patient presenting with a pneumoperitoneum, the diagnosis and therapeutic management will depend on the type of surgery and the risk of GI tract lesions, with the existence or no existence of intestinal anastomosis that may form a fistula, on the extent of the pneumoperitoneum related to the time since surgery and to a possible drainage, and finally on the presence of localized inflammatory signs, orienting the diagnosis toward GI tract lesions. In doubtful cases and if the patient's clinical condition allows it, CT may be repeated within 8–12 h, with an increase or a decrease of the pneumoperitoneum being strong arguments in favor or not in favor of a postoperative perforation.

In postcolonoscopy follow-up, GI tract perforation is a very rare complication (Anderson et al. 2000; Tulchinsky et al. 2006), complicating 0.005–0.002% of diagnostic colonoscopies and 0.2–0.4% of colonoscopies with polypectomy. Nevertheless, the development of mucosectomy has increased the risk of perforation. The mechanisms of perforations from colonoscopy are various and include hyperpressure either from the endoscope or from excessive insufflations, and lesions from parietal electrocoagulation due to polypectomy. Perforations generally affect abnormal, inflammatory, and/or stenosed colon. The diagnosis of postendoscopy colic perforation will be made by the presence of a pneumoperitoneum. The therapeutic management, whether surgical or not, will depend on both the presence of peritoneal signs and colic preparation. Indications for surgical treatment include poor colic preparation, a blunt parietal rupture on colonoscopy or CT signs of peritonitis, or the presence of an obstruction downstream of the perforation, and, obviously, deterioration of clinical features when conservative treatment was chosen. Of note, such a pneumoperitoneum revealing a macroscopic perforation is only of value when there are acute symptoms after colonoscopy. Indeed, according to a few authors, a pneumoperitoneum can be related to up to 1% of colonoscopies. Although this percentage is likely to be overestimated (Pearl et al. 2006), a true benign pneumoperitoneum may form after colonoscopy, either from transparietal diffusion or from a microperforation favored by forced mobilization of the intestine and air insufflations, requiring no surgical treatment.

References

Ames JT, Federle MP, Pealer KM (2009) Perforated duodenal diverticulum: clinical and imaging findings in eight patients. Abdom Imaging 34:135–139

Anderson ML, Pasha TM, Leighton JA (2000) Endoscopie perforation of the colon: lessons from a 10-year study. Am J Gastroenterol 95:3418–3422

Behrman SW (2005) Management of complicated peptic ulcer disease. Arch Surg 140:201–208

Bixby SD, Lucey BC, Soto JA et al (2006) Perforated versus nonperforated acute appendicitis: accuracy of multidetector CT detection. Radiology 241:780–786

Byun HJ, Ah HK, Kim AY et al (2003) CT findings in peripheral T-cell lymphoma involving the gastrointestinal tract. Radiology 227:59–67

Catel L, Lefèvre F, Laurent V et al (2003) Occlusion du grêle sur bride: quels critères scanographiques de gravité rechercher? J Radiol 84:27–31

Cazejust J, Castaglioli B, Bessoud B et al (2007) Perforation gastro-duodénale: le rôle de la TDM multicoupe. J Radiol 88:53–57

Chen HS, Sheen-Chen SM (2000) Obtruction and perforation in colorectal adenocarcinoma: an analysis of prognosis and current trends. Surgery 127:370–376

Chen CC, Huang HS, Yang CC, Yeh YH (2001) The features of perforated peptic ulcers in conventional computed tomography. Hepatogastroenterology 49:1393–1396

Cho KC, Baker SR (1994) Extraluminal air diagnosis and significance. Radiol Clin North Am 32:829–844

Choi A, Jang KM, Kim MJ et al. (2009) What determines the periportal free air, and ligamentum teres and falciform ligament signs on CT: can these specific air distributions be valuable predictors of gastroduodenal perforation? Eur J Radiol. doi:10.1016/j.ejrad.2009.07.033

Chung SY, Ha HK, Kim JH et al (2001) Radiologic findings of Behçet syndrome involving the gastro-intestinal tract. Radiographics 21:911–926

Druart ML, Van Hee R, Etienne J et al (1997) Laparoscopic repair of perforated duodenal ulcer. A prospective multicenter clinical trial. Surg Endosc 11:1017–1020

Earls JP, Dachman AH, Colon E et al (1993) Prevalence and duration of postoperative pneumoperitoneum: sensitivity of CT vs left lateral decubitus radiography. AJR Am J Roentgenol 161:781–785

Facy O, Radais F, Chalumeau C (2007) Perforation stercorale du côlon. Physiopathologie et stratégie thérapeutique. Gastroenterol Clin Biol 31:1069–1070

Feliciano DV, Ojukwo JC, Rozycki GS et al (1999) The epidemic of cocaine-related juxtapyloric perforations. Ann Surg 229:801–806

Flamant Y (1995) Association de recherche en chirurgie et association universitaire de recherche en chirurgie. Douleurs abdominales aiguës de l'adulte. Encycl Med Chir (Paris), Gastro-entérologie, 9001-B-10

Furukawa A, Saotome T, Yamasaki M et al (2004) Cross-sectional imaging in Crohn disease. Radiographics 24:689–702

Gayer G, Jonas T, Apter S et al (2000) Postoperative pneumoperitoneum as detected by CT: prevalence, duration, and relevant factors affecting its possible significance. Abdom Imaging 25:301–305

Ghai S, Pattison J, Ghai S, O'Malley M, Khalili K, Stephens M (2007) Primary gastrointestinal lymphoma: spectrum of imaging findings with pathologic correlations. Radiographics 27:1371–1388

Ghekiere O, Lesnik A, Hoa D et al (2007a) Value of CT in the diagnosis of the cause of non-traumatic gastro-intestinal perforation. J Comput Assist Tomogr 31:169–176

Ghekiere O, Lesnik A, Millet I et al (2007b) Direct visualization of perforation sites in patients with a non-traumatic free pneumoperitoneum: added diagnostic value of thin transverse slices and coronal and sagittal reformations for multi-detector CT. Eur Radiol 17:2302–2309

Goh B, Tan YM, Lin SE et al (2006) CT in the preoperative diagnosis of fish bone perforation of the gastrointestinal tract. AJR Am J Roentgenol 187:710–714

Grassi R, Romano S, Pinto A, Romano L (2004) Gastro-duodenal perforations: conventional plain film, US and CT findings in 166 consecutive patients. Eur J Radiol 50:30–36

Ha HK, Ko GY, Yu Es et al (1999) Intestinal tuberculosis with abdominal complications: radiologic and pathologic features. Abdom Imaging 24:32–38

Hainaux B, Agneessens E, Bertinotti R et al (2006) Accuracy of MDCT in predicting site of gastrointestinal tract perforation. AJR Am J Roentgenol 187:1179–1183

Heffernan C, Pachter HL, Megibow AJ, Macari M (2005) Stercoral colitis leading to fatal peritonitis: CT findings. AJR Am J Roentgenol 184:1189–1193

Heinzerling JH, Huerta S (2006) Bowel perforation from bevacizumab for the treatment of metastatic colon cancer: incidence, etiology, and management. Curr Surg 63:334–337

Hibben JF, Gorodetsky AA, Wilbur AC (1995) Perforated jejunal diverticulum: CT diagnosis. Abdom Imaging 20:29–30

Hinchey EJ, Schaal PG, Richards GK (1978) Treatment of perforated diverticular disease of the colon. Adv Surg 12:85–109

Horrow MM, White DS, Horrow JC (2003) Differentiation of perforated from non perforated appendicitis at CT. Radiology 227:46–51

Imuta M, Awai K, Nakayama Y et al (2007) Multidetector CT findings suggesting a perforation site in the gastrointestinal tract: analysis in surgically confirmed 155 patients. Radiat Med 25:113–118

Kim SH, Shin SS, Jeong YY et al (2009) Gastrointestinal tract perforation: MDCT findings according to the perforations sites. Korean J Radiol 10:63–70

Kimchi NA, Broide E, Shapiro M, Scapa E (2002) Nontraumatic perforation of the small intestine. Report of 13 cases and review of the literature. Hepatogastroenterology 49:1017–1022

Korn O, Onate JC, Lopez R (2007) Anatomy of the Boerhaave syndrome. Surgery 141:222–228

Lau WY, Leung KL, Kwong KH et al (1996) A randomized study comparing laparoscopic versus open repair of perforated peptic ulcer using suture or sutureless technique. Ann Surg 224:131–138

Liu SI, Siewert B, Raptopoulos V, Hodin RA (2002) Factors associated with conversion to laparotomy in patients undergoing laparoscopic appendectomy. J Am Coll Surg 194:298–305

Livingston EH, Woodward WA, Sarosi GA, Haley RH (2007) Disconnect between incidence of non perforated and perforated appendicitis Implications for pathophysiology and management. Ann Surg 245:886–892

Loiseau D, Borie F, Agostini H, Millat B (2005) Diverticulite sigmoïdienne. Gastroenterol Clin Biol 29:809–816

Lorhmann C, Ghanem N, Pache G et al (2005) CT in acute perforated sigmoid diverticulitis. Eur J Radiol 56:78–83

Mabrut JY, Buc E, Zins M et al (2007) Prise en charge thérapeutique des formes compliquées de la diverticulite sigmoïdienne (abcès, fistule et péritonite). Gastroenterol Clin Biol 31:3527–3533

Ongolo-Zogo P, Borson O, Garcia P et al (1999) Acute gastroduodenal peptic ulcer perforation: contrast-enhanced and thin-section spiral CT findings in 10 patients. Abdom Imaging 24:329–332

Pagnoux C, Mahr A, Guillevin L (2003) Manifestations abdominales et digestives au cours des vascularites systématiques. Ann Med Interne 154:457–467

Park JJ, Wolff BG, Tollefson MK et al (2005) Meckel diverticulum: the Mayo Clinic experience with 1476 patients (1950–2002). Ann Surg 241:529–533

Pearl JP, McNally MP, Elster EA, Denobile JW (2006) Benign pneumoperitoneum after colonoscopy: a prospective pilot study. Mil Med 171:648–649

Ramakrishinan K, Salinas RC (2007) Peptic ulcer disease. Am Fam Physician 76:1005–1012

Rubesin SE, Levine MS (2003) Radiologic diagnosis of gastrointestinal perforation. Radiol Clin North Am 41:1095–1115

Saif MW, Elfiky A, Salem RR (2007) Gastrointestinal perforation due to bevacizumab in colorectal cancer. Ann Surg Oncol 14:1860–1869

Siu WT, Leong HT, Law BKB et al (2002) Laparoscopic repair for perforated peptic ulcer: a randomized controlled trial. Ann Surg 235:313–319

Tagliacozzo S, Tocchi A (1997) Antimesenteric perforations of the colon during diverticular disease: possible pathogenetic role of ischemia. Dis Colon Rectum 40:1358–1361

Taourel P, Garibaldi F, Arrigoni J et al (2004) Cecal pneumatosis in patients with obstructive colon cancer: correlation of CT findings with bowel viability. AJR Am J Roentgenol 183:1667–1671

Tsuboi M, Takase K, Kaneda I et al (2008) Perforated and nonperforated appendicitis: defect in enhancing appendiceal wall—depiction with multi-detector row CT. Radiology 246:142–147

Tulchinsky H, Madhala-Givon O, Wasserberg N et al (2006) Incidence and management of colonoscopic perforations: 8 years' experience. World J Gastroenterol 12:4211–4213

Yagan N, Auh YH, Fischer A (2009) Extension of air into the right perirenal space after duodenal perforation: CT findings. Radiology 250:740–748

Zins M, Bruel JM, Pochet P et al (2007) Quelle est la valeur diagnostique des différents examens dans la diverticulite simple et compliquée? Quelle doit être la stratégie diagnostique? Gastroenterol Clin Biol 31:3515–3519

Zissin R, Hertz M, Osadchy A, Even Sapir E, Gayer G (2008) Abdominal CT findings in nontraumatic colorectal perforation. Eur J Radiol 65:125–132

Acute Gastrointestinal Bleeding

Benoit Paul Gallix

Contents

1	**Introduction**	329
2	**Epidemiology**	330
3	**Physiopathology and Clinical Findings**	330
4	**CT for Acute GI Bleeding**	331
4.1	CT Technique	331
4.2	CT Findings	334
5	**Potential Pitfalls of MDCT**	336
5.1	False-Positive Results	336
5.2	False-Negative Results	336
6	**Diagnostic Strategies and CT Impact on the Management of Patients with GI Bleeding**	338
6.1	Place of MDCT in the Management of Acute UGIB	338
6.2	Place of MDCT in the Management of Acute LGIB	338
7	**Conclusion**	340
	References	340

B. P. Gallix (✉)
Department of Abdominal Imaging,
Saint Eloi University Hospital-CHU de Montpellier,
80 Avenue Augustin Fliche,
34295 Montpellier Cedex 5, France
e-mail: b-gallix@chu-montpellier.fr

Abstract

Gastrointestinal (GI) bleeding can be subdivided into two categories: acute and clinically overt GI bleeding (hematemesis, melena, and hematochezia) or occult bleeding, identified by an unexplained iron deficiency or positive fecal occult blood testing result, or both. This chapter gives an overview of the epidemiology, clinical findings, and available diagnostic modalities in assessing GI bleeding. We discuss and illustrate the technique, advantages, and limitations of contrast-enhanced multidetector computed tomography for the diagnosis of acute GI bleeding.

1 Introduction

Gastrointestinal (GI) bleeding can be subdivided into two categories: acute and clinically overt GI bleeding (hematemesis, melena, and hematochezia) or occult bleeding, identified by an unexplained iron deficiency or positive fecal occult blood testing result, or both.

Acute GI bleeding is a common and severe clinical disease. The evaluation and treatment of acute GI bleeding are complex and often require a multispeciality approach involving emergency physicians, gastroenterologists, radiologists, and surgeons. Acute GI bleeding is typically classified as either upper GI bleeding (UGIB) or lower GI bleeding (LGIB) based on the suspected location of the bleeding site (Barkun et al. 2003).

The key factor in the management of acute GI bleeding is the assessment and adequate resuscitation of the patient. This must be achieved before diagnosis and specific therapy can be performed.

P. Taourel (ed.), *CT of the Acute Abdomen*, Medical Radiology. Diagnostic Imaging,
DOI: 10.1007/174_2010_139, © Springer-Verlag Berlin Heidelberg 2011

For GI bleeding, endoscopy is the most accurate diagnostic test and upper GI endoscopy should always be performed first after adequate resuscitation in all cases of hematemesis and also in a patient who presents with melena or hematochezia because severe UGIB can present in this way. In patients with LGIB, it is generally accepted that colonoscopy is usually appropriate when bleeding has stopped spontaneously and bowel preparation is possible. However, the usefulness of colonoscopy for the diagnosis of acute massive bleeding is still controversial.

Until recently, computed tomography (CT) was not widely used as a primary diagnostic modality for detection and localization of acute GI bleeding. The introduction of multidetector CT (MDCT) has led to increased image resolution and decreased scanning time. MDCT has the capacity to acquire arterial and portal venous phase images separately, and allows identification of contrast medium extravasation (Yoon et al. 2006).

This chapter gives an overview of the epidemiology, clinical findings, and available diagnostic modalities in assessing GI bleeding. We discuss and illustrate the technique, advantages, and limitations of contrast-enhanced MDCT for the diagnosis of acute GI bleeding.

2   Epidemiology

The incidence of acute UGIB ranges from 48 to 160 per 100,000 adults per year, and acute UGIB is twice as common in men as in women. Acute LGIB is less common, with an incidence of 20 per 100,000 (Lewis et al. 2002; Zhao and Encinosa 2008).

The mortality rate from UGIB ranges from 10 to 14% in patients presenting to the hospital with a bleed, but the mortality rate is 3 times as great when UGIB develops during hospitalization (Lewis et al. 2002). These rates have remained stubbornly high despite the introduction of earlier therapeutic endoscopy and more accurate monitoring of high-risk patients. The mortality rate of acute UGIB is correlated with age and the severity of comorbid disease, as well as the cause of the bleeding. These factors have been unaffected by improvements in endoscopic and surgical treatments, so the number of truly preventable deaths may be quite small (Rockall et al. 1997).

Table 1 Sources of upper gastrointestinal bleeding (Rockall et al. 1995)

Source/findings	Frequency (%)
Peptic ulcer (or gastric erosion)	46
Esophagitis	10
Mallory–Weiss tear	5
Neoplasm	4
Varices	4
Other	6
None	25

The incidence of LGIB ranges from nine to 27 cases per 100,000 adults. The age range of patients with LGIB is 63–77 years. Acute LGIB is 200 times more likely to occur in an 80-year-old than in a 20-year-old (Farrell and Friedman 2005). LGIB occurs more often in men than in women (Hebert et al. 1999). Compared with patients acute UGIB, patients with acute LGIB are significantly less likely to experience shock (19 vs. 35%, respectively) and require fewer blood transfusions (36 vs. 64%). Colonic bleeding necessitates fewer blood transfusions compared with bleeding from the small intestine (Duggan 2001). Acute bleeding in the lower GI tract stops spontaneously in most patients (80%). The overall mortality rate ranges from 2 to 4%. The mortality rate of LGIB ranges from 2 to 4% and is markedly higher when the bleed occurs in an inpatient setting than when patients present with this problem (Longstreth 1997).

3   Physiopathology and Clinical Findings

Bleeding from the upper GI tract invariably presents with hematemesis and/or melena. The vomitus can be bright red (fresh) or the color of ground coffee (altered blood). Melena consists of the passage of black tarry stools caused by bacterial degradation of hemoglobin and is generally due to upper GI sources of bleeding, although small bowel and proximal colonic lesions can also be the cause. Common causes of UGIB are listed in Table 1. Although varices and bleeding from upper GI malignancy account for only 8% of cases, they account for 17% of deaths from upper GI hemorrhage (Rockall et al. 1995).

Table 2 Sources of hematochezia (Zuckerman and Prakash 1999)

Source/finding	Frequency (%)
Diverticulum	17–40
Angiodysplasia	9–21
Colitis (ischemic, infectious, chronic irritable bowel disease, and radiation injury)	2–30
Neoplasia, postpolypectomy bleeding	11–14
Anorectal disease (including rectal varices)	4–10
Upper gastrointestinal bleeding	0–11
Small bowel bleeding	2–9

The passage of bright or dark-red blood via the rectum is usually due to a lower GI cause of bleeding, but this distinction is not absolute, and in a study of patients presenting with significant per rectum bleeding via the rectum, 11% were found to have an upper GI cause (Jensen and Machicado 1998). To distinguish between the two by stool color is not always possible and a diagnostic approach is to perform upper GI endoscopy first if the patient has bright or altered blood passed via the rectum and signs of significant blood loss.

The sources of acute LGIB and their frequency as reported in the literature are listed in Table 2. Colonic diverticula seem to be the most frequent source of hematochezia, followed by angiodysplasias, inflammatory or ischemic colitis, and postpolypectomy bleeding (Zuckerman and Prakash 1999).

Most often, acute GI bleeding have an arterial origin. The arterial supply of the upper GI tract is provided by the celiac axis and the superior mesenteric artery (SMA). Extensive collateralization between the celiac artery and the SMA protects the upper GI tract from ischemic insult and allows embolization procedures to be performed with a low risk of ischemic injury.

Peptic ulcer bleeding has remained the commonest cause of upper GI hemorrhage. Severe ulcer bleeding typically occurs when the ulcer base erodes through the wall of an artery. Arterial erosion can also be due to malignancy of the stomach or duodenum.

The arterial supply of the lower GI tract is provided by branches of both the SMA and the inferior mesenteric artery that are interconnected through a series of arcades. Colonic diverticula, angiodysplasia, solitary rectal ulcer, and postpolypectomy bleeding are generally due to arterial lesion.

GI bleeding can also have a venous origin. Venous bleeding from the upper GI tract is typically due to gastric or esophageal in the setting of portal hypertension, and hemorrhoids are the source of acute LGIB in 5% of patients.

4 CT for Acute GI Bleeding

4.1 CT Technique

The CT diagnosis of acute GI bleeding relies on the ability to identify extravasated intravenous contrast medium within the lumen of the GI tract. Then intravenous contrast medium injection is essential when evaluating a patient with suspected acute GI bleeding. In many cases, bleeding is intermittent and might be slow, thereby limiting detection of the causative lesion. It is essential that the CT be performed while the patient is actively bleeding (Laing et al. 2007). Literature series scanning protocols are summarized in Table 3.

4.1.1 Oral Contrast Medium

If acute GI bleeding is suspected, the CT scan should be performed without prior positive oral contrast medium as it will obscure the ability to detect contrast medium extravasated into the GI lumen. A negative oral contrast medium such as water or PEG is typically not used in the acute setting as the patient may require an urgent CT scan. Negative intraluminal oral contrast medium may also lead to a dilution of the extravasated contrast medium (Stuber et al. 2008).

4.1.2 Unenhanced Scans

Most investigators agree that a preliminary unenhanced CT scan is necessary to detect preexisting high-density material in the bowel lumen, such as pills, sutures, metallic clips, or contrast medium in intestinal lumen (Table 3) (Figs. 1, 2). Jaeckle et al. (2008) published the only original series without using unenhanced acquisition prior to injection. Dose reduction justified this technical approach. However, potential misinterpretation can easily be avoided using an unenhanced scan. Moreover, an unenhanced scan should be performed using low-dose protocols and a relatively thick slice (3–5 mm) to reduce radiation exposure.

Table 3 Scanning protocols from literature studies

Authors	n	Scanner	Flow rate (mL/s)	Oral contrast medium	Scan phases			
					Plain	Arterial	Portal venous	Delayed
Ernst et al. (2003)	24	DSCT	4	None	+	+	0	+
Tew et al. (2004)	13	4 MDCT	3–4	None	+	+	0	0
Yoon et al. (2006)	26	4 MDCT	3.5	None	+	+	0	0
Scheffel et al. (2007)	18	4–64 MDCT	NA	None	+	+	±	0
Jaeckle et al. (2008)	26	16–40 MDCT	4	None	0	+	+	0
Zink et al. (2008)	55	8–64 MDCT	4	None	+	+	0	0
Kennedy et al. (2010)	86	64 MDCT	4–5	None	+	+	0	0

DSCT dual-source computed tomography, *MDCT* multidetector computed tomography, *NA* not available

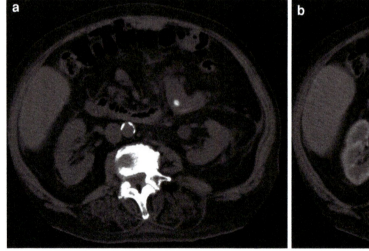
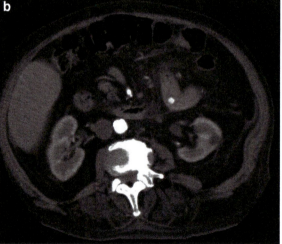

Fig. 1 Pseudo finding of active bleeding. Transverse unenhanced (**a**) and arterial phase (**b**) multidetector computed tomography (MDCT) images in a 82-year-old man who presented with severe hematochezia. An area of hyperat-tenuation is depicted in the small bowel after injection (*arrow*) (**b**). However, this is consistent with a foreign body (probably pills) as is demonstrated on the unenhanced image (*arrow*) (**a**)

4.1.3 Intravenous Contrast Medium Injection

It has been proven that the sensitivity of CT in depicting active GI bleeding is directly correlated with the peak aortic enhancement level (Kuhle and Sheiman 2003). Therefore, dose, flow rate, and scanning time should be optimized for this setting.

For CT imaging of the abdomen in the adult, it is generally accepted that the total dose of iodine necessary to obtain a good-quality injection for both arterial and venous phases is between 500 and 700 mg/kg. Recently published series used high-concentration contrast medium with 350 mg of iodine per milliliter or more. Therefore, 120–150 mL of contrast medium with 350 mg of iodine per milliliter is routinely used. The total amount of contrast medium injected could also be adapted to the patient weight using a dose of 2 mL/kg.

Acute Gastrointestinal Bleeding

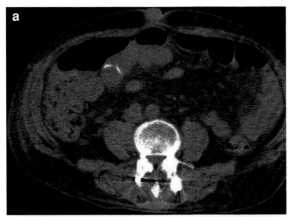

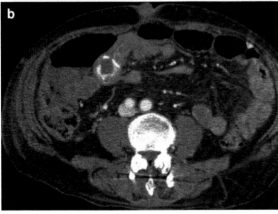

Fig. 2 Bleeding near a surgical suture. Transverse unenhanced (**a**) and arterial phase (**b**) MDCT images in a 63-year-old man with a marked lowering of the hemoglobin level with a history of duodenopancreatectomy with Roux-en-Y anastomosis 8 days before the MDCT. Bleeding from the pancreatojejunal anastomosis was suspected by the surgeon. Suture material of the inferior bowel loop anastomosis (*arrow*) can be mistaken for gastrointestinal (GI) bleeding, but this hyperattenuating area is clearly identified on unenhanced images (*arrow*) (**a**). The arterial phase demonstrates bleeding within the small bowel adjacent to the anastomosis (*arrow*) (**b**). Comparison of images acquired before and after contrast medium injection demonstrates the modification of the preexisting hyperdensity that confirms the bleeding near the surgical suture

Rapid injection is crucial. As shown in Table 3, in most investigations contrast medium is injected at a rate of 4 mL/s or more.

4.1.4 Scanning Phases

CT should be performed during the arterial phase to identify active extravasation of contrast medium. Arterial phase CT was performed in all published series (Table 3). Some authors used an empiric delay, whereas others advocated the use of automatic bolus triggering software with a region of interest placed in the abdominal aorta and a predefined enhancement threshold. The capacity of CT to depict low-grade bleeding is directly related to the level of peak aortic enhancement (Kuhle and Sheiman 2003). With use of MDCT and a contrast medium injection rate of 4 mL/s or more, a peak aortic enhancement of 200 HU can be easily obtained and allows optimal depiction of intravenous contrast medium extravasation. In animal models, the contrast medium extravasation is maximum 8 s after the peak aortic enhancement (Kuhle and Sheiman 2003). In our institution, we use a predefined 150-HU enhancement threshold, and the acquisition starts 5 s after this threshold is obtained in the aorta.

Some authors performed a single postinjection arterial phase acquisition, whereas others performed two acquisitions, frequently arterial and portal venous, or arterial and delayed (Table 3). On the basis of experiments in pig, Dobritz et al. (2009) demonstrated that dual-phase MDCT with arterial and portal venous acquisitions provided higher sensitivity than single-phase CT for detection of small intestinal bleeding. Therefore, they recommended arterial and portal venous acquisitions for the diagnostic workup of patients with acute GI hemorrhage (Fig. 3).

Scanning protocols varied considerably in the published series depending on the type and the generation of the CT scanner. With the latest generation of MDCT scanners (16–64-detector row or more), the following parameters are generally used: detector configuration from 0.5 to 0.625 mm; slice thickness of 1 mm or less; 100 or 120 kV; rotation time less than 0.5 s; a maximum of 200 mA using dose modulation software to reduce exposure to ionizing radiation.

4.1.5 Image Reconstruction and Reading

The acquired data are generally reconstructed into a 2–3-mm-thick axial and coronal section for workstation review and the picture archiving and communication system. The thin slices are also sent to a 3D workstation for review in order for the radiologist to be able to perform multiplanar and maximum intensity projection reconstructions (Figs. 4, 5).

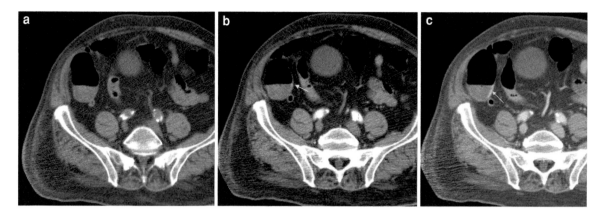

Fig. 3 Active right colonic angiodysplasia hemorrhage. Axial 3-mm maximum MDCT images were acquired before injection (**a**), during the arterial phase (**b**), and during the portal venous phase (**c**). During the arterial phase (**b**) a very subtle area of hyperattenuation is identified at the air–fluid level in the right colon (*arrow*). With only the arterial phase image it is very difficult to affirm this is consistent with a focus of bleeding. During the portal venous phase (**c**) the extravasation increases in volume and confirms active bleeding. The GI bleeding originated from an angiodysplasia of the cecum. The patient underwent repeated and oriented colonoscopy that confirmed the diagnosis. The bleeding area was treated with an argon laser during the colonoscopy

4.2 CT Findings

4.2.1 Positive Diagnosis of GI Bleeding

The CT diagnosis of acute GI bleeding depends on the ability to identify the presence of extravasation of contrast medium within the bowel lumen. An active contrast medium extravasation is defined as a focal area of high attenuation (generally higher than 100 HU) located within the bowel lumen. To avoid potential misinterpretation caused by preexisting high-density material in the bowel lumen, the area of high attenuation should not be visible on the unenhanced scan (Fig. 1). In the case of active extravasation, the area of attenuation generally increases in size but decreases in density on portal or delayed phase images owing to diffusion and dilution of the extravasated contrast medium (Fig. 3).

A variety of patterns have been described, linear, jetlike, swirled, ellipsoid, and pooled configurations, or the entire bowel lumen may be filled, resulting in a hyperattenuating loop (Laing et al. 2007). Some authors have applied attenuation criteria for the diagnosis of acute GI bleeding. Willmann et al. (2002) reported that the focal attenuation of active extravasation on MDCT ranged from 91 to 274 HU and Yoon et al. (2006) used a threshold value of 90 HU. Like Laing et al. (2007), we prefer to compare unenhanced images with arterial and/or portal images to confirm the bleeding.

Evaluation with CT angiography may also demonstrate the cause of the bleed such as GI tract tumor, GI ulcer, hemorrhoid bleeding rectal ulcer (Fig. 4), and colon diverticular bleed (Fig. 6) (Kennedy et al. 2010). In addition to detection of active bleeding, an advantage of contrast-enhanced MDCT is the ability to demonstrate morphologic changes in the GI tract, which could suggest specific conditions causing acute GI bleeding such as intestinal tumors or small bowel diverticula (Fig. 7) (Yoon et al. 2006; Ernst et al. 2003).

4.2.2 Performances of CT for the Diagnostic Workup of a Patient Suffering from Acute GI Bleeding

Kuhle and Sheiman (2003) showed in a porcine model that active colonic hemorrhage is detectable by single-detector-row helical CT, if contrast-enhanced blood is extravasating at a rate of 0.3 mL/min or higher. More recently, Dobritz et al. (2008) demonstrated that dual-phase MDCT provides high sensitivity and specificity in the detection of intestinal bleeding with bleeding velocities of 0.5–1.0 mL/min. They suggested that MDCT has the ability to depict acute LGIB which may exceed the lower limit of 0.5 mL/s classically cited for mesenteric angiography.

Numerous studies (Table 4) have shown that MDCT angiography is sensitive and highly specific for diagnosing acute GI bleeding. MDCT seems to be

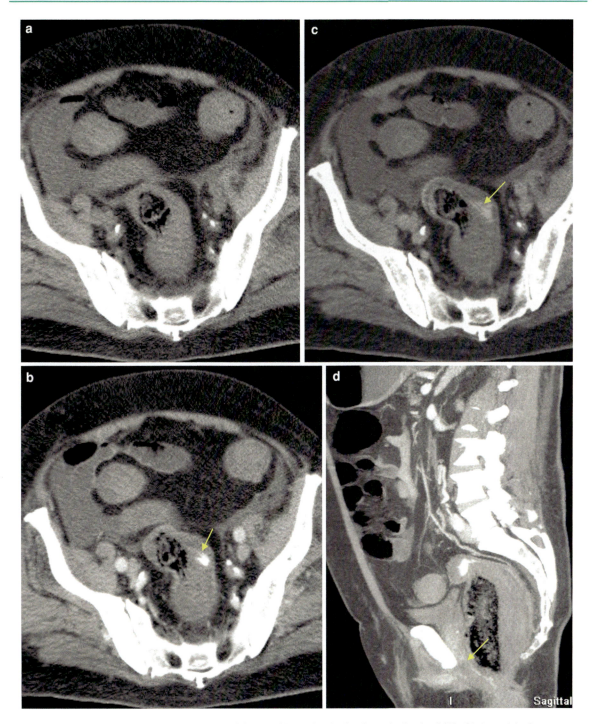

Fig. 4 Bleeding due to rectal ulcer in a 67-year-old man with prior history of liver gastric surgery and severe hematochezia. The patient received anticoagulants and anastomosis bleeding was suspected. A first colonoscopy was inconclusive owing to the presence of blood in the colon. Transverse unenhanced (**a**), arterial phase (**b**), portal venous phase (**c**), and sagittal maximum intensity projection (MIP) (**d**) images demonstrate rectal distension with blood. In the arterial phase image a high-density focal area is clearly visible (**b**) (*arrow*) in the upper part of the rectum compatible with active bleeding. During the portal venous phase (**c**) the extravasation decreases in density but increases in volume and confirms active bleeding. Sagittal MIP allows precise localization of the bleeding (**d**). Repeated colonoscopy after stabilization and preparation demonstrates the presence of a solitary ulcer with active bleeding that was treated with a clip and epinephrine injection

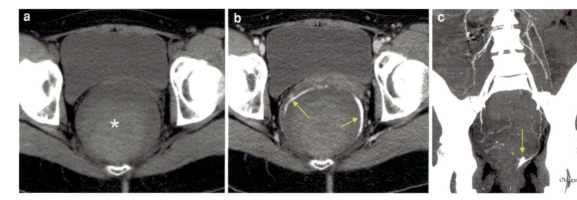

Fig. 5 Hemorrhoidal rectal bleeding. Computed tomography (CT) images in a 55-year-old woman who presented with bright-red blood passed via the rectum. **a** Axial unenhanced MDCT shows the rectum full of a hyperattenuatting clot (*asterisk*). **b** During the portal phase, the CT image demonstrates extravasated contrast medium (*arrows*) in the rectal lumen at the peripheral part of the clot. **c** Coronal MIP from portal phase acquisition allows precise localization of the bleeding (*arrow*) and the dilation of both hemorrhoidal arteries and veins. Surgery confirmed the hemorrhoidal rectal bleeding

superior to global visceral angiography in the detection of acute GI hemorrhage. Recently, a large retrospective evaluation of the performance of CT in detection and localization of clinically active GI bleeding was published by Kennedy et al. (2010). The overall sensitivity, specificity, accuracy, and positive and negative predictive values of CT were 79, 95, 91, 86, and 92%, respectively. Kennedy et al. concluded that MDCT provides valuable information for the localization of the bleeding source and that CT should be performed first to determine the appropriateness of catheter angiography and guide mesenteric catheterization.

5 Potential Pitfalls of MDCT

Several potential pitfalls should be recognized in order to reliably analyze MDCT examination performed for suspected acute GI bleeding.

5.1 False-Positive Results

Preexisting hyperattenuating material can be present within the GI lumen and mimic contrast medium extravasation. These pitfalls can easily be avoided by performing an unenhanced scan before intravenous contrast medium injection, and by comparing very carefully images obtained before and after contrast medium injection. Multiplanar image registration could be helpful in order to clearly localize on multiplanar reconstruction the hyperdense area detected after injection on the images obtained before injection of contrast medium. This preexisting hyperdense material could have a different origin: GI tract surgical suture (Fig. 2), a foreign body such as pills (Fig. 1), contrast medium within the GI lumen from to previous CT examination.

Depiction of a false hyperattenuating area can be due to cone beam artifacts. These artifacts are observed at the air-fluid level interface and are commonly accentuated by movement artifacts. This artifact creates an area of hyperdensity that can be mistaken for acute extravasation (Stuber et al. 2008). This pitfall can be avoided by performing arterial and portal venous phase acquisitions after injection; the probability of the artifact being reproduced in both series is very poor.

Mucosal enhancement can also be mistaken for active extravasation, especially when the bowel loop is collapsed (Laing et al. 2007). Again, dual-phase acquisition after injection is helpful by demonstrating the absence of an increase in size of the hyperattenuating area, and the absence of contrast medium diffusing within the lumen on the portal venous phase image.

5.2 False-Negative Results

The most common cause for negative CT findings is the cessation of the bleeding at the time of the examination. It is known that even massive acute GI

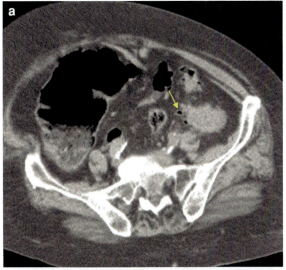
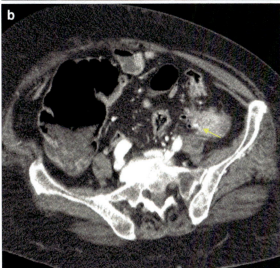

Fig. 6 Acute diverticular hemorrhage in an 84-year-old woman with hematochezia. **a** An unenhanced axial MDCT image through the level of the sigmoid colon demonstrates numerous diverticula (*arrow*). **b** A contrast-enhanced axial MDCT image at the same level shows a bleeding diverticulum (*arrow*). Subsequent colonoscopy performed after bowel preparation revealed multiple diverticula within the descending and sigmoid colon, with active bleeding identified at the junction between the descending and sigmoid colon. Local treatment (clip) was successful

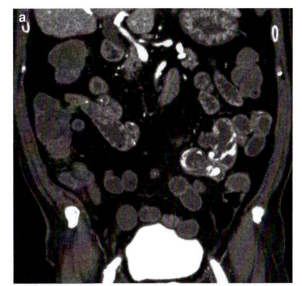
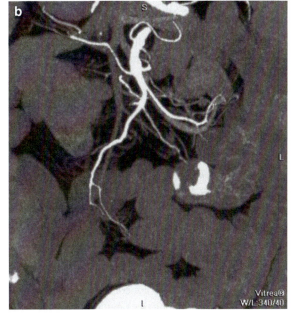

Fig. 7 Bleeding complicating an inflamed jejunal diverticulum. **a** A coronal arterial CT image obtained in a 22-year-old man with massive lower GI bleeding demonstrates extravasated contrast medium in the small bowel lumen. The extravasation was located at the distal part of the jejunum in a large diverticulum. Other diverticula were identified on CT in the jejunum. **b** Coronal arterial phase MIP reconstruction reveals massive intraluminal bleeding in the diverticulum and allows precise localization of the bleeding diverticulum. The patient underwent emergency bowel resection. Surgery revealed the presence of numerous jejunal diverticuli andthe bleeding source to be a large inflamed jenunal diverticulum

hemorrhage can be intermittent, and failure to demonstrate active bleeding may, therefore, not prove the absence of active foci of bleeding. This phenomenon of intermittent hemorrhage may explain some of the false-negative MDCT findings. It is crucial to perform CT acquisition at the time of active bleeding.

6 Diagnostic Strategies and CT Impact on the Management of Patients with GI Bleeding

The triage and evaluation of patients with GI hemorrhage remains variable and largely institution-specific. To best manage bleeding, it is useful to stratify patients on the basis of the severity of the hemorrhage and the suspected level of the bleeding.

6.1 Place of MDCT in the Management of Acute UGIB

The commonest cause of UGIB is peptic ulceration, which accounts for approximately 50% of cases where the cause of UGIB is identified. Other causes of severe UGIB are listed in Table 1. Varices and bleeding from upper GI malignancy can lead to very severe bleeding with a high mortality rate. In patients with hematemesis, early endoscopy should be performed as soon as the patient is stabilized. In most of cases upper GI endoscopy allows a precise diagnosis, by showing the bleeding area, and also permits the treatment of the bleeding foci by using clips, thermocoagulation, or sclerosant injection in combination with epinephrine injection.

As with other causes of upper GI hemorrhage, the initial management of acute variceal hemorrhage due to cirrhosis is resuscitation with endoscopy performed when the patient is hemodynamically stable.

The impact of MDCT in the management of UGIB is limited. MDCT should be reserved for patients for whom endoscopies were noncontributive, especially because massive bleeding does not allow the bleeding to be localized.

However, since percutaneous embolization can be considered as an alternative to surgery for patients for whom endoscopic therapy has failed to stop the bleeding, we think that MDCT should be performed before angiography in order to localize the site of bleeding and to guide mesenteric catheterization.

Hemorrhage from Roux-en-Y surgery after pancreaticoduodenectomy or gastric bypass is a critical condition because of difficult accessibility when using upper GI endoscopy. In this setting, postsurgical GI bleeding patients are also candidates for diagnostic MDCT. MDCT is the simplest technique available for bleeding localization in this specific condition. MDCT is also the first recommended imaging modality in the case of severe UGIB in patients with known gastroduodenal or pancreatic malignancy (Fig. 8).

Pancreatic pseudocysts are often combined with various complications, including hemorrhage with pseudoaneurysm formation, which may necessitate prompt embolization or surgery. In patients with GI bleeding and known pancreatitis (acute or chronic), MDCT should be the first recommended imaging modality.

6.2 Place of MDCT in the Management of Acute LGIB

In patients with hematochezia and concurrent hemodynamic instability, upper GI endoscopy should be performed first to exclude an UGIB source. If a patient with acute LGIB is a suitable candidate for colonoscopy, then colonoscopy should be the first test. Since colonoscopy requires a minimum of 6 h bowel preparation in order for it to be safe and effective (without preparation, the view through the endoscope will be obscured by feces and blood), this only applies to patients whose bleeding is not so acute and can safely wait at least 6 h before treatment. MDCT should be the next test used if the patient is not a suitable candidate for colonoscopy, or if colonoscopy fails to diagnose the cause and site of bleeding. This is because MDCT is available at all hours without advanced preparation. If the CT findings are positive, and if CT localizes the bleeding site, the patient should be referred to the interventional radiology department for embolization of the bleeding source.

If CT fails to localize the bleeding site and the bleeding is continuing, the patient should be explored using a nuclear imaging procedure using ^{99m}Tc-labeled red blood cells. However, this technique has numerous limitations, such as imprecise anatomic localization of bleeding, time-consuming procedure, and limited availability for timely after-hours studies.

Table 4 Performances of CT for the depiction of gastrointestinal bleeding

Authors	n	Bleeding site location sensitivity	Specificity	Overall accuracy
Ernst et al. (2003)	24	(15/24) 79%	NA	NA
Tew et al. (2004)	13	(7/13) 53%	NA	NA
Yoon et al. (2006)	26	(20/22) 91%	99%	88%
Scheffel et al. (2007)	18	(15/18) 83%	NA	NA
Jaeckle et al. (2008)	26	(24/26) 93%	NA	81%
Zink et al. (2008)	55	50%	100%	NA
Kennedy et al. (2010)	86	(19/22) 86%	95%	91%

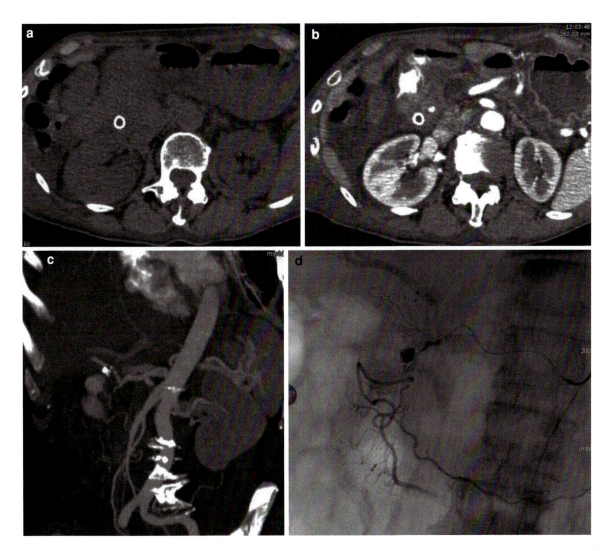

Fig. 8 Bleeding from an erosion of the gastroduodenal artery in a 48-year-old man with acute mild upper GI bleeding following pancreatic malignancy and metallic stenting of the common bile duct. **a** Unenhanced and **b** contrast-enhanced axial CT images during the arterial phase demonstrate the massive contrast extravasation with a complete enhancement of the duodenum (*arrow*). **c** Coronal MIP from arterial phase acquisition allows precise localization of the bleeding (*arrow*) in order to guide selective angiography of the gastroduedenal artery (**d**). Subsequent coil embolization was performed

For patients whose bleeding is so severe that definitive therapy is required in 2 h or less, the only available test is MDCT. Once MDCT results are available, positive or negative, the interventional radiology and emergency surgery attending physicians should work together to determine the appropriate treatment for the patient.

7 Conclusion

Acute GI bleeding occurs increasingly with age and can be associated with substantial morbidity and mortality. Recent advances have improved the endoscopic, radiologic, and surgical management of patients with LGIB. However, treatment decisions are still often based on local expertise and preference.

The first choice investigation for both UGIB and LGIB bleeding is endoscopy. It allows accurate diagnosis and specific treatment in most cases. However, there are times when endoscopy will be unsuccessful and it will be necessary to use other modalities. In these circumstances MDCT has become the modality of choice: it has the advantage of being readily available at all hours without advanced preparation, is noninvasive, and is rapid. Moreover, CT scanning of the abdomen can be performed immediately during hemorrhagic episodes, and bleeding can be depicted within the small bowel, an anatomic region not readily accessible to endoscopy. MDCT also provides valuable information that can be used to determine the appropriateness of catheter angiography and to guide mesenteric catheterization if a bleeding source is localized.

References

Barkun A, Bardou M, Marshall JK (2003) Consensus recommendations for managing patients with nonvariceal upper gastrointestinal bleeding. Ann Intern Med 139:843–857

Dobritz M, Engels HP, Schneider A, Wieder H, Feussner H, Rummeny EJ, Stollfuss JC (2008) Evaluation of dual-phase multi-detector-row CT for detection of intestinal bleeding using an experimental bowel model. Eur Radiol 19(4):875–881

Dobritz M, Engels HP, Schneider A, Bauer J, Rummeny EJ (2009) Detection of intestinal bleeding with multi-detector row CT in an experimental setup. How many acquisitions are necessary? Eur Radiol 19(12):2862–2869

Duggan JM (2001) Transfusion in gastrointestinal Haemorrhage, when and how much? Aliment Pharmacol Ther 15(8): 1109–1113

Ernst O, Bulois P, Saint-Drenant S, Leroy C, Paris JC, Sergent G (2003) Helical CT in acute lower gastrointestinal bleeding. Eur Radiol 13(1):114–117

Farrell JJ, Friedman LS (2005) The management of lower gastrointestinal bleeding. Aliment Pharmacol Ther 21(11): 1281–1298

Hebert PC, Wells G, Blajchman MA, Marshall J, Martin C, Pagliarello G et al (1999) A multicenter, randomized, controlled clinical trial of transfusion requirements in critical care. Transfusion Requirements in Critical Care Investigators, Canadian Critical Care Trials Group. N Engl J Med 340(6):409–417

Jaeckle T, Stuber G, Hoffmann MH, Jeltsch M, Schmitz BL, Aschoff AJ (2008) Detection and localization of acute upper and lower gastrointestinal (GI) bleeding with arterial phase multi-detector row helical CT. Eur Radiol 18(7):1406–1413

Jensen DM, Machicado GA (1998) Diagnosis and treatment of severe hematochezia. The role of urgent colonoscopy after purge. Gastroenterology 95(6):1569–1574

Kennedy DW, Laing CJ, Tseng LH, Rosenblum DI, Tamarkin SW (2010) Detection of active gastrointestinal hemorrhage with CT angiography: a 4(1/2)-year retrospective review. J Vasc Interv Radiol 21(6):848–855

Kuhle WG, Sheiman RG (2003) Detection of active colonic hemorrhage with use of helical CT: findings in a swine model. Radiology 228(3):743–752

Laing CJ, Tobias T, Rosenblum DI, Banker WL, Tseng L, Tamarkin SW (2007) Acute gastrointestinal bleeding: emerging role of multidetector CT angiography and review of current imaging techniques. Radiographics 27:1055–1070

Lewis JD, Bilker WB, Brensinger C, Farrar JT, Strom BL (2002) Hospitalization and mortality rates from peptic ulcer disease and GI bleeding in the 1990s: relationship to sales of nonsteroidal anti-inflammatory drugs and acid suppression medications. Am J Gastroenterol 97:2540–2549

Longstreth GF (1997) Epidemiology and outcome of patients hospitalized with acute lower gastrointestinal hemorrhage: a population-based study. Am J Gastroenterol 92(3):419–424

Rockall TA, Logan RF, Devlin HB, Northfield TC (1995) Incidence and mortality from acute upper gastrointestinal haemorrhage in the United Kingdom. Steering Committee and members of the National Audit of Acute Upper Gastrointestinal Haemorrhage. Br Med J 1311(6999):222–226

Rockall TA, Logan RF, Devlin HB, Northfield TC (1997) Influencing the practice and outcome in acute upper gastrointestinal haemorrhage. Steering Committee of the National Audit of Acute Upper Gastrointestinal Haemorrhage. Gut 41(5):606–611

Scheffel H, Pfammatter T, Wildi S, Bauerfeind P, Marincek B, Alkadhi H (2007) Acute gastrointestinal bleeding: detection of source and etiology with multi-detector-row CT. Eur Radiol 17(6):1555–1565

Stuber T, Hoffmann MH, Stuber G, Klass O, Feuerlein S, Aschoff AJ (2009) Pitfalls in detection of acute gastrointestinal bleeding with multi-detector row helical CT. Abdom Imaging 34(4):476–482

Tew K, Davies RP, Jadun CK, Kew J (2004) MDCT of acute lower gastrointestinal bleeding. AJR Am J Roentgenol 182(2):427–430

Willmann JK, Roos JE, Platz A, Pfammatter T, Hilfiker PR, Marincek B, Weishaupt D (2008) Multidetector CT: detection of active hemorrhage in patients with blunt abdominal trauma. AJR Am J Roentgenol 179(2):437–444

Yoon W et al (2006) Acute massive gastrointestinal bleeding: detection and localization with arterial phase multidetector row helical CT. Radiology 239:160–167

Zhao Y, Encinosa W (2008) Hospitalizations for gastrointestinal bleeding in 1998 and 2006. HCUP Statistical Brief 65. Agency for Healthcare Research and Quality, Rockville. http://www.hcup-us.ahrq.gov/reports/statbriefs/sb65.pdf. Accessed 23 Nov 2009

Zink SI, Ohki SK, Stein B, Zambuto DA, Rosenberg RJ, Choi JJ, Tubbs DS (2008) Noninvasive evaluation of active lower gastrointestinal bleeding: comparison between contrast-enhanced MDCT and 99mTc-labeled RBC scintigraphy. AJR Am J Roentgenol 191(4):1107–1114

Zuckerman GR, Prakash C (1999) Acute lower intestinal bleeding. Part II: etiology, therapy, and outcomes. Gastrointest Endosc 49(2):228–238

Intra- and Retroperitoneal Hemorrhages

Philippe Otal, Julien Auriol, Marie-Charlotte Delchier, Marie-Agnès Marachet, and Hervé Rousseau

Contents

1	**Introduction**.. 343
2	**Intraperitoneal Bleeding**............................ 344
2.1	Common CT Features of Intraperitoneal Bleeding................................ 344
2.2	Intraperitoneal Bleeding of Hepatic Origin.............. 344
2.3	Intraperitoneal Bleeding of Splenic Origin 347
2.4	Intraperitoneal Bleeding of Miscellaneous Gastrointestinal Origin 348
2.5	Intraperitoneal Bleeding of Gynecological Origin... 348
3	**Retroperitoneal Bleeding** 348
3.1	Ruptured AAA.. 349
3.2	Perirenal Bleeding 350
3.3	Periadrenal Bleeding 352
3.4	Peripancreatic Bleeding.................................. 354
3.5	Systemic Causes of Spontaneous Retroperitoneal Bleeding.............................. 355
4	**Conclusion** 356
	References.. 356

P. Otal (✉) · J. Auriol · M.-C. Delchier · M.-A. Marachet · H. Rousseau
Service de radiologie, Hôpital Rangueil,
1, Avenue Jean-Poulhès, TSA 50032,
31059 Toulouse Cedex 9, France
e-mail: otal.p@chu-toulouse.fr

Abstract

Spontaneous intraperitoneal or retroperitoneal hemorrhage can result from a vast variety of causes. When exception is made for hemoperitoneum caused by gynecological conditions, best explored by transvaginal ultrasonography, computed tomography (CT) is, in most cases, the best imaging modality, allowing not only the localization of the bleeding, but also the analysis of the underlying cause. Despite the high diagnostic performance of magnetic resonance imaging in most of the diseases described in this chapter, CT offers many advantages, such as its high availability in an emergency and a much shorter scan time.

1 Introduction

Spontaneous intraperitoneal or retroperitoneal hemorrhage can result from a vast variety of causes. When exception is made for hemoperitoneum caused by gynecological conditions, best explored by transvaginal ultrasonography (US), computed tomography (CT) is, in most cases, the best imaging modality, allowing not only the localization of the bleeding, but also the analysis of the underlying cause. Despite the high diagnostic performance of magnetic resonance imaging (MRI) in most of the diseases described in this chapter, CT offers many advantages, such as its high availability in an emergency and a much shorter scan time.

P. Taourel (ed.), *CT of the Acute Abdomen*, Medical Radiology. Diagnostic Imaging,
DOI: 10.1007/174_2010_87, © Springer-Verlag Berlin Heidelberg 2011

2 Intraperitoneal Bleeding

Hemoperitoneum is a common finding in abdominal traumatism. Nontraumatic hemoperitoneum is a less frequent situation, requiring prompt diagnosis and treatment. Hemoperitoneum induced by a hepatic, splenic, or peritoneal tumor or gynecological disorders (such as ectopic pregnancy or ruptured ovarian cyst) is more common than intraperitoneal bleeding associated with syndromic hemolysis, elevated levels of liver enzymes, and low platelet counts (HELLP syndrome), blood dyscrasia, or anticoagulation therapy. An unsuspected diagnosis is often made because the clinical symptoms are not specific, consisting of abdominal pain and hypovolemic shock. Thus, imaging plays a determinant role in the management of such situations. Although US is an efficient technique in the diagnosis of hemoperitoneum, its performance is limited in the workup of the cause. CT is able to detect a small amount of intraperitoneal blood and allows the diagnosis of most nontraumatic causes. US remains the modality of choice for the diagnosis of hemorrhage arising from the pelvis, particularly ectopic pregnancy.

2.1 Common CT Features of Intraperitoneal Bleeding

Intraperitoneal effusion of blood from the site of bleeding depends both on gravity and on anatomy. The most dependent compartments of the peritoneal cavity are the hepatorenal fossa (Morison pouch) and the pelvic cul-de-sac (pouch of Douglas). Although blood effusion originating from the liver usually reaches the pelvis along the right paracolic gutter, the communication between the perisplenic space and the left paracolic gutter is limited by the left phrenicocolic ligament.

The CT density of intraperitoneal blood depends on several factors. First, when a clot forms, hemoglobin concentrates and densities increase up to 90 HU (New and Aronow 1976). Nevertheless, intraperitoneal blood appears with low attenuation in the case of low hematocrit (Levine et al. 1996). The hematocrit effect designates the dependent sedimentation of red blood cells. The CT appearance of intraperitoneal blood also depends on its age. Clot

lysis starts within several days and results in density attenuation reduction toward that of water. When clot resorption is inhomogeneous or in the case of intermittent rebleeding, the CT appearance becomes more heterogeneous (Wolverson et al. 1983).

When the diagnosis of intraperitoneal bleeding is made, localization of its source is a challenging issue for CT because an emergent radiological or surgical hemostasis may be obtained. The sentinel clot sign describes the relatively higher attenuating hematoma that tends to form near the bleeding site (Fig. 1). Visualization of the images with a narrow window width is helpful in the case of a low-attenuation gradient between the hematoma and the surrounding structures. Localization of the bleeding source is sometimes indicated by an active arterial extravasation of the intravenous contrast material. A delayed acquisition sometimes reveals a low-grade extravasation or allows a better understanding of the distribution of the extravasated contrast material. Even when no extravasation is depicted, contrast material injection is essential in the diagnosis of the bleeding source because it may reveal solid abdominal organ abnormalities.

2.2 Intraperitoneal Bleeding of Hepatic Origin

Hepatic conditions resulting in spontaneous intraperitoneal bleeding are dominated by hypervascular neoplasm.

2.2.1 Hepatocellular Carcinoma

Spontaneous rupture of hepatocellular carcinoma (HCC) is less frequent in Europe and America than in Asia and Africa, where it occurs in up to 14% of cases, probably owing to the size of the tumor at diagnosis. Several theories have been advanced to explain spontaneous rupture of HCC (Mortele et al. 2003): (1) rupture of a parasitic artery or vein (e.g., inferior phrenic vessel), (2) laceration of superficial HCC, occurring spontaneously or as a consequence of a minor trauma, and (3) complete hepatic vein occlusion by vascular invasion. Large peripheral HCC, with no overlying parenchyma, is more prone to bleed (Kanematsu et al. 1992). The manifestation of HCC bleeding ranges from intratumoral minor bleeding to intraperitoneal tumoral rupture through

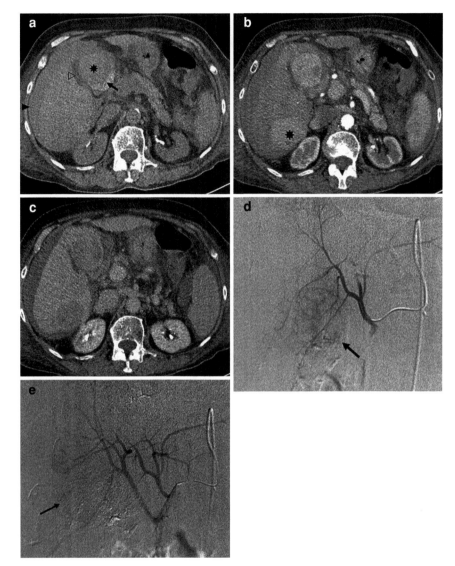

Fig. 1 Intraperitoneal bleeding caused by a ruptured hepatocellular carcinoma (HCC). a On unenhanced computed tomography (CT) with appropriate windowing, a subcapsular sentinel clot (*arrow*) is present around a hepatic mass (*star*) in the caudate lobe. Fluid in the peritoneal space (*closed triangle*) is hyperdense compared with bile in the gallbladder (*open triangle*). b On enhanced CT, the hepatic mass shows the usual enhancement of HCC in the arterial phase. A second lesion is present in the posterior aspect of the right lobe (*star*). Fibrotic changes of liver manifest themselves as capsular irregularity. c In the portal phase, both hepatic lesions show typical washout. d The arterial feeding of the hepatic mass is confirmed by selective angiography performed before chemoembolization. e Devascularization of the HCC after injection of an emulsion of doxorubicin and lipiodol followed by Gelfoam particles. The second lesion appears on this nonselective angiogram (*arrow*)

subcapsular hematoma. Right hypochondrial pain and shock dominate the symptoms. Diagnosis relies more on CT than on depiction of blood-stained ascites. A subcapsular sentinel clot is often present (Fig. 1). Even when contrast material injection does not reveal the specific enhancement pattern of HCC (early enhancement and washout), diagnosis can be advanced when a subcapsular mass is visible in a cirrhotic liver. When vital prognosis is not threatened, MRI can be considered as a very reliable diagnostic tool for both HCC and hemorrhagic complications. Angiography has no role to play in the diagnosis of ruptured HCC, but transarterial catheter embolization is often the best therapeutic option in patients with very high risk of postoperative morbidity and mortality (Kim et al. 2006).

Hemoperitoneum can be encountered in a cirrhotic patient without HCC, usually attributed to the rupture of intraperitoneal varices from portal hypertension. Nevertheless, no specific cause is found in one third of patients (DeSitter and Rector 1984).

2.2.2 Benign Hepatocellular Tumor

Although intraperitoneal bleeding from a hepatic origin suggests the diagnosis of HCC when the liver is cirrhotic, adenoma is the more frequent cause of

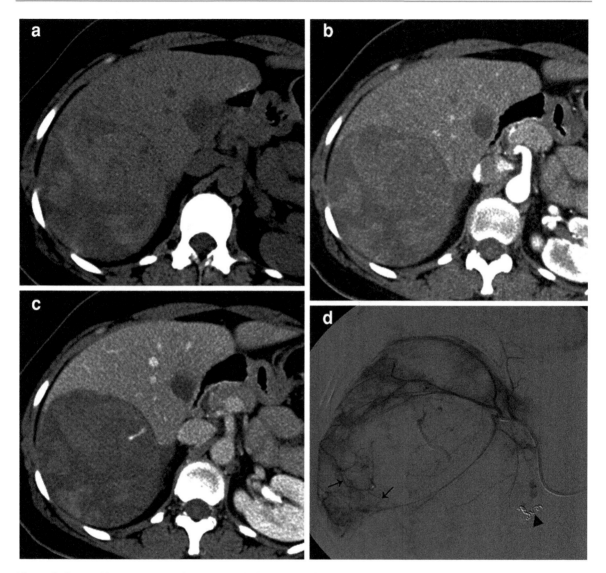

Fig. 2 Patient with spontaneous intraperitoneal bleeding caused by hepatocellular adenoma in a 22-year-old woman. a Precontrast CT shows a focal intrahepatic bleeding. b In the arterial phase of contrast enhancement, no change is visible in the hematoma. c In the portal phase, an extravasation appears inside the lesion. Otherwise, no tumor staining is depicted. d An angiogram is obtained during the embolization procedure. Coils (*closed triangle*) are seen in the feeding vessels of the inferior aspect of the tumor. Selective opacification of another arterial branch feeding the mass shows peripheral centripetal vessel (*arrows*) characteristics of adenoma

hepatic tumor bleeding in women of childbearing age with a prolonged use of oral contraceptives (Meissner 1998). Metabolic disorders such as type 1 glycogen storage disease or Gaucher disease are far less common. Although adenoma is solitary in most cases, it is not uncommonly associated with focal nodular hyperplasia. The status of adenomatosis is a rare condition, defined by the presence of at least ten lesions. The risk of spontaneous bleeding of hepatic adenoma is high enough, besides the potential transformation in HCC, to indicate a preventive treatment, either surgery or embolization. Recent advances in pathology have allowed the individualization of subgroups of hepatic adenomas more prone to spontaneous bleeding (Bioulac-Sage et al. 2007). Imaging suggests the diagnosis when intrahepatic, subcapsular, or intraperitoneal hemorrhage is related to a hypervascular tumor and when the liver does not show

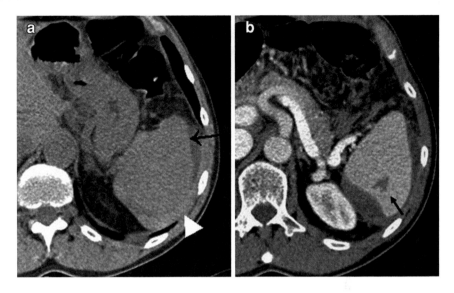

Fig. 3 Spontaneous splenic rupture in a young patient with mononucleosis infection. **a** Precontrast CT shows a perisplenic peritoneal effusion with a sentinel clot (*arrow*). **b** Splenic fracture appears after intravenous contrast material injection (*arrow*)

fibrotic changes (Fig. 2). Selective embolization of the hepatic artery can be proposed as the first approach in the management of patients with hemorrhaging hepatocellular adenomas (Stoot et al. 2007). Follow-up of small (less than 5 cm) steatotic adenomas in female patients is recommended by some teams because the risk of complication is low in that particular group (Dokmak et al. 2009).

Unlike adenoma, focal nodular hyperplasia is usually discovered incidentally, and spontaneous rupture has rarely been reported (Becker et al. 1995).

2.2.3 Hemangioma

Hemangioma is the most common benign hepatic tumor. It rarely becomes symptomatic. Local compression signs (pain, vomiting) are more frequent than spontaneous hemorrhage (Casillas et al. 2000). Pregnancy is an established condition of higher risk of rupture, in association or not in association with consumptive coagulopathy, HELLP syndrome, or cocaine abuse.

2.2.4 Metastasis

Spontaneous rupture of liver metastases is rare (Casillas et al. 2000). In most of the reported cases, primary cancer originates from lung, kidney, and melanoma. Colon, pancreas, gallbladder, testicular cancers, and choriocarcinoma also produce hepatic metastases prone to spontaneous bleeding. Bleeding is favored by different factors, such as necrosis (spontaneous or chemotherapy-induced), increased abdominal pressure (caused by straining, coughing), subcapsular location, and local venous congestion resulting from tumor obstruction. In this situation of palliative care, angiographic embolization is a valuable tool.

2.2.5 HELLP Syndrome

This syndrome was first described by Weinstein (1982). It is a serious obstetric condition, in preeclamptic or eclamptic women, associated with hemolysis, elevated levels of liver enzymes, and low platelet count, and is able to evolve quickly toward hepatic necrosis or infarction, and disseminated intravascular coagulopathy. US is often the first imaging modality used to rule out gallbladder disease in a patient presenting with right upper quadrant pain. Even if subcapsular and intrahepatic hematoma can be diagnosed by US, contrast-enhanced CT is the best modality to depict not only the hemorrhagic complications (hematoma, liver rupture, hemoperitoneum) but also the ischemic ones, with hepatic infarction and their characteristic peripheral wedge-shaped areas (Nunes et al. 2005).

2.3 Intraperitoneal Bleeding of Splenic Origin

Spontaneous splenic rupture is known to occur in pathological conditions such as infection (mononucleosis, malaria) and metabolic disorders (amyloidosis, Gaucher disease) (Fig. 3). Uncommonly, the

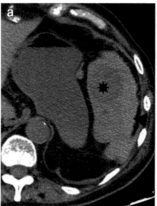 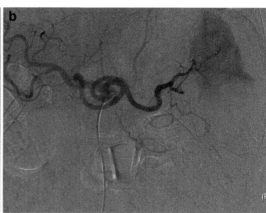

Fig. 4 Spontaneous splenic rupture in a patient with melanoma and splenic metastases. **a** Precontrast CT shows hemoperitoneum (*closed triangle*) around the spleen. A spontaneously hypointense splenic mass is visible (*star*). **b** Celiac artery opacification demonstrates a poorly enhanced lesion of the inferior lesion of the spleen, responsible for splenic rupture

underlying pathological process is a tumor, either a congenital cyst or neoplasm (hemangiomatosis, angiosarcoma, leukemia, lymphoma, metastasis) (Fig. 4). CT is obviously the modality of choice for the diagnosis of splenic rupture and the depiction of an underlying mass. Rupture of an accessory spleen has rarely been reported and is also best depicted by CT.

In the differential diagnosis of bleeding splenic tumor, particularly hemangioma, the possibility of peliosis must be kept in mind: this rare condition of unknown cause results in the development of blood-filled cavities in the spleen and, more rarely, the liver, lymph nodes, and bone marrow. These masslike lesions demonstrate contrast pooling and may also rupture into the peritoneal cavity.

Spontaneous rupture of splenic artery aneurysm yields a high rate of mortality, estimated to be approximately 36% (Shanley et al. 1996). Splenic artery aneurysms are much more frequent in women, and the risk of rupture is particularly increased during pregnancy. Even if plain film may reveal the classic "signet ring" in the left upper quadrant, CT angiography is the best diagnostic modality prior to percutaneous embolization.

Intraperitoneal hemorrhage may be the manifestation of vascular complication of pancreatitis when a pseudoaneurysm ruptures in the peritoneal cavity. Because retroperitoneal complications are more frequent, this condition is detailed in Sect. 3.4.

2.5 Intraperitoneal Bleeding of Gynecological Origin

Ectopic pregnancy or ruptured ovarian cyst is the most common cause of intraperitoneal hemorrhage from gynecological origin. If a diagnosis is made on the basis of clinical and biological features, transvaginal US is the best modality to depict both the hemoperitoneum and its underlying cause. If the clinical findings are nonspecific, CT is often the first imaging modality applied, but the depiction of a hemoperitoneum associated with adnexal abnormalities, cystic or not, should result in the realization of transvaginal US, which allows a better characterization of the lesions, unless the hemodynamic status of the patient requires an emergent laparoscopy.

3 Retroperitoneal Bleeding

2.4 Intraperitoneal Bleeding of Miscellaneous Gastrointestinal Origin

Peptic ulcer is very uncommonly responsible for intraperitoneal hemorrhage. CT is able to describe the gastric origin of the bleeding unless radiopaque oral contrast material has been given.

Retroperitoneal hemorrhage is a rare clinical situation, originating in most cases from a ruptured abdominal aortic aneurysm (AAA). Rupture of an aortic branch and spontaneous hemorrhage of a retroperitoneal organ are less common. The urological causes are dominated by renal neoplasms. Clinical diagnosis is difficult for many reasons. No specific clinical sign exists because lumbar pain is the dominating symptom. Even in the case of ruptured AAA, the classic triad associated with sudden abdominal or flank pain, shock, and pulsatile abdominal mass is encountered in a minority of cases. Furthermore, bleeding may be insidious and progressive, over days, making diagnosis more difficult. Similarly, biological tests lack specificity, consisting in deglobulinization signs.

Thus, diagnosis always relies on imaging evaluation. Despite its availability, US plays a minor role. Acoustic windows to the retroperitoneum may be limited by overlying bowel gas, and a small amount of retroperitoneal hematoma is easily missed. Even when the retroperitoneal hematoma is demonstrated, its origin remains difficult to identify, an AAA or large enough renal masses excepted. In contrast, CT has several advantages: it is readily available, fast to perform, both sensitive and specific in the diagnosis of retroperitoneal blood effusion, and very effective in the evaluation of most of the local causes of spontaneous bleeding. As a consequence, the role of MRI is of limited value, but its high resolution is useful in rare cases where CT lacks contrast for depicting a neoplasm within the blood suffusion. Another option in this situation is to perform serial CT to detect a causative lesion. Angiography is of limited value from a diagnostic point of view, except in rare cases where small vessels, beyond the domain of CT angiography, are to be depicted, such as in cases of panarteritis nodosa or arteriovenous malformations. Inversely, angiography plays an important therapeutic role, through embolization and stent-graft placement.

3.1 Ruptured AAA

AAA is frequent, encountered in 2–4% of the population older than 50 years (Bengtsson et al. 1992). Most AAAs are true aneurysms and involve the aortic segment below the renal arteries. Conventionally, diagnosis relies on an abdominal aorta diameter of 3 cm or more. When the rupture involves the anterior aortic wall, death by intraperitoneal hemorrhage is sudden. Patients who reach the emergency department present in most cases with rupture of the posterolateral wall, resulting in a retroperitoneal hemorrhage. The clinical triad is associated with sudden abdominal or flank pain, shock, and pulsatile abdominal mass.

Rupture into the inferior vena cava is much less common, resulting in an aortocaval fistula. Rupture into the duodenum is very rare in the case of native AAA and involves almost exclusively patients with a history of aortic bypass.

US is of limited value in the diagnosis of ruptured AAA: even a large amount of retroperitoneal hematoma can be missed. Furthermore, in the absence of retroperitoneal hematoma, US is unable to detect signs of impendent rupture. Despite its high diagnostic performance in this field, MRI has no role to play in an emergency because of its limited availability and its long acquisition time. Furthermore, even in the case of contraindication to the injection of iodinated contrast material, unenhanced CT allows accurate diagnosis of ruptured AAA. Owing to its widespread availability in the emergency department and its high speed of realization, CT is the imaging modality of choice for the diagnosis not only of AAA but also of acute aortic syndrome. CT also has high diagnostic performance in other emergent situations with clinical symptoms that are sometimes confused with those of abdominal disorders such as pancreatitis, appendicitis, and bowel obstruction.

Diagnosis of rupture is evident when a retroperitoneal hematoma is seen near an AAA (Rakita et al. 2007). Retroperitoneal hematoma appears as a hyperattenuating collection involving one or more retroperitoneal compartments, with a predilection for perirenal and pararenal spaces and psoas muscle (Fig. 5). Intraperitoneal effusion is usually delayed.

A direct sign of ruptured AAA, consisting in the extravasation of intravenous contrast material into the retroperitoneal space, is uncommon but not mandatory to establish the diagnosis. Otherwise, contrast material injection is useful for locating the digestive and renal branches of the aorta and defining their relationships with the aneurysmal neck (Fig. 5). This information, of limited value for the vascular surgeon, becomes of crucial importance for the interventional radiologist when an endoluminal stent-graft placement is planned. The endovascular repair of ruptured AAA plays an increasing role in patients at high risk of surgery as long as they remain relatively stable.

The draped aorta sign is encountered in cases of contained ruptures of AAA and refers to the presence of thrombus of the aneurysmal sac leaking toward the adjacent vertebral bodies (Halliday and al-Kutoubi 1996).

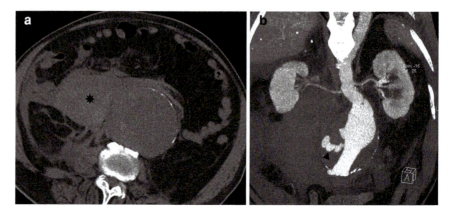

Fig. 5 Ruptured abdominal aortic aneurysm (AAA). **a** Axial unenhanced CT shows a heterogeneous hyperattenuating collection (*star*) in the right retroperitoneal space. **b** Frontal reformation of contrast-enhanced CT allows evaluation of the length of the aneurysmal proximal neck. Active extravasation is seen inside the aneurysmal thrombus (*closed triangle*)

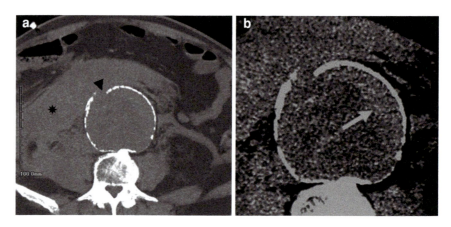

Fig. 6 Ruptured AAA. **a** Hemoretroperitoneum is visible around an AAA presenting a focal interruption (*closed triangle*) of otherwise circumferential wall calcifications. **b** A different windowing of the same slice depicts the hyperattenuating crescent sign (*arrow*)

This sign is present when the posterior wall of the aorta closely follows the contour of an adjacent vertebral body.

When the diagnosis of ruptured AAA is made clinically and retroperitoneal hemorrhage is absent, attention must be paid to radiological findings predictive of impending rupture. The value of the depiction of a focal interruption of otherwise circumferential wall calcifications is enhanced when a previous CT scan demonstrating a continuous calcification wall is available (Siegel and Cohan 1994) (Fig. 6).

The hyperattenuating crescent sign, even if not specific, is an early sign of impending or acute rupture, best depicted on unenhanced CT. It reveals the recent hemorrhage within either the peripheral wall or the aneurysm wall, appearing as a hyperdense cleft (Fig. 6). The sensitivity and specificity of the crescent sign for the diagnosis of complicated AAA are 77 and 93%, respectively (Mehard et al. 1994).

Spontaneous rupture of an iliac aneurysm is less frequent than AAA rupture, and can be clinically misleading. Diagnosis relies on CT angiography, with imaging features similar to those of AAA rupture (Fig. 7).

3.2 Perirenal Bleeding

Spontaneous perirenal hemorrhage is, according to an old literature review, related to a renal mass in almost 90% of cases (McDougal et al. 1975). In that review, 57.7% of perirenal hematomas arose from a renal tumor, 33.4% of them were malignant [most of them were renal cell carcinoma (RCC)], and 24.3% were benign [dominated by angiomyolipoma (AML)]. Vascular disease (17.9% of cases) included periarteritis nodosa, ruptured renal artery aneurysm, renal vein thrombosis, arteriovenous malformation, and renal infarction. The remaining causes were infection

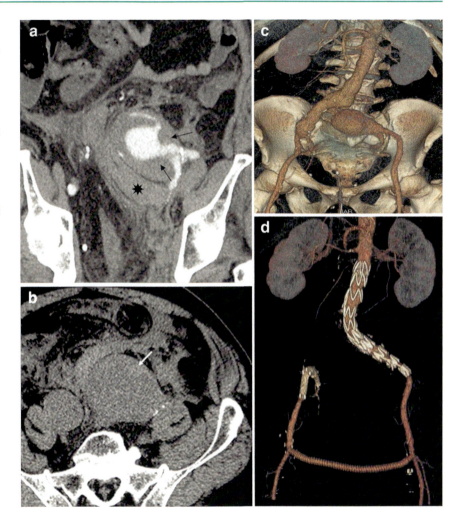

Fig. 7 Spontaneous rupture of an iliac artery aneurysm. **a** The left common iliac artery aneurysm is partially thrombosed (*arrows*) and surrounded by retroperitoneal blood effusion (*star*). **b** The precontrast slice reveals a hyperattenuating crescent sign (*arrow*). Volume rendering image of the aorta and iliac arteries before (**c**) and after (**d**) endovascular repair (aorto-uni-iliac stent graft, occlusion of the right external and internal iliac arteries) completed by a femorofemoral bypass

(10.3%), nephritis, blood dyscrasias, lithiasis, and hydronephrosis.

A higher incidence (30%) of AML was noted in a more recent series (Sebastia et al. 1997). Retroperitoneal bleeding is the first manifestation of approximately 15% of AMLs (Mouded et al. 1978; Pode and Caine 1992), particularly those of 4 cm or more, which are prone to bleed once in 50% of cases (Oesterling et al. 1986). The differing degree of vascularity of these masses, composed of fat, smooth muscle, and vessels, explains partly the differing risk of spontaneous bleeding. Pregnancy is a recognized facilitating factor of bleeding. CT provides an almost specific diagnosis when depicting fat within the lesion (Fig. 8).

Among malignant neoplasms, RCC yields most of the spontaneous renal bleeding. Despite its low incidence of spontaneous bleeding, RCC is in some series the most common renal neoplasm associated with spontaneous perirenal bleeding, owing to its high prevalence. Renal metastases prone to bleed arise from choriocarcinoma, melanoma, and lung carcinoma.

Hemorrhages from vascular origin are rare, dominated by the rupture of a renal artery aneurysm. Renal parenchyma infection (pyelonephritis, abscess, tuberculosis), renal cystic diseases, hydronephrosis, and lithiasis are more rarely involved in retroperitoneal hemorrhage. Infectious renal processes such as cortical abscesses may induce spontaneous perirenal hemorrhage by arterial erosion (Murray et al. 1979).

Fig. 8 Spontaneous bleeding of an angiomyolipoma of the right kidney. **a** A large fatty mass of the right kidney is surrounded by a subcapsular hematoma (*arrow*) and a hemoretroperitoneum (*star*). **b** The relationships between the subcapsular hematoma (*arrow*) and the retroperitoneal bleeding (*star*) are well depicted on the coronal reformation. Large pseudoaneurysms (*closed triangle*) are present within the renal mass. **c** Selective renal angiography confirms the presence, at the upper pole of the kidney, of radiolucent mass containing several peripheral pseudoaneurysms. **d** The result of selective coil embolization

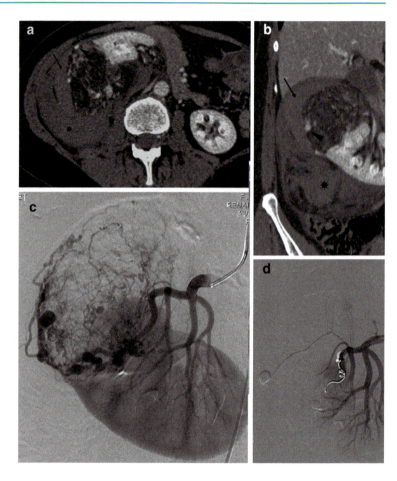

Table 1 Causes of spontaneous adrenal hemorrhage (Kawashima et al. 1999)

Stress[a]: surgery, sepsis, burns, hypotension, pregnancy, exogenous adrenocorticotropic hormone, exogenous steroids

Neonatal stress[a]: difficult labor or delivery, asphyxia, hypoxia, septicemia, hemorrhagic disorders, extracorporeal membrane oxygenation, associated renal vein thrombosis

Hemorrhagic diathesis or coagulopathy[a]: anticoagulants, antiphospholipid syndrome, systemic lupus erythematosus, disseminated intravascular coagulopathy

Underlying adrenal tumors[a]: pseudocyst, myelolipoma, hemangioma, pheochromocytoma, adrenocortical adenoma, adrenocortical carcinoma, metastases (bronchogenic carcinoma, angiosarcoma, melanoma)

Idiopathic disease

[a] Causes of bilateral adrenal hemorrhage

Rupture of a renal cyst as a local cause of perirenal hemorrhage is very rare because a renal cyst usually ruptures into the pyelocaliceal system. It has been demonstrated that end-stage kidney disease favors perirenal hemorrhage by cumulating factors such as platelet function alteration and heparinization for hemodialysis.

3.3 Periadrenal Bleeding

Conditions facilitating spontaneous adrenal bleeding are rare and are summarized in Table 1. From a clinical point of view, the risk of adrenal insufficiency, even if rare, must be kept in mind because associated with bilateral massive adrenal hemorrhage,

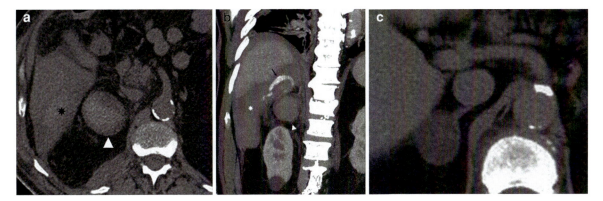

Fig. 9 Spontaneous bleeding of an adrenal adenoma as a complication of anti-vitamin K treatment. **a** On precontrast CT, the right adrenal gland appears enlarged and hyperdense (*open triangle*). A hematoma (*star*) is present at the posterior face of the liver, extending from the retroperitoneal space through the area nuda hepatis. **b** After intravenous contrast material injection, active bleeding is visible in the perihepatic hematoma (*arrow*). **c** A CT scan performed 6 months earlier confirms the typical hypodense pattern of an adrenal adenoma

adrenal insufficiency destroys more than 90% of each gland.

Stress-induced adrenal hemorrhage is seen in surgery, sepsis, burns, fulminant meningococcemia (Waterhouse–Friderichsen syndrome), pregnancy, and with administration of adrenocorticotropic hormone or steroids. Adrenal hemorrhage results in the combination of hypervascularity (induced by an increase in local secretion of adrenocorticotropic hormone) and elevated adrenal venous pressure (secondary to venoconstriction). General processes such as disseminated intravascular coagulopathy may also participate in adrenal hemorrhage. In antiphospholipid syndrome, the *primum movens* for adrenal hemorrhage is adrenal vein thrombosis.

Adrenal hemorrhage in neonates may result from hypoxia, septicemia, coagulopathy, or a difficult delivery, particularly if the mother is diabetic. The association of adrenal hemorrhage with renal vein thrombosis in neonates must also be remembered.

Adrenal hematoma is round or oval, usually associated with a periadrenal fat stranding, which may also involve the perirenal space. The possible extension of spontaneous perirenal or perihepatic hematoma to the periadrenal fat makes it sometimes difficult to determine from which organ the hemorrhage arises.

One imaging challenge concerns patients without a general risk factor for spontaneous adrenal bleeding, raising the question of a possible underlying cystic or solid mass. Comparison of unenhanced and enhanced

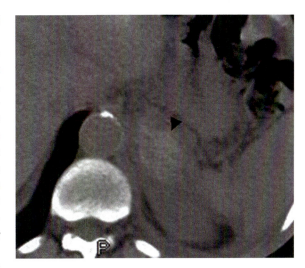

Fig. 10 Spontaneous hemorrhage of an adrenal metastasis from lung cancer: enlarged spontaneously hyperdense left-sided adrenal mass (*closed triangle*)

CT scans is essential. MRI may play a role in difficult cases. Otherwise, serial CT may reveal the underlying mass, whereas the clot resolves (Kawashima et al. 1999).

Nevertheless, some cases remain unsolved. For example, it is almost impossible to distinguish a hemorrhagic cyst from a hemorrhagic neoplasm in the case of a cystic lesion with an irregular thick wall. Similarly, the characteristic fatty component of a myelolipoma may be obscured by the superimposed hematoma.

Fig. 11 Spontaneous retroperitoneal bleeding of a peripancreatic pseudoaneurysm in a patient with acute pancreatitis. **a** On precontrast CT, a hyperdense crescent sign (*closed triangle*) is depicted. **b** After intravenous contrast material injection, the pseudoaneurysm (*star*) is enhanced between the superior mesenteric artery and the gastroduodenal artery. The pseudoaneurysm is best depicted on the coronal maximum intensity (MIP) projection (**c**). **d** Selective angiography of the superior mesenteric artery confirms the presence of the pseudoaneurysm, which appears excluded after coil embolization (**e**)

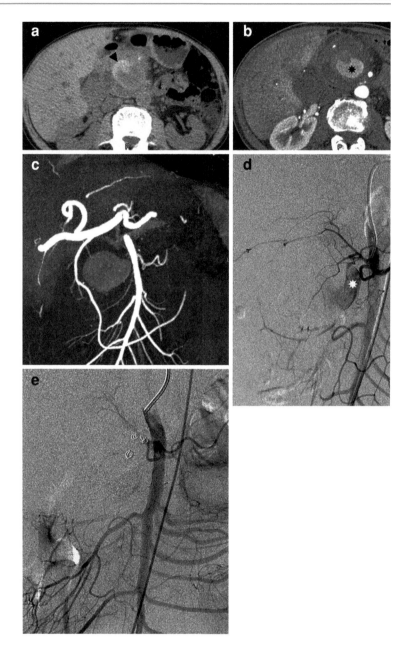

Despite its high prevalence, adrenal adenoma is exceptionally complicated by a hemorrhage (Fig. 9). Pheochromocytoma is the commonest adrenal neoplasm revealed or complicated by spontaneous bleeding. Liquefaction of former intraglandular hematoma is thought to explain the classic, although uncommon, presentation of a pheochromocytoma as a cystic mass. Intratumoral hemorrhage is a common feature of adrenocortical carcinoma. Among secondary adrenal neoplasms, metastases from lung and melanoma origin are the most prone to bleed and hemorrhage can be the initial manifestation of the metastasis (Fig. 10).

3.4 Peripancreatic Bleeding

Owing to their mainly retroperitoneal location, pathological processes affecting the pancreas, particularly acute or chronic pancreatitis, may induce a

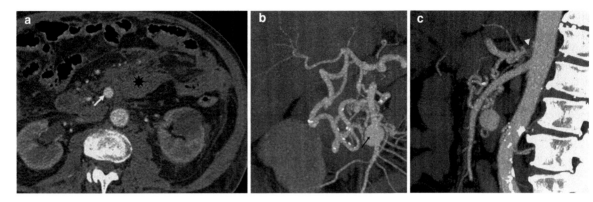

Fig. 12 Ruptured aneurysm of a pancreaticoduodenal artery in a patient with occlusion of the celiac trunk. **a** The pseudoaneurysm (*arrow*) is complicated by a blood effusion within the root of the mesentery (*star*). Its relationships with the pancreaticoduodenal arcades are best demonstrated on the coronal MIP projection (**b**). **c** Sagittal MIP projection confirms the occlusion of the celiac trunk (*open triangle*)

retroperitoneal bleeding. Pseudoaneurysm is observed as a complication of acute or chronic pancreatitis. The erosion of the artery may be biological (resulting from the autodigestion of the pancreatic or peripancreatic artery by elastase and trypsin) or mechanical (by erosion of a pancreatic pseudocyst into a neighboring visceral artery, converting a pseudocyst into a pseudoaneurysm) or both. Rupture of the pseudoaneurysm may involve the pancreatic ducts (resulting in wirsungorrhagia), the bile ducts (resulting in hemobilia), the gastrointestinal tract, the retroperitoneal spaces, or the peritoneal cavity. Splenic, pancreaticoduodenal, and gastroduodenal arteries are the most frequently involved vessels. CT is the best imaging tool, able to depict the pseudoaneurysms associated with features of chronic or acute pancreatitis (Fig. 11). Information obtained from CT simplifies the approach to the targeted vessel during subsequent angiographic embolization. CT may also reveal other causes of hemorrhage such as rupture of gastric varices in the case of segmental portal hypertension or splenic rupture.

Another condition favoring a retroperitoneal bleeding is the rupture of a pancreaticoduodenal artery developing as the complication of a celiac trunk or superior mesenteric artery stenosis (Fig. 12). As opposed to the false aneurysms, developing as a consequence of a local injury, such as pancreatitis, the lesion in that particular case is a true aneurysm. This is a much more uncommon situation, described for the first time by Sutton and Lawton (1973). A literature review in 1999, gathering 52 cases, found a prevalence of celiac trunk lesion of 63% (De Perrot et al. 1999). The theory originally proposed by Sutton and Lawton, based on the increased blood flow in the collateral network developing at the expense of the pancreaticoduodenal arcades, is supported by the description of cases where the treatment of the celiac trunk stenosis (direct revascularization or arcuate ligament section) allowed complete aneurysm regression. The same hypothesis is supported by another series that demonstrated 80% of peripancreatic artery dilatation in the group with celiac trunk stenosis and none in the control group (Patten et al. 1991). In a more recent review of 36 cases of aneurysm of the pancreaticoduodenal arteries associated with a celiac trunk stenosis, the size of the aneurysm did not appear as a factor for rupture because most ruptured aneurysms measured less than 10 mm, whereas all nonruptured aneurysms measured 10 mm or more (Ducasse et al. 2004). When ruptured, the pancreaticoduodenal artery aneurysm requires an emergent radiological arterial embolization. Later, to prevent recurrence, a surgical resection of the arcuate ligament and treatment of the celiac artery stenosis are recommended by several authors.

3.5 Systemic Causes of Spontaneous Retroperitoneal Bleeding

Systemic causes of retroperitoneal bleeding are dominated by polyarteritis nodosa. In this systemic vasculitis, fragility of the media of small and medium-sized arteries results from the deposition of immune complexes in the arterial wall and leads to microaneurysms and hemorrhage. Multiorgan involvement is common. Kidney is involved in approximately 80% of cases, with a risk of perirenal hemorrhage (Maes et al. 2000). Abdominal complications may also occur because the mesenteric arteries are involved in 60% of cases (Adajar et al. 2006).

4   Conclusion

Spontaneous intraperitoneal and retroperitoneal hemorrhages can result from a vast variety of causes. CT plays an essential role in the positive and etiological diagnoses of most of the situations. It also affords important data for the interventional radiologist when hemostatic embolization or stent-graft placement is planned. MRI is of very limited value in this clinical situation, whereas US remains an essential tool in the evaluation of gynecological disorders.

References

Adajar MA, Painter T, Woloson S, Memark V (2006) Isolated celiac artery aneurysm with splenic artery stenosis as a rare presentation of polyarteritis nodosum: a case report and review of the literature. J Vasc Surg 44(3):647–650

Becker YT, Raiford DS, Webb L, Wright JK, Chapman WC, Pinson CW (1995) Rupture and hemorrhage of hepatic focal nodular hyperplasia. Am Surg 61(3):210–214

Bengtsson H, Bergqvist D, Sternby NH (1992) Increasing prevalence of abdominal aortic aneurysms. A necropsy study. Eur J Surg 158(1):19–23

Bioulac-Sage P, Balabaud C, Bedossa P, Scoazec JY, Chiche L, Dhillon AP et al (2007) Pathological diagnosis of liver cell adenoma and focal nodular hyperplasia: Bordeaux update. J Hepatol 46(3):521–527

Casillas VJ, Amendola MA, Gascue A, Pinnar N, Levi JU, Perez JM (2000) Imaging of nontraumatic hemorrhagic hepatic lesions. Radiographics 20(2):367–378

De Perrot M, Berney T, Deleaval J, Buhler L, Mentha G, Morel P (1999) Management of true aneurysms of the pancreaticoduodenal arteries. Ann Surg 229(3):416–420

DeSitter L, Rector WG Jr (1984) The significance of bloody ascites in patients with cirrhosis. Am J Gastroenterol 79(2):136–138

Dokmak S, Paradis V, Vilgrain V, Sauvanet A, Farges O, Valla D et al (2009) A single-center surgical experience of 122 patients with single and multiple hepatocellular adenomas. Gastroenterology 137(5):1698–1705

Ducasse E, Roy F, Chevalier J, Massouille D, Smith M, Speziale F et al (2004) Aneurysm of the pancreaticoduodenal arteries with a celiac trunk lesion: current management. J Vasc Surg 39(4):906–911

Halliday KE, al-Kutoubi A (1996) Draped aorta: CT sign of contained leak of aortic aneurysms. Radiology 199(1):41–43

Kanematsu M, Imaeda T, Yamawaki Y, Seki M, Goto H, Sone Y et al (1992) Rupture of hepatocellular carcinoma: predictive value of CT findings. AJR Am J Roentgenol 158(6):1247–1250

Kawashima A, Sandler CM, Ernst RD, Takahashi N, Roubidoux MA, Goldman SM et al (1999) Imaging of nontraumatic hemorrhage of the adrenal gland. Radiographics 19(4):949–963

Kim PT, Su JC, Buczkowski AK, Schaeffer DF, Chung SW, Scudamore CH et al (2006) Computed tomography and angiographic interventional features of ruptured hepatocellular carcinoma: pictorial essay. Can Assoc Radiol J 57(3):159–168

Levine CD, Patel UJ, Silverman PM, Wachsberg RH (1996) Low attenuation of acute traumatic hemoperitoneum on CT scans. AJR Am J Roentgenol 166(5):1089–1093

Maes K, Billiet I, Haerens M, Mattelaer J (2000) Massive bilateral renal and perirenal hemorrhage due to polyarteritis nodosa: a life-threatening urologic condition. Eur Urol 38(3):349–351

McDougal WS, Kursh ED, Persky L (1975) Spontaneous rupture of the kidney with perirenal hematoma. J Urol 114(2):181–184

Mehard WB, Heiken JP, Sicard GA (1994) High-attenuating crescent in abdominal aortic aneurysm wall at CT: a sign of acute or impending rupture. Radiology 192(2):359–362

Meissner K (1998) Hemorrhage caused by ruptured liver cell adenoma following long-term oral contraceptives: a case report. Hepatogastroenterology 45(19):224–225

Mortele KJ, Cantisani V, Brown DL, Ros PR (2003) Spontaneous intraperitoneal hemorrhage: imaging features. Radiol Clin North Am 41(6):1183–1201

Mouded IM, Tolia BM, Bernie JE, Newman HR (1978) Symptomatic renal angiomyolipoma: report of 8 cases, 2 with spontaneous rupture. J Urol 119(5):684–688

Murray HW, Soave R, Collins MH (1979) Fatal retroperitoneal hemorrhage. An unusual complication of renal cortical abscess. JAMA 241(17):1823–1824

New PF, Aronow S (1976) Attenuation measurements of whole blood and blood fractions in computed tomography. Radiology 121(3 Pt. 1):635–640

Nunes JO, Turner MA, Fulcher AS (2005) Abdominal imaging features of HELLP syndrome: a 10-year retrospective review. AJR Am J Roentgenol 185(5):1205–1210

Oesterling JE, Fishman EK, Goldman SM, Marshall FF (1986) The management of renal angiomyolipoma. J Urol 135(6):1121–1124

Patten RM, Coldwell DM, Ben-Menachem Y (1991) Ligamentous compression of the celiac axis: CT findings in five patients. AJR Am J Roentgenol 156(5):1101–1103

Pode D, Caine M (1992) Spontaneous retroperitoneal hemorrhage. J Urol 147(2):311–318

Rakita D, Newatia A, Hines JJ, Siegel DN, Friedman B (2007) Spectrum of CT findings in rupture and impending rupture of abdominal aortic aneurysms. Radiographics 27(2): 497–507

Sebastia MC, Perez-Molina MO, Alvarez-Castells A, Quiroga S, Pallisa E (1997) CT evaluation of underlying cause in spontaneous subcapsular and perirenal hemorrhage. Eur Radiol 7(5):686–690

Shanley CJ, Shah NL, Messina LM (1996) Common splanchnic artery aneurysms: splenic, hepatic, and celiac. Ann Vasc Surg 10(3):315–322

Siegel CL, Cohan RH (1994) CT of abdominal aortic aneurysms. AJR Am J Roentgenol 163(1):17–29

Stoot JH, van der Linden E, Terpstra OT, Schaapherder AF (2007) Life-saving therapy for haemorrhaging liver adenomas using selective arterial embolization. Br J Surg 94(10):1249–1253

Sutton D, Lawton G (1973) Coeliac stenosis or occlusion with aneurysm of the collateral supply. Clin Radiol 24(1):49–53

Weinstein L (1982) Syndrome of hemolysis, elevated liver enzymes, and low platelet count: a severe consequence of hypertension in pregnancy. Am J Obstet Gynecol 142(2):159–167

Wolverson MK, Crepps LF, Sundaram M, Heiberg E, Vas WG, Shields JB (1983) Hyperdensity of recent hemorrhage at body computed tomography: incidence and morphologic variation. Radiology 148(3):779–784

Urological Emergencies

Patrice Taourel and Rodolphe Thuret

Contents

1	**Introduction**	359
2	**Colic Pain**	360
2.1	Clinical Findings and Problems	360
2.2	CT Findings	360
2.3	CT Pitfalls	361
2.4	CT Accuracy	362
2.5	Role and Impact of CT	363
3	**Urinary Tract Infection**	363
3.1	Clinical Findings and Problems	363
3.2	CT Findings	363
3.3	CT Pitfalls	365
3.4	CT Accuracy	366
3.5	Role and Impact of CT	366
4	**Fournier Gangrene**	367
4.1	Clinical Findings and Problems	367
4.2	CT Findings	367
4.3	CT Pitfalls	367
4.4	CT Impact	368
5	**Vascular Conditions**	368
5.1	Clinical Findings and Problems	368
5.2	CT Findings	368
5.3	CT Pitfalls	369
5.4	CT Accuracy	369
5.5	Role and Impact of CT	370
6	**Hemorrhagic Conditions**	370
6.1	Clinical Findings and Problems	370
6.2	CT Findings	370
6.3	CT Pitfalls	372
6.4	CT Accuracy	372
6.5	Role and Impact of CT	372
7	**Bladder Perforation**	373
References		373

P. Taourel (✉)
Department of Imaging, Hôpital Lapeyronie,
34295 Montpellier Cedex 5, France
e-mail: p-taourel@chu-montpellier.fr

R. Thuret
Department of Urology, Hôpital Lapeyronie,
34295 Montpellier Cedex 5, France

Abstract

Renal colic pain due to an obstructing stone is the main renal cause of acute flank pain; however, other causes may be responsible for the same clinical findings, including acute pyelonephritis, acute vascular conditions, and hemorrhage. The purpose of this review is to describe the differential diagnosis, the CT findings and pitfalls, and the role and impact of CT in the diagnosis and management of the renal causes of acute flank pain.

1 Introduction

Renal colic pain due to an obstructing stone is the main renal cause of acute flank pain; however, other causes may be responsible for the same clinical findings, including acute pyelonephritis, acute vascular conditions, and hemorrhage. The purpose of this review is to describe the differential diagnosis, the CT findings and pitfalls, and the role and impact of CT in the diagnosis and management of the renal causes of acute flank pain.

Colic pain constitutes the most common cause of pain in patients with acute abdomen seen in an emergency department. However, in a patient referred for CT with suspicion of colic pain, 40–60% have an obstructing stone according to the clinical presentation

P. Taourel (ed.), *CT of the Acute Abdomen*, Medical Radiology. Diagnostic Imaging,
DOI: 10.1007/174_2010_88, © Springer-Verlag Berlin Heidelberg 2011

and to the experience of the referring physician. CT allows a wide spectrum of alternative genitourinary tract and non-genitourinary-tract diagnoses responsible for the symptoms. The goal of this review is to describe the CT features in the renal causes of non-traumatic acute flank pain.

2 Colic Pain

2.1 Clinical Findings and Problems

Flank pain due to urolithiasis is a common problem in patients presenting to the emergency department. Up to 12% of the population will have a urinary stone during their lifetime, and recurrence rates approach 50% (Teichman 2004). The disease affects men 3 times as often as it does women. Some factors increase the risk of stones, such as genetics, diet, employment, and urinary tract infections, whereas specific entities such as idiopathic or secondary hypercalciuria and hyperuricosuria are associated with a high prevalence of stones.

Colic pain is often spasmodic and increases to a peak level of intensity and then decreases before increasing again. The pain is severe and may rapidly rise to a level of discomfort, needing narcotics for adequate control. As the stone approaches the ureteral junction, pain may radiate to the lower abdomen and into the scrotum, the labia, or the tip of the urethra, or may be associated with urinary urgency or dysuria, and may mimic cystitis.

Urinalysis is often the initial laboratory examination, and some investigators have suggested that dipstick or microscopic urinalysis that is negative for blood can effectively exclude the diagnosis of an obstructing ureteral stone and avoid additional testing (Press and Smith 1995). However, this assumption was challenged by the study of Luchs et al. (2002). This study included 950 patients with suspected renal colic and a stone on CT in 62% of patients and showed that microscopic hematuria had a sensitivity, specificity, positive predictive value, and negative predictive value of 84, 48, 72, and 65%, respectively. Consequently, the presence or absence of blood on urinalysis cannot be used to reliably determine which patients actually have ureteral stones, and additional tests are often necessary. It has been established for 10 years that the best modality to confirm the diagnosis of a urinary stone in a patient with acute

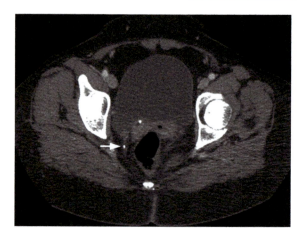

Fig. 1 Right ureterovesical junction stone. The stone is well individualized at the right uterovesical junction and must be differentiated from a posterior phlebolith (*arrow*), easily recognized because it is not located on the course of the ureter, and it is associated with a posterior tail of soft-tissue attenuation

flank pain is unenhanced helical CT of the abdomen (Teichman 2004; Vieweg et al. 1998).

2.2 CT Findings

CT shows direct and indirect findings of colic pain due to a stone. The direct finding is the visualization of the calculus itself. Regardless of composition, almost all renal and ureteral stones are detected by CT because the attenuation of stones is higher than that of surrounding tissue, even if attenuation of uric acid stones is lower than the attenuation of calcium. The most common locations for obstruction by a stone are at the three areas of the anatomic narrowing of the ureter: the ureteropelvic junction, the pelvic brim where the ureter crosses the iliac vessels, and the ureterovesical junction (Fig. 1). Secondary or indirect findings are hydronephrosis, hydroureter, perirenal edema, periureteral edema, and swelling of the kidney (Tamm et al. 2003; Ege et al. 2003).

The size of the stone is important information that should be included in the CT report because the likelihood of spontaneous stone passage decreases as the size of the stone increases. Most stones that are less than 5 mm in diameter are likely to pass spontaneously (Teichman 2004; Segura et al. 1997) and generally pass within 4 weeks after the onset of symptoms (Teichman 2004). The degree of functional

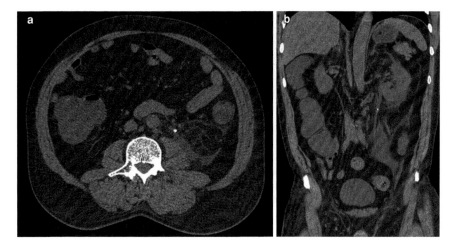

Fig. 2 Left ureteral stone. The left lumbar ureteral stone is well identified on the axial (**a**) and coronal (**b**) views. Note a significant fat stranding around the kidney in contrast to a lack of ureteral dilatation. This is in favor of a rupture of the collecting system

obstruction may be concluded from the degree of perirenal edema. It has been shown by comparing CT and intravenous urography in a population of patients with acute ureterolithiasis that with a qualitative assessment of perirenal edema on CT images, the degree of ureteral obstruction seen on intravenous urography was accurately predicted in 94% of patients (Boridy et al. 1999). Significant perirenal edema may imply severe obstruction with rupture of the collecting system (Fig. 2). However, the degree of obstruction is not a key point in the treatment of a patient with a ureteral stone; the treatment of choice (noninterventional management, shock-wave lithotripsy, or ureteroscopy) depends on the size and the location of the stone, and on the duration of the symptoms (Teichman 2004, Tamm et al. 2003). In pure uric acid stone, oral dissolution therapy is efficient even for a big stone. The characteristic of the stone may be suspected on the basis of the history of the patient, of a low urinary pH, and on a calculus visible on CT but radiolucent on plain imaging or on the scout view.

2.3 CT Pitfalls

The most common difficulty is the differentiation of phleboliths from ureteral calculi. Some findings may be helpful to differentiate these two entities: a soft-tissue rim sign, which refers to a soft-tissue ring surrounding the calcification representing the edematous wall of the ureter, is in favor of a stone, whereas an associated tail of soft-tissue attenuation (representing the associated vein) that extends to the calcification is in favor of a phlebolith (Fig. 1) (Tamm et al. 2003;

Rucker et al. 2004). In clinical practice, viewing on a workstation in interactive cine mode is helpful to follow the ureter on its entire course and to localize the origin of a calcification. We do not find that coronal reformations are helpful in differentiating stone from phlebolith and improving urinary stone detection. In a study including more than 200 uroliths in 72 patients, the only added value of coronal reformation performed with 1.25-mm axial acquisitions was to reduce the evaluation time; furthermore, coronal reformation was less sensitive than axial sections to diagnose alternative conditions (Memarsadeghi et al. 2007). In clinical practice, the main advantage of coronal reformatting is to give more readable views for physicians (Fig. 2).

False-negative CT findings may be due to the size and the composition of the calculus. In our experience, a 1-mm slice may exceptionally be helpful to diagnose a very tiny stone, even if our usual interpretation mode is 3 mm thick. In a study assessing the effect of section width, it was shown that overlapping 3-mm sections were sufficient for the detection of urinary stone disease. Sections measuring 1.5 mm thick did not have any added value, whereas small calculi (3 mm or less) might be missed on 5-mm-thick sections (Memarsadeghi et al. 2005). Stones radiolucent on CT are matrix stones that are made of organic material and are occasionally seen in patients with urease-producing bacteria (Liu et al. 2003) and indinavir stone; indinavir stone may be encountered in patients with the human immunodeficiency virus (HIV) who are undergoing treatment with this protease inhibitor, and for whom the medication can crystallize in the urine (Gentle et al. 1997).

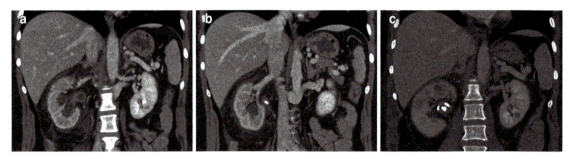

Fig. 3 a–c Pyonephrosis. Findings of obstruction of the right kidney with asymmetric nephrography and pyelic dilatation (**a**). There is also an abnormal enhancement of the pyelic wall, meaning pyelitis (**a**). The obstruction was due to a stone located at the ureteropelvic junction. A JJ tube well shown on a follow-up CT was set in an emergency with passage of infected urine. Note, at this time, there is development of infection of the parenchyma

In these two cases, stones may be or may not be detected with CT. In patients with colic pain, hydronephrosis, and/or hydroureter, and when no ureteral calcification can be identified, the differential diagnosis will include calcification too small to detect, indinavir stone in a HIV patient, but more often a pyelonephritis or a passed stone. In the case of perirenal edema and renal swelling without either calcification or hydroureteronephrosis, renal infarction and renal vein thrombosis should be considered in the differential diagnosis, and a CT scan should be immediately repeated with intravenous contrast material (Tamm et al. 2003; Rucker et al. 2004).

An obstructing stone at the ureteral insertion can be difficult to differentiate from a stone that has recently passed into the bladder. In this case, prone imaging may be added to determine whether the calculus is free within the bladder lumen or fixed within the ureterovesical junction (Levine et al. 1999).

In patients with obstruction, enlargement of the kidney (Fig. 3), thickening of the renal pelvic wall, or nonhomogeneous filling of the collecting system after administration of intravenous contrast material is suggestive of pyonephrosis (Craig et al. 2008). However, CT evaluation generally does not allow one to distinguish simple hydronephrosis from pyonephrosis on the basis of fluid attenuation measurements (Fig. 3) (Fultz et al. 1993).

2.4 CT Accuracy

The sensitivity and specificity of CT for the diagnosis of stone are above 95%, superior to those of intravenous urography, which was the previous gold standard. Consequently, CT is becoming the new gold standard in the diagnosis of colic pain in the evaluation of other tests, which may be biological, such as hematuria testing (Luchs et al. 2002), or radiological, such as plain film (Poletti et al. 2006), or a combination of abdominal plain film and ultrasonography (US) (Catalano et al. 2002).

In addition to having a high accuracy in the diagnosis of colic pain, CT enables significant alternative or additional diagnoses to be made. In a large two-center study including 1,000 patients (Katz et al. 2000), with a diagnosis of ureteral calculi in 557 patients and a diagnosis of recently passed stone, CT permitted an alternative diagnosis to be established in 101 examinations (10%). There were 62 genitourinary tract and 39 non-genitourinary-tract diagnoses. Among the 62 genitourinary tract diagnoses, there were 23 adnexal masses and nine cases of pyelonephritis, whereas other causes of urinary tract obstructions were encountered in 12 cases, including three cases of ureteropelvic junction obstruction, one case of ureteral obstruction due to adenopathy, four cases of ureterovesical junction obstruction, and four cases of bladder outlet obstruction. Among the 39 non-genitourinary-tract diagnoses, the diseases were very diverse, with a predominance of colic disease (eight cases) and of appendicitis (five cases). There was only one case of aortic dissection and two cases of muscle hemorrhage. The disease pattern was remarkably similar in another study (Ahmad et al. 2003), including 233 consecutive patients with helical CT for suspicion of ureteral colic and that showed a ureteral calculus in 64% of patients, findings of recent passage of calculi in 4% of patients, and significant additional or alternative diagnoses in 12% of patients with a 50% rate of genitourinary tract and non-genitourinary-tract diagnoses.

2.5 Role and Impact of CT

CT is rightly considered by urologists (Katz et al. 2000) as the technique providing the most rapid and most accurate information for both patients and the referring physician in patients with suspicion of colic pain. Despite the additional cost, they claim that the only reason for not using it is its lack of availability. More important than the cost are concerns about radiation exposure. It is now considered that CT is the major cause of radiation exposure. Consequently, in patients younger than 30 years, especially because they have a personal or a family history of urolithiasis, we believe that abdominal plain film and US must be used first. The stones missed by these techniques generally do not require any invasive treatment (Catalano et al. 2002). If CT is performed, a low-dose protocol must be used, especially in thin patients because it has been shown that low-dose CT (30 mA) achieves sensitivities and specificities close to those of standard-dose CT (180 mA) in assessing the diagnosis of renal colic, depicting ureteral calculi of 3 mm or larger (Poletti et al. 2007) in patients with a body mass index of 30 or below. CT without intravenous contrast material is sufficient to diagnose colic pain. However, in some suspicions of alternative conditions, intravenous contrast material is mandatory. It must be kept in mind in patients with vascular risks that the clinical findings of acute aortic and splanchnic arterial conditions may overlap with those or renal colic. Even if unenhanced CT may diagnose a ruptured abdominal aortic aneurysm and aortic dissection (Rucker et al. 2004), intravenous contrast material is always required to exclude the latter. Furthermore, according to the results of the unenhanced CT scan, injection must be performed when there is suspicion of bleeding in the urinary tract or of the kidney, and when unenhanced CT shows unilateral perirenal stranding or nephromegaly without a stone to look for pyelonephritis or a serious vascular condition such as renal infarction, renal vein thrombosis, or renal artery aneurysm (Rucker et al. 2004).

3 Urinary Tract Infection

3.1 Clinical Findings and Problems

Urinary tract infections constitute the second most common urological disease after the colic pain responsible for emergency department visits. In adults, diagnosis of urinary tract infection is typically based on characteristic clinical features and abnormal laboratory values. In cystitis, diagnosis is performed on the basis of dysuria and urinary frequency and urgency. In pyelonephritis, symptoms include an abrupt onset of chills, fever, and unilateral flank pain with costovertebral tenderness, which may be accompanied by the "lower tract signs" present in cystitis.

Cystitis is due to the action of an infectious organism, the usual urinary pathogens being *Escherichia coli* and *Proteus mirabilis*. Most infections are uncomplicated and involve only the urinary bladder, but in some cases the infection migrates up the ureter to the central collecting system, even in the absence of reflux, with the constitution of a ureteropyelitis, and then the bacteria may enter the renal tubules with the constitution of nephritis. Besides the ascending pyelonephritis, some infection may seed hematogenously.

Even if acute cystitis is generally noncomplicated, some conditions must be associated with complicated cystitis and the lack of pyelonephritis: diabetes, neurogenic bladder, bladder outlet obstruction, and enterovesical fistulization. The main feature of complicated cystitis is emphysematous cystitis, a rare condition that is characterized by gas collections inside the bladder wall with varied clinical presentations from an incidental finding of abdominal-to-severe sepsis, with a mortality of 7% in a meta-analysis including 135 cases (Thomas et al. 2007). Two thirds of patients are women and two thirds of patients have diabetes mellitus.

3.2 CT Findings

CT is the imaging modality of choice in the evaluation of patients with acute bacterial pyelonephritis. As recently recommended (Stunell et al. 2007), we use precontrast imaging, followed by postcontrast imaging at approximately 50–90 s when the normal

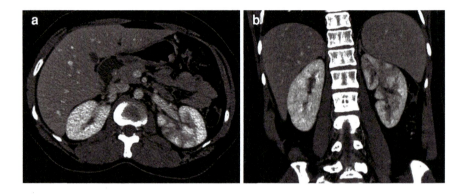

Fig. 4 Pyelonephritis of the left kidney. A striated nephrogram involving the whole left kidney is well shown on the axial slice (**a**) as well as on coronal reformatting (**b**)

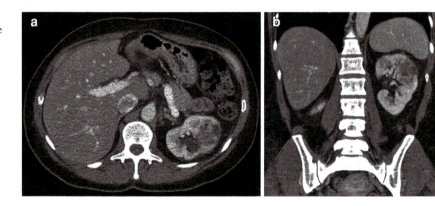

Fig. 5 Abscess of the left kidney. Hypodense mass in the upper part of the left kidney with a bean appearance, well seen on axial (**a**) and coronal (**b**) views. Note that the fat stranding around the kidney is very subtle

kidney is homogeneously enhanced and delayed imaging if urinary tract obstruction is suspected. We believe that vascular and corticomedullary phases recommended in some protocols (Browne et al. 2004) may be avoided.

Unenhanced CT is sufficient for identifying urinary tract gas, calculi, hemorrhage, renal enlargement, inflammatory masses, and obstruction.

The diagnostic features of acute bacterial nephritis after administration of intravenous contrast material are consecutive to the pathological state of the disease (Craig et al. 2008). The striated nephrogram is due to obstruction of the tubules by edema with intervening normal tubules, seen as linear bands of alternating hypodense and hyperdense striations parallel to the tubules. The striations have a lobar distribution, and may be unifocal or multifocal, and unilateral or bilateral (Fig. 4). The wedge-shaped hypodense areas radiating from the papilla to the cortical surface represent areas of poorly functioning parenchyma due to vasospasm, tubular obstruction, and/or interstitial edema. These disturbances lead to a decrease of the flow through the tubule and explain the pattern of delayed and persistent enhancement seen 3–6 h after intravenous contrast material administration (Fig. 4). Pelvic and caliceal wall thickening and enhancement may be the only finding of an affected kidney if the patient has pyelitis. However, diffusion of the inflammatory process leads to stranding or obliteration of perirenal fat and thickening of fascias. Unenhanced fluid collections within the abnormal renal parenchyma indicate the development of abscesses (Fig. 5) that are more common in diabetic patients. When these collections are round and bilateral, hematologic seeding must be suspected, and in such cases, blood and urine cultures grow the same organism. The presence of air within the kidney results in the diagnosis of emphysematous pyelitis or pyelonephritis. In emphysematous pyelitis, CT shows gas bubbles or gas–fluid levels within the renal calices or sinus (Craig et al. 2008). Emphysematous pyelitis has a better prognosis than emphysematous pyelonephritis, where gas is located within the parenchyma. Emphysematous pyelonephritis is a life-threatening necrotizing infection of the kidney associated in 90% of cases with poorly controlled diabetes;

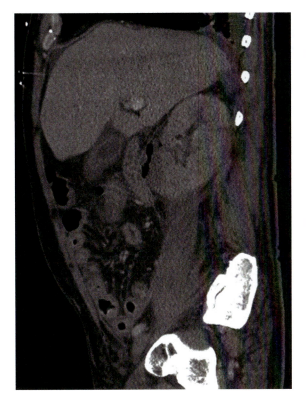

Fig. 6 Emphysematous pyelonephritis. Sagittal reformatting shows air that dissects the anterior perirenal space with fluid collection

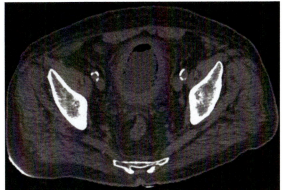

Fig. 7 Emphysematous cystitis. Air within the wall of the bladder, which is characteristic of emphysematous cystitis because of the lack of bladder instrumentation

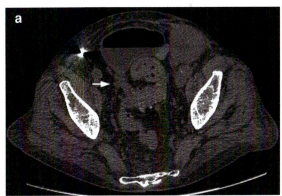

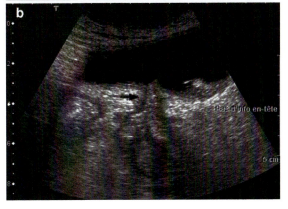

Fig. 8 Colovesical fistula complicating diverticulitis. The colovesical track (*arrow*) is well seen on CT (**a**) as well as on ultrasonography (**b**). Note the thickening of the sigmoid wall, the colic diverticula, and the presence of air in the bladder

a classification with a prognosis value is based on CT findings (Wan et al. 1996) The type 1 and 2 diseases are characterized by a parenchymal destruction that manifests itself as either streaky or mottled areas of gas, but in type 1 diseases (Fig. 6), intrarenal or extrarenal collection is missing, whereas they are present in type 2 diseases associated with a more fulminant course and a higher mortality rate, and the necessity of an aggressive treatment with percutaneous drainage (Narlawar et al. 2004) and/or partial or total nephrectomy.

Emphysematous cystitis is easily detected by CT that shows intraluminal or intramural gas (Fig. 7). The differential diagnosis must be established with other causes of intraluminal gas such as consequences of urinary tract instrumentation or enteric fistula formation from adjacent bowel carcinoma or inflammatory disease (sigmoid diverticulitis, Crohn disease) (Fig. 8). Crohn disease constitutes the most common cause of enterovesical fistula; these fistulas occur more often from the ileum than from the colon (Wong-You Cheong et al. 2006).

3.3 CT Pitfalls

The main difficulties in CT diagnosis are because the findings encountered are not specific to infection.

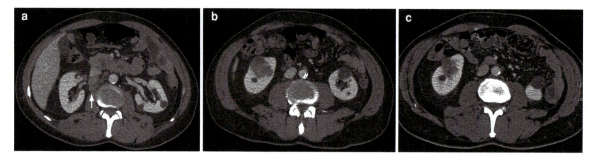

Fig. 9 a–c Chronic abscess of the kidney. A first CT examination shows retroperitoneal lymph nodes (**a**) and a mass in the lower part of the right kidney (**b**). There is no fat stranding around the kidney. The biopsy of the mass did not confirm a renal tumor but diagnosed an abscess. One month later, the renal mass has decreased in size (**c**)

Striations that are a subtle finding of a moderate pyelonephritis may be seen in normal kidneys when low-osmolarity contrast materials are used or in poorly hydrated patients (Stunell et al. 2007). Low-enhancement areas within the parenchyma are the consequence of an interstitial nephritis, but there are other noninfectious causes of nephritis, such as drugs, granulomatous disease (e.g., sarcoidosis), and immunologic or metabolic disease. Perirenal stranding may be related to previous infection, trauma, or vascular disease. Air within the collecting system may have a noninfectious origin such as trauma, instrumentation, and fistula. Consequently, these different findings must be interpreted according to the clinical conditions and have a great value in patients with clinical findings consistent with pyelonephritis.

In practice, the most difficult question may be to differentiate pyelonephritis from pyonephrosis because pelvic and ureteral wall thickness, perirenal fat stranding, and a striated nephrogram can occur in these two diseases. Obstruction is, of course, a reason for pyonephrosis, but dilatation of the pelvis and ureter may be present in pyelonephritis because endotoxin may inhibit ureteral peristalsis (Stunell et al. 2007). This distinction is of great importance because pyonephrosis requires emergent drainage of the collecting system to prevent permanent loss of function and life-threatening Gram-negative septicemia.

In the same way, in patients with obstruction, parenchymal or perirenal changes, thickening of the renal pelvic wall, or nonhomogeneous filling of the collecting system after intravenous contrast material administration are the reasons for pyonephrosis (Craig et al. 2008). However, CT evaluation generally does not allow one to distinguish simple hydronephrosis from pyonephrosis on the basis of fluid-attenuation measurements.

Other pitfalls may be due to the confusion between a tumoral mass and an infectious mass. Fever may be due to either the inflammatory process or a paraneoplastic syndrome. Inflammatory changes around the mass and pyuria are the reasons for an infection. However, in some cases, the diagnosis of infection is a good surprise of the biopsy (Fig. 9).

3.4 CT Accuracy

CT is considered superior to intravenous urography and US in detecting parenchymal abnormalities, delineating disease, and detecting perirenal collections. In patients with consistent clinical findings, all regions of hypoattenuating parenchyma on CT are considered acute pyelonephritis, and the disease is specifically described in terms of unilateral/bilateral, focal/diffuse, focal swelling/no focal swelling, or renal enlargement/no renal enlargement (Talner et al. 1994). Consequently, because CT is used as the gold standard for the diagnosing and staging of pyelonephritis, its accuracy cannot be evaluated.

3.5 Role and Impact of CT

Diagnosis of acute pyelonephritis in the adult patient is still predominantly a clinical diagnosis. However, CT has a great role in selected clinical scenarios:
– When the diagnosis is doubtful on the basis of the symptoms or urinalysis or if other diseases such as ureteric colic or renal infarction are suspected

- To assess those patients at significant risk of severer life-threatening complications (diabetic, elderly, or immunocompromised patients)
- To assist in the diagnosis of acute pyelonephritis when the patient fails to respond to appropriate therapy within the first 72 h, which occurs in about 5% of patients
- When there is a possibility of pyonephrosis that would require urgent drainage. In this case, US may be an alternative to CT.

4   Fournier Gangrene

4.1   Clinical Findings and Problems

Fournier gangrene represents a urologic emergency with a potentially high mortality rate. It is a rapidly progressing, microbial necrotizing fasciitis of the perineal, perianal, and genital regions, with a mortality rate ranging from 15 to 50% (Levenson et al. 2008). The infection is most often polymicrobial, with clostridia, streptococci, and staphylococci species and coliform bacteria commonly cultured. Synergistic effects of the bacteria lead to thrombosis of small subcutaneous vessels, and rapid gangrenous involvement of the surrounding skin and deep fascia ensues. Bacterial sources originate from the adjacent skin, the rectum and anus, and the lower urinary tract. The disease is most often due to a local infection adjacent to a point of entry (including abscesses in the perianal, perirectal, and ischiorectal regions), or anal fissures. However, bowel perforation and urological causes including urinary tract infection, neurogenic bladder, recent instrumentation, and epididymitis must be systematically looked for.

Predisposing factors reflect impaired host resistance from reduced cellular immunity. These factors include diabetes mellitus (seen in up to 60% of cases), alcoholism, and HIV infection.

The most common presenting symptoms of Fournier gangrene include scrotal swelling, pain, hyperemia, pruritus, and fever. Crepitus identified on physical examination is very suggestive of the diagnosis.

Although the diagnosis of Fournier gangrene is most often made clinically, the role of imaging is to help in cases of early manifestation or ambiguous physical findings, and to better discern the extent of the disease.

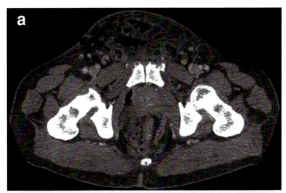

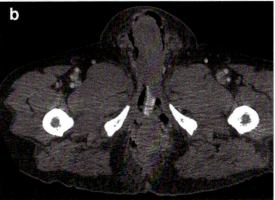

Fig. 10 **a**, **b** Fournier gangrene. Subcutaneous emphysema around the penis and the scrotum dissecting the perianal and periprostatic space

4.2   CT Findings

CT patterns (Levenson et al. 2008; Grayson et al. 2002) include suggestive findings, pathognomonic findings, and causal findings.

Suggestive findings are the presence of fascial thickening, fat stranding, fluid collection, or abscess around the scrotum and perineum and extending to the inguinal regions, thighs, abdominal wall, and retroperitoneum. The pathognomonic finding in this setting is a subcutaneous emphysema that dissects along fascial planes (Fig. 10). Causal factors may be a perianal abscess, a fistulous tract, an intra-abdominal or retroperitoneal infectious process, or a bowel perforation that is generally located in the infraperitoneal space.

4.3   CT Pitfalls

In early Fournier gangrene, CT can depict progressive soft-tissue infiltration, possibly with no evidence of subcutaneous emphysema (in about 10% of patients). In Fournier gangrene due to bowel perforation, the extraluminal air consecutive to the bowel perforation must not be confused with the diffusion of the emphysema.

4.4 CT Impact

The impact of CT is threefold: it can favor an early diagnosis and a differentiation between Fournier gangrene and other less aggressive entities such as soft-tissue edema or cellulitis; it can allow one to diagnose the cause of the gangrene; and, overall, it plays an important role in the evaluation of disease extent for appropriate surgical treatment (Yanar et al. 2006) because complete surgical debridement of all necrotic tissue is the most important factor in improving survival of patients with Fournier gangrene.

5 Vascular Conditions

5.1 Clinical Findings and Problems

Symptoms of nontraumatic acute renal infarction may mimic exactly those of stone colic or acute pyelonephritis. Fever and leukocytosis are common if the volume of infarcted parenchyma is substantial, but generally they occur 1 or 2 days after the pain. An elevated serum lactate dehydrogenase level is characteristic of infarction and helps to distinguish it from infection. Classically, renal infarct is the consequence of renal embolism that generally occurs in the setting of cardiac disease, notably atrial fibrillation. It may also be the consequence of an aortic dissection because more than one third of patients with aortic dissection have involvement of the visceral or iliac arterial branches. Other diseases may be responsible for renal infarction: vasculitis such as polyarteritis nodosa, systemic lupus erythematosus, drug-induced vasculitis, paraneoplastic syndrome, hypercoagulable state, or acute venous occlusion (Kawashima et al. 2000). However, in numerous cases, acute renal infarction may occur in previously apparently healthy individuals; in a study including 27 consecutive patients presenting with nontraumatic CT-documented renal infarction, 11 patients (41%)

had obvious cardiac disease, whereas 16 patients (59%) had no discernible structural or arrhythmic cardiac disease (Bolderman et al. 2006). These patients were younger and besides smoking had fewer cardiovascular risk factors. Among these unknown causes of infarct, renal artery dissection should be considered. Renal artery dissection is usually the natural extension of aortic dissection, the consequence of percutaneous angioplasty, or the result of percutaneous angioplasty. However, isolated dissection of the renal artery must be kept in mind (Ramamoorthy et al. 2002). Spontaneous isolated dissection of visceral arteries such as the celiac artery, superior mesenteric artery, or renal artery has recently been described (D'Ambrosio et al. 2007; Kanofskh and Lepor 2007), and it is likely that the incidence has been underestimated in the past because the diagnosis, now facilitated by the development of cross-sectional imaging, was previously not established.

The clinical manifestations of renal vein thrombosis depend on the age of the patient, the specific disease process, and the speed with which it occurs. When the clinical manifestations are acute, the presentation includes gross hematuria, flank pain, and loss of renal function, and the most common abnormality is membranous glomerulonephritis (Kawashima et al. 2000; Liach et al. 1980). In renal vein thrombosis associated with tumor, the clinical findings depend on the tumor, and thrombosis is often discovered in the staging of the renal tumor.

5.2 CT Findings

In renal infarct, contrast-enhanced CT readily shows absence of enhancement in the affected renal tissue. Acute infarcts appear as wedge-shaped areas of decreased attenuation within an otherwise normal-appearing kidney, which may be numerous and bilateral. In the acute phase, the infarct has an edematous appearance (Fig. 11a), with a retraction of the involved infarcted kidney in the chronic phase (Fig. 11b). When large areas of the kidney are involved, an increase in the size of the kidney due to edema can be seen (Kawashima et al. 2000). When no cardiac disease is known, special care must be taken on the examination of the renal arteries: identification of intimal flap or thrombosed false lumen seen as a linear filling defect, and the presence of segmental fat

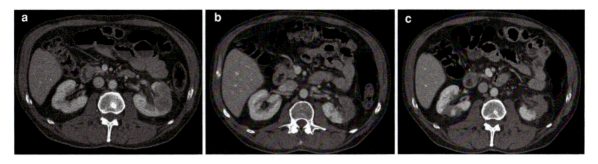

Fig. 11 Bilateral renal infarct. Poorly enhanced area in the anterior part of the left kidney (**a**). On a follow-up CT scan, the involved infarcted left kidney was retracted (**b**), whereas findings of right ischemia appeared with a wedge-shaped unenhanced area (**c**)

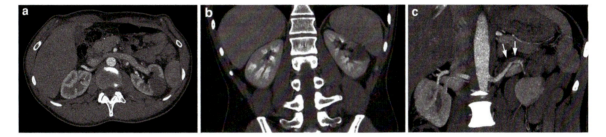

Fig. 12 Left renal infarct due to dissection of the renal artery. The infarct of the medial part of the left kidney is well seen on axial (**a**) and coronal (**b**) views as a wedge-shaped hypodense area. There is a segmental fat infiltration (*arrows*) around the left renal artery that is thinned (**c**)

infiltration around the artery is the reason for the diagnosis of dissection of the renal artery (Fig. 12).

In renal vein thrombosis, CT shows direct and indirect findings. The direct finding is the identification of the thrombus in the renal vein with or without extension into the inferior vena cava. Indirect findings are the consequences of the thrombus on the kidney with enlargement of the ipsilateral kidney, edema in the renal sinus and perirenal space, and the coarse striations of a diminished nephrogram (Kawashima et al. 2000).

specific to infarct, usually appears several days after onset of the infarction, as shown in a study assessing the cortical rim sign in posttraumatic renal infarction (Kamel and Berkowitz 1996). Furthermore, this finding may be encountered in long-standing hydronephrosis, renal vein obstruction, and acute renal failure. Spontaneous renal artery dissection is a good example of *misknowledge* of a disease that may be diagnosed by CT with the interpretation of the thin slices and the attention focused on the wall and content of the renal arteries.

5.3 CT Pitfalls

CT pitfalls are due to errors in the examination protocol, errors in the interpretation of findings present on CT, and lack of knowledge of the disease responsible for renal infarct. The CT protocol needs intravenous contrast material for renal infarct to be diagnosed, which may be lacking in the clinical setting of a presumed colic pain. For CT interpretation one must know that the cortical rim, considered as

5.4 CT Accuracy

In a study including 44 cases of renal infarction in patients with atrial fibrillation (Hazanov et al. 2004), over a period of nearly 20 years, renal isotope scan was performed in 37 cases, US in 27 cases, and contrast-enhanced CT in only 15 cases. US, CT, and renal isotope scan had a sensitivity of 11, 80, and 97%, respectively, so renal isotope scan was considered as the most sensitive diagnostic technique.

However, as concluded by the authors, CT requires further assessment because of the improvement of CT technology, and we believe that CT now has high predictive values to diagnose or rule out a renal infarct.

5.5 Role and Impact of CT

Classically, unenhanced helical CT is the ideal diagnostic test for patients with acute flank pain. It is highly accurate for the diagnosis of a stone, and it may diagnose extrarenal causes of abdominal pain such as appendicitis and diverticulitis. However, in patients in whom there is doubt regarding a vascular cause of the pain, contrast-enhanced CT is recommended. It must be performed in patients at risk of thromboembolic occlusion of the renal artery, or if there is an elevated level of serum lactate dehydrogenase. In 50-year-old male smokers, with a clinical presentation consistent with colic pain but without a past history of a stone, we recommend intravenous injection if unenhanced slices did not show a stone, to look for a renal infarct due to a spontaneous renal artery dissection.

6 Hemorrhagic Conditions

6.1 Clinical Findings and Problems

Spontaneous (nontraumatic) bleeding may affect the perirenal and subcapsular spaces, the renal parenchyma, or the collector system.

The main causes of spontaneous perirenal bleeding are tumors, vasculitis, and arteriovenous malformations. Long-term renal hemodialysis increases the risk of spontaneous hemorrhage, with or without an associated tumor. In a meta-analysis including 165 cases of spontaneous renal hemorrhage, the most common cause was benign or malignant neoplasm (101 cases, 61%), with angiomyolipoma being predominant (48 cases), followed closely by renal cell carcinoma (43 cases). Vascular disease was the next most common offender (28 cases, 17%), with polyarteritis

nodosa occurring more frequently (20 cases) (Zhang et al. 2002). Adrenal tumors are rarer causes of bleeding than renal tumors. However, pheochromocytoma (Fig. 13) corticosurrenaloma, myelolipoma, and metastases may be responsible for a unilateral cause of perirenal hematoma (Kawashima et al. 1999). Other causes of adrenal hemorrhage include stress and coagulopathy with other bilateral bleeding.

Hematuria has rarely hemodynamic consequences, and the task is often to identify its cause because hematuria can have a wide range of causes, including neoplasms, infection, trauma, drug toxicity, coagulopathies, vascular diseases, varices, and prolonged exercise, with infection and nephrolithiasis accounting for about 50% of cases (Joffe et al. 2003). However, some causes are more often responsible for severe bleeding with potentially shock: bladder tumors, hemorrhagic cystitis encountered, for instance, in an oncologic setting in patients with administration of ifosfamide and cyclophosphamide or as a complication of bone marrow transplantation, and vascular lesions.

6.2 CT Findings

CT without the use of contrast material will show the site of the bleeding, which may be an intraluminal bleeding, a subcapsular hematoma, or a perirenal hematoma. Because angiomyolipoma and renal cell carcinoma are the most common causes of spontaneous hemorrhage from a renal cause, CT must be use to look for this underlying tumor. Renal angiomyolipomas (Fig. 14) more than 4 cm in diameter have a greater tendency to bleed spontaneously, whereas for carcinomas, tumor size is not a good indicator of bleeding risk because tumors smaller than 4 cm are nearly as likely to bleed as larger tumors (Zhang et al. 2002). These small tumors may be obscured by hemorrhage, and when the initial imaging examination does not demonstrate the cause of renal hemorrhage, repeat CT following resolution or evacuation of the hematoma is essential (Prando et al. 2006). In bilateral renal hemorrhage, reconstructions on the intrarenal vessels to look for aneurysm are

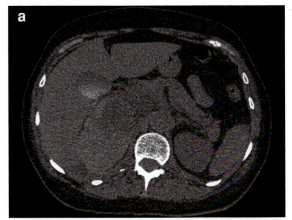
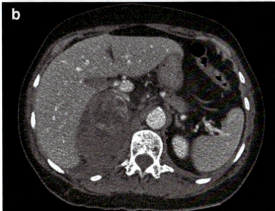
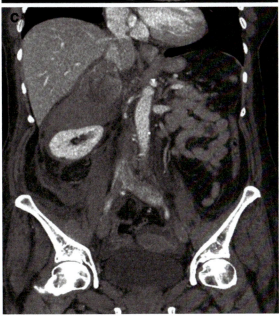

Fig. 13 **a–c** Perirenal hematoma due to bleeding by pheochromocytoma. A right perirenal mass is well seen on the axial slices before (**a**) and after (**b**) intravenous contrast material administration and on the coronal reformatting (**c**). The mass has a double component: spontaneously hyperdense without contrast and not enhanced for the one corresponding to the hematoma, and hypodense and heterogeneously enhanced for the adrenal tumor. Surgery revealed a pheochromocytoma

particularly helpful because renal vasculitis (polyarteritis nodosa) is the most common cause of this condition. Autosomal dominant polycystic kidney disease often presents clinically with acute flank pain caused by cyst hemorrhage or rupture. A clot or hematocrit effect within a cyst suggests that hemorrhage is recent, whereas calcified and hyperdense cysts likely indicate older hemorrhage (Talner and Vaughan 2003, Levine and Grantham 1985). Subepithelial hemorrhage is encountered most often as a complication of anticoagulation therapy. CT shows diffuse thickening of the pelvic and ureteral wall (Fig. 15).

CT urography is helpful in the evaluation of hematuria (Joffe et al. 2003). It is used to look for renal masses, papillary, caliceal, pelvic, and ureteral abnormalities, and bladder diseases. For hematuria responsible for an emergent setting, CT will generally show bladder thickening generally in the context of advanced bladder cancer or of hemorrhagic cystitis such as from administration of ifosfamide and cyclophosphamide or a complication of bone marrow transplantation. In some cases, hematuria is caused by life-threatening vascular diseases (Muraoka et al. 2008). CT can show an iliac artery–ureteral fistula in patients with predisposing factors such as pelvic or vascular surgery, ureteral stent or pelvic irradiation, a renal arteriovenous malformation, or a ruptured renal artery aneurysm (Muraoka et al. 2008). In these conditions, arterial phase, thin section, and reformatting are often needed to identify the vascular abnormality, its relationship with the surrounding vessels, and to establish a vascular map before an eventual embolization.

Nutcracker syndrome is a cause of repeated bouts of gross hematuria and left flank pain. It is defined by the compression of the left renal vein between the superior mesenteric artery and the aorta with an

Fig. 14 a, b Perirenal hematoma due to bleeding by an angiomyolipoma. Mass containing fat developed in the upper part of right kidney with perirenal hyperdense collection. The tumor is poorly enhanced when comparing before (**a**) and after (**b**) intravenous contrast material reformatting

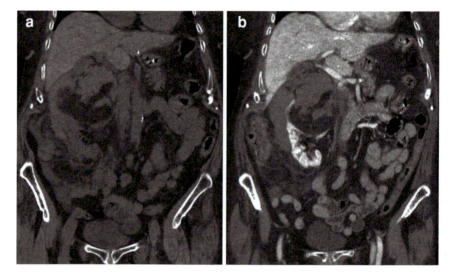

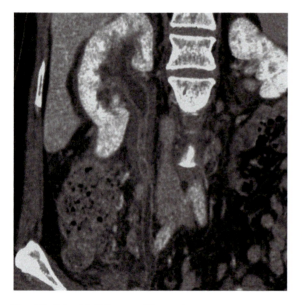

Fig. 15 Subepithelial ureteral hemorrhage

increase in left renal pressure and rupture of collateral veins into the collecting system. CT can show the stenosis of the left renal vein with proximal distention and the presence of collateral pathways (Fig. 16) (Muraoka et al. 2008).

6.3 CT Pitfalls

Subcapsular soft-tissue attenuation, such as encountered in lymphoma, may mimic subcapsular hemorrhages on unenhanced scans, and intravenous contrast material is helpful to enable exclusion of a subcapsular soft-tissue mass (Rucker et al. 2004). As shown previously, a tumor may be masked by hematoma when the tumor is small and the hemorrhage large. In the same way, in patients with hematuria, the clot sometimes responsible for colic pain (clot colic) may mask a urothelial tumor, and the use on the unenhanced CT examination with a very narrow window may be helpful to identify the underlying tumor.

Aneurysm of the intrarenal arteries or arteriovenous fistula needs to be identified with thin slices and scanning in the adequate arterial phase, when they are tiny. Last, association of disease may be confusing. For instance, at least 10% of patients with autosomal dominant polycystic disease develop stones and therefore may present with classic ureteral stone colic.

6.4 CT Accuracy

CT is the best imaging examination to diagnose renal bleeding and its cause. However, to our knowledge, no study has focused on its accuracy in this clinical setting, and failure in the acute phase in the identification of a small tumor responsible for the bleeding must be kept in mind.

6.5 Role and Impact of CT

Nontraumatic catastrophic hemorrhage from the urinary tract is uncommon and is rarely clinically

Urological Emergencies

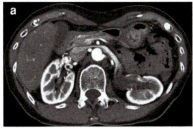
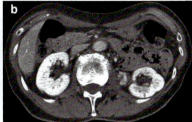
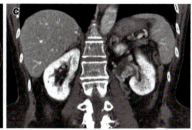

Fig. 16 a–c Nutcracker syndrome. The axial slice (**a**) shows compression of the left renal vein between the aorta and the superior mesenteric vein, with the development of the collateral vein within the left side of the pelvis well shown on a lower axial slice (**b**) and on the coronal reformatting (**c**)

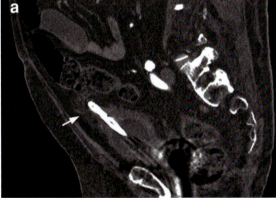

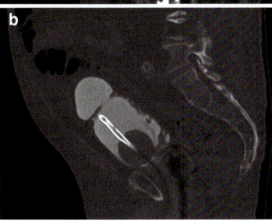

Fig. 17 a, b Pseudoperforation of the bladder. Sagittal reformatting shows the bladder probe crossing the bladder wall with some fat stranding around the bladder dome (**a**). On the same view in a delayed phase, a bladder diverticulum is filled by the contrast material, explaining this pseudopattern of the bladder perforation

suspected, except if there is hematuria. Consequently, the diagnosis is often revealed by CT, which has a great diagnostic impact. Besides its diagnostic impact, CT has a great impact on the management of the bleeding by allowing one to choose between a medical option, an embolization, or surgery, and by pointing out the bleeding vessel or vessels, which is helpful in the case of an embolization as well as in the case of a surgical option.

7 Bladder Perforation

Spontaneous rupture of the urinary bladder is an uncommon and life-threatening event. Prompt diagnosis followed by surgical intervention is the key for a successful outcome. The most common causes of atraumatic rupture of the urinary bladder are chronic inflammation, bladder outflow obstruction, cancer (Ahmed et al. 2009), and overall bladder augmentation cystoplasty because it is encountered in about 10% of children with an augmented urinary bladder (DeFoor et al. 2003). Clinically, most patients present with lower abdominal pain with associated symptoms of dysuria, being unable to void, anuria, and hematuria.

CT will show fluid around the bladder, extraluminal air close to the bladder due to the migration of air after a bladder intubation, and will be used to look for the cause of perforation. Additionally, the identification of the bladder probe crossing the bladder wall is an argument for a bladder perforation by keeping in mind that such a feature may be mimicked in the setting of bladder diverticula (Fig. 17).

References

Ahmad NA, Ather MH, Rees J (2003) Incidental diagnosis of diseases on un-enhanced helical computed tomography performed for ureteric colic. BMC Urol 3:2

Ahmed J, Mallick IH, Ahmad SM (2009) Rupture of urinary bladder: a case report and review of literature. Cases J 2:7004

Bolderman R, Oyen R, Verrijcken A et al (2006) Idiopathic renal infarction. Am J Med 119:356.e9–12

Boridy IC, Kawashima A, Goldman SM, Sandler CM (1999) Acute ureterolithiasis: nonenhanced helical CT findings of perinephric edema for prediction of degree of ureteral obstruction. Radiology 213:663–667

Browne RFJ, Zwirewich C, Torreggiani WC (2004) Imaging of urinary tract infection in the adult. Eur Radiol 14: 168–183

Catalano O, Nunziata A, Altei F et al (2002) Prima, helical CT versus selective helical CT after unenhanced radiography and sonography. AJR Am J Roentgenol 178:379–387

Craig WD, Wagner BJ, Travis MD (2008) Pyelonephritis: radiologic-pathologic review. Radiographics 28:255–276

D'Ambrosio N, Friedman B, Siegel D et al (2007) Spontaneous isolated dissection of the celiac artery: CT findings in adults. AJR Am J Roentgenol 188:W506–W511

DeFoor W, Tackett L, Minevich E, Wacksman J, Sheldon C (2003) Risk factors for spontaneous bladder perforation after augmentation cystoplasty. Urology 62:737–741

Ege G, Akman H, Kuzucu K, Yildiz S (2003) Acute ureterolithiasis: incidence of secondary signs on unenhanced helical CT and influence on patient management. Clin Radiol 58:990–994

Fultz PJ, Hampton WR, Totterman SM (1993) Computed tomography of pyonephrosis. Abdom Imaging 18:82–87

Gentle DL, Stoller ML, Jarrett TW et al (1997) Protease inhibitor-induced urolithiasis. Urology 50:508–511

Grayson DE, Abbott RM, Levy AD, Sherman PM (2002) Emphysematous infections of the abdomen and pelvis: a pictorial review. Radiographics 22:543–561

Hazanov N, Somin M, Attali M et al (2004) Acute renal embolisms. Forty-four cases of renal infarction in patients with atrial fibrillation. Medicine 83:292–299

Joffe SA, Servaes S, Okon S, Horowitz M (2003) Multidetector row CT urography in the evaluation of hematuria. Radiographics 23:1441–1456

Kamel IR, Berkowitz JF (1996) Assessment of the cortical rim sign in posttraumatic renal infarction. J Comput Assist Tomogr 20:803–806

Kanofskh JA, Lepor H (2007) Spontaneous renal artery dissection. Urology 9:156–160

Katz DS, Scheer M, Lumerman JH et al (2000) Alternative or additional diagnoses on unenhanced helical computed tomography for suspected renal colic: experience with 1000 consecutive examinations. Urology 56:53–57

Kawashima A, Sandler CM, Ernst RD et al (1999) Imaging of nontraumatic hemorrhage of the adrenal gland. Radiographics 19:949–963

Kawashima A, Sandler CM, Emst RD et al (2000) CT evaluation of renovascular disease. Radiographics 20: 1321–1340

Levenson RB, Singh AK, Novelline RA (2008) Fournier gangrene: role of imaging. Radiographics 28:519–528

Levine E, Grantham JJ (1985) High-density renal cysts in autosomal dominant polycystic kidney disease demonstrated by CT. Radiology 154:477–482

Levine J, Neitlich J, Smith RC (1999) The value of prone scanning to distinguish ureterovesical junction stones from ureteral stones that have passed into the bladder: leave no stone unturned. AJR Am J Roentgenol 172:977–981

Liach F, Paper S, Massry SG (1980) The clinical spectrum of renal vein thrombosis: acute and chronic. Am J Med 69:819–827

Liu CC, Li CC, Shih MC et al (2003) Matrix stone. J Comput Assist Tomogr 27:810–813

Luchs JS, Katz DS, Lane MJ et al (2002) Utility of hematuria testing in patients with suspected renal colic: correlation with unenhanced helical CT results. Urology 59:839–842

Memarsadeghi M, Heinz-Peer G, Helbich TH et al (2005) Unenhanced multidetector row CT in patients suspected of having urinary stone disease: effect of section width on diagnosis. Radiology 235:530–536

Memarsadeghi M, Schaefer-Prokop C, Prokop M et al (2007) Unenhanced MDCT in patients with suspected urinary stone disease: do coronal reformations improve diagnostic performance? AJR Am J Roentgenol 189:60–64

Muraoka N, Sakai T, Kimura H et al (2008) Rare causes of hematuria associated with various vascular diseases involving the upper urinary tract. Radiographics 28:855–867

Narlawar RS, Raut AA, Nager A et al (2004) Imaging features and guided drainage in emphysematous pyelonephritis: a study of 11 cases. Clin Radiol 59:192–197

Poletti PA, Platon A, Rutschmann OT et al (2006) Abdominal plain film in patients admitted with clinical suspicion of renal colic: should it be replaced by low-dose computed tomography? Urology 67:64–68

Poletti PA, Platon A, Rutschmann OT et al (2007) Low-dose versus standard-dose CT protocol in patients with clinically suspected renal colic. AJR Am J Roentgenol 188: 927–933

Prando A, Prando D, Prando P (2006) Renal cell carcinoma: unusual imaging manifestations. Radiographics 26: 233–244

Press SM, Smith AD (1995) Incidence of negative hematuria in patients with acute urinary lithiasis presenting to the emergency room with flank pain. Urology 45:753–757

Ramamoorthy SL, Vasquez JC, Taft PM et al (2002) Nonoperative management of acute spontaneous renal artery dissection. Ann Vasc Surg 16:157–162

Rucker CM, Menias CO, Bhalla S (2004) Mimics of renal colic: alternative diagnoses at unenhanced helical CT. Radiographics 24:S11–S33

Segura JW, Preminger GM, Assimos DG et al (1997) Ureteral Stones Clinical Guidelines Panel summary report on the management of ureteral calculi. J Urol 158:1915–1921

Stunell H, Buckley O, Feeney J et al (2007) Imaging of acute pyelonephritis in the adult. Eur Radiol 17:1820–1828

Talner LB, Davidson AJ, Lebowitz RL et al (1994) Acute pyelonephritis: can we agree on terminology? Radiology 192:297–305

Talner L, Vaughan M (2003) Nonobstructive renal causes of flank pain: findings on noncontrast helical CT (CT KUB). Abdom Imaging 28:210–216

Tamm EP, Silverman PM, Shuman WP (2003) Evaluation of the patient with flank pain and possible ureteral calculus. Radiology 228:319–329

Teichman JMH (2004) Acute renal colic from ureteral calculus. N Engl J Med 350:684–693

Thomas AA, Lane BR, Thomas A et al (2007) Emphysematous cystitis: a review of 135 cases. Journal Compilation 100:17–20

Vieweg J, The C, Freed K et al (1998) Unenhanced helical computerized tomography for the evaluation of patients with acute flank pain. J Urol 160:679–684

Wan YL, Lee TY, Bullard MJ et al (1996) Acute gas-producing bacterial renal infection: correlation between imaging findings and clinical outcome. Radiology 198:433–438

Wong-You Cheong J, Woodward PJ, Manning MA, Davis CJ (2006) From the archives of the AFIP: inflammatory and nonneoplastic bladder masses: radiologic-pathologic correlation. Radiographics 26:1847–1868

Yanar H, Taviloglu K, Ertekin C et al (2006) Fournier's gangrene: risk factors and strategies for management. World J Surg 30:1750–1754

Zhang JQ, Fielding JR, Zou KH (2002) Etiology of spontaneous perirenal hemorrhage: a meta-analysis. J Urol 167:1593–1596

Gynecologic Emergencies

Patrice Taourel, Fernanda Curros Doyon, and Ingrid Millet

Contents

1	**Introduction**	377
2	**Premenopausal Patients**	378
2.1	Pelvic Inflammatory Disease	378
2.2	Endometriosis	380
2.3	Adnexal Torsion	381
2.4	Hemorrhagic or Ruptured Ovarian Cysts	383
2.5	Ovarian Hyperstimulation Syndrome	384
2.6	Ectopic Pregnancy	385
2.7	Uterine Causes	385
3	**Patients Whose Pregnancy Is Known**	387
4	**Postpartum Patients**	388
4.1	Endometritis and Pelvic Abscess	388
4.2	Ovarian Vein Thrombosis and Thrombophlebitis	388
4.3	Retained Product of Conception	388
4.4	Uterine Rupture	389
4.5	Pelvic Hematomas	389
5	**Postmenopausal Patients**	390
References		390

P. Taourel (✉) · F. C. Doyon · I. Millet
Department of Imaging,
CHU Montpellier, Hospital Lapeyronie,
371 Avenue du Doyen Gaston-Giraud,
34295 Montpellier Cedex 5, France
e-mail: p-taourel@chu-montpellier.fr

Abstract

Acute pelvic pain is a routine situation in an emergency department. Ultrasonography is classically the first and sometimes the only necessary imaging tool. MRI is the preferred technique in young woman. However, in clinical practice CT is being performed more and more often as the first-line imaging in patients for whom the clinical hypotheses are often not good ones. Many gynaecologic disorders, including pelvic inflammatory disease, endometriosis, adnexal torsion, hemorrhage or rupture, leiomyoma complications, and pregnancy or postpartum complications, demonstrate suggestive CT findings. However, interpretation of these CT findings must take into account the age of the patient and the patient's hormonal status.

1 Introduction

Although ultrasonography (US) is classically the modality of choice for diagnosing gynecologic emergencies, gynecologic disease is detected or suspected with increasing frequency by CT. However, CT is being performed more and more often as the first-line imaging in patients with acute pain of the lower quadrants. In clinical practice, a gastrointestinal cause is often evoked for explaining acute abdomen, making a CT scan indicated. Furthermore, CT may be performed if US findings are equivocal or if the abnormalities extend beyond the field of view achievable with the endovaginal probe (Bennett et al. 2002; Potter and Chandrasekhar 2008).

P. Taourel (ed.), *CT of the Acute Abdomen*, Medical Radiology. Diagnostic Imaging,

The two main causes of a surgical gynecologic emergency are ectopic pregnancy and ovarian torsion. The diagnostic argument must take into account the epidemiological context and particularly the age of the patient. So we will review the contribution of CT with regard to the age of the patient.

2 Premenopausal Patients

2.1 Pelvic Inflammatory Disease

2.1.1 Clinical Context

Pelvic inflammatory disease (PID) refers to infection and resultant inflammation of the upper female genital tract, including the endometrium, fallopian tubes, and ovaries. It constitutes one of the most common diseases in women. The source of the disease is typically an ascending lower genital tract infection, even though hematogenous spread and direct extension of an infection (e.g., from an adjacent abscess) are also possible. *Neisseria gonorrhoeae* or *Chlamydia trachomatis* is believed to be the offending agent in two thirds of cases, but polymicrobial infection has also been reported. PID is one of the most common diseases in women, representing about one quarter of visits to the emergency department for gynecologic pain. Prompt diagnosis and treatment of PID are important because of the severity of long-term sequelae of untreated PID, which include infertility due to fallopian tubal occlusion, ectopic pregnancy, recurrence of PID, and chronic pelvic pain. Patients usually present with a myriad of nonspecific symptoms, including fever, abdominal or pelvic pain, vaginal discharge, uterine bleeding, dyspareunia, dysuria, adnexal or cervical tenderness, nausea, vomiting, and other vague constitutional symptoms (McCormack 1994; Sam et al. 2002). The reference standard for diagnosing PID is laparoscopy, however, this is an expensive and invasive procedure that is seldom used in a clinical setting, making imaging useful for diagnosis. Furthermore, imaging is useful to stage the disease and to identify patients who require hospitalization as opposed to antibiotic therapy on an outpatient basis.

2.1.2 CT Findings

The CT findings in PID differ according to the stage of the disease.

In early PID, CT findings may be normal or may only show a nonspecific mild pelvic edema that results in thickening of the uterosacral ligaments and haziness of the pelvic fat with obscuration of the pelvic fascial planes. Suggestive findings show the presence of inflammatory thickening of the fallopian tubes with, in some cases, the identification of mural nodules corresponding to thickened endosalpingeal folds, which helps to differentiate fallopian tubes from a digestive structure such as appendicitis. Findings are usually bilateral, although one side may be affected more than the other. Early oophoritis may manifest itself as enlarged and abnormally enhanced ovaries that may demonstrate a polycystic appearance (Sam et al. 2002). Other findings include abnormal endometrial thickening, abnormal endometrial enhancement and endometrial fluid consistent with endometritis, enlargement of the cervix consistent with cervicitis, and periovarian stranding.

In more advanced PID, the fallopian tubes exhibit a greater degree of wall thickening and enhancement and are filled with complex fluid, findings that usually indicate pyosalpinx. Then frank tubo-ovarian abscess is shown by the presence of a thick-walled, complex fluid collection that may contain internal septa, a fluid–debris level, or gas. In pelvic peritonitis complicating PID, a peritoneal collection is present and salpinx involvement is generally bilateral (Fig. 1). Coronal and sagittal reformatting may be helpful in demonstrating continual fluid-filled cystic structures, thereby confirming a dilated fallopian tube rather than a complex multilocated cystic mass (Yitta 2009); they are also helpful to differentiate pyosalpinx, with its tubular form, from ovarian abscess (Fig. 2).

Occasionally in mild and in advanced PID, bacteria may spread by means of direct extension along the right paracolic gutter or through the lymphatic system, causing inflammation of the right upper quadrant peritoneal surfaces and the right lobe of the liver (Romo and Clarke 1992). This corresponds to the clinical finding of perihepatitis, known as Fitz–Hugh–Curtis syndrome. CT is used to look for a thickening of the perihepatic peritoneum which is abnormally enhanced in the arterial phase because of the inflammation or in the delayed phase because of an early capsular fibrosis (Kim et al. 2009; Cho et al. 2008). Other involvements of adjacent structures in PID include a bowel with small or large bowel obstruction or ileus and ureters with hydronephrosis (Cho et al. 2008).

Gynecologic Emergencies

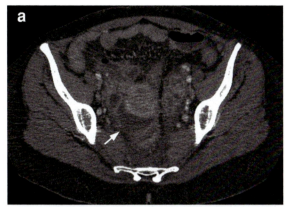

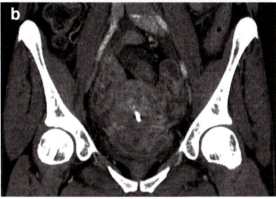

Fig. 1 Pelvic peritonitis complicating a bilateral pyosalpinx. Bilateral solid and cystic masses are well seen on the axial slice (**a**) and coronal reformatting (**b**). Note the peritoneal collection (*arrow*) behind the uterus with an enhanced wall suggestive of peritonitis. Note also the presence of an intrauterine device

2.1.3 CT Pitfalls

CT pitfalls may be due to unusual causes of tubo-ovarian abscess, difficulties in differentiating tubo-ovarian abscesses from other pelvis abscesses of other origin, or atypical forms of common causes of PID.

Unusual causes of tubo-ovarian abscess mainly include actinomycosis and tuberculosis (Kim et al. 2004).

Actinomycosis is a chronic suppurative infection by *Actinomyces israelii*. On CT, tubo-ovarian actinomycosis usually appears as a predominantly solid mass or a solid and cystic mass in the adnexal region, with contrast enhancement very prominent in the solid portion (Ha et al. 1993). The other key point in actinomycosis is the presence of thick, linear, and well-enhanced lesions extending directly from the mass into the adjacent tissue planes, which reflects the invasive

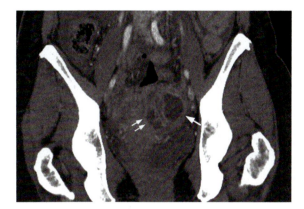

Fig. 2 Tubo-ovarian abscess. The coronal reformatting well differentiates the left ovarian abscess (*arrow*) from the salpinx (*double arrows*) with its characteristic tubular shape

nature of actinomycosis. These inflammatory extensions sometimes form perirectal masses or masses in the cul-de-sac, may mimic seeding masses from ovarian malignancies (Cho et al. 2008). The presence of an intrauterine device (IUD) is an ancillary diagnostic finding, by keeping in mind that IUDs are also commonly found with other causes of tubo-ovarian abscess and the absence of an IUD on CT scans does not mean the absence of a history of IUD use (Kim et al. 2004).

Genital involvement is rare in tuberculosis; the affected sites are predominantly the endometrium (72%) and the salpinx (34%) and less frequently ovaries (12.9%) and the cervix (2.4%) (Namavar Jahromi et al. 2001). CT findings mimic peritoneal carcinomatosis with thickened salpinges or nodularities along tubo-ovarian surfaces, cystic or both solid and cystic adnexal masses, usually bilateral, accompanied by ascites, omental or mesenteric infiltrations, and peritoneal thickening (Kim et al. 2004).

General pelvic abscess, resulting from an adjacent infection in the appendix, colon, or uncommonly bladder, may mimic tubo-ovarian abscess. An arguments for tubo-ovarian abscess is the anterior displacement of the broad ligament because of the posterior position of the mesoovarium, whereas an argument against is obviously the identification of normal ovaries.

In some cases, diagnosis may be difficult because salpinx involvement, adnexal involvement, or rarely a myometrium involvement is the consequence of a gastrointestinal tract infection, mainly diverticulitis and appendicitis (Fig. 3).

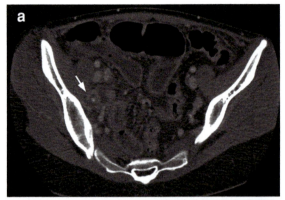
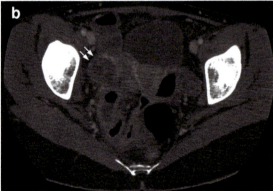
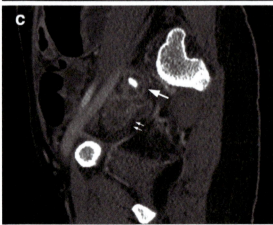

Fig. 3 Appendicitis involving the right ovary. The upper axial slice (a) shows findings of appendicitis (*arrow*) with dilatation of the appendix, thickening and increased enhancement of the appendicular wall, and an appendicolith. The lower axial slice (b) shows an abscess of the right ovary (*double arrows*). Sagittal reformatting (c) shows the contiguity between appendicitis (*arrow*) and the involved right ovary (*double arrows*)

2.1.4 CT Impact

Endovaginal US is classically the modality of imaging recommended to diagnose PID. However, in clinical practice, CT indications for PID are common:

Table 1 Indications for hospitalization of patients who have pelvic inflammatory disease

Presence of abscess
Pregnancy
All adolescents (compliance with therapy unpredictable)
Immunodeficiency
Uncertain diagnosis and surgical emergencies
Gastrointestinal tract symptoms (nausea and vomiting)
History of operative or diagnostic procedures
Inadequate response to outpatient therapy
Peritonitis in upper quadrants
Presence of an intrauterine device

1. Because a nongynecologic abnormality was suspected to be the cause of lower abdominal pain
2. To stage the full extent of the disease especially when patients fail to respond to antibiotic therapy or when complications of PID such as abscess are suspected
3. When US is difficult to perform or the findings are equivocal

By giving a complete assessment of the disease, it can provide arguments for hospitalization of patients who have PID (the indications for which as summarized by McWilliams et al. 2008 are given in Table 1) and can be used to monitor an eventual surgical treatment.

2.2 Endometriosis

Endometriosis results from the ectopic location of endometriosis glands and stroma outside the uterus. It affects an estimated 10% of premenopausal women, with as much as 80% of ectopic endometrial tissue found in the ovaries. Other sites include the uterine serosal surface, rectovaginal septum, fallopian tubes and bowel, most commonly the rectosigmoid colon. Although endometriosis is a common cause of chronic abdominal pain, an acute setting is rare but can occur in four clinical complications:

1. Small or large bowel obstruction due to the site of endometriosis implantation in the bowel.
2. Acute appendicitis resulting from endometriosis deposits in the appendix and obstructing its lumen.
3. Acute parietal pain due to an endometrioma in the abdominal wall within the rectus muscle or extending into the subcutaneous fat. It complicates

previous abdominal surgery (cesarian) or amniocentesis. Clinically, a peri-incisional abdominal wall hernia may be suspected. CT shows a mass within the abdominal wall with a marked contrast enhancement, which may be confused with a tumoral mass such as a dermoid tumor or a hypervascular metastasis (Bennett et al. 2010)
4. Secondary rupture or infection of an endometrioma is very rare. It may be responsible for a complex adnexal mass that may simulate on CT PID, hemorrhagic cyst, or even malignancies (Potter 2008).

2.3 Adnexal Torsion

2.3.1 Clinical Context

Adnexal torsion is a gynecologic emergency caused by partial or complete twisting of the ovary, ispsilateral fallopian tube or both, resulting in vascular compromise. Adnexal torsion is frequently associated with a large ipsilateral ovarian tumor or with large cystic ovaries seen in ovarian hyperstimulation syndrome (McWilliams et al. 2008). Tumoral causes are benign, including predominantly teratomas, ovarian cysts, and cystadenomas and less often fibromas. Although, it can also occur in normal ovaries, usually in adolescents, this is very rare and was never present in a retrospective study of 135 adnexal torsions (Bouguizane et al. 2003). Early surgical intervention is needed to save the affected ovary in young women. So in the setting of acute pelvic pain, ovarian torsion is often a leading diagnostic consideration, especially when an ovarian mass is discovered.

Adnexal torsion accounts for about 3% of gynecologic emergencies in the USA (Schraga et al. 2007). It may occur in women of all ages, with the highest prevalence in women in their reproductive years and particularly in pregnant women. The classic presentation includes sharp, localized right or left lower abdominal pain, tenderness and peritoneal findings, and a pelvic mass; gastrointestinal complaints with nausea and vomiting are encountered in 70% of patients (McWilliams et al. 2008), whereas fever constitutes an argument for a necrosis complicating the ovarian torsion.

US constitutes the primary imaging modality when adnexal torsion is suspected. However, CT is often performed because adnexal torsion was not the first diagnosis envisaged by the physician since it may

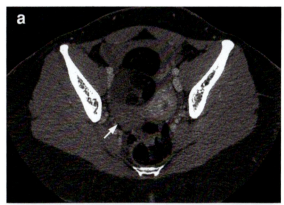

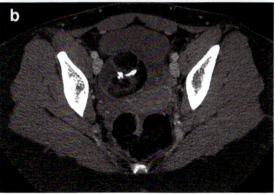

Fig. 4 Torsion of an ovary with a teratoma: Axial slices (**a**, **b**) show a fat-containing mass on the right side. Note some fluid collection around the teratoma. The normal right ovary is well seen (*arrow*). The uterus is deviated to left side. Surgery confirmed torsion of the left ovary with teratoma

mimic other causes of acute abdominal pain such as appendicitis or colic pain, because US findings are equivocal, or because further characterization of the pelvic disease is necessary.

2.3.2 CT Findings

The main finding of adnexal torsion is the presence of an adnexal mass, which is generally totally or partially cystic with or without fat and which measures more than 5 cm in diameter (Hiller et al. 2007; Ghang et al. 2008; Lee et al. 2009) (Fig. 4).

Several intra-adnexal as well as extra-adnexal CT findings are helpful to differentiate adnexal torsion from a common tumor of the ovary:

- The presence of a thickening of the fallopian tube seen between the uterus and the ovarian mass. It appears on CT as a tubular masslike lesion or a target lesion (Fig. 5).

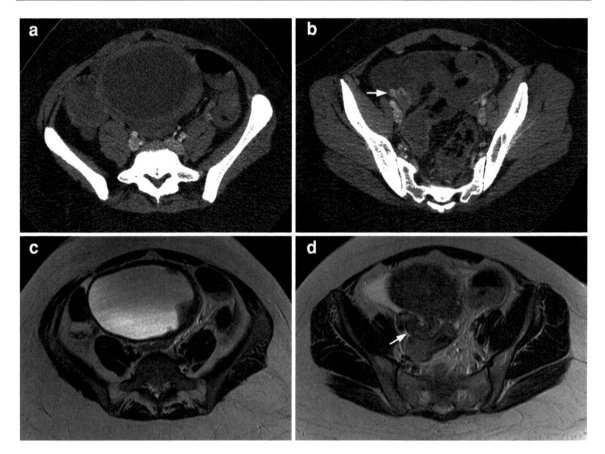

Fig. 5 Torsion of an ovary with a serous cystadenoma. The axial CT slice (a) show a cystic medial mass with a smooth wall thickening more pronounced on its right side. A thickened and enhanced right fallopian tube is well seen on a lower slice (b) (*arrow*). Axial T2-weighted MRI slices show clearly the cystic mass with a smooth thickened wall and some papillary projections (c) and, better visualized, the abnormal right fallopian tube as a tubular masslike lesion (d) (*arrow*). Surgery confirmed the torsion of the right fallopian tube and of the right ovary with a serous cystadenoma

- The identification of a smooth wall thickening without nodularity on the cystic mass. This thickening is more often eccentric than concentric (Rha et al. 2002) (Fig. 5).
- The displacement of adnexa which may be on the controlateral side of the pelvis (Fig. 4) or on the midline in a far anterior position abutting the anteropelvic fascia or posterior in the pouch of Douglas (Fig. 6).
- The deviation of uterus to side of the involved ovary (Fig. 4).
- The noncontinuity of the ipsilateral gonadal vein with the twisted adnexal mass.

Other findings such as ascites or infiltration of pelvic space are less helpful in the setting of acute pelvic pain, but the site of the infiltration is a good indicator of the torsion side (Fig. 6).

2.3.3 CT Pitfalls

In clinical practice, the identification of an ovarian mass is a clue to diagnosing ovarian torsion in adults. However, most ovarian tumors are not complicated by torsion. So the identification of the location of the involved ovary (normal location, contralateral displacement, midline displacement) is important and needs the visualization of the uninvolved ovary, which is not constant. If serial CT is available, a change in the configuration of the ovary may aid in the diagnosis (Ghossian et al. 1997). Otherwise, visualization of the fallopian tube is challenging when a large complex adnexal mass is present on CT, explaining why tubal involvement may be found less commonly on CT than on pathologic examination (Hiller et al. 2007). Finally, if fat density characteristic of teratoma is missing, the underlying pathologic process causing

Gynecologic Emergencies

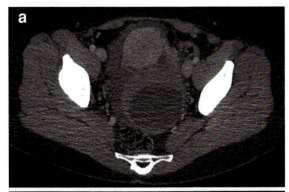

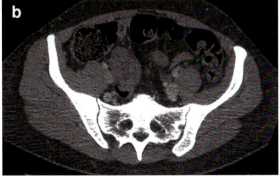

Fig. 6 Torsion of an ovary with a serous cystadenoma. The lower CT slice (**a**) shows a cystic mass with an eccentric wall thickening. The mass is posterior in the pouch of Douglas and there is some fluid around the mass. The upper CT slice (**b**) shows a mass on the right side in front of the iliac vessels. On surgery, there was torsion of the right ovary with a serous cystadenoma

torsion may not be characterized by CT. Fluid especially may mean either a cystic tumor or a necrosis complicating the torsion.

The differentiation between patients with hemorrhagic infarction and those without is difficult. Adnexal hemorrhage which can manifest itself on unenhanced images as an area of increased attenuation is in favor of infarction (Ghang et al. 2008) but this needs unenhanced CT, which is not commonly performed in the setting of acute abdomen. The lack of enhancement of the adnexa could theoretically be an argument for necrosis, but CT is not reliable to assess the flow within it.

2.3.4 CT Impact

Diagnosis of ovarian torsion remains difficult and is often made by ruling out other causes and by having a strong clinical suspicion (McWilliams et al. 2008). US is usually the first examination performed for this diagnosis, with an overall accuracy allowing an expeditious diagnosis (Ghang et al. 2008), and in most cases there is no need for CT (Hiller et al. 2007). However, CT may be helpful in the case of indeterminate US findings or for a better assessment of the mass responsible for the torsion. Furthermore, the CT diagnosis of adnexal torsion must be known since CT is often the first imaging performed in the clinical setting of acute abdomen. An early diagnosis can help prevent irreversible structural damage and may allow conservative, ovary-sparing treatment, with instead of performing a salpingo-oophorectomy a laparoscopic evaluation with a gentle untwisting of the ovary, the removal of the adnexal tumor, and an oophoropexy against the pelvic sidewall.

2.4 Hemorrhagic or Ruptured Ovarian Cysts

2.4.1 Clinical Context

Significant hemorrhage of an ovarian cyst is a common cause of acute pelvic pain. If there is cyst rupture, it can be life-threatening because of associated hemoperitoneum and hypotension, particularly in patients being treated with anticoagulation (Ghang et al. 2008). Hemorrhage is more frequent in a corpus luteum cyst than in a follicular cyst owing to the increased vascularity of the ovary during the luteal phase. Other ovarian masses, such as endometrioma, may rarely rupture. For instance, the content of a teratoma may spill into the peritoneum with chemical peritonitis and fat-containing peritoneal implants.

2.4.2 CT Findings

Hemorrhagic ovarian cyst before rupture often appears unilocular on CT images with an interval attenuation of 40–100 UH. A fluid–fluid level may be observed. If there is cyst rupture, hemoperitoneum will also be present and the ovary may even be normal if rupture has totally decompressed the cyst (Fig. 7). Contrast-enhanced CT may delineate the cyst wall with a ring of peripheral contrast enhancement, and delayed CT may be useful in demonstrating the site of pooling of contrast-enhanced blood in the pelvis if imaging is performed during active bleeding (Hertzberg et al. 1999).

A ruptured ectopic pregnancy could manifest itself with a similar clinical picture, so correlation with

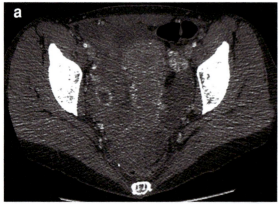

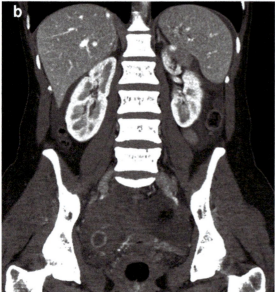

Fig. 7 Ruptured corpus luteum with hemoperitoneum. Axial (**a**) and coronal (**b**) views show a corpus luteum with an enhanced wall in the right ovary and a significant amount of high-attenuation pelvic fluid surrounding the corpus luteum. The free peritoneal fluid in Morrison's pouch is hypodense and well seen on the coronal view

Table 2 Hemoperitoneum of gynecologic origin

Ectopic pregnancy

Rupture of a hemorrhagic ovarian cyst

Adnexal torsion

Endometriosis

Rupture of a uterine leiomyoma

Rupture of the uterus

need not be immediately evaluated with US for further comparisons.

The differentiation by imaging between hemorrhagic follicular and corpus luteum cyst is impossible. In uncomplicated cysts, the wall of luteal cysts is thicker than that of follicular cysts, but it is likely that in a complicated follicular cyst the wall becomes thicker. So, temporal correlation of a symptomatic cyst with the luteal phase of the menstrual cycle or with a positive β-HCG level favors the diagnosis of hemorrhagic corpus luteum (Potter 2008).

Consequently, in clinical practice, even if the CT diagnosis of hemorrhagic or ruptured cyst is a common occurrence, strict rules need to be followed in such a setting, including correlation with β-HCG levels to rule out an ectopic pregnancy, temporal correlation with the phase of the cycle, and second-look US for further comparisons.

β-HCG levels prior to imaging to exclude this possibility is essential. Hemorrhagic ovarian cyst and ectopic pregnancy constitute the two most common causes of hemoperitoneum of gynecologic origin (Table 2).

2.4.3 CT Impact

Management of hemorrhagic or ruptured cyst is conservative in the lack of hemodynamic instability with the need for follow-up US performed within one or two menstrual cycles to determine whether the cyst has resolved (Borders et al. 2004). So when hemorrhagic ovarian cysts are detected initially on CT, they

2.5 Ovarian Hyperstimulation Syndrome

Ovarian hyperstimulation syndrome is a rare, potentially fatal, syndrome; it is usually iatrogenic secondary to ovarian stimulant drug therapy for infertility and occurs during the luteal phase or early pregnancy (Delvigne and Rozenberg 2003). But in some rare cases it may also be present as a spontaneous event in pregnancy. The syndrome consists of ovarian enlargement with abdominal discomfort through extravascular accumulation of exudates, leading to weight gain, ascites, pleural effusions, intravascular volume depletion with hemoconcentration, and oliguria in differing degrees. Pain, abdominal distention, nausea, and vomiting are frequently seen.

CT shows bilaterally enlarged ovaries due to multiple distended, peripherally located corpora lutea cysts of various sizes, producing the "spoke wheel" appearance with stromal ovarian tissue located centrally with surrounding cysts (Kim and Lee 1997).

The appropriate clinical setting makes the differential diagnosis easy with a bilateral cystic ovarian neoplasm.

2.6 Ectopic Pregnancy

Ectopic pregnancy accounts for approximately 2% of all pregnancies and is the most common cause of pregnancy-related mortality in the first trimester. The main risk factors for ectopic pregnancy include a history of ectopic pregnancy, tubal surgery, and PID. Ninety-five percent of ectopic pregnancies are tubal, whereas other types of ectopic pregnancies include interstitial, cornual, ovarian, cervical, scar, intra-abdominal, and heterotopic pregnancy (Lin et al. 2008).

Early diagnosis and treatment of ectopic pregnancy are essential in reducing maternal mortality and preserving future fertility and workup of a patient with possible ectopic pregnancy entails hormonal assays and endovaginal pelvic US. However, with increased use of CT in the emergent setting, pregnant women may inadvertently undergo CT scanning when the pregnancy is not known at the time of the emergency.

CT findings of tubal ectopic pregnancy described in the few cases reported in the literature, as well as in our experience of three recent cases, are univocal.

CT shows an adnexal area of low attenuation with a dramatic enhanced ring (Pham and Lin 2007) (Fig. 8). This enhanced ring is equivalent to the ring of fire described by Pellerito et al. (1992) with color Doppler imaging to describe the high-velocity, low-impedance flow of trophoblastic tissue surrounding an ectopic adnexal pregnancy. The adnexal cystic structure is adjacent to the ipsilateral ovary and is often associated with hyperdense fluid in the peritoneum consistent with a hemoperitoneum.

The main CT differential diagnosis of ectopic pregnancy is a corpus luteum cyst for three reasons: the wall of a corpus luteum may have a strong enhancement, a corpus luteum cyst may rupture in the peritoneum, and a corpus luteum cyst may occur in the setting of early pregnancy. If clinical symptoms and β-HCG levels do not permit one to differentiate these two entities, the location of the adnexal cystic mass may be a clue, with an intraovarian location suggesting a corpus luteum cyst, since intraovarian ectopic pregnancy is very rare.

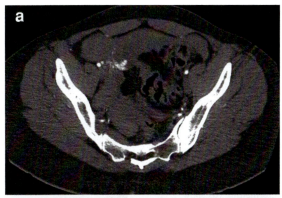

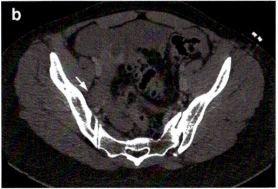

Fig. 8 Ruptured ectopic pregnancy: The axial slice in the arterial phase (**a**) shows an enhanced rim. Note also a huge amount of peritoneal fluid. In a delayed phase at the same level (**b**), the normal right ovary is well shown (*arrow*), proving that the cause of bleeding was not an ovarian cyst

2.7 Uterine Causes

Uterine causes of acute abdominal pain may be linked to a complication of leiomyomas or in particular conditions to rupture or torsion of the uterus itself.

2.7.1 Complications of a Leiomyoma

Leiomyomas, also known as myomas or fibroids, are the most common gynecologic neoplasm, occurring in 20–30% of women of reproductive age. However, acute pelvic pain is rare in leiomyoma. It may be due to different complications, including acute degeneration and particularly hemorrhagic degeneration, torsion of a pedunculated subserosal leiomyoma, prolapse of pedunculated submucosal leiomyomas, or rupture within the peritoneum.

Acute degeneration is the most common cause of acute pain due to leiomyomas. It can occur spontaneously or following an interventional procedure such

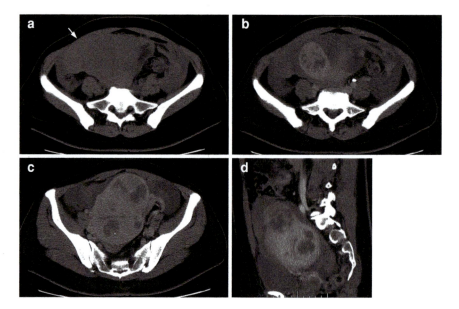

Fig. 9 Rupture of uterine leiomyoma with hemoperitoneum. Axial slices before (**a**) and after (**b**) intravenous contrast material administration show a hyperdense collection consistent with hemoperitoneum (*arrow*), in front of an enhanced mass. Note also free hypodense peritoneal fluid in the paracolic gutters. The lower axial slice (**c**) and sagittal reformatting (**d**) show multiple leiomyomas. Surgery confirmed the diagnosis of rupture of uterine leiomyoma within the peritoneum

as uterine embolization. It is typically seen on CT as a low-attenuation mass in the uterus. Hemorrhagic or red degeneration of a uterine leiomyoma is attributed to obstruction of peripheral veins and is most likely to happen during the period of gestation. Usually, it does not require surgical treatment in an emergency. It is characterized on CT by a hypodense and heterogeneous central component (Bennett et al. 2003).

Torsion may complicate pedunculated subserosal leiomyomas and constitutes a surgical emergency. Clinical symptoms depend on the degree of the rotation and the speed at which the torsion develops. CT shows a mass contiguous to the uterus, which is hypodense with small higher attenuation on unenhanced images indicating hemorrhagic infarction; enhancement of the wall of the mass as a regular rim corresponds to obstructed peripheral veins. In some cases (Roy et al. 2005), a shaggy localized zone within the myometrium against the mass is identified, representing the twisted pedicle.

Pedunculated submucosal leiomyomas may prolapse or abort into the vaginal canal. This may lead to acute pelvis pain due to uterine contractions and vaginal bleeding. Although aborting submucosal leiomyomas are better analyzed with MRI, sagittal and coronal multiplanar reformation images are useful in demonstrating the prolapse of the submucosal leiomyoma and its relationship to the cervix and vagina (Yitta 2009).

Rupture of a uterine leiomyoma is a very rare complication of leiomyoma and may be the result of trauma, torsion, or spontaneous rupture of superficial blood vessels. CT can show the myometrial mass. Leiomyomas may have a variety of appearances depending on their degeneration, with the most specific finding, solid "mass-type" calcifications, being rarely encountered. However, the great majority of myometrial masses are leiomyomas, making this diagnosis likely in patients with myometrial masses. CT diagnosis of rupture of uterine leiomyoma is performed on the presence of a myometrial mass, a sentinel clot with its characteristic high attenuation closed to the mass and which permits one to identify the source of hemoperitoneum (Lubner et al. 2007) (Fig. 9), and helps one to differentiate rupture of uterine leiomyoma from other causes of bleeding due to gynecologic conditions (Lotterman 2008; Gupta et al. 2008).

2.7.2 Rupture and Torsion of the Uterus

Rupture and torsion of the uterus are very rare events, especially in the nonpregnant woman. Rupture of the uterus in the nonpregnant woman is usually iatrogenic, resulting from dilatation or curettage. Uterine rupture may be complete, involving the full thickness of the wall and potentially life-threatening, or incomplete, as is generally the case in the 0.1% of perforations complicating IUD placement. In uterine perforation, CT with, in particular, sagittal and coronal reconstructions

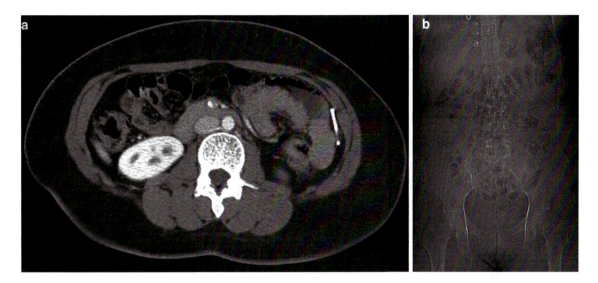

Fig. 10 Migration of an intrauterine device. The axial CT slice (**a**) shows a metallic foreign body within the greater omentum, with its characteristic T shape displaying an intrauterine device well demonstrated on the scout view (**b**). This migration means a perforation of the uterus which was not symptomatic

is helpful for the diagnosis and staging by showing a myometrial defect and assessing its location, size, and depth. In perforation complicating IUD placement, which may be not symptomatic, CT easily shows the hyperdense IUD outside the uterine lumen (Fig. 10).

Torsion of a nonpregnant uterus is exceptional, with fewer than ten cases reported. Uterine torsion is always along the transition between the corpus and cervix uteri and is defined as rotation of more than 45° around the long axis of the uterus. It is favored by the presence of a big leiomyoma. CT can show a nonenhancement of the uterine corpus in contrast with a normal enhancement of the cervix and a whorled enhanced structure in the cervix suggesting the mechanism of torsion (Jeong et al. 2003; Matsumoto et al. 2007).

3 Patients Whose Pregnancy Is Known

All the diseases seen in nonpregnant women may be encountered in pregnant women, with an increased occurrence of some of these diseases. Complications of leiomyomas are more frequent with a predisposition for hemorrhagic degeneration, especially during the period of greatest increase in myometrial volume, generally before 10 weeks of gestation (Eyvazzadeh and Levine 2006). Uterine leiomyoma torsion and uterine torsion are less rare in pregnant women than in nonpregnant women. For ovarian torsion, it has been shown that patients with ovarian hyperstimulation syndrome have a greater risk of torsion (16%) than those who do not become pregnant (Mashiach et al. 1990). Last pregnancy increases the risk of rupture of a corpus puteum (Hallatt et al. 1984). However, during pregnancy, the risk of exposure of the fetus to radiation is increased, so more than the usual benefit is necessary to justify CT. Consequently, gynecologic acute diseases are not investigated by CT. In a retrospective study including 78 pregnant women who underwent CT for abdominal pain (Lazarus et al. 2007), CT established the diagnosis in 35% of cases. The main diagnoses performed by CT were appendicitis, urinary tract calculi, bowel obstruction, and cholelithiasis and there were no cases of gynecologic emergencies, demonstrating that for performing gynecologic diagnoses, CT had not been indicated. It must be kept in mind that some nongynecologic common acute diseases have an incidence that is even increased during pregnancy (Augustin and Majerovic 2007; Rooholamini et al. 1993): colic pain, cecal and sigmoid volvulus, acute cholecystitits, liver disease including acute fatty liver of pregnancy, HELLP syndrome, hepatic rupture, and acute pancreatitis. It may be necessary to perform a CT examination for diagnosis; CT findings in these diseases are dealt with in the corresponding chapters.

4 Postpartum Patients

Conversely to pregnancy, in which CT is of limited use, CT is the primary modality in making the diagnosis or determining the severity of peripartum and postpartum complications, including endometritis, abscess, ovarian vein thrombosis and thrombophlebitis, retained product of conception, and hemorrhage.

4.1 Endometritis and Pelvic Abscess

Endometritis is the most common cause of fever during the postpartum period. The incidence of postpartum endometritis after a vaginal delivery in comparison with cesarean delivery is low (2–3%). The incidence of endometritis is particularly high when there is a delay between membrane rupture and cesarean delivery. Other risk factors for endometritis are prolonged labor, premature rupture of the membranes, clot, and retained product of conception (Zuckerman et al. 1997). CT may show fluid or air in the cavity as well as endometrial enhancement on postcontrast images (Menias et al. 2007). However, these findings are nonspecific, and it has been shown by both US and CT that intrauterine air may be present in about 20% of healthy postpartum women and it may persist for as long as 3 weeks after delivery.

Pelvic abscesses may complicate endometritis. They are more frequent after cesarean delivery for several reasons: endometritis is more common, infection may occur in the region of incision, and infection can spread to the parametrium after a cesarean delivery because the parametrial space between the leaves of the broad ligaments may be entered during the development of the bladder flap (Zuckerman et al. 1997). CT shows classic findings suggesting an abscess with a thick-walled, rim-enhanced, fluid-filled structure with adjacent inflammatory stranding and in some cases air–fluid levels and internal septations (Menias et al. 2007).

4.2 Ovarian Vein Thrombosis and Thrombophlebitis

Although ovarian vein thrombosis is classically seen as a postpartum complication, with an overall incidence of about 1 in 1,000 deliveries, it may occur in the setting of PID, oncologic patients, and recent pelvic surgery. The enlarging uterus compresses the ovarian veins, causing venous stasis and thrombosis. Ovarian vein thrombosis is unilateral in most patients on the right (80%) more commonly than on the left (6%) and bilateral in 15% of patients (Munsik and Gillanders 1981). The predilection for right-sided involvement results from uterine dextroversion during pregnancy and from retrograde flow from the left renal vein preventing the left ovarian vein from the stasis. CT shows a tubular structure with wall enhancement corresponding to the dilated gonadal vein with central low-attenuation thrombus. Following the course of the gonadal vein from the pelvis to the inferior vena cava for the right ovarian vein and to the left renal vein for the left ovarian vein helps one to distinguish it from the ureter or appendix. In some cases, thrombosis of ovarian vein collateral vessels when they are retrocecal in location may mimic retrocecal appendicitis (Fig. 11).

Thrombophlebitis may complicate a bland thrombus, particularly in postpartum patients with endometritis. Patients with thrombophlebitis usually present with fever and acute frank pain. Perivascular stranding associated with an enlarged gonadal vein helps to support the diagnosis of thrombophlebitis and distinguish it from bland thrombus (Zuckerman et al. 1997).

4.3 Retained Product of Conception

Uterine atony and retained product of conception constitute the most common causes of postpartum hemorrhage. Less often, hemorrhage reveals a trophoblastic disease. The differentiation between these entities is essential since uterine atony is medically treated, a retained product of conception needs curettage, and a choriocarcinoma needs chemotherapy. US remains the radiological investigation of choice for initial diagnosis, whereas MRI is of invaluable use in assessing extrauterine tumor spread (Allen et al. 2006, Green et al. 1996). If performed, CT gives strong arguments for differentiating placental tissue from a clot by showing an enhancement of retained product of

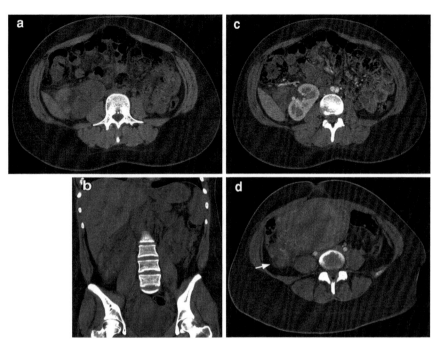

Fig. 11 Thrombosis of periovarian collaterals in a postpartum woman. The axial slice (**a**) and coronal reformatting (**b**) before intravenous contrast matarial administration show a tubular structure which is spontaneously hyperdense lateral to the right kidney. This structure was not enhanced after contrast material administration (**c**). Note also the big uterus related to the postpartum condition and the structure (*arrow*) corresponding to ovarian collaterals with thrombosis, posterolaterally to the uterus (**d**)

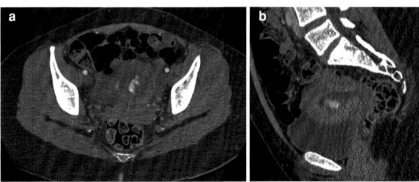

Fig. 12 Retained product of conception responsible for postpartum hemorrhage: The axial slice (**a**) in the arterial phase and sagittal reformatting (**b**) in a portal phase show a dilatation of the uterine lumen, with enhanced structure displaying the presence of placental tissue within the uterus

conception (Fig. 12), whereas a clot, often hyperdense, is not enhanced. The presence of calcification, also well seen on US, is an ancillary finding for placental tissue. The imaging appearance of retained product of conception may overlap with that of gestational trophoblastic neoplasia. Myometrial or extrauterine invasion shown by MRI or CT and overall a high and persistent level of β-HCG are key points for the diagnosis of gestational trophoblastic neoplasia.

4.4 Uterine Rupture

This rare complication may occur before or during labor or during the delivery. It occurs most frequently in patients with previous surgery of the uterus (myomectomy, cesarean section). Uterine rupture may occur before or during labor or during delivery. The clinical presentation is often alarming, with severe abdominal pain and intraperitoneal and vaginal bleeding making the diagnosis clinical with an immediate laparotomy. However, less severe cases may prompt CT evaluation. CT will show a low-attenuation defect within the normally enhanced myometrium, meaning the disruption of the uterine wall, and a periuterine hematoma (Has et al. 2008).

4.5 Pelvic Hematomas

Hemorrhage is a classic complication of cesarean section. Bleeding generally occurs at the site of the lower uterine incision with the development of a hematoma in the potential extraperitoneal space between the bladder and the lower uterine segment, the so-called bladder flap hematoma. Broad-ligament and rectus sheath hematomas (Rooholamini et al. 1993) or intraperitoneal hemorrhage is more rarely encountered.

5 Postmenopausal Patients

In postmenopausal patients, gynaecologic emergencies are rarer but remain possible.

Findings of PID must be due to the propagation to the fallopian tube or to the ovaries of a bowel inflammation, and in postmenopausal patients, pyosalpinx or ovarian abscesses must lead to a search for diverticulitis or a bowel perforation within the salpinx or the ovaries.

In a retrospective series including 14 women with adnexal involvement from diverticulitis, a gas collection within the adnexa was both sensitive and a specific sign of colosalpingeal fistula, allowing differentiation between fistula and contiguous periadnexal inflammation without fistula (Panghaal et al. 2009). In the same way, ovarian abscess may be the consequence of a perforated sigmoid cancer within the ovary (Fig. 13).

Women of reproductive age and particularly pregnant women have the highest prevalence of ovarian torsion. However, ovarian torsion can occur in women of all ages and consequently in postmenopausal women. In a study focused on CT features of adnexal torsion (Hiller et al. 2007), it occurred in 29% of the 35 patients included in the study who were postmenopausal.

Complications of a leiomyoma with acute clinical findings are relatively uncommon, whatever the age of the patient, without any specificity in postmenopausal patients. By contrast, in a postmenopausal patient with acute pelvic pain and a pelvic mass, the acute revelation of a malignant tumor of the ovary must be kept in mind. Acute abdomen may be due to a hemorrhage within the tumor, a rupture, or torsion (Genevois 2008). However, these conditions are rare, and, for instance, in a series including 135 ovarian torsions (Bouguizane et al. 2003), the torsion was due to a malignancy only in two cases. In our experience,

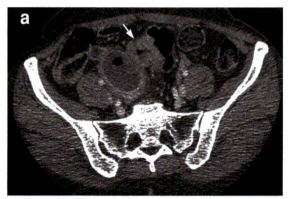

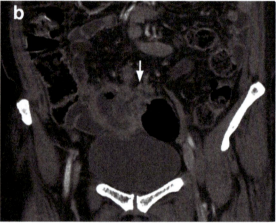

Fig. 13 Perforated sigmoid cancer within the right ovary. The axial slice (**a**) and coronal reformatting (**b**) show a hypodense mass above the bladder on the right side of the pelvis with a thick wall; the mass contains an air bubble. The relationship between the mass and the sigmoid colon (*arrow*) with a thickened and irregular wall is clearly demonstrated by a perforation of the tumoral colon within the ovary

ovarian malignancies are more often responsible for acute abdomen by extension to the bowel or by peritoneal carcinomatosis with, in both cases, a bowel obstruction.

References

Allen SD, Lim AK, Seckl MJ, Blunt DM, Mitchell AW (2006) Radiology of gestational trophoblastic neoplasia. Clin Radiol 61:301–313

Augustin G, Majerovic M (2007) Non-obstetrical acute abdomen during pregnancy. Eur J Obstet Gynecol Reprod Biol 131:4–12

Bennett GL, Slywotzky CM, Giovanniello G (2002) Gynecologic causes of acute pelvic pain: spectrum of CT findings. Radiographics 22:785–801

Bennett GL, Harvey WB, Slywotzky CM, Birnbaum BA (2003) CT of the acute abdomen: gynecologic etiologies. Abdom Imaging 28:416–432

Bennett GL, Slywotzky CM, Cantera M, Hecht EM (2010) Unusual manifestations and complications of endometriosis. Spectrum of imaging findings: pictorial review. AJR Am J Roentgenol 194:34–46

Borders RJ, Breiman RS, Yeh BM, Qayyum A, Coakley FV (2004) Computed tomography of corpus luteal cysts. J Comput Assist Tomogr 28:340–342

Bouguizane S, Bibi H, Farhat Y et al (2003) Les torsions des annexes de l'utérus. Aspects cliniques et thérapeutiques: à propos d'une série de 135 cas. J Gynecol Obstet Biol Reprod 32:535–540

Cho HJ, Kim HK, Suh JH, Lee GJ, Shim JC, Kim YH (2008) Fitz-Hugh-Curtis syndrome: CT findings of three cases. Emerg Radiol 15:43–46

Delvigne A, Rozenberg S (2003) Review of clinical course and treatment of ovarian hyperstimulation syndrome (OHSS). Hum Reprod Update 9:77–96

Eyvazzadeh AD, Levine D (2006) Imaging of pelvic pain in the first trimester of pregnancy. Radiol Clin North Am 44:863–877

Genevois A, Marouteau N, Lemercier E, Dacher JN, Thiebot J (2008) Imagerie de la douleur pelvienne aiguë. J Radiol 89:92–106

Ghang HG, Bhatt S, Dogra VS (2008) Pearls and pitfalls in diagnosis of ovarian torsion. Radiographics 28:1655–1668

Ghossian MA, Buy JN, Sciot C, Jacob H, Hugol D, Vadrot D (1997) CT findings before and after adnexal torsion: rotation of a focal solid element of a cystic adjunctive sign in diagnosis. AJR Am J Roentgenol 169:1343–1346

Green CL, Angtuaco TL, Shah HR, Parmley TH (1996) Gestational trophoblastic disease: a spectrum of radiologic diagnosis. Radiographics 16:1371–1384

Gupta N, Dadhwal V, Misra R, Mittal S, Kiran S (2008) Atypical presentation of a leiomyoma as spontaneous massive haemoperitoneum. Eur J Obstet Gynecol Reprod Biol 138:114–124

Ha HK, Lee HJ, Kim H et al (1993) Abdominal actino-mucosis: CT findings in 10 patients. AJR Am J Roentgenol 161: 791–794

Hallatt JG, Steele GH Jr, Snyder M (1984) Ruptured corpus luteum with hemoperitoneum: a study of 173 surgical cases. Am J Obstet Gynecol 149:5–9

Has R, Topuz S, Kalelioglu I, Tagrikulu D (2008) Imaging features of postpartum uterine rupture: a case report. Abdom Imaging 33:101–103

Hertzberg BS, Kliewer MA, Paulson EK (1999) Ovarian cyst rupture causing hemoperitoneum: imaging features and the potential for misdiagnosis. Abdom Imaging 24: 304–308

Hiller N, Appelbaum L, Simanovsky N, Lev-Sagi A, Aharoni D, Sella T (2007) CT features of adnexal torsion. AJR Am J Roentgenol 189:124–129

Jeong YY, Kang HK, Park JG, Ghoi HS (2003) CT features of uterine torsion. Eur Radiol 13:249–250

Kim IY, Lee BH (1997) Ovarian hyprestimulation syndrome: US and CT appearances. Clin Imaging 21:284–286

Kim SH, Kim SH, Yang DM, Kim KA (2004) Unusual causes of tubo-ovarian abscess: CT and MR imaging findings. Radiographics 24:1575–1589

Kim JY, Kim Y, Jeong WK, Song SY, Cho OK (2009) Perihepatitis with pelvic inflammatory disease (PID) on MDCT: characteristic findings and relevance to PID. Abdom Imaging 34:737–742

Lazarus E, Mayo-Smith W, Mainiero MB, Spencer PK (2007) CT in the evaluation of nontraumatic abdominal pain in pregnant women. Radiology 244:784–790

Lee JH, Park SB, Shin SH et al (2009) Value of intra-adnexal and extra-adnexal computed tomographic imaging features diagnosing torsion of adnexal tumor. J Comput Assist Tomogr 33:872–876

Lin EP, Bhatt S, Dogra VS (2008) Diagnostic clues to ectopic pregnancy. Radiographics 28:1661–1671

Lotterman S (2008) Massive hemoperitoneum resulting from spontaneous rupture of uterine leiomyoma. Am J Emerg Med 26:974e1–974e2

Lubner M, Menias C, Rucker C (2007) Blood in the belly: CT findings of hemoperitoneum. Radiographics 27:109–125

Mashiach S, Bider D, Moran O, Goldenberg M, Ben-Rafael Z (1990) Adnexal torsion of hyperstimulated ovaries in pregnancies after gonadotropin therapy. Fertil Steril 53:76–80

Matsumoto H, Ohta T, Nakahara K, Kojimahara T, Kurachi H (2007) Torsion of a nongravid uterus with a large ovarian cyst: usefulness of contrast MR image. Gynecol Obstet Invest 63:163–165

McCormack WM (1994) Pelvic inflammatory disease. N Engl J Med 330:115–119

McWilliams G, Hill MJ, Dietrich CS (2008) Gynecologic emergencies. Surg Clin N Am 88:265–283

Menias CO, Elsayes KM, Peterson CM et al (2007) CT of pregnancy-related complications. Emerg Radiol 13: 299–306

Munsik R, Gillanders L (1981) A review of the syndrome of puerperal ovarian vein thrombophlebitis. Obstet Gynecol Surv 36:57–66

Namavar Jahromi B, Parsanezhad ME, Ghane-Shirazi R (2001) Female genital tuberculosis and infertility. Int J Gynaecol Obstet 75:269–272

Panghaal VS, Chernyak V, Patlas M, Rozenblit AM (2009) CT features of adnexal involvement in patients with diverticulitis. AJR Am J Roentgenol 192:963–966

Pellerito JS, Taylor KJ, Quedens-Case C et al (1992) Ectopic pregnancy: evaluation with endovaginal color flow imaging. Radiology 183:407–411

Pham H, Lin EC (2007) Adnexal ring of ectopic pregnancy detected by contrast-enhanced CT. Abdom Imaging 32:56–58

Potter W, Chandrasekhar CA (2008) US and CT evaluation of acute pelvic pain of gynecologic origin in nonpregnant premenopausal patients. Radiographics 28:1645–1659

Rha SE, Byun JY, Jung SE et al (2002) CT and MR imaging features of adnexal torsion. Radiographics 22:283–294

Romo LV, Clarke PD (1992) Fitz-Hugh-Curtis syndrome: pelvic inflammatory disease with an unusual CT presentation. J Comput Assist Tomogr 16:832–833

Rooholamini SA, Hansen GC, Kioumehr F et al (1993) Imaging of pregnancy related complications. Radiographics 13:753–770

Roy C, Bierry G, El Ghali S, Buy X, Rossini A (2005) Acute torsion of uterine leiomyoma: CT features. Abdom Imaging 30:120–123

Sam JW, Jacobs JE, Birnbaum BA (2002) Spectrum of CT findings in acute pyogenic pelvic inflammatory disease. Radiographics 22:1327–1334

Schraga ED, Kulkarni R, Blanda M (2008) Ovarian torsion. http://www.emedicine.com/emerg/topic353htm. Accessed 14 Mar 2007

Yitta S, Hecht ME, Sliwotzky CM, Bennett GL (2009) Added value of multiplanar reformation in the multidetector CT evaluation of the femal pelvis: a pictorial review. Radiographics 29:1987–2005

Zuckerman J, Levine D, McNicholas MJ et al (1997) Imaging of pelvic postpartum complications. AJR Am J Roentgenol 168:663–668

Acute Diseases Related to Intra-abdominal Fat in Adults

Etienne Danse

Contents

1   Introduction 393
2   Primary Epiploic Appendagitis 393
3   Acute Torsion of the Greater Omentum 395
4   Mesenteric Panniculitis 395
References 397

Abstract

Acute disease related to intra-abdominal fat are due to inflammation of this fat and include mainly primary epiploic appendagitis, torsion of the greater omentum and mesenteric panniculitis.

1 Introduction

Normal fatty structures of the abdominal cavity include fat around the kidneys (perirenal space and pararenal space), fat close to and around the intestines (the mesenteric folds, the great omentum, and the epiploic appendages), and fat of the falciform ligament and around the rectum (the mesorectum).

In the abdominal cavity, fatty tissue is present in a variable amount depending on the status of the patient. Changes of the fatty tissues around the intestines are indicative of local or diffuse processes.

This chapter is dedicated to the most common situations related to inflammation of the fatty tissues of the intestines.

2 Primary Epiploic Appendagitis

Primary epiploic appendagitis, so-called acute torsion of an epiploic appendage, is an acute abdominal disorder due to spontaneous torsion of a fatty appendix adherent to the tenia coli. Most authors consider this disorder as equivalent to an ischemic event (Danse et al. 2001). The frequence of this affection is 1.3% and its incidence is 8.8 cases per million population per year (De Brito et al. 2008).

E. Danse (✉)
Diagnostic Radiology Department,
Université Catholique de Louvain,
St-Luc University Hospital,
Brussels, Belgium
e-mail: etienne.danse@uclouvain.be

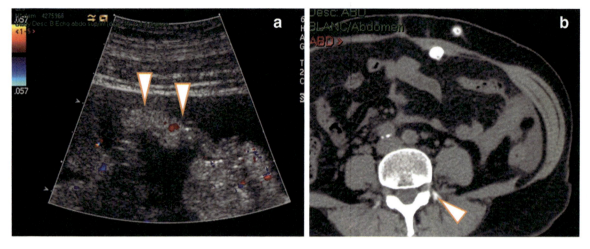

Fig. 1 Normal epiploic appendage in a patient having ascites related to peritoneal dialysis. **a** On sonography, the normal epiploic appendage (*arrowheads*) is visible because of the presence of ascites; it is an hyperechoic mass, with presence of color Doppler sonography flow. **b** On CT, a normal epiploic appendage appears as an elongated fatty tissue mass, connected to the anterior colic wall (*arrowhead*)

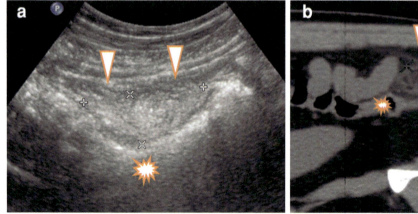
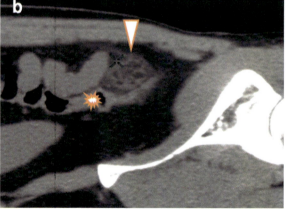

Fig. 2 Primary epiploic appendagitis of the descending colon. **a** On sonography, a hyperechoic ovoid mass (*arrowheads*) is compressing the colon (*asterisk*). **b** On CT, with multiplanar reformation, a fatty mass with hyperattenuating areas (*arrowhead*) is visible close to the colon (*asterisk*)

Epiploic appendages are composed of well-vascularized fatty tissue spreading along the tenia coli, visible from the cecum to the distal colon. The length ranges from 0.5 to 5 cm (mean, 3 cm). In normal situations, they are invisible. In patients having enough ascites, normal epiploic appendages can be seen, more frequently along the sigmoid colon. On sonography, they appear as hyperechoic elongated structures, but they are easier to detect on CT as tubular fatty structures (Fig. 1).

Acute torsion of such appendages is a cause of acute abdominal pain. This condition appears spontaneously without predisposing factors (De Brito et al. 2008). Most of the primary appendagites are reported in the right iliac fossa (in 55% of the cases), the rest being located in 30% of cases in the left iliac fossa and uncommonly in the hypogastric area (Danse et al. 2001).

Pain is increased with movement, when the patient coughs, and during deep inspiration. Nausea and vomiting are present in 25% of cases.

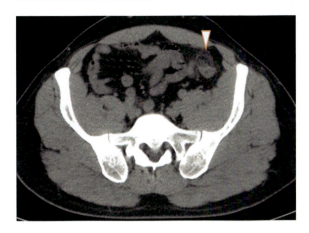

Fig. 3 Typical CT findings in a case of primary epiploic appendagitis: fatty mass with a peripheric hyperattenuating halo, close to the descending colon (*arrowheads*)

Examination of the abdomen reveals a palpable and painful mass. The findings of blood tests are normal or associated with moderate signs of inflammation (a slight increase of the C-reactive protein level and moderate hyperleukocytosis). Spontaneous resolution is the common evolution within 8 days (De Brito et al. 2008).

Sonographic findings include a round hyperechoic mass, ranging from 3 to 5 cm in its long axis, located close to the colic wall (Danse et al. 2001). A thin hypoechoic rim is visible around this hyperechoic mass (Fig. 2a). A hypoechoic millimeter-sized nodule can be seen in the center of the hyperechoic mass. Focal thickening of the peritoneum can be seen close to the lesion.

On CT, primary epiploic appendagitis appears as a round zone of increased density of fatty tissue, adherent to the colon. A focal zone of increased density of the peritoneum is often visible, more frequently than with sonography (Fig. 2b). Some nodules, into the mass, can have a more increased density, related to thrombosis of the small epiploic vessels. The adjacent colon looks normal.

In both techniques (sonography and CT), the absence of colic wall changes is helpful for making a distinction between primary epiploic appendagitis (Fig. 3) and the secondary form, related to local inflammation (appendicitis, diverticulitis, acute gynecologic disorders, etc.).

3 Acute Torsion of the Greater Omentum

Acute and spontaneous torsion of the greater omentum is another form of fatty tissue disorder. The greater omentum is composed of fat and vessels and is located anteriorly to the bowel loops, arising from the great curvature of the stomach and then from the transverse colon. Its lower free borders are the common sites of spontaneous torsion. This acute disorder can be followed by necrosis and is called omental infarct.

Compared with primary epiploic appendagitis, omental infarct is uncommon. It can be seen in the subhepatic area and in the iliac fossa.

On sonography and CT, a round or oval fat tissue area is demarcated, looking hyperechoic with sonography and of increased density compared with the normal fat seen on CT. The mass is commonly larger than that in primary appendagitis (Hollerweger et al. 1996; Puylaert 1992) (Fig. 4).

4 Mesenteric Panniculitis

This disorder is characterized by inflammation of the fatty tissue of the mesenteric root. This condition is observed more frequently in men than in women. It is reported in 0.6% of CT examinations (Zissin et al. 2006). No relevant cause is noted for this disorder, other than predisposing factors: previous abdominal surgery (cholecystectomy or appendicectomy), previous abdominal trauma, an autoimmune disease, or use of drugs (Zissin et al. 2006; Patel et al. 1999). Ischemic disorders of the intestine are also associated with this condition (Seo et al. 2001). Apparition of a lymphoma in the follow-up has been reported (Kipfer et al. 1974). Mesenteric panniculitis has been reported in association with previous malignancy, or in combination with, particularly, gastrointestinal and urogenital malignancies (Zissin et al. 2006; Daskalogiannaki et al. 2000).

The disease is included in the group of sclerosing mesenteritis, with three stages being reported combining inflammation, fibrosis, and necrosis of the fatty tissues of various degrees (Federle and Anne 2004):

1. Mesenteric panniculitis *sensu stricto*: inflammation > necrosis > fibrosis

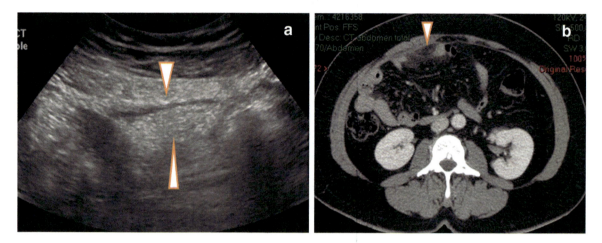

Fig. 4 Omental Infarct **a** Sonography: hyperechoic mass (*arrowheads*), adjacent to the small bowel and with thickening of the peritoneum. **b** CT: focal area of fatty infiltration and combined with thickening of the adjacent peritoneum

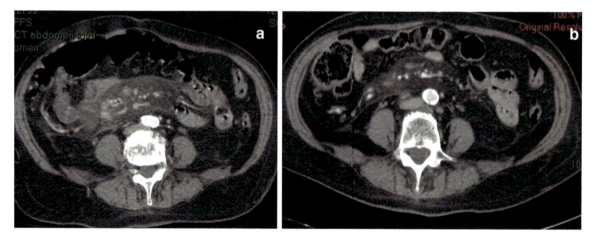

Fig. 5 Mesenteric panniculitis **a** At the initial stage of the disease: tubular infiltration of the fatty tissue around the superior mesenteric artery and vein, including enlarged nodes. **b** After therapy (corticoids), moderate infiltration of the fatty tissue is seen

2. Mesenteric lipodystrophia: necrosis > inflammation > fibrosis
3. Retractile mesenteritis: fibrosis > inflammation > necrosis

The first stage is usually nonsymptomatic. The degeneration of the fatty tissue is reversible and includes infiltration of the mesenteric root or isolated or multiple inflammatory masses. The second stage is related to increased inflammation, with plication of the mesenteric roots with at least one inflammatory mass. The inflammation is extended to the mesos and the adjacent organs: mesocolon, omentum, and retroperitoneum. The symptoms are nonspecific and include abdominal pain, nausea, vomiting, fever, weight loss, and transit modification.

Retractile mesenteritis, quite uncommon, is based on fibrotic and collagenous deposits, leading to obstructive mesenteric masses, rarely causing vascular involvement (Kipfer et al. 1974). In this late stage, treatment with steroids is the first option. Surgery is required in the case of mechanical bowel obstruction (Patel et al. 1999; Kipfer et al. 1974; Goth et al. 2001).

Mesenteric panniculitis is the most common form of sclerosing mesenteritis detected with sonography and CT. Sonographic signs for mesenteric panniculitis include increased echogenicity of the fatty tissue around the superior mesenteric veins and arteries, together with hypoechoic nodules in this hyperechoic fat tissue.

With CT, hyperattenuation of the perivascular tissue is confirmed, as is the presence of small mesenteric masses (lymph nodes). CT has a relevant role to confirm the diagnosis, and to exclude infiltration of the mesenteric fat due to other causes, such as pancreatitis, inflammation of the bowel, a subjacent lymphoma, or a desmoid tumor (Patel et al. 1999) (Fig. 5).

Mesenteric panniculitis is commonly evoked with CT by showing a well-defined, inhomogeneous fatty mass with higher attenuation than the normal retroperitoneal fat, occasionally with preserved perivascular fat (fat CT sign), which contains small nodules and is surrounded by a tumoral pseudocapsule (Zissin et al. 2006).

The retractile form of panniculitis is uncommon: we see ill-defined masses in the mesenteric root, with calcifications and spiculations. The differential diagnosis has to be made with carcinoid tumor and peritoneal carcinomatosis and can be oriented with the fat CT sign suggesting a benign process. In carcinoid tumor, bowel wall thickening and liver metastases are detected. In patients with carcinomatosis, ascites is frequent, and nodules are seen in places other than the mesenteric root: on the liver surface and in the falciform ligament, in the rectovaginal recess, and around the spleen.

In patients with preexisting malignancy or a combination of malignancy, PET–CT has been reported as contributive for making the distinction between true mesenteric panniculitis and tumoral involvement of mesenteric nodes with malignancy (Zissin et al. 2006).

The combination of increased fatty attenuation of the mesenteric fat and small mesenteric nodules is called "misty mesentery" (Mindelzun et al. 1996).

This aspect can be seen in other diseases infiltrating the mesentery, such as inflammation, edema, hemorrhage, and metastases (Zissin et al. 2006).

References

Danse EM, Van Beers BE, Baudrez V et al (2001) Epiploic appendagitis: color Doppler sonographic findings. Eur Radiol 11:183–186

Daskalogiannaki M, Voloudaki A, Prassopoulos P, Magkanas E, Stefanaki K, Apostolaki E et al (2000) CT evaluation of mesenteric panniculitis: prevalence and associated diseases. AJR Am J Roentgenol 174:427–431

De Brito P, Gomez MA, Besson M, Scotto B, Huten N, Alison D (2008) Frequency and epidemiology of primary epiploic appendagitis on CT in adults with abdominal pain. J Radiol 89:235–243

Federle MP, Anne VS (2004) Sclerosing mesenteritis. In: Federle MP (ed) Diagnostic imaging abdomen. Amyris, Salt Lake City

Goth J, Otridge B, Brady H, Breatnach E, Dervan P, MacMathuna P (2001) Aggressive multiple myeloma presenting as mesenteric panniculitis. Am J Gastroenterol 96:238–241

Hollerweger A, Rettenbacher Th, Macheiner P, Gritsmann N (1996) Spontaneous fatty tissue necrosis of the omentum and epiploic appendices: clinical, ultrasonic and CT findings. ROFO 165:529–534

Kipfer RE, Moertel CG, Dahlin DC (1974) Mesenteric lipodystrophy. Ann Intern Med 80:582–588

Mindelzun RE, Jeffrey RB Jr, Lane MJ, Silverman PM (1996) The misty mesentery on CT: differential diagnosis. AJR Am J Roentgenol 167:61–65

Patel N, Saleeb SF, Teplick SK (1999) Mesenteric panniculitis with extensive inflammatory involvement of the peritoneum and intraperioneal structures. Radiographics 19:1083–1085

Puylaert JB (1992) Rightsided segmental infarction of the omentum: clinical, US and CT findings. Radiology 84:169–172

Seo M, Okada M, Okina S, Ohdera K, Nakashima R, Sakisaka S (2001) Mesenteric panniculitis of the colon with obstruction of the inferior mesenteric vein. Dis Colon Rectum 44:885–889

Zissin R, Metser U, Hain D, Even-Sapir E (2006) Mesenteric panniculitis in oncologic patients: PET-CT findings. Br J Radiol 79(937):37–43

Acute Disease of the Abdominal Wall

Catherine Cyteval

Contents

1	**Normal Anatomy of the Abdominal Wall**	399
2	**Hernia**	402
2.1	Types of Abdominal Wall Hernias	403
2.2	Causes of Acute Symptoms in Abdominal Wall Hernias	405
2.3	Complications of Surgical Repair Procedures in Abdominal Wall Hernias	407
3	**Hematoma**	407
4	**Abscess**	408
5	**Unspecific Muscular Disease**	408
6	**Conclusions**	408
References		408

Abstract

Various acute diseases, including hernia, hematoma, and abscess, can occur within the abdominal wall. Different imaging modalities have been used to confirm suspected abdominal wall lesions or postsurgical complications; adequate visualization of intra-abdominal organs and the abdominal wall, fast imaging acquisition, three-dimensional data sets, multiplanar reformation capabilities, and contrast material injection allowing visualization of vascularization in the abdominal wall are important advantages of multidetector row computed tomography compared with other modalities.

1 Normal Anatomy of the Abdominal Wall

The abdominal wall represents the boundaries of the abdominal cavity (Salmons 1995). It consists of skin, subcutaneous tissues, and a muscular layer that is divided into anterior, anterolateral, and posterior groups (Fig. 1). The abdominal wall is separated from the peritoneum by a layer of fascia that has different names depending on where it covers (e.g., fascia transversalis, psoas fascia) (Fisch and Brodey 1981).

The anterior muscle group consists of rectus abdominis muscles lying within the rectus sheath. The rectus abdominis muscle is a paired muscle running vertically on each side of the anterior wall of the human abdomen. There are two parallel muscles, separated by a midline band of connective tissue

---

C. Cyteval (✉)
Service d'imagerie médicale, Hôpital Lapeyronie,
371 Avenue du Doyen Gaston Giraud,
34295 Montpellier Cedex 5, France
e-mail: c-cyteval@chu-montpellier.fr

P. Taourel (ed.), *CT of the Acute Abdomen*, Medical Radiology. Diagnostic Imaging,
DOI: 10.1007/174_2010_91 © Springer-Verlag Berlin Heidelberg 2011

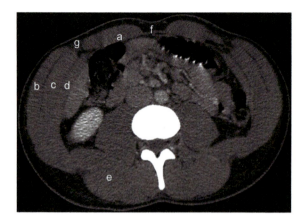
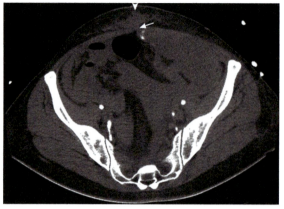

Fig. 1 Axial computed tomography (CT) scan of the lower abdomen shows the abdominal muscles, which are as follows: *a* rectus abdominis muscle, *b* external oblique muscle, *c* internal oblique muscle, *d* transverse abdominal muscle, *e* posterior muscle group, *f* linea alba, and *g* Spiegel line

Fig. 2 The axial contrast-enhanced reformatted CT image of the abdomen shows herniation of omental fat through the umbilical orifice (*arrow*) with stranding of herniated fat (*arrowhead*)

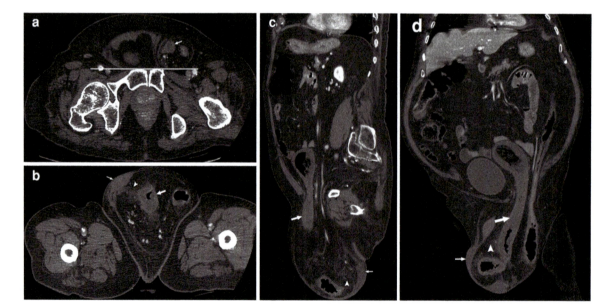

Fig. 3 Incarceration of an inguinal hernia in an 80-year-old man. **a, b** Axial contrast-enhanced reformatted CT images of the abdomen show a strangulated left direct inguinal hernia located entirely anterior to the orthogonal lines drawn at the pubic tubercle (**a**) with wall thickening and reduction of the mural enhancement of herniated bowel, severe fat stranding (*arrow*), mesenteric engorgement (*arrowhead*), and extraluminal fluid confined to the hernial sac (*thin arrow*), findings that suggest strangulation (**b**). **c, d** Sagittal and coronal contrast-enhanced reformatted CT images of the abdomen more clearly show mural thickening and reduction of the mural enhancement of herniated bowel (compare with that of intra-abdominal bowel loops)

called the linea alba (white line). It extends from the pubic symphysis inferiorly to the xiphoid process and lower costal cartilages superiorly. The rectus abdominis muscle is usually crossed by three fibrous bands linked by the tendinous inscriptions.

The anterolateral muscle group is formed by external and internal oblique and transversus abdominis muscles:

– The external oblique muscle is the largest and the most superficial (outermost) of the three flat

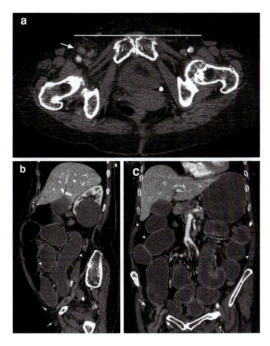

Fig. 4 Strangulated femoral hernia in a 75-year-old woman. **a** The axial contrast-enhanced reformatted CT image of the abdomen shows a strangulated right hernia entirely located posterior to the orthogonal lines drawn at the pubic tubercle. Mural enhancement of herniated bowel is normal (similar to that of intra-abdominal bowel loops). **b, c** Sagittal and coronal contrast-enhanced reformatted CT images of the abdomen more clearly show the amplitude of the wall defect (*arrows*), air–fluid levels, and dilatation of intra-abdominal bowel loops secondary to small bowel obstruction (*arrowhead*)

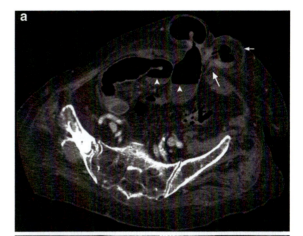

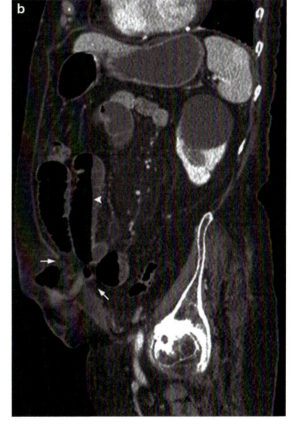

Fig. 5 Hypogastric paramedial hernia in an 85-year-old woman who presented with abdominal distension. **a, b** Axial and sagittal contrast-enhanced reformatted CT images of the abdomen show a strangulated hernia (*arrows*) causing small bowel obstruction (*arrowheads*). A herniated bowel loop with a C-shaped configuration and fat stranding around the herniation are also seen. The sagittal contrast-enhanced reformatted CT image (**b**) of the abdomen more clearly demonstrates the amplitude of the wall defect (*thin arrows*), air–fluid levels, and dilatation of intra-abdominal bowel loops secondary to small bowel obstruction (*arrowhead*)

muscles of the lateral anterior abdomen. It arises from the external surfaces and inferior borders of the fifth through 12th ribs. It ends at the linea alba, pubic crest, tubercle, anterior superior iliac spine, and anterior half of the iliac crest. The aponeurosis of the external oblique muscle forms the inguinal ligament. The muscle also contributes to the inguinal canal.

- Just deep to the external oblique is the internal oblique muscle. Its fibers run perpendicular to the external oblique muscle, beginning in the thoracolumbar fascia of the lower back, the anterior two thirds of the iliac crest, and the lateral half of the inguinal ligament. The muscle fibers run from these points superiomedially (up and toward the midline) to the muscle's insertions on the inferior borders of the tenth through 12th ribs and the linea alba.
- The transverse abdominal muscle is the deepest muscle layer of the lateral abdominal wall. It lies

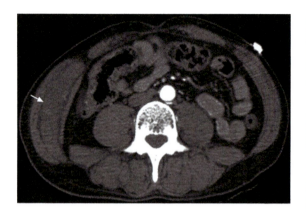
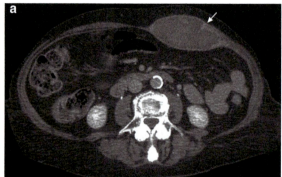

Fig. 6 The axial unenhanced CT scan of the abdomen shows a hematoma of the right internal oblique muscle (*arrow*) in a 33-year-old hemophilic patient. The muscle appears thickened and hypoattenuating relative to surrounding tissues

just below the internal oblique muscle. The muscle runs laterally from the front of the inside part of the hip bone (anterior iliac crest and inguinal ligament) to the last rib of the rib cage and ends by joining with the rectus abdominis muscle.

The inguinal canal is a short, narrow, diagonal passage in the lower anterior abdominal wall that is lined by the aponeuroses of these three muscles. It has openings at either end: the deep and superficial inguinal rings. The deep inguinal ring is an oval gap in the fascia transversalis and lies 1 cm superior to the inguinal ligament and lateral to the inferior epigastric vessels. The superficial inguinal ring is a triangular opening in the aponeurosis of the external oblique muscle. In males, the inguinal canal transmits the spermatic cord, spermatic artery, and the genital branch of the genitofemoral nerve from the pelvic cavity to the scrotum that includes the vas deferens and the testicular artery. In females, it transmits the round ligament of the uterus and the ilioinguinal nerve to the labia majora (Bhosale et al. 2008).

Latissimus dorsi, quadratus lumborum, and paraspinal muscles make up the posterior muscle group.

2 Hernia

Abdominal wall hernias are frequent, and although most of them are asymptomatic, they may develop acute complications that necessitate emergent surgery. In the USA, complications related to external hernias represent one of the most common reasons for

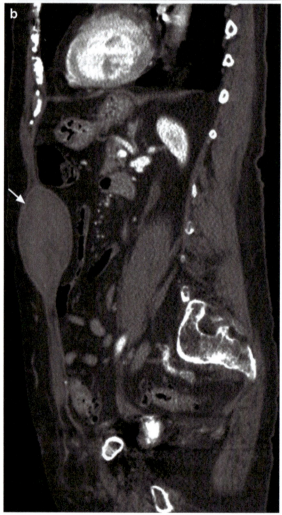

Fig. 7 Rectus sheath hematoma in a 78-year-old woman receiving anticoagulation therapy. **a** The axial enhanced CT scan of the abdomen shows a hematoma contained in the left rectus sheath with a roughly oval form (*arrow*) hypoattenuating relative to surrounding tissues. **b** The sagittal unenhanced reformatted CT image of the abdomen more clearly shows the hematoma developed above the level of the arcuate line

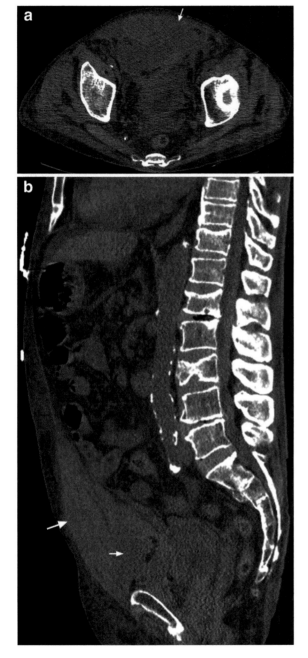

Fig. 8 Rectus sheath hematoma in a hemodialysis patient. a The axial unenhanced CT scan of the abdomen shows a hematoma of the rectus (*arrow*). b The sagittal reformatted CT image of the abdomen more clearly shows the hematoma developed below the level of the arcuate line and breaks back through the fascia transversalis into the Retzius space (*thin arrow*)

emergent surgery performed in patients over 50 years old (Rutkow 2003). Prompt diagnosis is desirable because delay is associated with greater morbidity.

Because of its superior anatomic detailing, multidetector row computed tomography (CT) may detect subtle signs of complication within the hernial sac, including bowel obstruction, incarceration, and strangulation, as well as traumatic wall hernias and postsurgical complications (e.g., hernia recurrence, fluid collections, infection, mesh-related complications). Axial CT imaging performed with the patient in the supine position is typical. If hernias are seen, a thin reconstruction (sections of 2.5-mm or less) may improve multiplanar reformation. Postural maneuvers (e.g., prone or lateral decubitus patient positioning) and maneuvers that increase intra-abdominal pressure (e.g., straining, Valsalva maneuver) can help depict subtle hernias that would otherwise be missed (Emby and Aoun 2003). Intravenous administration of contrast material is necessary for characterization of the vascular supply. Positive oral contrast material or water may be used to better visualize bowel loops.

2.1 Types of Abdominal Wall Hernias

2.1.1 Groin Hernias

Groin hernias include inguinal hernias (direct or indirect) and femoral hernias.

Inguinal hernias are the most common type of abdominal wall hernia. They occur in children (most commonly indirect-type hernias) and adults (both direct and indirect types), manifesting themselves medial (direct type) or lateral (indirect type) to the inferior epigastric vessels (Ghahremani et al. 1987). Regardless of the patient's age, inguinal hernias are more common in males than in females. In boys, most inguinal hernias develop because the peritoneal extension accompanying the testis fails to obliterate. In adults, inguinal hernias are caused by acquired weakness and dilatation of the internal inguinal ring.

Femoral hernias are less common than inguinal hernias. They occur medial to the femoral vein and posterior to the inguinal ligament, usually on the right side. Unlike inguinal hernias, they are more common in females.

Both types of hernias are defined by their relationships relative to the inguinal ligament. Inguinal hernias are superior to the ligament, whereas femoral hernias lie below the ligament. Indirect inguinal hernias and femoral hernias are more prone to obstruction than direct inguinal hernias (Wechsler et al.

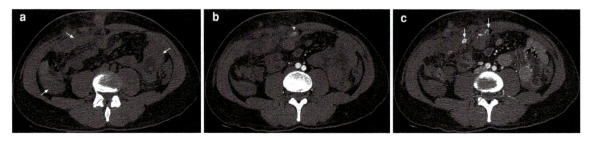

Fig. 9 Acute arterial hemorrhage in a 34-year-old woman after fibrinolysis for pulmonary embolism. **a** The axial unenhanced CT scan shows an intra-abdominal hematoma (*arrows*). **b, c** Two-phase contrast-enhanced reformatted CT images show extravasation of contrast material (*arrowhead*) into the hematoma. On the arterial phase image (**b**) only a small amount of contrast material is evident underneath the abdominal wall, whereas the venous phase images (**c**) show active bleeding (*arrows*) into the hematoma

1989), and are frequently responsible for incarceration of a short segment of bowel herniating through a narrow hernia neck.

Although the inguinal ligament may not be visible on CT, the pubic tubercle, corresponding to the anteroinferior insertion site of this ligament, is easily detected on CT (Wechsler et al. 1989). Inguinal hernias, anatomically situated above the ligament, are located entirely anterior to (direct inguinal hernia) or partially anterior to (indirect inguinal hernia) orthogonal lines drawn at the pubic tubercle from an axial image. Femoral hernias that are situated below the ligament are located posterior to orthogonal lines drawn at the pubic tubercle on an axial image.

2.1.2 Ventral Hernias

Ventral hernias include all hernias within the anterior and lateral abdominal walls. Midline defects affect umbilical, paraumbilical, epigastric, and hypogastric hernias (Fig. 2). Umbilical hernias are by far the most common type of ventral hernias; they are usually small and are particularly common in women. Paraumbilical hernias are large abdominal defects through the linea alba in the umbilicus region and are usually related to diastasis of the rectus abdominis muscles. Epigastric hernias and hypogastric hernias occur in the linea alba above and below the umbilicus, respectively.

Paramedian or lateral defects may also occur, although they are less common. Spiegel hernia is located between the rectus abdominis muscle and the aponeurosis of the oblique muscles below the umbilicus. Typically, omentum and short segments of bowel protrude through the defect. These entities have a high prevalence of incarceration.

2.1.3 Lumbar Hernias

Lumbar hernias occur through defects in the lumbar muscles or the posterior fascia, below the 12th rib and above the iliac crest. They usually occur after surgery or trauma. Herniation may occur through the superior (Grynflett–Lesshaft) or, less commonly, the inferior (petit) lumbar triangle. The superior lumbar triangle is bordered by the internal oblique muscle anteriorly, the 12th rib superiorly, and the erector spinal muscle posteriorly. The inferior lumbar triangle is bordered by the external oblique muscle anteriorly, the iliac crest inferiorly, and the latissimus dorsi muscle posteriorly. Diffuse lumbar hernias may also occur, usually after flank incisions in kidney surgery, and may contain bowel loops, retroperitoneal fat, kidneys, or other viscera.

2.1.4 Hernias Due to an Incision or a Traumatism

Incisional hernias are delayed complications of abdominal surgery. They may manifest themselves anywhere in the abdominal wall and are more commonly encountered in association with vertical than with transverse incisions. Incisional hernias usually manifest themselves during the first few months after surgery. Their reported prevalence ranges from 0.5 to 13.9% for most abdominal surgical operations (Ghahremani et al. 1987).

Abdominal trauma can result in a wide variety of abdominal wall hernias, ranging from small defects caused by direct injury to more extensive defects resulting from compression injury to the abdomen. The most common locations are areas of relative anatomic weakness: the lumbar region and the lower abdomen.

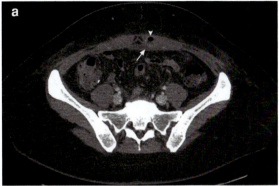

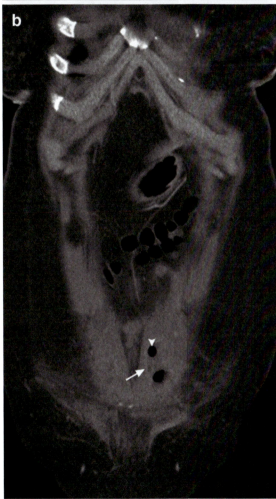

Fig. 10 Infected fluid collection within the abdominal wall in a 30-year-old woman 3 weeks after conservative surgery for endometriosis. **a, b** Axial and coronal contrast-enhanced reformatted CT scans of the lower abdomen show gas within the rectus sheath fluid collection (*arrowhead*), enhancement of the collection wall, and fat stranding around the collection that was suspicious of an infection (*arrow*)

2.1.5 Other Hernias

Less common hernias include interparietal, Richter, and Littre hernias of the abdominal wall, and sciatic, obturator, and perineal hernias in the pelvis.

"Interparietal (interstitial) hernia" refers to a hernial sac located in the fascial planes between the abdominal wall muscles that does not exit into the subcutaneous tissue. This type of hernia occurs most frequently in the inguinal region. "Richter hernia" refers to herniation of the antimesenteric wall of the bowel that does not compromise the entire wall circumference. It most frequently occurs in association with femoral hernias. "Littre hernia" refers to an inguinal hernia that contains a Meckel diverticulum. All of these uncommon abdominal hernias are particularly prone to incarceration and strangulation (Harrison et al. 1995).

Pelvic hernias most frequently occur in elderly women and are secondary to acquired weakness of the pelvic floor. Sciatic and obturator hernias are rare and usually manifest themselves as herniation of small bowel loops or a ureter through the sciatic or obturator foramen, respectively. Perineal hernias are more common than sciatic or obturator hernias and occur adjacent to the anus or labia majora or in the gluteal region.

2.2 Causes of Acute Symptoms in Abdominal Wall Hernias

The most common complications of abdominal wall hernias lead to acute abdominal pain. Early diagnosis of hernia complications is feasible with multidetector row CT, potentially improving the patient's outcome by preserving bowel viability (Yu et al. 2004).

2.2.1 Incarceration

"Incarceration" refers to an irreducible hernia and is diagnosed clinically when a hernia cannot be reduced or pushed back manually. The diagnosis of incarceration cannot be made with imaging alone, but can be suggested when herniation occurs through a small defect and the hernial sac has a narrow neck. Detection is important because incarceration predisposes a patient to complications such as obstruction, inflammation, and ischemia. Axial and multiplanar reformation images improve visualization of the hernia defect and permit assessment of the size and content (Aguirre et al. 2004). Impending strangulation of

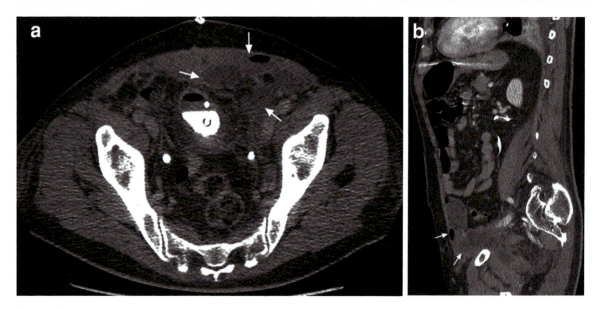

Fig. 11 Abscess within the abdominal wall after prostatic surgery in a 74-year-old man. **a**, **b** Axial and sagittal contrast-enhanced reformatted CT scans of the lower abdomen show large fluid collections into the Retzius space spreading through the fascia transversalis into the abdominal wall containing gas

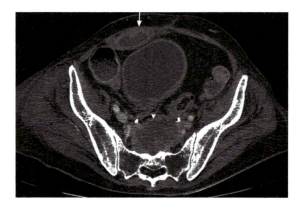

Fig. 12 Infected fluid collection (*arrow*) in a 62-year-old man who had undergone colonic surgery for cancer 2 weeks before. The CT scan shows a second collection just before the spine (*arrowhead*). Infection was confirmed by microbiologic analysis of the wall fluid collection obtained using imaging-guided aspiration

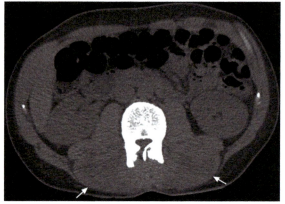

Fig. 13 Myositis in a 34-year-old man with HIV infection for 5 years. The axial unenhanced reformatted CT image of the abdomen shows diffuse hypoattenuation of the posterior muscle group with increased volume

these hernias should be suspected when there is free fluid within the hernial sac, bowel wall thickening, or luminal dilatation (Fig. 3). If fatty tissue or fluid but no bowel is present in an incarcerated hernia, time is not a limiting factor in preparing the patient for surgery. In contrast, incarcerated bowel requires immediate surgery to prevent bowel necrosis and subsequent resection of the affected bowel loop (Rettenbacher et al. 2001).

2.2.2 Strangulation

"Strangulation" refers to ischemia caused by a compromised blood supply. It usually occurs when the hernia defect obstructs the afferent and efferent bowel loops, creating a closed loop within the herniated bowel. Multidetector row CT findings include closed loop obstruction and ischemia (Yu et al. 2004). Findings in closed loop obstruction include dilated, fluid-filled U-shaped or C-shaped loops of bowel entrapped within the hernial sac and proximal obstruction. Ischemia findings include wall thickening, abnormal mural hypoattenuation or hyperattenuation and enhancement, mesenteric vessel engorgement, fat obliteration, mesenteric haziness, and ascites (Fig. 4). The afferent and efferent limbs may have a "serrated beak" appearance at the transition point. Strangulated abdominal wall hernias are associated with a high surgical fatality rate (6–23%) secondary to the strangulated viscus (Bendavid 1998). Normal mural enhancement does not exclude strangulation, whereas abnormal enhancement strongly suggests it.

2.2.3 Bowel Obstruction

After adhesions, abdominal wall hernias are the second leading cause of small bowel obstruction (10–15% of cases) (Macari and Megibow 2001). Colonic obstruction caused by abdominal wall hernia is uncommon. Most cases of bowel obstruction secondary to abdominal wall hernia occur after incarceration and strangulation. In these cases, bowel obstruction occurs with the transition point at the level of the hernia. Key CT findings include dilated bowel proximal to the hernia associated with normal-caliber, reduced-caliber, or collapsed bowel distal to the obstruction (Fig. 5). The degree of change in caliber helps predict the grade of obstruction. Other findings may include tapering of the afferent and efferent limbs at the hernia defect, dilatation of the herniated bowel loops, and fecalization of small bowel contents proximal to the obstruction (Furukawa et al. 2001).

2.3 Complications of Surgical Repair Procedures in Abdominal Wall Hernias

Several different surgical procedures are used to repair abdominal wall hernias, ranging from open or laparoscopic suture repair to the use of mesh. Two main types of mesh with different principal components are used: polypropylene mesh, which is not visible on CT because it is isoattenuating relative to surrounding tissues and expanded polytetrafluoroethylene mesh which is hyperattenuating relative to surrounding tissues.

Complications after surgical hernia repair may occur in up to 50% of cases. Half of them may require surgical reintervention and immediate accurate diagnosis with multidetector row CT. In addition to complications due to hernia recurrence or infection, some complications are mesh-specific. Inflammatory reactions may create fibrosis of surrounding tissues or intraperitoneal adhesions and can lead to small bowel obstruction (Bendavid 1998). Less frequently, meshes may detach from supporting tissues and migrate within the abdominal wall or within the peritoneum (Parra et al. 2004).

3 Hematoma

Abdominal wall hematomas may be associated with trauma, anticoagulation therapy (especially subcutaneous injection of heparin), and blood dyscrasia, or may occur spontaneously because of muscular strain. These commonly involve the anterior or anterolateral muscle groups and may dissect along fascial planes or involve the muscle itself. Acute hematomas are hyperdense because of clot formation, and attenuation values decrease with time as breakdown of blood products occurs (Fig. 6).

Hematomas of the rectus sheath developed above the level of the arcuate line are mostly contained within the rectus sheath and take a roughly oval form (Fig. 7). Hematomas below the level of the arcuate line in the lower third of the abdominal wall tend to break back through the fascia transversalis into the Retzius space (Fig. 8). This failure often results in large collection of blood, with fluid–fluid level, occupying much of the pelvis (Blum et al. 1995).

Although hematomas are typically treated nonsurgically, a residual mass may persist for several weeks. Malignant tumors of the abdominal wall are uncommon and are usually metastases (especially lung tumors and pancreatic tumors). Primary sarcomas may also develop and are sometimes found when bleeding occurs.They should be discussed when the patient is not receiving anticoagulation therapy, or when blood dyscrasia is found. High attenuation on unenhanced images, lack of enhancement, and resolution on follow-up studies help to confirm the diagnosis of simple hematoma (Moreno Gallego 1997).

In patients with blood pressure instability, a CT scan with injection of contrast material (without injection, arterial time, portal time, and late time) has to be carried out to identify the artery responsible for bleeding and allow the planning of a possible embolization (Fig. 9).

4 Abscess

Inflammatory disease of the abdominal wall commonly results from postsurgical wound infection or extension of an intra-abdominal abscess. Infected fluid collections may involve subcutaneous (superficial) or mesh-surrounding (deep) tissues. Differentiation is important because superficial infections are managed conservatively, whereas deep infections require intervention such as percutaneous drainage or prosthesis removal. When the usefulness of physical examination is limited, particularly in obese patients, CT is the method of choice to evaluate suspected abdominal wall infection. Imaging is used to confirm the presence and define the location and volume of collections, to guide aspiration, and to monitor treatment. At the beginning of the infection, CT can visualize diffuse edema with cellulitis. When a fluid collection is found, an abscess can be suspected in front of the following: fat stranding in surrounding tissues, an enhanced rim, thick septa, gas or gas–fluid level (the latter reported to be present in approximately 30% of abscesses), and the development of a new collection 1 week or more after surgical repair (Pandolfo et al. 1986). When imaging findings alone do not adequately help one to predict the nature of a fluid collection, imaging-guided aspiration is often necessary to establish the diagnosis (Figs. 10, 11, 12).

5 Unspecific Muscular Disease

Seldom unspecific muscular disease can cause acute pain (e.g., myositis or muscular tears when coughing) and has to be sought when no abdominal or retroperitoneal lesion explains the symptoms (Fig. 13).

6 Conclusions

A CT scan is especially crucial in acute abdominal wall diseases because it allows excellent anatomic delineation and vascular approach of the findings. In addition to visualizing the abdominal wall, it allows intra-abdominal exploration, which is essential for planning the optimal treatment.

References

Aguirre DA, Casola G, Sirlin C (2004) Abdominal wall hernias: MDCT findings. AJR Am J Roentgenol 183(3):681–690

Bendavid R (1998) Complications of groin hernia surgery. Surg Clin North Am 78(6):1089–1103

Bhosale PR et al (2008) The inguinal canal: anatomy and imaging features of common and uncommon masses. Radiographics 28(3):819–835; quiz 913

Blum A et al (1995) Imaging of severe forms of hematoma in the rectus abdominis under anticoagulants. J Radiol 76(5):267–273

Emby DJ, Aoun G (2003) CT technique for suspected anterior abdominal wall hernia. AJR Am J Roentgenol 181(2):431–433

Fisch AE, Brodey PA (1981) Computed tomography of the anterior abdominal wall: normal anatomy and pathology. J Comput Assist Tomogr 5(5):728–733

Furukawa A et al (2001) Helical CT in the diagnosis of small bowel obstruction. Radiographics 21(2):341–355

Ghahremani GG et al (1987) CT diagnosis of occult incisional hernias. AJR Am J Roentgenol 148(1):139–142

Harrison LA et al (1995) Abdominal wall hernias: review of herniography and correlation with cross-sectional imaging. Radiographics 15(2):315–332

Ianora AA et al (2000) Abdominal wall hernias: imaging with spiral CT. Eur Radiol 10(6):914–919

Macari M, Megibow A (2001) Imaging of suspected acute small bowel obstruction. Semin Roentgenol 36(2):108–117

Moreno Gallego A et al (1997) Ultrasonography and computed tomography reduces unnecessary surgery in abdominal rectus sheath haematoma. Br J Sep 84(9):1295–1297

Pandolfo I et al (1986) CT findings in palpable lesions of the anterior abdominal wall. J Comput Assist Tomogr 10(4):629–633

Parra JA et al (2004) Prosthetic mesh used for inguinal and ventral hernia repair: normal appearance and complications in ultrasound and CT. Br J Radiol 77(915):261–265

Rettenbacher T et al (2001) Abdominal wall hernias: cross-sectional imaging signs of incarceration determined with sonography. AJR Am J Roentgenol 177(5):1061–1066

Rutkow IM (2003) Demographic and socioeconomic aspects of hernia repair in the United States in 2003. Surg Clin North Am 83(5):1045–1051 v–vi

Salmons S (1995) Muscles of the abdomen. In: Gray's anatomy. Churchill Livingstone, New York, pp 819–829

Wechsler RJ et al (1989) Cross-sectional imaging of abdominal wall hernias. AJR Am J Roentgenol 153(3):517–521

Yu CY et al (2004) Strangulated transmesosigmoid hernia: CT diagnosis. Abdom Imaging 29(2):158–160

Complications of Abdominal Surgery (Abdominal, Urologic and Gynecologic Emergencies)

Marc Zins and Isabelle Boulay-Coletta

Contents

1	**Introduction**	409
2	**CT Technique**	410
3	**Normal Postoperative CT Appearance After Abdominal Surgery**	410
3.1	Pneumoperitoneum	410
3.2	Fluid Collection	410
3.3	Postoperative Ileus	411
4	**CT Appearance of Complications After Abdominal Surgery**	411
4.1	Peritonitis	411
4.2	Abcesses	411
4.3	Postoperative Bowel Obstruction	412
4.4	Postoperative Abdominal Wall Complications	413
5	**Specific Complications**	414
5.1	Biliary Surgery	414
5.2	Anastomotic Leaks After Gastrointestinal Tract Surgery	415
5.3	Gynecologic Surgery	415
5.4	Urologic Surgery	415
References		417

M. Zins · I. Boulay-Coletta
Department of Radiology,
Saint Joseph Hospital,
Paris, France

M. Zins (✉)
Department of Radiology,
Groupe Hospitalier Paris Saint Joseph,
185 rue Raymond Losserand,
75674 Paris Cedex 14, France
e-mail: mzins@hpsj.fr

Abstract

CT has become the standard reference technique for the diagnosis of most common complications following abdominal, urologic, or gynecologic surgery. An adapted CT technique and knowledge of normal postoperative anatomy are essential for accurate interpretation of CT scans. The main complications following abdominal, urologic, or gynecologic surgery include peritonitis, abscesses, hemorrhage, small-bowel obstruction, abdominal wall wound or hematoma, and anastomotic leaks.

1 Introduction

Despite many improvements in perioperative morbidity related to the development of the laparoscopic approach, complications are still commonly observed after abdominal, gynecologic, or urologic surgery and remain a challenging problem for both the physician and the radiologist. Cross-sectional imaging and particularly CT play a crucial role in the diagnosis and the therapeutic management of most common postoperative complications (Gore et al. 2004). Postoperative imaging of the abdomen in an emergency condition remains difficult and should be integrated in a multidisciplinary approach where physical examination and laboratory tests play a major role (Zins and Ferretti 2009). In this chapter, we will review the CT features of common acute complications following abdominal, gynecologic, or urologic surgery.

P. Taourel (ed.), *CT of the Acute Abdomen*, Medical Radiology. Diagnostic Imaging,
DOI: 10.1007/174_2011_203 © Springer-Verlag Berlin Heidelberg 2011

2 CT Technique

CT examination of the postoperative abdomen should start from the level of the dome of the diaphragm and end at the level of the pelvic floor. Associated examination of the thorax may be indicated if pulmonary embolism or pneumonia is suspected. The use of multidetector CT allows such extended study. A first unenhanced scan is recommended (1) to look with a focus on spontaneously increased density consistent with bleeding and (2) to detect a large amount of free intraperitoneal air that could contraindicate rectal contrast medium enema. A second scan is performed after intravenous administration of iodinated contrast medium for exploration of the entire abdominal cavity in the portal phase. The portal phase is perfectly suited for assessment of bowel wall enhancement, as well as for the diagnosis of abdominal collection or abscesses with peripheral enhancement (Zappa et al. 2009). In the case of suspicion of an anastomotic bowel leak, CT should be associated with oral or rectal water-soluble enema, depending on the location of the gastrointestinal anastomosis (Zappa et al. 2009; Power et al. 2007).

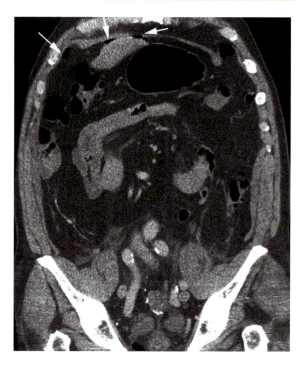

Fig. 1 Postoperative CT 3 days after left-sided colectomy in a 65-year-old woman. Presence of a small amount of free intraperitoneal air (*arrows*) representing normal residual pneumoperitoneum

3 Normal Postoperative CT Appearance After Abdominal Surgery

3.1 Pneumoperitoneum

Free intraperitoneal air after abdominal surgery is a common finding on CT in the early postoperative period and represents residual postoperative pneumoperitoneum (Gayer et al. 2004). A small amount of free air can be seen during the first week following surgery, but it should not exceed a few milliliters after 3 or 4 days (Fig. 1). Many factors influence the importance of postoperative pneumoperitoneum: a high body weight index is associated with smaller postoperative pneumoperitoneum in obese patients; conversely, in male patients, the presence of postoperative drains and the type of abdominal surgery (colectomy, gastrectomy, and cholecystectomy) seem to be associated with larger postoperative pneumoperitoneum (Gayer et al. 2004).

3.2 Fluid Collection

The presence of a moderate amount of reactive intraperitoneal fluid is commonly observed during the early postoperative period. It is usually not collected and resolves spontaneously and progressively in less than 2 weeks. Small postoperative fluid collections predominate the surgical bed. Larger volumes of fluid collections can be observed in all peritoneal compartments of the abdominal cavity (Gore et al. 2004; Zappa et al. 2009). Some pitfalls must be known and recognized:
- After Whipple resection, transient fluid collections may be observed in the pancreatic bed or around the three anastomoses, simulating an anastomotic leak (Lepanto et al. 1994). A small amount of gas bubbles can be observed in these collections and should not necessarily indicate infection (Fig. 2) (Lepanto et al. 1994).
- After left-sided hemicolectomy, accumulation of fluid around the pancreatic tail can be observed and is commonly related to the mobilization of the

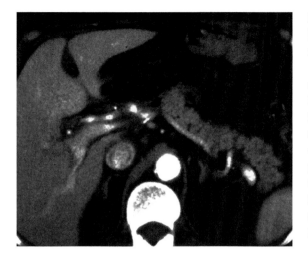

Fig. 2 Postoperative CT 3 days after a Whipple procedure in a 75-year-old man. Presence of a transient fluid collection with a small amount of gas

splenic flexure. This feature should not be mistaken for a posttraumatic pancreatitis (Zappa et al. 2009).

3.3 Postoperative Ileus

Postoperative Ileus is a common finding on CT in the early postoperative period and can develop after all types of surgery, including extraperitoneal surgery. Surgical manipulation of the gut induces an intestinal muscularis inflammatory response resulting in postsurgical ileus. Distended bowel loops with air and fluid may persist for 2–4 days after surgery. If the inhibition of bowel activity lasts more than 3 days, it is referred to as postoperative paralytic ileus and may need specific treatment (Baig and Wexner 2004). The CT appearance includes distended loops of small bowel and/or large bowel without any clear transition zone between dilated and collapsed bowel loops.

4 CT Appearance of Complications After Abdominal Surgery

4.1 Peritonitis

Seventy percent of complications following abdominal surgery are septic complications (Bartels 2009). Post-operative peritonitis usually results from intraoperative or delayed injury to a digestive organ; it is accompanied by a high mortality rate. Prognosis is directly related to early diagnosis and appropriate re-intervention.

The diagnosis of peritonitis is mainly based on clinical and laboratory signs. In case of discrepancy between CT results and clinical and laboratory signs, the latter should be preponderant in therapeutic decision making. In fact, clinical and laboratory signs of gravity impose prompt re-operation. If CT has been performed, CT features suggestive of peritonitis are: (a) persistence or enlargement of a diffuse fluid collection, (b) enhancement of the parietal peritoneum and (c) presence of gas bubbles within a fluid collection (Zappa et al. 2009).

4.2 Abscesses

Postoperative abscesses still remain a difficult diagnostic challenge for the radiologist. The abscesses may develop locally, in the surgical bed, or distantly, related to the spread of septic material along the anatomic pathways between various intraperitoneal compartments (Gore et al. 2004). The subphrenic spaces and the pouch of Douglas are common localizations of postoperative abscesses. CT is considered the standard reference technique, and has an accuracy of over 90% for the diagnosis of postoperative abscesses (Benoist et al. 2002; Harrisinghani et al. 2002; Van Sonnenberg et al. 2001; Fulcher and Turner 1996). Abscesses appear as a well-circumscribed, rounded or ellipsoid fluid collection with an attenuation value around 0–25 Hounsfield units (HU). They show peripheral rim enhancement and may be associated with internal air–fluid levels or gas bubbles (Gore et al. 2004) (Fig. 3). Stranding of the peritoneal fat planes around the abscess is also a common finding. Absence of communication with the gastrointestinal tract is easily demonstrated using multidetector CT with multiplanar reformations. In contrast to the presence of air in the fluid collection, the presence of a peripheral rim enhancement is not a specific sign for the diagnosis of abscess. Differential diagnosis may be difficult and includes loculated sterile hematomas, pseudocyst, and sterile fluid collection. One of the main advantages of CT over ultrasonography (US) or MRI is its very high negative predictive value for the diagnosis of localized postoperative abscess (Negus and Sidhu 2000). In practice, the CT features described above have

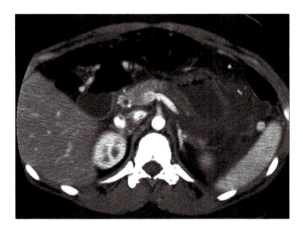

Fig. 3 Postoperative CT 8 days after left-sided pancreatectomy in a 64-year-old man. Presence of a fluid collection containing small gas bubbles with peripheral enhancement and representing an abscess

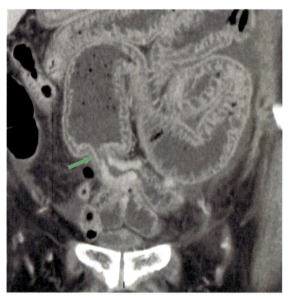

Fig. 4 Mechanical small-bowel obstruction on CT performed 14 days after appendicectomy associated with peritonitis in a 34-year-old man

moderate specificity, and in the case of clinical suspicion of sepsis, any significant intraabdominal collection will be managed with a CT-guided puncture with associated drainage if necessary (Akinci et al. 2005).

4.3 Postoperative Bowel Obstruction

Adhesions are the most common cause of small-bowel obstruction after abdominal or gynecologic surgery and more than 90% of patients who have undergone abdominal surgery will have enteric adhesions (Sandrasegaran et al. 2005). Adhesion-related small-bowel obstruction is presumed to exist on CT when there is a narrow zone of transition without an identifiable obstructive lesion. However, adhesion-related small-bowel obstruction is a rare condition in the immediate postoperative period. Early postoperative small-bowel obstruction is mainly related to an inflammatory process (hematoma, abscess, anastomotic leak) (Zappa et al. 2009). In the immediate postoperative period, CT is the method of choice for diagnosing mechanical small-bowel obstruction and distinguishing it from paralytic ileus (Taourel et al. 1995). In the case of mechanical small-bowel obstruction, the CT diagnosis is based on the presence of dilated small-bowel loops proximal to the suspected site of obstruction and collapsed or normal-appearing loops of small bowel distal to the obstruction (Fig. 4). Multiplanar reformations increase accuracy and confidence in the identification of the transition zone (Hodel et al. 2009). Although these patients rarely require surgery, those with complete, closed-loop, or strangulating obstruction with CT signs of ischemia (decreased bowel wall enhancement, thickening of the bowel wall) require emergent surgery (Sandrasegaran et al. 2005; Zalcman et al. 2000).

4.3.1 Transmesenteric Hernias

Internal hernia is a very uncommon cause of small-bowel obstruction but that may be increasing in frequency owing to the development of gastric bariatric surgery (Blachar et al. 2001) Transmesenteric hernia is the most common type of acquired internal hernia and is usually related to prior abdominal surgery, especially with the creation of a Roux-en-Y anastomosis (e.g., liver transplantation, gastric bypass). Transmesenteric hernias occur through the tear in the mesocolon through which the Roux loop is brought during a retrocolic anastomosis (Sandrasegaran et al. 2005). CT may allow confident diagnosis in most cases in showing a cluster of dilated bowel loops anterior to the transverse mesocolon associated with a deviation and an engorgement of the mesenteric vessels as they pass through the transverse mesocolon (Sandrasegaran et al. 2005; Blachar et al. 2001) (Fig. 5).

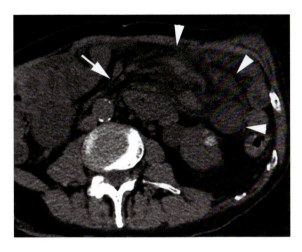
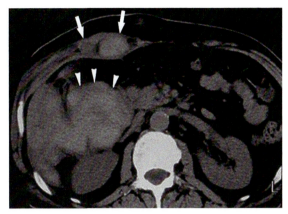

Fig. 5 Transmesenteric hernia in a 64-year-old man with history of total gastrectomy for cancer. Presence of a cluster of dilated bowel loops anterior to the transverse mesocolon (*arrowheads*) associated with an engorgement of the mesenteric vessels (*arrows*)

Fig. 6 Rectus sheath hematoma above the arcuate line in a 65-year-old man with abdominal pain and a drop in hematocrit after cholecystectomy: CT demonstration. The unenhanced CT scan shows spindle-shaped, hyperattenuating rectus sheath hematoma (*arrows*) and associated hematoma in the gallbladder fossa (*arrowheads*)

4.4 Postoperative Abdominal Wall Complications

Postoperative complications involving the abdominal wall and presenting as acute abdomen include wound infection, abdominal wall hematoma, and complicated incisional hernias (Gore et al. 2004).

4.4.1 Wound Infection

Wound infections following abdominal, gynecologic, or urologic surgery remain a major source of postoperative morbidity, accounting for about a quarter of the total number of nosocomial infections (Nichols 1991). Today, many of these infections are first recognized in the patient's home because of the large number of operations done in the outpatient setting. As the presence of wound infection is most often clinically apparent, CT plays a minor role in establishing the diagnosis. In some cases, CT performed for another indication will demonstrate a fluid collection containing gas bubbles or an air–fluid level, deep within the incision area, and allows earlier diagnosis and management. US is also an excellent alternative imaging technique for diagnosing such occult abdominal wall abscess.

4.4.2 Abdominal Wall Hematoma

Clinical diagnosis of abdominal wall hematoma is often easy when a patient presents with abdominal pain, swelling, a palpable mass, and a drop in hemoglobin level and hematocrit. Rectus sheath hematomas result from intraoperative injury of the epigastric vessels and are associated with paramedian incision or cesarean section (Gore et al. 2004). Rectus sheath hematomas above the level of the arcuate line are easy to diagnose with CT or US and are treated conservatively. On unenhanced CT, they appear as a spindle-shaped, hyperattenuating formation developed in the rectus sheath (Fig. 6). Below the arcuate line, these hematomas extend posteriorly through the thin fascia transversalis into the prevesical space and large hyperattenuating collections, displacing the peritoneal contents, as often seen (Blum et al. 1995); therefore, precise diagnosis with CT is mandatory.

4.4.3 Complicated Incisional Hernias

Incisional hernias develop in approximately 5% of patients after abdominal surgery and represent a significant iatrogenic problem. Most incisional hernias are recognized by careful inspection and palpation and can be easily confirmed by US examination when the findings of clinical examination are equivocal. However, 10% of incisional hernias cannot be detected on physical examination (obese patients, interparietal hernias) and remain clinically silent for several years. Therefore, CT evaluation of the postsurgical abdomen often shows unsuspected incisional hernias. The main complication occurring with incisional hernias is incarceration and strangulation of

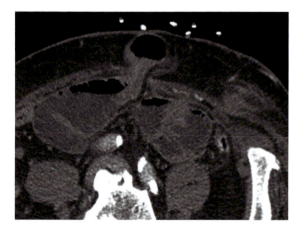

Fig. 7 Incarcerated incisional hernia in a 76-year-old man following jejunostomy

bowel loops. This situation is uncommon in the early postoperative period. CT is accurate in establishing a precise diagnosis of incarceration and strangulation, and helps in therapeutic management, in indicating the need for prompt surgical intervention (Fig. 7).

5 Specific Complications

5.1 Biliary Surgery

Specific complications following hepatobiliary surgery include bile leakage, bile duct injury, and dropped gallstones. US and MRI with magnetic resonance cholangiopancreatography (MRCP) sequences are the preferred modalities for assessment of the postoperative biliary tract (Hoeffel et al. 2006). MRI is particularly well suited in patients with jaundice or biliary tract stenosis. In patients with a nondistended biliary tract and suspected bile leak, MRCP should be completed by the injection of a liver-specific contrast medium with biliary excretion to achieve noninvasive biliary tract opacification. CT is mainly performed in patients with bile peritonitis or biloma, with suspected hepatic artery or portal vein injury in addition to biliary tract injury, and in patients with suspicion of dropped gallstones. On CT, bilomas appear as well-defined fluid collections in the perihepatic spaces, with low attenuation value (Gore et al. 2004) (Fig. 8). Percutaneous aspiration associated with drainage under CT or sonographic guidance will confirm the

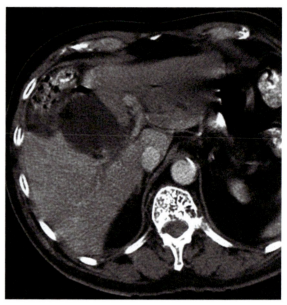

Fig. 8 Large biloma on CT following cholecystectomy in a 63-year-old man

diagnosis of bile leakage. Abscesses related to dropped gallstones result from gallbladder perforation during laparoscopic cholecystectomy. This condition is rare in the early postoperative period, with a mean duration of 2 years from the time of surgery to the development of clinical symptoms (Morrin et al. 2000). But in some cases, the dropped gallstones will result in early abscess formation or inflammatory reaction and indicate a requirement for prompt reintervention because simple drainage without removal of the calculi by surgery will be inadequate (Morrin et al. 2000; Bennett et al. 2000).

5.2 Anastomotic Leaks After Gastrointestinal Tract Surgery

CT is the preferred technique for diagnosis of a postoperative lower gastrointestinal tract leak (Khoury et al. 2009). However, the accuracy and sensitivity of CT for diagnosing anastomotic bowel leakage are moderate (Khoury et al. 2009; Power et al. 2007). In fact, the presence of fluid collection and/or free gas around the anastomosis is a common finding after gastrointestinal tract surgery and does not represent a specific sign of anastomotic leak (Power et al. 2007).

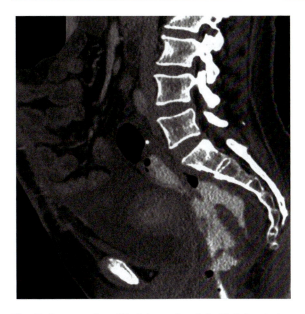

Fig. 9 Postoperative CT 6 days after left-sided hemicolectomy showing a large anastomotic leakage with extraluminal accumulation of rectally administered contrast medium anterior to the sacrum

The most specific sign of anastomotic leakage is extraluminal accumulation of the orally or rectally administered contrast medium (Fig. 9) but this sign seems to have a low sensitivity (Power et al. 2007). Thus, CT findings should be carefully interpreted in combination with clinical symptoms.

5.3 Gynecologic Surgery

Surgery remains the main treatment option for most gynecologic diseases. Total hysterectomy, myomectomy, and cesarean section represent the most frequent interventions. In the early postoperative period, specific risks and complications related to those interventions include bladder injury, ureteral injury, bowel injury, vesicovaginal or rectovaginal fistulas, hemorrhage, and abscesses (Paspulati and Dalal 2010). CT is ideally suited for diagnosis of visceral injuries, hemorrhage, and sepsis, whereas MRI is the preferred technique for assessment of postoperative fistulas.

Hemorrhage is the most common complication following gynecologic surgery and the diagnosis is based on physical signs and laboratory tests. When CT is performed, a high attenuation (60–90 HU) is demonstrated within the surgical bed (Fig. 10). Extravasation of contrast medium is diagnostic for active bleeding, which may necessitate transcatheter arterial embolization.

Bowel perforation occurs mainly in the small bowel or the rectosigmoid colon. The presence of an important pneumoperitoneum after the first postoperative week is an indicator of bowel perforation.

Bladder and ureteral injuries may be revealed by urinoma, ureteral obstruction and ureterovaginal or vesicovaginal fistulas (Paspulati and Dalal 2010). CT urography is now the preferred imaging technique for assessment of urinary tract injuries.

5.4 Urologic Surgery

Surgery remains the major treatment option in patients with malignant renal or bladder tumors, and radical prostatectomy with a retropubic, perineal, or laparoscopic approach is the most frequently used treatment for prostate cancer confined to the prostate (Catalá et al. 2009; Israel et al. 2006; Yablon et al. 2004). In the early postoperative period, CT plays a major role in the diagnosis and management of postoperative complications. Multidetector CT with the use of the CT urography technique is now the preferred modality for postoperative assessment in patients who have had urinary tract surgery (Catalá et al. 2009; Israel et al. 2006). Moreover, the excretory phase images are well suited for diagnosis of urinary leaks and should be part of the CT protocol for assessment of any fluid collection following urinary tract surgery.

5.4.1 Cystectomy and Prostatectomy

In the early postoperative period, specific risks and complications related to cystectomy or prostatectomy include urinomas related to anastomotic leaks (vesicourethral, ureteroileal, or ileourethral), fistulas, and rectum injury (Fig. 11) (Catalá et al. 2009; Yablon et al. 2004).

Urinary leakage occurs in nearly 4% of patients after urinary diversion; it is more frequent at the site of the ureteroileal anastomosis and is well demonstrated with excretory phase images (Catalá et al. 2009). Leaks at the site of the intestinal anastomotis are currently

Fig. 10 Hematoma following caesaran section. CT appearance with **a** the axial view and **b** the sagittal view

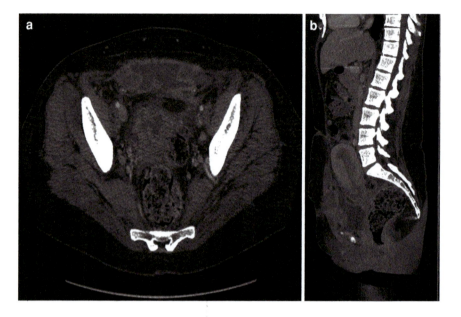

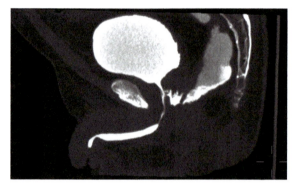

Fig. 11 CT urography following prostatectomy showing a vesicourethral leak

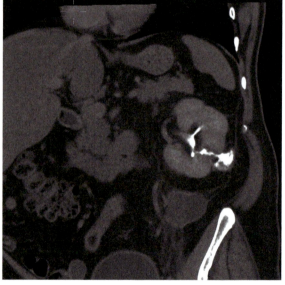

Fig. 12 Postoperative CT in the excretory phase, 8 days after left-sided partial nephrectomy in a 54-year-old man showing urinary leakage

associated with urinary-enteric, enterocutaneous, or enterogenital fistulas (Catalá et al. 2009).

5.4.2 Nephrectomy and Partial Nephrectomy

Partial nephrectomy using a laparoscopic approach is being performed with increased frequency for the treatment of renal cell carcinoma. This is a complex procedure compared with radical nephrectomy, with a major complication rate of about 10% (Israel et al. 2006).

In the early postoperative period, specific risks and complications related to partial nephrectomy include vascular complications (hematoma, renal infarction, pseudoaneurysm) and urinary leakage related to failure of calyceal repair. Multidetector CT with use of the arterial phase is perfectly suited for assessment of a pseudoaneurysm, whereas the use of an excretory phase is mandatory for positive diagnosis of urinary leakage as well as precise location of the leak (Fig. 12) (Israel et al. 2006).

References

Akinci D, Akhan O, Ozmen MN et al (2005) Percutaneous drainage of 300 intraperitoneal abscesses with long-term follow-up. Cardiovasc Intervent Radiol 28:744–750

Baig MK, Wexner SD (2004) Postoperative ileus: a review. Dis Colon Rectum 47:516–526

Bartels H (2009) Special aspects of postoperative complications following visceral surgery. Chirurgie 80:780–789

Bennett AA, Gilkeson RC, Haaga JR et al (2000) Complications of "dropped" gallstones after laparoscopic cholecystectomy: technical considerations and imaging finding. Abdom Imaging 25:190–193

Benoist S, Panis Y, Pannegeon V et al (2002) Can failure of percutaneous drainage of postoperative abdominal abscesses be predicted? Am J Surg 184:148–153

Blachar A, Federle MP, Brancatelli G, Peterson MS, Oliver JH III, Li W (2001) Radiologist performance in the diagnosis of internal hernia by using specific CT findings with emphasis on transmesenteric hernia. Radiology 221:422–428

Blum A, Bui P, Boccaccini H et al (1995) Imaging of severe forms of hematoma in the rectus abdominis under anticoagulants. J Radiol 76:267–273

Catalá V, Solà M, Samaniego J et al (2009) CT findings in urinary diversion after radical cystectomy: postsurgical anatomy and complications. Radiographics 29:461–476

Fulcher AS, Turner MA (1996) Percutaneous drainage of enteric-related abscesses. Gastroenterologist 4:276–285

Gayer G, Hertz M, Zissin R (2004) Postoperative pneumoperitoneum: prevalence, duration and possible significance. Semin Ultrasound CT MR 25:286–289

Gore RM, Berlin JW, Yagmai V, Mehta U, Newmark GM, Ghahremani GG (2004) CT diagnosis of post operative abdominal complications. Semin Ultrasound CT MR 25:207–221

Harrisinghani MG, Gervais DA, Hahn PF et al (2002) CT guided transgluteal drainage of deep pelvic abscesses: indications, technique, procedure-related complications, and clinical outcome. Radiographics 22:1353–1367

Hodel J, Zins M, Desmottes L et al (2009) Location of the transition zone in CT of small-bowel obstruction: added value of multiplanar reformations. Abdom Imaging 34:35–41

Hoeffel C, Azizi L, Lewin M et al (2006) Normal and pathologic features of the postoperative biliary tract at 3D MR cholangiopancreatography and MR imaging. Radiographics 26:1603–1620

Israel GM, Hecht E, Bosniak MA (2006) CT and MR imaging of complications of partial nephrectomy. Radiographics 26:1419–1429

Khoury W, Ben-Yehuda A, Ben-Haim M, Klausner JM, Szold O (2009) Abdominal computed tomography for diagnosing postoperative lower gastrointestinal tract leaks. J Gastrointest Surg 13:1454–1458

Lepanto L, Gianfelice D, Dery R et al (1994) Post operative changes, complications and recurrent disease after Wipple's operation CT features. AJR Am J Roentgenol 163:841–846

Morrin MM, Kruskal JB, Hochman MG et al (2000) Radiologic features of complications arising from dropped gallstones in laparoscopic cholecystectomy patients. AJR 174:1441–1445

Negus S, Sidhu PS (2000) MRI of retroperitoneal collections: a comparison with CT. Br J Radiol 73:907–912

Nichols RL (1991) Surgical wound infection. Am J Med 91:54S–64S

Paspulati RM, Dalal TA (2010) Imaging of complications following gynecologic surgery. Radiographics 30:625–642

Power N, Atri M, Ryan S, Haddad R, Smith A (2007) CT assessment of anastomotic bowel leak. Clin Radiol 62:37–42

Sandrasegaran K, Maglinte DD, Lappas JC, Howard TJ (2005) Small-bowel complications of major gastrointestinal tract surgery. AJR Am J Roentgenol 185:671–681

Taourel PG, Fabre JM, Pradel JA et al (1995) Value of CT in the diagnosis and management of patients with suspected acute SBO. AJR Am J Roentgenol 165:1187–1192

Van Sonnenberg E, Wittich GR, Goodacee BW et al (2001) Percutaneous abscess drainage: update. World J Surg 25: 362–369

Yablon CM, Banner MP, Ramchandani P, Rovner ES (2004) Complications of prostate cancer treatment: spectrum of imaging findings. Radiographics 24:S181–S194

Zalcman M, Sy M, Donckier V, Closset J, Gansbeke DV (2000) Helical CT signs in the diagnosis of intestinal ischemia in small-bowel obstruction. AJR Am J Roentgenol 175:1601–1607

Zappa M, Sibert A, Vullierme MP, Bertin C, Bruno O, Vilgrain V (2009) Postoperative imaging of the peritoneum and abdominal wall. J Radiol 90:969–979

Zins M, Ferretti G (2009) Postoperative imaging of the abdomen and chest: humility and multidisciplinary approach. J Radiol 90:887

Part V

CT Diagnosis in Traumatic Abdomen

Abdominal Trauma

Ingrid Millet and Patrice Taourel

Contents

1 Background.. 422
1.1 Lesion Mechanisms.. 422
1.2 Divergent Issues 422

2 Intra-abdominal Effusions 425
2.1 Intraperitoneal Effusions 425
2.2 Retroperitoneum 427

3 Splenic Traumas... 428
3.1 CT Findings... 428
3.2 CT Pitfalls... 430
3.3 Impact on Management...................................... 431

4 Hepatic Traumas 432
4.1 CT Findings... 432
4.2 CT Pitfalls... 436
4.3 Impact on Management...................................... 437

5 Pancreatic Traumas...................................... 437
5.1 CT Findings... 438
5.2 CT Pitfalls... 439
5.3 Impact on Management...................................... 439

6 Intestinal and Mesenteric Traumas............. 440
6.1 CT Findings... 440
6.2 CT Pitfalls... 443
6.3 Impact on Management...................................... 445

7 Renal and Urinary Tract Trauma................. 445
7.1 CT Findings... 446
7.2 CT Pitfalls... 450
7.3 Impact on Management...................................... 450

8 Adrenal Gland Injury 451
8.1 CT Findings... 452
8.2 CT Pitfalls... 452
8.3 Impact on Management...................................... 452

9 Vesical Traumas 453
9.1 CT Findings... 453
9.2 CT Pitfalls... 455
9.3 Impact on Management...................................... 455

10 Urethral Injury.. 455
10.1 CT Findings... 456
10.2 Impact on Management...................................... 456

11 Genital Organ Injury 456

12 Abdominal Vessel Injury 456
12.1 Pelvic Vessels.. 457
12.2 Abdominal Aorta.. 458
12.3 Inferior Vena Cava.. 459

13 Parietal Injury... 460
13.1 CT Findings... 460
13.2 Impact on Management...................................... 461

14 Diaphragmatic Injury................................... 461
14.1 CT Findings... 461
14.2 CT Pitfalls... 462
14.3 CT Impact 463

References.. 463

I. Millet · P. Taourel (✉)
Imagerie Médicale, Hôpital Lapeyronie,
371 Avenue du Docteur Gaston Giraud,
34000 Montpellier, France
e-mail: patricetaourel@wanadoo.fr;
p-taourel@chu-montpellier.fr

Abstract

Abdominal injuries are more often observed in the setting of polytrauma. Detection and accurate description of hemoperitoneum, solid organ injuries (contusion, hematoma, laceration, fracture), bowel perforation, and arterial bleeding allow optimal multidisciplinary management. Mesenteric and bowel injuries are often difficult to diagnose and may be masked by the presence of more frequent injuries (spleen, liver). Multidetector CT is the gold standard imaging modality for the diagnosis of traumatic abdominal injuries, but also to evaluate their seriousness and consequently for the management of abdominal trauma. This chapter deals with CT findings and CT pitfalls in traumatic abdominal lesions and underlines the key points with impact on the management.

1 Background

Approximately one third of trauma patients presents with signs of abdominopelvic injury.

1.1 Lesion Mechanisms

Traumas can be classified into two categories, open and blunt traumas:

1. A trauma is referred to as open trauma in the case of cutaneous effraction and is usually caused by cold weapons or firearms. The aim of the CT scan is to precisely determine the extent of organic lesions along the trajectory of the injuring object and appreciate the depth of the trauma, notably by searching for injury of the parietal peritoneum.

2. A trauma is referred to as a blunt trauma when there is no cutaneous effraction. A distinction is made between direct traumas due to contusion by compression (e.g., crushing of the abdomen against the steering wheel or the dashboard) and indirect traumas caused by blast injury or by deceleration, resulting in shear or traction injury to intraperitoneal organs, the severity of which is proportional to both the respective organ mass and the speed of the collision (e.g., wrenching of mesenteric vessels due to traction on the digestive structures).

If the patient's hemodynamic status is unstable in spite of appropriate measures being taken (usually defined as a lack of improvement following vascular filling of more than 2 l, including three to four red blood packs), many authors advocate the focused abdominal sonogram for trauma (FAST) procedure, which consists of quick ultrasonography performed at the patient's bedside. FAST evaluation allows visualization of the pericardium, the Morrison space, intersplenorenal space, parietocolic gutters, and the

Douglas pouch, and identification of a potential fluid collection, enabling optimal emergency treatment prior to a CT scan (hemothorax drainage, laparotomy in the case of hemoperitoneum, etc.).

In all of cases, as clinical abdominal examination is not very precise, a multislice CT scan is the investigation of first choice for abdominal trauma exploration (Shuman 1997; Stuhlfaut et al. 2007; Pal and Victorino, 2002).

1.2 Divergent Issues

1.2.1 Which Protocol Should Be Used?

The main subject of controversy concerns the CT scan protocol to be used, with some key questions:
- Is the use of an oral contrast medium necessary? (Stafford et al. 1999). No, because of its poor diagnostic performance.
- Is an initial acquisition without injection needed? Yes, as this allows the detection of hemorrhagic lesions in the mesentery (such as a sentinel blood clot, probably caused by a digestive injury) or in other solid organs (facilitated detection of intraparenchymal hematomas).
- Should a CT acquisition with intra-arterial injection be obtained? Yes, to detect arterial lesions and, in the presence of extravasations, to confirm their arterial or venous origin, which is likely to impact on the subsequent therapeutic management.
- Portal acquisition (70–100 s) is indispensable.
- Is a late-acquisition CT scan needed? Yes, on request, to characterize extravasations (blood, urine, or pseudoaneurysm) and detect lesions of the urinary tract.

1.2.2 What About Organ Classification?

To be pertinent and useful, a reliable classification system must be simple, easy to learn, applicable, and reproducible, and it must be understood by our correspondents, with a potential impact on either therapeutic management or prognosis. Given the multitude of trauma lesions that may be encountered in clinical practice at the same abdominal organ level, and because of intercenter therapeutic variations, no classification system currently meets all of these requirements. Knowledge of them is therefore not useful in emergency imaging. However, it is to the credit of these classification systems that they remind us of the

Abdominal Trauma

Table 1 American Association for the Surgery of Trauma (AAST) classification of splenic injury

Grade	Lesion description
1	Subcapsular hematoma, less than 10% of the surface area
	Capsular or parenchymal laceration less than 1 cm in parenchymal depth
2	Subcapsular hematoma, 10–50% of the surface area
	Intraparenchymal hematoma less than 5 cm in diameter
	Laceration, 1–3 cm parenchymal depth, with no trabecular vessel involvement
3	Subcapsular hematoma, 50% of the surface area or expanding hematoma
	Intraparenchymal hematoma more than 5 cm in diameter
	Laceration more than 3 cm in parenchymal depth or involving a trabecular vessel
4	Laceration involving a segmental vessel or hilar vessel with splenic devascularization of more than 25%
5	Lacerated spleen with multiple ruptures

Table 2 AAST classification of hepatic injury

Grade	Lesion description
1	Subcapsular hematoma, less than 10% of the surface area
	Capsular or parenchymal laceration less than 1 cm in depth
2	Subcapsular hematoma, 10–50% of the surface area
	Intraparenchymal hematoma less than 10 cm in diameter
	Laceration, 1–3 cm in parenchymal depth, and less than 10 cm in length
3	Subcapsular hematoma, more than 50% of the surface area, expanding hematoma, or ruptured hematoma with active bleeding
	Intraparenchymal hematoma more than 10 cm in diameter, expanding hematoma, or ruptured hematoma
	Laceration more than 3 cm in depth
4	Intraparenchymal ruptured hematoma with active bleeding
	Laceration involving 25–75% of the hepatic lobe or one to three segments of the same lobe
5	Laceration involving more than 75% of the hepatic lobe or more than three segments of the same lobe
	Vascular lesions of hepatic veins or retrohepatic inferior vena cava
6	Avulsion of hepatic vascular pedicle

significant points that must figure in each posttrauma CT scan report. Furthermore, these systems may also be useful for the comparison of lesions in the setting of scientific studies. The international classification currently used is the American Association for the Surgery of Trauma (AAST) classification, described by organ here, but the Mirvis classification for liver injuries and Fullen's classification for gastrointestinal tract injuries are also commonly used. It is obvious that this type of classification cannot replace the precise emergency trauma.

AAST classification of splenic injuries (Table 1). Based on both surgical observations and CT scan findings, this classification takes into account the size and the location of contusions and hematomas, as well as the depth of lacerations and signs of devascularization. The lesion's severity increases with the grade.

AAST classification of hepatic injuries (Table 2). This classification takes into account the size of subcapsular and intraparenchymal hematomas, the depth of lacerations, and signs of devascularization.

It should be noted that Mirvis et al. (1989) have proposed another CT scan classification of hepatic injuries, partly based on the ASAT classification, with only five grades.

AAST classification of pancreatic injuries (Table 3). This classification is based on the lesions'

Table 3 AAST classification of pancreatic injury

Grade	Lesion description
1	Medium-sized hematoma without duct involvement
	Superficial laceration without duct involvement
2	Voluminous hematoma without duct involvement
	Voluminous laceration with neither duct involvement nor parenchymal tissue loss
3	Laceration distal transection or parenchymal injury with duct involvement
4	Laceration proximal transection or parenchymal injury with involvement of the ampulla
5	Massive fragmentation of the pancreas head

Table 4 Fullen's classification of gastrointestinal injury

Grade	Ischemia	Digestive segment
I	Maximum	Jejunum, ileum, and ascending colon
II	Moderate	Major segment of small intestine and/or ascending colon
III	Minimal	Minor segment(s) of small intestine or ascending colon
IV	No	Absence of ischemia

Zone	Superior mesenteric artery segment
I	Proximal trunk until the first branch (inferior pancreaticoduodenal artery)
II	Trunk between inferior pancreaticoduodenal artery and middle colic artery
III	Distal trunk below the middle colic artery
IV	Segmental jejunal, ileal, and colic branches

Table 5 AAST classification of renal injury

Grade	Lesion description
1 (by far the most common)	Renal contusion
	Non expanding subcapsular hematomas with no parenchymal laceration
2	Non expanding perirenal hematoma, confined to the retroperitoneum
	Superficial cortical lacerations less than 1 cm in depth without collecting system injury
3	Renal lacerations more than 1 cm in parenchymal depth without collecting system injury
4	Renal lacerations extending through the renal cortex, medulla, and collecting system with urinary loss
	Injuries involving the main renal artery or vein with continuous bleeding
	Segmental artery thrombosis with segmental infarction without associated lacerations
5	Shattered kidney
	Involvement of the main renal artery or vein that devascularizes the kidney (occlusion or arterial or venous avulsion)

size and topography, as well as on the concomitant duct involvement; it appears to correlate with mortality and posttraumatic complication rates.

Fullen's classification of gastrointestinal injuries (Table 4). This old classification, which is still commonly used, is based on the digestive territory that is ischemic (grades) and the lesion's distance from the superior mesenteric artery (zones).

AAST classification of renal injuries (Table 5). This classification was validated by an international consensus conference in 2004 (Santucci et al. 2004), allowing the classification of renal injuries depending

Abdominal Trauma

on the trauma severity and seriousness. However, owing to the potential coexistence of vascular, parenchymal, and urinary tract injuries, especially in the case of grade 4 and 5 lesions, functional prognosis and/or therapeutic management may differ. Therefore, this classification system does permit a prognostic or therapeutic approach.

2 Intra-abdominal Effusions

2.1 Intraperitoneal Effusions

2.1.1 Hemoperitoneum

Hemoperitoneum is commonly observed in the case of abdominopelvic trauma.

2.1.1.1 Typical Imaging Results

Images typically consist of a spontaneously hyperdense intraperitoneal fluid collection, with densities reaching approximately 30–50 HU for free hemoperitoneum, and 45–70 HU for clotted blood (Lubner et al. 2007).

The presence of a liquid level (sedimentation of red blood cells), occurring within a few hours, may help confirm the bloody nature of the fluid. In the case of free extravasation of contrast medium in the peritoneal cavity, the density is superior to 100 HU.

Radiology findings suggesting a diffuse hemoperitoneum do not provide any clues as to its origin, as they may reflect solid-organ or hollow-organ injury, or even bone injury. In the case of splenic or hepatic trauma, the effusion tends to migrate caudally toward the Douglas pouch by passing along the left or right parietocolic gutters, according to the physiological movements of intraperitoneal fluids. When moderate, the presence of a triangular fluid collection trapped between the intestinal loops guides the diagnosis toward a digestive or mesenteric injury. A localized effusion restricted to the omental bursa (previously termed "the posterior cavity of the epiploon") guides the diagnosis toward pancreatic or bile duct injury.

A hemoperitoneum has a good localizing value if it is focal and dense around an organ, suggesting a traumatic lesion of this organ, the so-called sentinel clot sign.

In the presence of an abundant, low-density, free fluid collection, without any apparent cause, late CT

Table 6 Density of intra-abdominal liquid effusions expressed in Hounsfield units (*HU*)

0–20 HU	Preexisting ascites
	Bile
	Urine
	Digestive fluid
	Diluted or old blood
30–45 HU	Free nonclotted intraperitoneal blood
45–70 HU	Clotted blood/sentinel clot sign hematoma
>100 HU	Extravasation of contrast medium (vascular or urinary)

acquisition is essential to exclude bladder perforation into a free peritoneal cavity (Drasin et al. 2008).

The clinical relevance of a hemoperitoneum may be classified according to the number of compartments that are involved, taking into account the perihepatic and perisplenic compartments, the Morrison space, each of the parietocolic gutters, the inframesocolic space, and the pelvic space. Hemoperitoneum is considered minor (volume less than 200 ml) if only one compartment is involved, moderate (volume between 200 and 500 ml) when two compartments are involved, and major (volume more than 500 ml) when more than two compartments are affected.

2.1.1.2 Pitfalls and Diagnostic Difficulties

False-negative results. In one quarter of cases, the fluid collection is not found to be hyperdense owing to low hematocrit or bleeding that has continued for over 48 h. In these cases, the density is close to 20 HU because of dilution, and the hemoperitoneum cannot be distinguished from other causes of intraperitoneal liquid effusions (Table 6).

False-positive results. A limited fluid accumulation in the Douglas pouch in a woman of childbearing age may be simply due to recent ovulation and unrelated to the trauma.

Differential diagnosis. Posttraumatic intraperitoneal fluid accumulation is not necessarily blood. It may be urine (in the case of intraperitoneal bladder rupture) (Fig. 1) or digestive fluid (in the case of digestive tract perforation).

2.1.1.3 Therapeutic Impact

The spontaneous trend is toward slow regression within 7–10 days. Specific treatment depends on the injured organ.

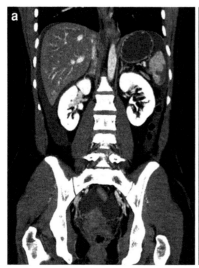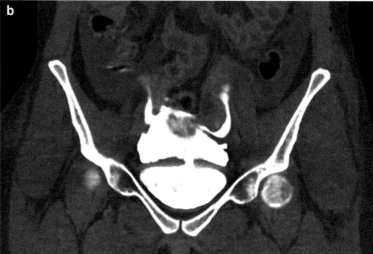

Fig. 1 Posttraumatic intraperitoneal fluid in relation to urine. Coronal reformatting in the portal phase (**a**) shows hypodense peritoneal fluid close to the liver, close to the spleen, and in the pelvic space. Note also the presence of hypodensity within the spleen (cf. Fig. 4). Delayed coronal reformatting (**b**) clearly shows a peritoneal leak from the bladder responsible for the presence of urine in the peritoneal space

2.1.2 Pneumoperitoneum

In the case of blunt trauma, accumulation of air in the peritoneal cavity is indicative of digestive tract rupture.

2.1.2.1 Typical Imaging Results

Findings typically include the presence of air outside the digestive tract, within the peritoneal cavity. Its detection is facilitated by a CT scan obtained using the pulmonary window setting.

Pneumoperitoneum may be diffuse and free, or focal and embedded between the intestinal loops and mesenteric recesses, usually in contact with the injured loop, which has a high localization value.

2.1.2.2 Pitfalls and Diagnostic Difficulties

Differential diagnosis. Air within the peritoneal cavity is not necessarily indicative of digestive tract perforation, as this may also occur under other circumstances:
- Open abdominal trauma: the air usually originates from outside, and thus presents no diagnostic value in favor of digestive tract perforation.
- Subdiaphragmatic origin by diffusion from a pneumomediastinum or pneumothorax (notably via a diaphragmatic leak), specifically if the patient is being mechanically ventilated.
- Vesical origin following intraperitoneal bladder rupture in a urinary bladder catheterized patient.
- Trauma of female internal genital organs.

A pneumoperitoneum of digestive origin tends to expand steadily on CT scans taken at subsequent times, whereas it usually regresses in the case of other origins.

Lastly, a pneumoperitoneum may be caused by digestive microperforations due to barotraumas, without any macroscopic counterpart, responsible for negative laparotomies. However, this is an exclusion diagnosis; its treatment is conservative with clinical surveillance and CT scan monitoring.

False-positive results. Is the location of the visualized air intraperitoneal, retroperitoneal, or subperitoneal? To answer this question, perfect knowledge of CT radioanatomy of the peritoneum is necessary (Taourel et al. 1999). Diagnostic errors are common, mainly due to air bubbles in the anterior abdominal cavity, the topography of which may be either intraperitoneal (behind the anterior parietal peritoneum) or preperitoneal (outside the anterior parietal peritoneum). The presence of a liquid–air level along with a hemoperitoneum is indicative of an intraperitoneal location.

False-negative results. In more than half of all digestive tract perforation cases, a pneumoperitoneum is absent during the first hours, which may be due to both the small size of the perforations involving the small intestine and the low air content in the small

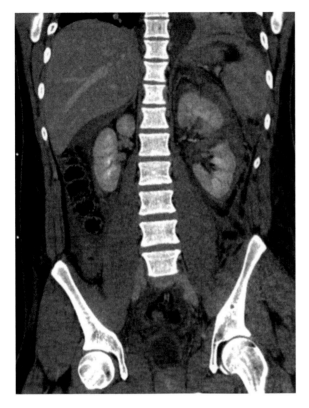

Fig. 2 Diffusion of a perirenal hematoma due to left renal fracture in the peritoneal perisplenic, Morrison, and right laterocolic spaces

intestinal loops. In this case, the patient must be examined for other indirect signs of digestive tract perforation.

2.1.2.3 Therapeutic Impact

In blunt trauma cases, the patient must be routinely examined for digestive tract perforation. When the diagnosis is based on CT scans or is made peroperatively, treatment for a digestive leak is always surgical, consisting of excision–suture or resection–anastomosis.

2.2 Retroperitoneum

As the retroperitoneum is divided into three compartments, fluid accumulation in one of these compartments guides the diagnosis toward the traumatic injury of an organ located in this compartment:
1. The perirenal space contains the kidneys, the adrenal glands, and the proximal ureter. A hematoma of the perirenal space pushes the duodenum forward, the kidney inside, forward, and upward, and the colon laterally
2. The anterior pararenal space contains the pancreas, the second and third duodenal segments, the adjacent segments of the colon, and the part of the liver not covered by peritoneum (with hepatic veins). A hematoma of the pararenal space pushes the kidney outward and upward, and the duodenum and colon forward.
3. The posterior pararenal space only contains fat. A hematoma of the posterior pararenal space pushes the kidney forward and outside, and the colon forward and inside. Only in very rare cases does such a hematoma lead to compression, as this space is open upward and downward. It is mandatory to look not only for bone (rachis/pelvis), vessel, ureter, or muscle (psoas) lesions, but also for extrapleural thoracic (diaphragmatic lesion) or abdominoparietal injury because the posterior pararenal space communicates with the pelvic subperitoneal spaces and because of the continuity with the anterior abdominal and the extrapleural thoracic spaces.

2.2.1 Hemoretroperitoneum

Images typically show a spontaneous hyperdensity of retroperitoneal topography.

Any retroperitoneal fluid accumulation is not necessarily blood, as it may be urine originating from a urinoma due to injury of the collecting duct system. Furthermore, it may also be caused by intensive resuscitation with massive vascular filling.

A retroperitoneal hematoma usually progresses toward spontaneous tamponade. It may diffuse within the peritoneal cavity, meaning that the presence of peritoneal fluid does not mean there is a peritoneal lesion (Fig. 2).

Treatment depends on the causal lesions.

2.2.2 Retropneumoperitoneum

Retropneumoperitoneum is defined by the presence of extradigestive and retroperitoneal air. Air in the anterior pararenal space is indicative of duodenal perforation, whereas air in the posterior pararenal space suggests colic (perforation of ascending or descending colon) or rectal perforation. Retropneumoperitoneum may also be caused by simple air diffusion originating from a pneumomediastinum via the physiological

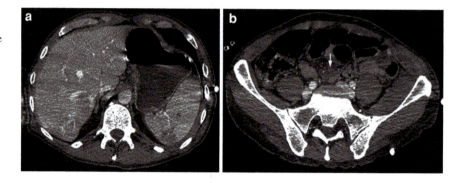

Fig. 3 Splenic contusion. Axial slice (**a**) showing a splenic contusion without free peritoneal fluid. On a lower axial slice (**b**) some weak infiltration of the mesenteric fat around the mesenteric vessels was prospectively underestimated (*arrow*) (see Fig. 18)

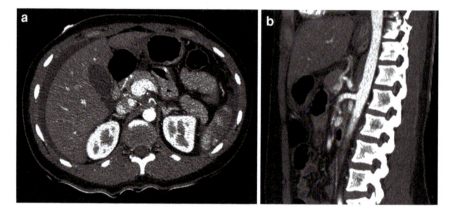

Fig. 4 Splenic infarct due to dissection of the celiac trunk (same patient as in Fig. 1). The axial slice (**a**) shows peripheric triangular hypodensities within the spleen, whereas sagittal reformatting (**b**) shows dissection of the celiac trunk. Surgery performed for the bladder peritoneal rupture confirmed the lack of splenic injury

diaphragmatic spaces; it does not have any diagnostic value when associated with an open trauma.

The main diagnostic difficulty is its differentiation from a pneumoperitoneum. Another pitfall is to confuse a duodenal diverticulum with a retropneumoperitoneum. There is no specific treatment for a retropneumoperitoneum, as its management depends on the causal lesion (Taourel et al. 2008).

3 Splenic Traumas

Following an abdominal trauma, the spleen is the most commonly injured organ (approximately 40% of cases) because of its parenchymal spongy structure and its fragile and fine capsule. In the presence of a preexisting disease associated with splenomegaly, the spleen is even more exposed.

Currently, conservative treatment is preferred, and is possible in most cases, as the spleen has significant restoration capacities.

3.1 CT Findings

CT scan diagnosis is based on the lack of splenic parenchymal enhancement during the portal phase, which may present different features depending on the lesion. An adjacent strip of hemoperitoneum is almost always present, and the perisplenic hematoma pushes the spleen back without causing any deformation. In some cases, only a sentinel blood clot or a simple thickening of the anterior pararenal fascia and left lateroconal fascia are observed. When this occurs, fractures of the first left ribs must be considered (Marmery and Shanmuganathan 2006).

3.1.1 Parenchymal Contusion

Parenchymal contusion appears as a hypodense intraparenchymal area with irregular contours (Fig. 3). This must be differentiated from parenchymal infarction, which usually presents a triangular shape with clear delineation (Fig. 4).

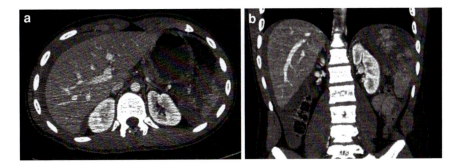

Fig. 5 Scattered spleen seen on the axial slice (**a**) as well as on coronal reformatting (**b**)

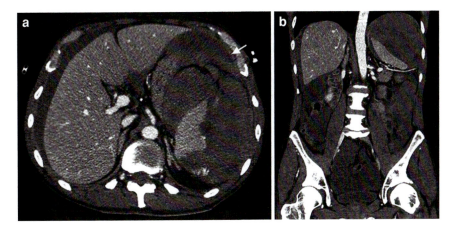

Fig. 6 Splenic subcapsular hematoma with rupture in the peritoneum. The axial slice (**a**) and coronal reformatting (**b**) clearly show the subcapsular hematoma which compresses the splenic parenchyma with rupture within the peritoneal space. Note the peritoneal fluid is hyperdense close to the rate (sentinel clot) (*arrow*), whereas it is hypodense in the right subphrenic space

3.1.2 Parenchymal Laceration

This lesion appears as a superficial, linear hypodensity, usually less than 3 cm in length, which is at times linked to the splenic parenchyma. If the lesion involves two visceral surfaces, or if its length is more than 3 cm, it is referred to as a fracture. If there are multiple fractures, it is referred to as a scattered spleen, from which several, more or less vascularized fragments can detach (Fig. 5).

3.1.3 Subcapsular Hematoma

The CT scan typically shows a crescent-shaped perisplenic hyperdensity on slices from noninjected series, and a hypodensity in relation to the spleen on slices from injected series. The lesion compresses the splenic parenchyma, pushing it back. Rupture of the splenic capsule may follow, caused by its volume, possibly accounting for two-time traumatic ruptures, with massive intraperitoneal bleeding (Fig. 6).

3.1.4 Intraparenchymal Hematoma

This lesion first appears as a spontaneous hyperdensity, usually rounded, with irregular contours, on slices from noninjected series, then, following injection, as a hypodensity in relation to the enhanced splenic parenchyma.

3.1.5 Vascular Trauma

The most dangerous vascular traumatic lesions are arterial lesions (Marmery et al. 2008).

3.1.5.1 Dissection/Thrombosis

Intraparenchymal arterial lesions are shear injuries, with intimal lacerations of small intraparenchymal arteries, resulting in thromboses and distal ischemia. The exact location and the extent of the ischemic area vary, depending on both the number of small arteries injured and the importance of the collateral arterial network. CT scans reveal a lack of parenchymal enhancement, usually of triangular shape with a peripheral basis, with well-defined contours, remaining hypodense, even on delayed imaging following injection.

Hilar dissection of the splenic artery or more proximal dissection (Fig. 4) is often associated with thrombosis, reflected by an interruption of arterial contrast enhancement on the series obtained during

Table 7 CT characteristics of the main types of rupture and differential diagnosis

Rupture type	Shape	Enhancement in the arterial and portal phases	Feature in the delayed phase
Pseudoaneurysm	Regular outline Round Unchanged according to the phase (arterial, portal, delayed)	Similar to the aorta Sometimes hypodense rim	Washout
Free rupture	Irregular outline Not well limited Changed according to the phase	Increased density in the portal phase in comparison with other arteries	Increase of the size
Parenchymal fragments	Variable Non modified according to the phase	Same as normal parenchyma	Same as normal parenchyma

the arterial phase, along with a partial or total absence of splenic enhancement. At times, the absence of splenic enhancement may only concern the inferior splenic pole, the superior splenic pole being supplied by blood flow from the short gastric arteries.

3.1.5.2 Arterial Rupture

In the case of arterial rupture, bleeding may be confined within a pseudoaneurysm, an intraparenchymal hematoma, or a subcapsular hematoma; bleeding may also occur into the free peritoneal cavity. In any case, extravasations of contrast medium may be visualized during arterial time as a hyperdensity in the form of a "blush" at the splenic level. A precise analysis during the other acquisition times is crucial to differentiate a pseudoaneurysm from contrast medium extravasations in the free peritoneal cavity and healthy parenchymal fragments. For this differential diagnosis, the delayed phase is of paramount importance (Table 7) (Anderson et al. 2007).

Splenic arteriovenous fistulas may occur following concomitant arterial and venous injuries. CT scan findings mimic a pseudoaneurysm, and the diagnosis is confirmed using arteriography.

It should be noted that the spleen may differ in size (up to a 50% increase) on successive examinations, as the adrenergic response that immediately follows the trauma results in an initial reflex contraction.

3.2 CT Pitfalls

3.2.1 False-Negative Results

Standard errors occur when the lesions involve the upper parts of the abdomen and are not detected on axial slices (a phenomenon known as partial volume effect with the diaphragm). For this reason, coronal reformatting on CT scanning should be routinely used to identify these lesions.

3.2.2 False-Positive Results

- Spotted spleen: Early heterogeneity of the splenic parenchyma is physiological, resulting in a spotted spleen, which may be mistaken for a laceration. Therefore, one must wait for the necessary time to achieve homogenization (portal time 70–100 s).
- Congenital lobulation: A physiological splenic indentation must not be interpreted as a laceration. In most cases, the indentation involves the medial splenic border and is very thin at the difference of splenic injury (Fig. 7), it is classically not associated with hemoperitoneum, and presents smooth and regular contours. Furthermore, its features do not change with time, whereas lacerations tend to decrease in number and size on subsequent CT scans.
- Tonguelike projection of left liver lobe: The interface between the tonguelike projection of the left liver lobe and the spleen should not be mistaken for a fracture. Coronal and sagittal reconstructions allow physicians to correct the diagnosis.
- Movement artifacts: Movement or metallic (extrinsic material) artifacts may produce false images of laceration or subcapsular hematomas. Recognizing these artifacts is crucial, and in the case of poor-quality imaging, this does not permit any formal conclusions regarding the organ's integrity, and the examination should be repeated immediately.

3.2.3 Differential Diagnosis

- Focal enhancement area: This may represent a pseudoaneurysm, a fragment of normal spleen within the contusion area, or active bleeding.

Abdominal Trauma

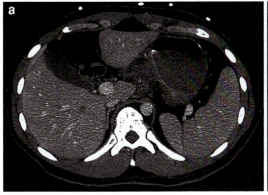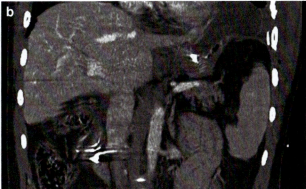

Fig. 7 Pseudofeature of splenic indentation due to a splenic fracture. The axial slice (**a**) shows a linear hypodensity crossing the spleen. Although slightly thick, this hypodensity was prospectively considered as an indentation because of the lack of perisplenic fluid. Surgery, performed for left diaphragmatic rupture well shown on the coronal reformatting (**b**) with passage of the stomach through the thorax, diagnosed splenic fracture

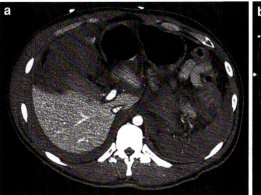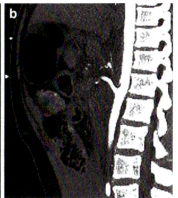

Fig. 8 Hypodense spleen because of vasoconstriction complicating a dissection of the celiac trunk. The axial slice (**a**) shows a hypodense and homogenous spleen, and sagittal reformatting (**b**) shows a dissection of the celiac trunk, which was posttraumatic in this young patient

- Overall splenic hypodensity: This finding may be linked to a shock spleen due to reflex vasoconstriction of the splenic artery, celiac or splenic artery dissection (Fig. 8), or splenic artery rupture with downstream devascularization, resulting in a massive hemoperitoneum and hilar contrast medium extravasation.

3.3 Impact on Management

Therapeutic management comprises surgical, endovascular, or conservative treatments depending on the patient's age and comorbidities, the benefit–risk ratio of a splenectomy taking into account the risk of subsequent sepsis (likely to be multiplied by a factor of 50 in the case of splenectomy), the presence of arterial vascular lesions, associated lesions, and particularly the patient's hemodynamic status. The impact of these treatments on long-term morbidity and mortality rates still needs to be investigated.

Emergency splenectomy should be restricted to hemodynamically unstable patients (Kaseje et al. 2008; Savage et al. 2008), along with prevention of secondary infections by means of vaccinations and long-term antibiotherapy.

In all other cases, a CT scan allows guided therapeutic management, depending on various key parameters:

- The presence of a subcapsular hematoma requires careful clinical and biological surveillance in an intensive care unit or surgical unit over the course of several hours because of the risk of secondary rupture. This complication is observed in approximately 10% of subcapsular hematomas, and usually occurs during the first 10 days, particularly during the first 24 h, requiring emergency hemostatic splenectomy to be performed.

- The presence of arterial vascular lesions may necessitate an endovascular approach. In cases of venous bleeding, embolization is not indicated. Criteria for selecting appropriate candidates for this procedure have not yet been clearly defined. The patient must be hemodynamically stable or have responded to initial resuscitation measures. The CT scan must confirm that the bleeding is of arterial origin, determine whether the bleeding is confined, and if possible, find out which arterial branch is involved. The final therapeutic decision should be consensual and based on a multidisciplinary discussion involving the emergency radiologist, interventional radiologist, intensive care physician, and surgeon. This method is preferred over surgery in cases of pseudoaneurysms or arteriovenous fistulas. Its major advantage is to preserve the spleen, which decreases the risk of sepsis (Wei et al. 2008). Its main complications are the risk of secondary bleeding or the occurrence of intraparenchymal infarction with necrosis and abscess formation, requiring a secondary splenectomy (the risk of infarction appears to be higher with distal embolization than with proximal embolization).
- First-line conservative treatment will be used in all other patients. Intrasplenic hematomas tend to liquefy over time and may give rise to splenic cysts. Lacerations and contusions spontaneously disappear within a few weeks or months (2–3 months).

4 Hepatic Traumas

The liver is the second most commonly involved organ and hepatic traumas are the primary cause of death following abdominal traumas.

The main lesion mechanisms are as follows:

- Blunt traumas.
  - During acceleration–deceleration, shearing of the posterior attachments (between the Glisson capsule and the triangular ligaments) causes lesions of the posterior and superior parts of the right lobe of the liver, which may result in a disinsertion of the right hepatic vein at its confluence into the inferior vena cava.

Table 8 Features with impact on the management and the prognosis

Number of segments involved by the lacerations (significant if at least three segments are involved)

Central or subcapsular location of the lacerations and contusions

Extension of lesions within the porta hepatis or the gallbladder fossa

Importance of the hemoperitoneum

Vascular lesions with active bleeding or sentinel clot sign

  - Following a direct blow on the abdomen, there is a preferential involvement of the anterior segments of the right and left lobe, caught between the vertebrae and the impact area; this may result in a complete transection and a detachment of the left lobe (segments 2 and 3). These injuries of the left lobe of the liver are usually associated with lesions of the duodenopancreatic bloc and the transverse colon.
- Penetrating traumas: Preferential involvement of the right hepatic lobe is due to its larger size.

4.1 CT Findings

A hepatic trauma should be suspected in the presence of any abnormal hepatic contrast enhancement. The features of the lesions are well characterized and are described below. Hemoperitoneum is almost always present and is even more significant in cases of injury to the hepatic capsule (Yoon et al. 2005; Romano et al. 2004).

Certain elements of seriousness, if present, must necessarily be mentioned in the CT report (Table 8).

It should be noted that an isolated involvement of the caudate lobe of the liver is very rare.

4.1.1 Parenchymal Contusion

This lesion is characterized by a relative hypodense area in comparison with the enhanced healthy hepatic parenchyma, with irregular and poorly defined contours. This injury may be associated with hepatic perfusion problems due to sinusoid compression and obstruction by interstitial edema and increased resistance to portal blood flow. In addition, laceration and hematomas are frequently observed. The CT report

Abdominal Trauma

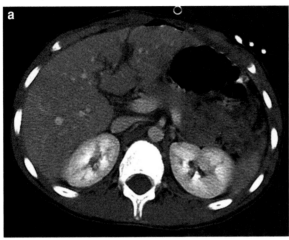
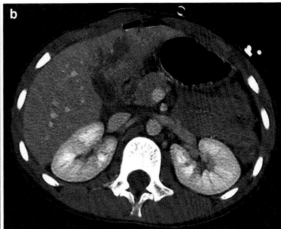

Fig. 9 Liver contusion and liver fracture. The upper axial slice (**a**) shows a liver fracture isolating a piece of segment 4 of the liver, whereas the lower slice (**b**) shows a liver contusion. There is no finding of seriousness for these liver injuries. By contrast, note the presence of a pneumoperitoneum and of fluid between the pancreas and the inferior vena cava related to a duodenal perforation

should precisely mention the lobar or segmental, superficial or central topography of the contusions, along with their extent and location in relation to the vascular elements.

4.1.2 Parenchymal Laceration

Parenchymal laceration is characterized by a linear, irregular, hypodense lesion in comparison with the enhanced adjacent liver, typically along the big vessels, particularly along the right and median hepatic veins and the posterior portal branches. These lesions are classified as superficial (less than 1 cm deep), medium (between 1 and 3 cm deep), and deep (more than 3 cm deep) lacerations, the latter being the least common.

If they involve two hepatic surface areas, they are referred to as fractures (Fig. 9). If they involve the posterior hepatic surface area, devoid of peritoneum, these lacerations are associated with a pericaval, retroperitoneal hematoma, which may extend to right adrenal fossa. If the injury is in proximity of the portal system and the hepatic hilus, there is a risk of concomitant bile duct trauma. If the lacerations are multiple and located close to the inferior vena cava, this is indicative of a severe hepatic trauma with risk of hepatic vein involvement, often associated with right hepatic vein avulsion.

In the worst-case scenario, hepatic fragmentation occurs, with devascularization of the different fragments. The CT report should always mention if the lesions extend to the capsules, vesicular bed, hilus, and vascular structures.

4.1.3 Subcapsular Hematoma

This perihepatic collection appears at first as hyperdense area on slices from noninjected series; it then becomes hypodense in relation to the adjacent enhanced liver tissue, presenting an almond shape or, more frequently, an ellipse, particularly in the case of an anteroposterior topography. This subcapsular hematoma exerts a mass effect on the adjacent liver tissue, with indentation and flattening, contrarily to a hemoperitoneum, which surrounds the liver without causing any deformation. If the hematoma is large, it may result in liver perfusion problems, caused by the portal flow obstruction, which may even result in portal flow inversion and subsequent arterial hypervascularization. The presence of perfusion problems, reflected by heterogeneous enhancement, should be mentioned in the report. Should arterial lesion embolization be required, the risk of hepatic necrosis is significantly increased in this case.

4.1.4 Intraparenchymal Hematoma

This lesion appears as a spontaneously hyperdense area in relation to the healthy adjacent liver tissue, then hypodense and nonenhanced on slices from

Table 9 CT findings of shock

Collapse of inferior vena cava: anteroposterior diameter at the stage of the left renal vein less than or equal to 1/4 the transverse diameter without extrinsic compression

Small aorta

Persistent nephrogram without excretion

Hypodense spleen, without enhancement and normal vascular pedicle

Increased enhancement of the small bowel wall

Increased enhancement of the adrenal glands

Sometimes findings of right cardiac insufficiency with reflux into the hepatic veins

injected series. The lesion's contours are more or less regular. In the absence of noninjected slices, it may be difficult to differentiate this lesion from that observed following contusion. However, caution is required, because, in the case of concomitant hepatic steatosis, the lesion diagnosis may not be made during injection, as the relative hypodensity of the hematoma may not be evident in comparison with the surrounding poorly enhanced liver tissue.

4.1.5 Shock Liver

CT findings in the case of shock liver typically consist of nonenhanced areas, scattered across the liver, with irregular peripheral contours, reflecting visceral artery spasms. In some cases, a linear capsular enhancement may be observed, reflecting the implementation of a new blood supply network. In the presence of other signs of hypovolemic shock (Table 9), these features should not be confused with traumatic lesions, as they tend to regress following appropriate resuscitation measures.

4.1.6 Periportal Edema

This lesion is characterized by periportal hypodensities running in parallel to the portal branches, which may be of various causes:

- Diffusion from intraparenchymal bleeding, along portal vessels
- Dilatation of periportal lymph vessels because of the increased central venous pressure due to massive vascular filling or obstructed venous return in relation with tamponade, hepatic vein obstruction, or massive pneumothorax
- Vascular or focal bile duct dissection, especially if the areas are focal rather than diffuse

Several authors consider this feature equivalent to a minimal hepatic traumatic lesion. Peripheral edema should not be confused with parenchymal lacerations, which are more irregular. If it is an isolated feature, periportal edema has no therapeutic or prognostic impact.

4.1.7 Vascular Lesions

4.1.7.1 Arterial Lesions

Segmental dissection. This injury is characterized by a segmental parenchymal devascularization area, which is hypodense for all injection times, triangularly shaped with peripheral basis, and due to thrombosis or distal arterial dissection (Taourel et al. 2007; Poletti et al. 2000).

Free artery rupture. The CT scan typically shows extravasation of contrast medium into an intraparenchymal or subcapsular hematoma or into the peritoneal cavity. It is crucial to obtain different acquisitions during the injection so as to determine whether the lesion is arterial (Fig. 10) or venous in origin, which has an impact on the therapeutic strategy (an endovascular approach is possible in the case of an arterial lesion). These different acquisition times are also necessary to confirm that the bleeding is free, and increasing in size over time. The blush's density is usually greater than 100 HU (approximately 150 HU on average), which allows the investigator to distinguish this lesion from a parenchymal fragment or hematoma, the densities of which lower (approximately 50 HU on average).

Pseudoaneurysm. Pseudoaneurysm is secondary to arterial wall rupture, with bleeding contained by fibrous capsular tissue or adventitial tissue. It may be primary in the case of intimal laceration, but more often it is delayed and secondary to vascular damage due to bile salts when it occurs near a laceration associated with bile duct injury. It appears as a rounded lesion presenting the same enhancement kinetics as the corresponding artery, to which it is connected, with a washout phase on late imaging. Its shape is not altered with the different acquisition times. It may undergo secondary rupture into the hepatic parenchyma or free peritoneal cavity, or even into the bile ducts, resulting in hemobilia and upper gastrointestinal tract bleeding. In exceptional cases, rupture occurs directly into the duodenum.

Fig. 10 Liver trauma with active bleeding from the right hepatic artery. The CT scan performed in the arterial phase (**a**) shows active bleeding in the posterior segment of the right lobe of the liver, with diffusion in the portal phase seen at the same level of the slice (**b**) and active bleeding within the peritoneum (**c**). An emergency angiography (**d**) with embolization was successful

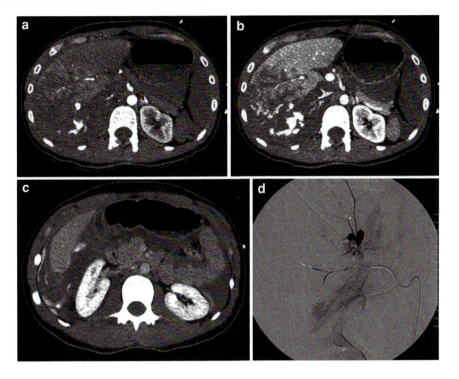

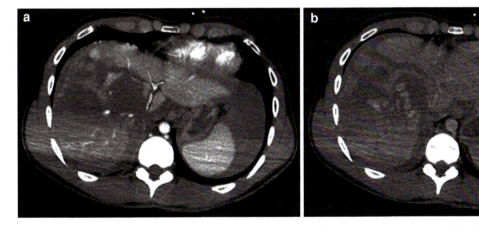

Fig. 11 Active bleeding with avulsion of the right hepatic vein. The CT scan in the portal phase (**a**) shows extravasation of contrast medium close to the site of the proximal right hepatic vein (which was not present in the arterial phase), which spreads out in a more delayed phase (**b**). The inferior vena cava is flat because of shock, and the insertion of the right hepatic vein was never seen

4.1.7.2 Venous Traumas

Traumas to the portal or hepatic venous system are characterized either by extravasation of contrast medium visualized in portal venous time but not in arterial time, or by partial or total lack of portal venous opacification.

If the contusion or laceration occurs near the hepatic venous system or inferior vena cava system, physicians must carefully examine the patient for major hepatic venous injury (Fig. 11), and especially if liver perfusion problems are observed.

In all cases, venous injury is considered to be a severe trauma, with very high mortality rates in the case of proximal lesions. When there are diagnostic doubts on CT examination, this should be brought to the attention of the surgeon (Liu et al. 2005).

In fact, should a laparotomy be envisaged, there is a significant risk of massive preoperative bleeding when the liver is being mobilized. The poor contractility of the hepatic venous system explains why spontaneous hemostasis is difficult to achieve.

4.1.8 Bile Duct Traumas

4.1.8.1 Gallbladder

The gallbladder is rarely injured during abdominal trauma except for cases of alcoholic patients, in whom the gallbladder is often distended and more vulnerable. Many patients present with associated injuries of the liver or the duodenum.

A large spectrum of gallbladder injuries may be encountered, such as contusion, laceration, perforation, and cholecystectomy with avulsion of the cystic duct and artery.

Typical CT signs are as follows:
- Focal or diffuse parietal thickening.
- Pericholecystic fluid.
- Parietal continuity solution.
- Hematoma, biloma, or choleperitoneum. The last lesion presents liquid density, theoretically less than that of water, but as it is often mixed with blood, it cannot be distinguished from simple ascites or an old hematoma using density measurements. The bile content of a collection can be diagnosed using direct fine-needle biopsy or by means of cholangio-MRI following mangafodipir (Teslascan®) administration, depicting bile leaks from the collection. During hepatic trauma monitoring, acute aggravation of an effusion or an intraparenchymal hematoma must evoke the possibility of a biloma, and should the intraperitoneal fluid collection increase in size, as reflected by enhanced peritoneal folds, the possibility of biliary peritonitis must be considered.
- Spontaneous intravesicular hyperdensity reflecting hemobilia (however, this is valid only in the absence of contrast medium injection during the previous 48 h).
- In rare cases, contrast medium extravasation by cystic artery disinsertion; in this case, the patient often has hemodynamic instability.

It should be noted that because the gallbladder is extraperitoneal, bile or blood leak from a ruptured gallbladder may be contained in the gallbladder fossa.

4.1.8.2 Common Bile Duct

Injury to the common bile duct usually occurs at the hepatic pedicle or where the bile duct enters the pancreatic head, which are sites of relative fixation. Lesions include either partial or complete ruptures, or more frequently, dissecting hematomas of the hepatic pedicle, resulting in cicatricial stenoses.

CT findings of bile duct injury are as follows:
- Edema in the hepatoduodenal ligament area
- Nonspecific free intraperitoneal fluid
- Associated liver or duodenal injuries

4.1.8.3 Intrahepatic Bile Ducts

The frequency of intrahepatic bile duct injuries is underestimated. They are more frequent when the hepatic injury occurs near the liver hilus, close to the portal branches. Most often they are asymptomatic, and the diagnosis is rarely made, except in the case of biloma or when focal dilatation of intrahepatic bile ducts, above the cicatricial stenosis, is observed during the control examination.

4.2 CT Pitfalls

The main diagnostic difficulty consists in the clear differentiation between shock liver, hepatic perfusion problems, and liver traumatic injuries. Abnormal perfusion patterns are usually diffuse and radial and tend to homogenize for late acquisitions, whereas contusion or laceration areas are more focal and nonenhanced.

Another diagnostic difficulty is encountered when injury occurs in a patient with liver steatosis. Should this be the case, intraparenchymal hematomas may be missed when using acquisitions during the portal venous phase, and a focal steatosis area may be confused with a lesion caused by ischemia or contusion. A precise analysis of the density evolution during the examination allows the investigator to correct the diagnosis, as enhancement is not observed for lesions due to ischemia or hematoma.

Other sources of confusion may be difficulty to distinguish periportal edema from laceration, or extravasation from healthy parenchyma within a contusion area, or laceration from a normal Arantius duct.

As for the spleen, technical deficiencies from the lack of several acquisition times, movement artifacts, beam hardening artifacts (extrinsic material) or

Table 10 Indications for surgical treatment in liver trauma

Shock

Active venous bleeding

Trauma of the gallbladder

Choleperitoneum

Abdominal surgery necessary for other causes

artifacts due to the position of arms in unmobilizable patients (Fig. 14) may render interpretation of findings unmobilizable difficult.

4.3   Impact on Management

Treatment is conservative in 90% of cases, in the absence of vascular involvement and hemodynamic instability. Surgical treatment is restricted to specific situations, which are summarized in the Table 10 (Poletti et al. 2000; Mattei-Gazagnes et al. 2001).

In cases of hepatic trauma with hemodynamic instability, the patient is directly transferred to the surgical ward for liver packing, allowing the patient to pass the critical period by providing rapid hemostasis. This procedure consists of pressing the liver against the diaphragm using compresses, then suturing the skin but not the aponeurosis. The reparation procedure consisting of suturing vascular lesions, hepatectomy, segmentectomy, embolization, or other procedures will be performed a second time.

If the patient is stable or has adequately responded to resuscitation measures, CT findings dictate the therapeutic strategy, depending on the lesions found. The primary objective is to detect active arterial bleeding sites, for which embolization is usually recommended. In this case, it is crucial to precisely describe the anatomical variations regarding the origin of the hepatic branches, as this facilitates the endovascular procedure. Should there be concomitant venous injuries, surgical treatment is recommended.

In all cases, treatment comprises careful monitoring in a specialized unit. In fact, although a secondary rupture is less likely than with splenic traumas, the morbidity rate is higher. However, there is currently no consensus on how often CT surveillance should be performed, as CT repetition does not appear to be required in low-grade injuries when there are no new clinical symptoms. On the other hand, CT repetition may be very useful for severe traumas with a high

frequency of secondary complications, which would allow early detection and improved therapeutic management.

The evolution is often favorable with restitution *ad integrum* of lesions within approximately 3 months.

The main complications of conservative treatment are vascular (arteriovenous fistula, false aneurysm, new bleeding, etc.), bilary (biloma formation, biliary peritonitis, etc.), infectious (infected hematoma), or mechanical (abdominal compartment syndrome).

It is of note that "abdominal compartment syndrome" refers to intra-abdominal hyperpression of various causes (occlusion, hemoperitoneum, pancreatitis, etc.), resulting in multisystem dysfunction (cardiovascular with hypotension, renal with oliguria, respiratory with hypercapnia and hypoxia, neurological, etc.) (Hunter and Damani 2004). As the intra-abdominal pressure is proportional to the intravesical pressure, clinical monitoring is based on this measurement. From CT findings, the diagnosis may be made if the anteroposterior abdominal diameter is 20% larger than the transverse diameter at the confluence of the left renal vein into the vena cava, with subcutaneous fat excluded from the measurement. The mean treatment is prevention, with the surgeon omitting skin suturing following laparotomy for patients who are at risk of developing this condition. In other cases, treatment is based on abdominal decompression using a large skin opening, in association with the management of the causal lesions.

5   Pancreatic Traumas

Pancreatic injury occurs in only about 3% of abdominal blunt trauma cases, and in slightly more than 10% of penetrating trauma cases.

The injury mechanism is direct impact (steering wheel, bicycle handlebar, seat belt, etc.) with compression and shear against the vertebral column. Associated shear forces account for the higher frequency of lesions at the isthmus level (transition zone between the pancreatic head, which is fixed, and the pancreatic body, which is more mobile) (Arvieux and Letoublon 2005).

Pancreatic injury is more common in young people, possibly due to less retroperitoneal fat, which acts as a protective buffer.

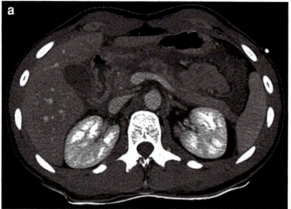 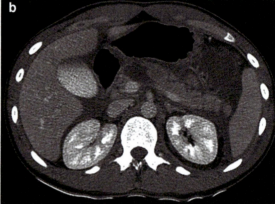

Fig. 12 Pancreas fracture with interruption of the main pancreatic duct. The axial slice (**a**) shows a linear parenchymal continuity solution located at the level of the pancreatic neck, with a transverse length more than 50% of the transverse pancreatic diameter. On the control CT scan performed 2 days later (**b**), there is clearly a complete interruption of the pancreas at the level of the pancreatic neck

5.1 CT Findings

The main CT findings include lack of pancreatic enhancement, particularly of the body, which is the most common site of injury, and other peripancreatic anomalies, which may be classified into direct and indirect signs (Linsenmaier et al. 2008).

The CT scan is primarily aimed at detecting main pancreatic duct injury, which constitutes a therapeutic emergency (surgical or endoscopic retrograde cholangiopancreatography). Other key CT findings allow the physician to quantify the degree of parenchymal necrosis and appreciate the integrity of the pancreatic papillae.

5.1.1 Direct Signs

5.1.1.1 Laceration/Pancreatic Rupture

Pancreatic laceration is revealed by a hypodense, linear, parenchymal continuity solution. If its length is more than 50% of the transverse pancreatic diameter, main pancreatic duct injury should be considered.

The lesion is referred to as pancreatic disruption when it transverses the pancreas, most commonly at the isthmus level. Its width appears to be a predictor of the likelihood of main pancreatic duct injury (Fig. 12). Multiplanar reconstructions and fine-slice CT facilitate the diagnosis. Multiple fractures may be observed, particularly at the pancreatic head, resulting in a burst fracture. The patient must be systematically examined for associated lesions of other organs, especially injury of the duodenum (very common), liver, gallbladder, choledochus, right kidney, and ascending colon.

5.1.1.2 Contusions/Hematomas

These lesions are characterized by a parenchymal hypodense area, resulting in a focal or global enlargement of the gland, presenting irregular contours. Hematoma injury must be differentiated from contusion injury on the basis of its spontaneously hyperdense aspect in association with the lack of enhancement.

5.1.2 Indirect Signs

These anomalies are frequently observed in the early stages, including:
- Edema with global pancreatic enlargement and loss of lobulation
- Peripancreatic fat infiltration
- Peripancreatic fluid, especially if it is located around the superior mesenteric artery or the omental bursa
- Hematic fluid between the dorsal face of the pancreas and the splenic vein
- Thickening of the left anterior pararenal fascia or fluid in the anterior pararenal space
- Concomitant duodenal injury (intramural hematoma or complete/incomplete perforation), which requires examination for injury to the pancreatic head.

Fig. 13 Pancreas contusion. The axial slice (**a**) shows a hypodense area in the proximal pancreatic body, located within its inferior part (*arrow*) as shown on the coronal reformatting (**b**). Control CT (not presented) showed a restitution *ad integrum* of the pancreas

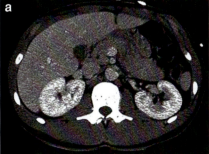
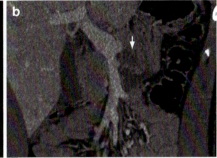

5.2 CT Pitfalls

There are no differential diagnoses, with the exception of hemorrhagic pancreatic tumors, which may mimic hematomas.

At the initial phase, diagnostic difficulties are essentially linked to associated lesions, which may interfere with or prevent an optimal parenchymal analysis because of significant fluid collections, movement artifacts, etc. Thus, a CT scan is likely to underestimate injury during the first 24 h, with the findings from 40% of all scans being normal. In cases of typical mechanism (accident history involving direct shock) or suspect associated lesions (duodenal or left hepatic lobe injury), physicians must examine patients for signs of minor pancreatic injury, and in their absence, the CT scan should be repeated, preferably with acquisition times relevant to the pancreatic paranchyma (45 s following injection), using fine millimeter slices.

Coronal reformatting may be helpful to investigate if contusion is located on the inferior or superior faces of the pancreas, making interruption of the main pancreatic duct unlikely (Fig. 13).

5.3 Impact on Management

Treatment largely depends on main pancreatic duct injury as well as associated organ injury, especially of the duodenum (Duchesne et al. 2008).

Laboratory analyses, including analysis of pancreatic enzyme levels such as amylase and lipase levels, are not very informative in the case of pancreatic injury. In fact, increased levels of pancreatic enzymes are only observed in half of pancreatic injury cases, with no correlation to the severity of the injury. As a result, increased pancreatic enzyme levels are

Table 11 Complications of conservative treatment in pancreatic trauma

Immediate complications	Delayed complications
Fistula	Ductal stenosis
Acute pancreatitis	Pseudocyst
Abscess/collection	Chronic pancreatitis

not predictive of main pancreatic duct injury, which dictates the therapeutic strategy.

In the case of diagnostic uncertainty as to main pancreatic duct injury, one of the following investigations should be performed:

- Magnetic resonance cholangiopancreatography, a noninvasive procedure aimed at examining the morphology and integrity of pancreatic and bile ducts using T2-weighted MRI. The accuracy of this procedure may be improved using intravenous secretin injection, which stimulates pancreatic fluid secretion, thereby allowing better pancreatic duct visualization.
- Endoscopic retrograde cholangiopancreatography, an invasive procedure, which is carried out under sedation. This technique allows the physician to confirm with certainty the diagnosis of pancreatic duct injury and to perform simultaneously a therapeutic procedure (pancreatic prosthesis) as necessary.

In the absence of pancreatic duct involvement, injury to the pancreas is simply monitored within a surgical environment using evolutive CT, allowing early detection of secondary complications, which are very common (Table 11).

If Wirsung injury is probable or certain, its treatment depends on the location of the pancreatic injury and may include endoprothesis, internal or external derivation, explorative laparotomy with resection of the injury (caudal splenopancreatectomy), or drainage. Pancreaticoduodenectomy should be restricted to very severe cases. The main postoperative risk is fistula

Table 12 Sites most often involved in the bowel injury	Small bowel	Ileocolic junction and Treitz angle
	Duodenum	Second and third segments by direct compression, common in children, and often associated with pancreatic lesion
		The perforation, if present, may be in the peritoneum or in the retroperitoneum
	Mesentery	Laceration/disinsertion with risk of ischemia
	Colon	Transverse > cecum > sigmoid
		Ascending and descending colon when there is avulsion of mesocolons
	Stomach	Rare and rarely isolated, generally involves lesser curvature

formation, which may lead to peritonitis and secondary sepsis. In the case of Wirsung rupture, a nonsurgical option can only be envisaged in a well-controlled clinical situation, with close daily monitoring.

6 Intestinal and Mesenteric Traumas

Bowel or mesentery injury occurs in 5% of patients with abdominal blunt trauma, but it is much more common following open trauma, especially in injuries caused by firearms. The diagnosis is often delayed, which markedly increases the mortality rate.

Following blunt traumas, injury is caused by two mechanisms:
1. Direct abdominal compression resulting in
   – Crushing of intestinal loops and mesentery against the spine, responsible for hematoma and parietal bowel contusion, usually located on the mesentery side, and responsible for mesentery contusion
   – Rapid increase in intraluminal pressure, similar to the blowout phenomenon, responsible for digestive perforations, occurring mainly along the antimesenteric border
2. Deceleration with shearing forces at points of fixations such as the ileocecal valve or duodenojejunal angle (Treitz angle), which causes stretching and tearing of the intestine and vessels

6.1 CT Findings

The main CT findings may be classified according to location into intestinal or peritoneomesenteric lesions, although though these lesions are often associated (Romano et al. 2006; Brofman et al. 2006; Ekeh et al. 2008).

Four CT findings should alert the radiologist:
1. Focal fat infiltration
2. Interloop hematoma (sentinel clot sign)
3. Bowel wall thickening
4. Free intraperitoneal air

The diagnosis is based on a precise CT analysis of the intestinal loops (parietal thickness, enhancement, diameter, content, etc.), mesentery, and vascular bundles (artery and vein permeability, escape of contrast medium, etc.).

The lesions are predominantly found in the duodenum and small bowel, whereas the other bowel segments are less frequently involved (Table 12).

If there is a strong suspicion of intestinal lesion on initial examination (focal bowel wall thickening, mesenteric infiltration, or focal and localized fluid collection), two strategies are possible:
1. Follow-up CT in 8–12 h to monitor any mesenteric anomaly or evolutive bowel injury
2. Immediate explorative laparoscopy depending on the clinical presumption and the surgeon's habits

6.1.1 Intestinal Lesions

6.1.1.1 Digestive Perforation

The direct CT sign is a transparietal continuity solution (Fig. 14), which may be either longitudinal or transverse, mainly located on the mesenteric side of the bowel. The perforation may occur intraperitoneally or retroperitoneally if there is involvement of retroperitoneal segments such as the ascending or descending colon, duodenum (Fig. 14), or rectum, leading to a pneumoperitoneum or retroperitoneum, respectively. Free intraperitoneal or retroperitoneal air may be missing if the perforation is small or is blocked and overall early after the trauma, making CT control necessary if there doubts regarding clinical or CT findings (Fig. 15). Other indirect signs (Table 13)

Abdominal Trauma

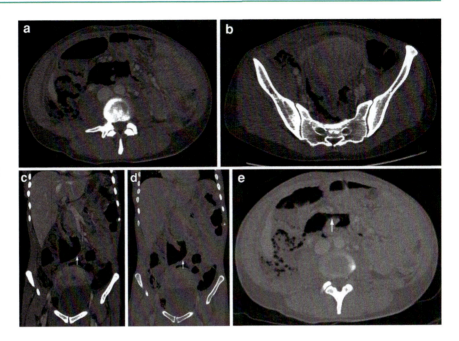

Fig. 14 Perforation of the third duodenual segment with retropneumoperitoneum. Axial slices at the abdominal (**a**) and pelvic (**b**) levels show extraluminal air within the retroperitonal and the subperitoneal spaces. The hole within the duodenum was large (*arrow*) and is clearly seen on the coronal reconstruction (**c**) as well as in coronal (**d**) and axial (**e**) views in the lung window

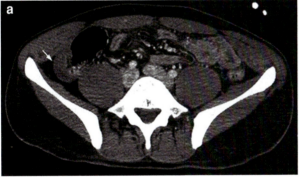
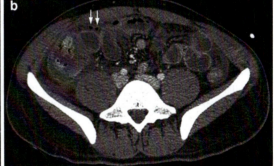

Fig. 15 Colic perforation undiagnosed on the initial CT. The initial CT scan (**a**) shows only a tiny collection (*arrow*) outside the colon, whereas on a control CT scan performed 12 h later because of worsening of the clinical condition of the patient (**b**) there are clearly findings of perforation with increase of the collection and overall extraluminal intraperitoneal air bubbles (*arrows*)

Table 13 Indirect findings of traumatic bowel perforation

Peritoneal findings	Digestive findings
Sentinel clot	Pneumoperitoneal bubbles localized within the mesentery
Focal mesenteric infiltration	Focal wall thickening

may support the diagnosis. The CT scan must determine the exact location of the perforation using multiplanar reconstructions to help the surgeon to select the best approach.

6.1.1.2 Contusion/Digestive Hematoma

The evolution of such injury is usually benign. On CT, an intramural hematoma appears as focal bowel wall thickening of greater than 3 mm for the small bowel, and 5 mm for the colon, located on a dilated or abnormally thickened intestinal loop, in relation to its normal features or to the adjacent intestinal loops. However, this wall thickening is not 100% specific to bowel injury (Table 14).

Contusion usually occurs on the subserosal side, with a trend toward spontaneous regression at variable delays ranging from a few weeks to a few months.

Table 14 Causes of bowel thickening related to trauma

Contusion/hematoma

Perforation

Distal ischemia due to mesenteric lesion

Bowel shock

Secondary to peritonitis

Bowel spasm

On CT, intramural hematoma appears as a spontaneously hyperdense area, on the mesenteric side of the bowel, which may be eccentric or concentric in appearance. If it is large, immediate or delayed mechanical obstruction may occur; rupture is also possible, due to the loss of necrotic tissue.

In children, duodenal hematoma may result from nonaccidental injury by direct epigastric injury, which must be considered in cases where accidental injury is uncertain or unlikely, more so if it is associated with inferior rib fractures (Strouse et al. 1999).

Blood content within the intestinal loops, which appears on slices from noninjected series as hyperdense intraluminal areas, may result from bowel wall injury regardless of its location.

6.1.1.3 Digestive Ischemia

Bowel ischemia is mostly segmental owing to distal branch vessel injury, but diffuse thickening of small bowel wall may also be observed in the case of hypotensive shock bowel indicating acute digestive dysfunction.

Typical CT signs include:

- Lack of parietal enhancement, which is the most specific sign, with late acquisitions required to confirm the enhancement abnormalities.
- Thickening of bowel wall in the case of venous ischemia or, on the contrary, thinning of the bowel wall in the case of arterial ischemia.
- Parietal pneumatosis with presence of air inside the bowel wall, which may at times be associated with air in the mesentery and portal venous system. This portal pneumatosis is not specific to digestive ischemia, as it may also be caused by parietal laceration, resulting in air dissection of the bowel wall. Furthermore, the presence of air in the portal venous system may be observed in the absence of digestive ischemia, as, for instance, in abdominal blunt trauma with increased intraluminal gastric pressure and laceration of the gastric mucosa; as a

result, air diffuses into the submucosa, then the gastric veins, and finally, the portal veins, leading to the presence of air in the portal system.

6.1.1.4 Reflex Ileus

Reflex ileus is common in trauma patients. It appears as a diffuse distention of the intestinal loops with air–fluid levels, without any transitional zone, with a trend toward spontaneous regression within a few days. Mechanical obstruction may be observed, due to a large hematoma or bowel herniation at the pelvic fracture site. This, however, is very rare, and the diagnostic strategy based on CT does not differ from that undertaken in nontraumatic mechanical occlusions.

6.1.1.5 Shock Bowel

Shock bowel is caused by hypotension resulting in systemic hypoperfusion. On CT, shock bowel appears as a diffuse thickening of the small bowel wall, along with intense enhancement because of the diffusion of the contrast medium into the interstitial sector caused by the increased vascular permeability, in association with low cardiac output. The intraluminal bowel content is usually liquid, and the colon is often normal. In this case, other CT findings associated with shock must be considered. All these signs rapidly disappear when appropriate treatment is initiated, with restoration of adequate blood volume.

6.1.2 Peritoneal Mesenteric Lesions

6.1.2.1 Air and Fluid Effusion

As a reminder, the presence of free air in the peritoneal cavity is a very specific but poorly sensitive sign, as it is missing in more than half of patients with digestive perforation. If focal, it has a good location value, with air bubbles embedded within the mesentery (Blayac et al. 2002).

The presence of air in the anterior pararenal space orients the diagnosis toward duodenal perforation; colic (with perforation of adjacent segments) or rectal perforation should be suspected when the air is in the posterior pararenal space.

An intraperitoneal air-fluid level is the most sensitive and specific sign that is indicative of digestive injury, but has no location value if it is diffuse. However, this air-fluid level has a location value if it is of small size and located between the intestinal loops, without any concomitant lesion of intra-abdominal solid organs. This diagnostic assumption is reinforced by the presence of a sentinel clot.

In the presence of a retroperitoneal, periduodenal air-fluid level, a traumatic lesion of the duodenum must be considered.

6.1.2.2 Mesenteric Edema

Mesenteric edema typically appears as increased fat density of the mesentery, which appears misty and infiltrated. This feature is caused by direct traumatic phenomena or indirect reactions, and had a good location value only if it is focal. It may be very subtle, but even in this case it keeps the same location value if it is focal (Fig. 3b).

It is the consequence of one of the following phenomena:

- Digestive injury: The radiologist must look for a thickening of the adjacent intestinal loops or bowel perforation.
- Vascular mesenteric injury: In this case, an active bleeding site or vascular thrombosis, with risk of intestinal devascularization downstream of the occluded vessel, must be considered.
- Mesenteric ecchymosis: Rarely isolated in clinical practice, this lesion necessitates urgent surgical exploration for occult perforation if there is the slightest clinical doubt.

6.1.2.3 Mesenteric Hematoma

This typically appears as a hyperdensity, with rather clear delineation, located between the intestinal loops, and is often referred to as the sentinel clot sign. It is situated within the mesentery, between the omentum and meso, usually in close contact with an injured intestinal loop or a vascular wound.

Should this be the case, the radiologist must examine the patient for vascular mesenteric escape of contrast medium, in addition to other potential signs of digestive injury (particularly significant parietal enhancement). In the case of distal branch vessel injury, a bowel ischemia syndrome may develop over several days, after which the abundant collateral vessel network usually comes into play. The arterial perforation may be incomplete, with bleeding contained by a normal adventitia, resulting in a mesenteric pseudoaneurysm. This situation, however, is rather exceptional.

The CT scan must clarify whether the active bleeding is of arterial or venous origin (Fig. 16),

which has a major impact on therapeutic management, as arterial bleeding is an indication for surgical intervention or embolization, whereas only close clinical surveillance is necessary for the other types of bleeding. In the worst-case scenario, a total disinsertion of the vascular pedicle of the mesentery or mesentery root is observed, necessitating emergency surgical hemostasis.

A hematoma of the greater omentum has no impact on the vitality of the intestinal loops.

6.1.3 Injury Occurring in Children

A seat belt syndrome has been described for children, and corresponds to an injury typically encountered in children wearing a seat belt and sitting in the middle of the rear seat of the car. This syndrome comprises periumbilical ecchymoses, vertebral column injury called a Chance fracture, and abdominal pelvic visceral organ and pelvic injuries. If the anamnesis is evocative, these lesions must be considered and looked for.

6.2 CT Pitfalls

Circumferential thickening of the bowel wall may be the consequences of several causes, such as a hematoma, a bowel perforation (Fig. 17), and an ischemia secondary to a mesenteric bleeding or when this is diffuse, it may be due to a shock bowel or a reaction to peritonitis.

The most critical diagnostic difficulty is related to the detection of extradigestive air bubbles, which necessitates careful reading and analysis as to their precise topography (intraperitoneal, retroperitoneal, or subperitoneal), with each location suggesting a different site of perforation. It must be known that extraluminal air may not be identified on the first CT scan, making a control CT scan necessary as soon as the clinical condition of the patient changes or in the case of unexplained peritoneal effusion.

In the same way, for the diagnosis of mesenteric bleeding, mesenteric fluid may be very subtle on the first CT scan and the active bleeding may be revealed on a control scan (Fig. 18).

Mesenteric calcifications, mostly related to sequelar lymph nodes, must not be confused with contrast medium extravasation. Yet, in CT acquisition without contrast medium injection, the high calcium density of more than 200 HU and the absence of

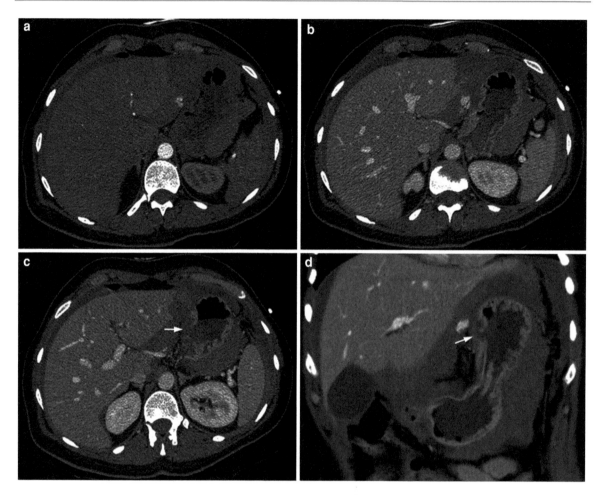

Fig. 16 Gastric injury of the lesser curvature with active bleeding and perforation. Axial slices in the arterial phase (**a**) and in the portal phase (**b**) show arterial active bleeding within the lesser omentum. At a different level, on the axial slice (**c**) as well as on the coronal reformatting (**d**), a bowel wall discontinuity (*arrow*) is seen in the lesser curvature characteristic of a perforation

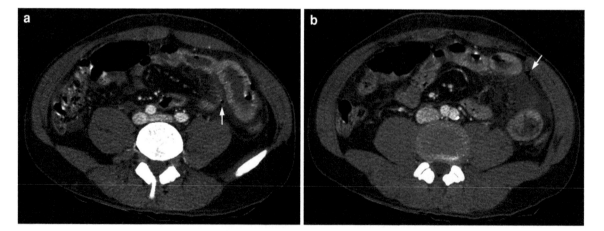

Fig. 17 Traumatic jejunal perforation responsible for jejunal wall thickening. Circumferential thickening of the jejunal loops is well seen on the lower slice (**a**), whereas localized mesenteric fluid is seen on the upper slice (**b**). Note the presence of extraluminal intraperitoneal air bubbles (*arrow*), meaning a perforation in this context of blunt trauma

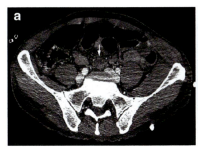 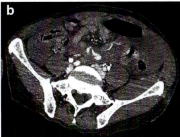 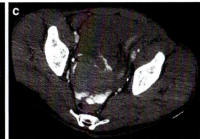

Fig. 18 Bleeding in the mesentery (same patient as in Fig. 3). On the initial CT scan (**a**), there was only some subtle fluid within the root mesentery (*arrow*). On a control CT scan performed because of worsening of the status of patient with findings of shock, CT shows active bleeding with extravasation of contrast medium within the mesentery (**b**) and diffusion of the contrast medium in the peritoneal cavity within the Douglas pouch (**c**)

lesion modifications over time should help correct the diagnosis in favor of sequelae.

Although mesenteric panniculitis may mimic mesenteric root hematoma, this condition may be differentiated from traumatic injury by its regular contours and by the presence of multiple lymph nodes surrounded by hypodense fat depositions.

6.3 Impact on Management

In the absence of treatment, the mortality and morbidity rates of these lesions are high because of the risk of peritonitis, abscess, sepsis, and mesenteric necrosis.

The therapeutic choice is based on the answer to three questions (Atri et al. 2008):
1. Is there evidence of bowel perforation?
2. Is there evidence of digestive dysfunction?
3. Is there evidence of active mesenteric bleeding? If so, is it arterial or venous?

In the presence of an obvious bowel perforation or signs indicative of bowel ischemia, urgent surgical treatment is required. Digestive wounds are sutured, and necrotic bowel segments are removed, with continuity reestablishment of the intestine using direct intestinal anastomosis.

In the case of distal venous vascular injury without signs of bowel ischemia, most patients are currently managed conservatively, with careful surveillance in a surgical ward. Arterial lesions are treated depending on their location and number, the patient's hemodynamic status, and any concomitant lesions. Treatment is mostly surgical, and usually consists of vascular ligature, and much less frequently embolization (Asayama et al. 2005), the latter being performed in the case of a pseudoaneurysm.

Hematomas and parietal contusions generally require conservative treatment, consisting of simple lesion surveillance, as spontaneous regression usually occurs within a few weeks. Mechanical bowel obstruction due to intramural hematoma or contusion is currently managed conservatively, patients being treated by fasting, nasogastric catheter insertion, and management of concomitant injuries.

For open traumas, the treatment is chiefly surgical, with explorative laparotomy performed in most patients with firearm injuries. For cold weapon injuries, therapeutic decisions largely depend on CT findings with respect to the depth of the injuring agent and injury screening.

7 Renal and Urinary Tract Trauma

Renal injury is common in trauma patients, with an incidence of approximately 10% in significant blunt abdominal injury, and 90% in minor blunt abdominal injury. The lesion mechanisms involved in renal and urinary tract injury are as follows:
- Direct impact by compression, with the right kidney being more vulnerable because of its low location, and therefore being relatively unprotected by the thoracic cage
- More rarely, deceleration of shearing forces passed to the renal pedicle, with the left kidney being more exposed in this particular case

In contrast to urinary tract lesions, renal lesions are less common in open abdominal traumas. The presence of a preexisting anomaly, such as horseshoe

Table 15 Renal criteria for performing CT in abdominal trauma

Macroscopic hematuria

Microscopic hematuria with shock

Important renal ecchymosis or fracture of the lumbar transverse process

Open trauma involving the retroperitoneum

Mechanism of deceleration (risk of pedicle injury)

In children all types of posttraumatic hematuria

Table 16 Anatomic lesions encountered in renal trauma

Parenchymatous lesions	Contusion
	Hematoma
	Laceration/fracture
Perirenal lesions	Subcapsular hematoma
	Perirenal hematoma
	Urinoma/urohematoma
	Hemoretroperitoneum
Urinary tract lesions	Caliceal rupture (often due to renal fracture)
	Avulsion of the pyeloureteral junction
Vascular lesions	Arterial: pedicle or segmental injury/dissection or rupture (contained or not contained bleeding)
	Venous pedicle: thrombosis or avulsion

kidney, junction syndrome, renal polykystosis, or renal tumor, increases the risk of developing traumatic injury.

It should be noted that in the case of isolated microscopic hematuria, associated with normal blood pressure, CT imaging does not seem justified, as this procedure is associated with a minimal risk of renal injury. The presence and severity of hematuria do not appear to correlate with the significance of renal injury. The indications for renal imaging are provided in Table 15.

7.1 CT Findings

The typical finding consists of a focal or diffuse enhancement of the kidney and/or urinary tract. The different types of lesion found on routine CT and described in this chapter are summarized in Table 16 (Uriot et al. 2005). In the case of renal/urinary tract injury, the radiologist must systematically look for concomitant injuries to adjacent organs, such as liver and adrenal gland injuries on the right side, and fractures of the lower ribs and lumbar vertebral apophyses on the left side (Harris et al. 2001; Lee et al. 2007; Kawashima et al. 2001).

7.1.1 Parenchymal Lesions

7.1.1.1 Contusion

Contusion appears as a hypodense, ill-defined, poorly enhanced region within the renal parenchyma, showing slight enhancement (less than the adjacent parenchyma), which allows one to differentiate this lesion from a segmental renal infarct, which does not show any enhancement. The lesion may be focal or diffuse; in the latter case, it exhibits the feature of a delayed nephrogram (diffuse renal striation as found

in the case of acute pyeloneophritis), which is indicative of interstitial edema and rupture of renal collecting tubules, responsible for urinary (and contrast medium) extravasation into the interstitial space, which may persist for days following the injury.

7.1.1.2 Hematoma

CT typically shows a round or ovular lesion, often small in size, with regular contours, which is spontaneously hyperdense in relation to the surrounding parenchyma, then becomes hypodense on the series following injection. In the absence of noninjection images, which allow its detection, a hematoma may mimic contusion injury or remain undetected if it is small and hidden within the parenchymal enhancement.

7.1.1.3 Laceration

CT findings consist of hypodense, irregularly linear areas, typically distributed along the vessels and filled with blood. They are best analyzed at arterial times. A perirenal hematoma is often associated. The radiologist must define the exact superficial (less than 1 cm from the renal cortex) or deep (more than 1 cm from the renal cortex) location of these lesions, and also determine whether the renal medulla and the collecting tubule system are involved.

If the laceration crosses the kidney, it is referred to as kidney fracture (Fig. 2). The ultimate stage is a fracture-shattering of the kidney, caused by multiple lacerations of the renal parenchyma and the urinary tract, resulting in several more or less vascularized renal fragments, associated with a urohematoma.

7.1.2 Perirenal Lesions

7.1.2.1 Subcapsular Hematoma

A subcapsular hematoma appears as an crescent-shaped, spontaneous hyperdensity, located in the periphery of the kidney, which becomes hypodense on the slices after injection. If the hematoma is large enough, it may exert a mass effect on the adjacent parenchyma, the hematoma becoming biconvex and resulting in a delay in the secretory and excretory phases due to venous compression. It may be difficult to differentiate it from a perirenal, extracapsular hematoma, limited by a renorenal bridging septum, which may give the same appearance but without exerting any compression on the renal parenchyma. A subcapsular hematoma may diffuse into the perirenal space, and then by contiguity into the other retroperitoneal spaces in the case of capsule rupture.

7.1.2.2 Perirenal Hematoma

The typical CT finding is a perirenal hypertense collection, which pushes the kidney back, but without causing any deformation. If the hematoma is large, it may leave a mark on the psoas muscle. It may diffuse into the anterior and posterior pararenal spaces and push the intestinal loops back. This is indicative of a more serious renal injury associated with a urohematoma, with concomitant renal and adrenal gland lesions.

7.1.2.3 Urinoma/Urohematoma

A urohematoma is defined as a lesion associating a urinoma and a perirenal hematoma, which develops in the presence of a more or less significant breach of the collecting tube system, with urine escape reflected by extravasation of contrast medium (eliminated by the kidney) on delayed imaging, in an extrarenal location. In this case, it is essential to obtain delayed CT acquisition (10–15 min), mobilize the patient (prone position) to detect the escape, and determine the precise extent and location of the urinoma (subcapsular, limited to the perirenal fascia, or extravasation beyond the fascia).

7.1.2.4 Hemoretroperitoneum

The natural progression of this lesion is toward spontaneous tamponade.

7.1.3 Vascular Lesions

7.1.3.1 Segmental Infarct

This lesion is defined as an area of arterial hypoperfusion due to dissection or thrombosis. On CT, it appears as a triangular parenchymal area, with a widest part at the cortex, which is not enhanced during the different phases, with clear delineation, contrarily to contusions. The lesion is segmental within a well-defined arterial territory (subsegmental/segmental/lobar).

7.1.3.2 Arterial Pedicle Injury

Arterial pedicle injury has been reported to occur more frequently on the left, involving the proximal third of the artery.

Dissection. This is due to a deceleration phenomenon with intimal laceration, which forms a flap protruding into the vessel lumen and leading to platelet aggregation, resulting in an obstructing thrombus of differing degrees (small-caliber renal artery) or extensive dissection. On the CT scan, dissection appears as a regular stenosis of variable length, with differing degrees of obstruction.

- In the case of a stenosing dissection, asymmetrical findings in secretion and parenchymography are observed.
- In the case of an occlusive lesion, the kidney is "dumb", with absence of enhancement (Fig. 19), which may be complete or partial according to the presence of a polar artery (Fig. 20). Renal arterial opacification stops abruptly, and there is retrograde opacification of the renal vein from the inferior vena cava (this sign is only observed on the right side, as on the left, the renal vein receives venous blood supply from the gonadic and adrenal gland veins, ensuring its opacification). Even if there is no renal enhancement on the first CT scan, some viable parenchyma may be seen on the control scan.

The classic "cortical rim sign", which corresponds to the opacification of the cortex corticis via the intermediary of the capsular arteries originating from the adrenal and inferior diaphragmatic branches, is often absent during the acute phase, owing to the systemic hypoperfusion and the delay in the implementation of the blood supply network. In most cases, no perirenal hematoma is observed.

Rupture. This injury is defined as a transparietal rupture caused by shearing forces. Rupture may be

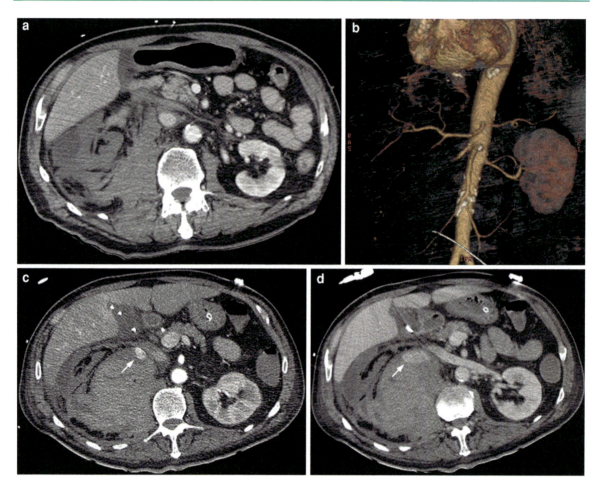

Fig. 19 Dissection of the right renal artery with delayed rupture responsible for hemoretroperitoneum. On the initial CT scan (**a**), there is a hemoretroperitoneum and a lack of enhancement of the right kidney, and with an obstruction of the right renal artery well seen on the 3D volume rendering (**b**). On a control CT scan performed because of clinical findings of shock, there is extravasation of contrast medium (*arrow*) (**c**), which spreads out in a more delayed phase (**d**), with an increase of the hemoretroperitoneum symptomatic of a rupture of the renal artery

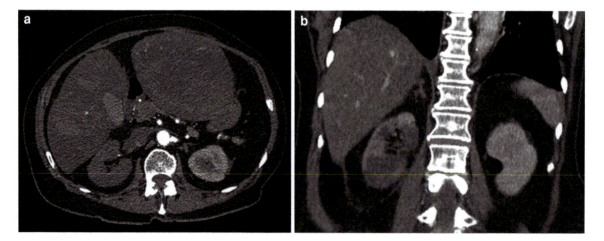

Fig. 20 Dissection of the right artery. The axial slice (**a**) shows a lack of enhancement of the right kidney, meaning there is an obstruction of the renal artery, whereas on the coronal reformatting (**b**) the upper part of the kidney remains enhanced because of the patency of a polar artery

Abdominal Trauma

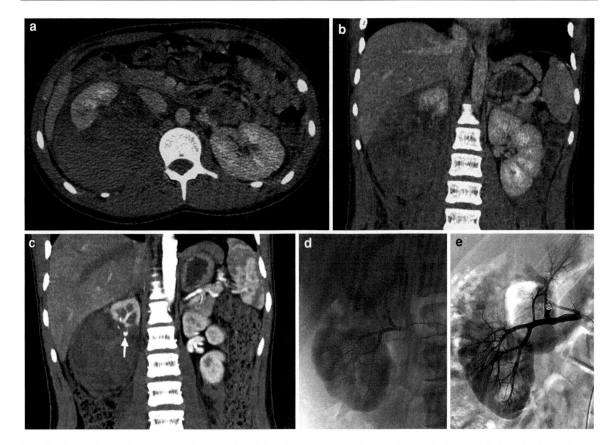

Fig. 21 Delayed pseudoaneurysm of a branch of the right renal artery. Axial (**a**) and coronal (**b**) slices in the portal phase show a hematoma in the renal fossa. On a control CT scan performed 1 week later, a pseudoaneurysm of a branch of the right renal artery is seen in the arterial phase (**c**) (*arrow*). This aneurysm was confirmed by angiography (**d**) and was embolized by coils (**e**)

complete and life-threatening in proximal artery rupture, with extravasation of contrast medium in the early phase and development of a hemoretroperitoneum, or may be better tolerated in traumatic branch renal artery injuries; it may also be contained and lead to a false aneurysm image, often seen secondary (Fig. 21). Rupture may complicate an arterial dissection and may be suspected if there are changes in the hemodynamic status of a patient with a known arterial dissection (Fig. 19).

In view of a potential therapeutic arteriography, it is essential to determine the precise location of the lesion and the supplying artery, as well as the vascular anatomical variations.

In this context, it should be noted that the absence of renal opacification may also be due to other causes, such renal pedicle avulsion, renal spasm following significant contusion, or vasoconstriction in relation to severe hypovolemic shock or major obstructive syndrome.

7.1.3.3 Vein Pedicle Injury

Traumatic injury of the renal vein is less frequent than that of the renal artery. The renal vein may be the seat of laceration, thrombosis, or rupture (exceptional). The CT findings are as follows:
- Incomplete or absent opacification of the renal vein
- Persistent nephrogram
- Reduction in excretion
- Nephromegaly

Concomitant perirenal hemorrhage is common. The prognosis is better in the case of left vein pedicle injury due to gonadic and adrenal venous blood supply than in the case of right vein pedicle injury.

7.1.4 Excretory Tract Injury

As previously mentioned, caliceal and pyelic lesions are associated with deep lacerations, resulting in the development of a perirenal urinoma, which may be detected on delayed CT images.

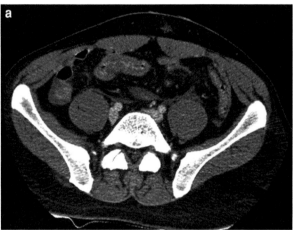 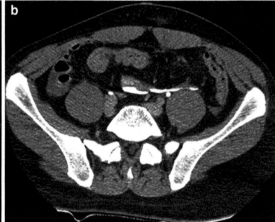

Fig. 22 Ureteral injury in an open trauma. The axial slice in the portal phase (**a**) shows fluid in the left retroperitoneum, immediately in front of the left psoas muscle. This effusion was opacified in a delayed phase (**b**) and consequently corresponded to urine. However the left ureter is still seen (*arrow*)

Ureteral injury is rare (less than 2% of urinary trauma cases), and is more frequently encountered in penetrating traumas, especially as iatrogenic postoperative complications. In the setting of abdominal blunt traumas, a distinction is made between lacerations that appear to be due to vertebral column hyperextension, resulting in a stretching of the urinary excretory system, and avulsions (shearing mechanism), which are predominantly seen at the pyeloureteral junction, and at times are associated with fracture of transversal apophyses of lumbar vertebra. Pyeloureteral junction lesions are usually secondary to pelvic fracture, resulting in the formation of a retroperitoneal urinoma, which rapidly increases in size over time, thereby lifting the bladder, without any evidence of bladder lesions.

Diagnosis is based on delayed or very delayed CT images (Fig. 22) (Uriot et al. 2005; Tezval et al. 2007).

In the case of pyeloureteral junction, a hematoma or urohematoma is observed on the medial side of the kidney or at the inferior kidney pole, with urine and thus contrast medium extravasation during the excretory phase. It is essential to obtain downstream opacification of the ureter (Fig. 22); in the absence of ureteral opacification or in the presence of signs of ureteral laceration, complete section must be suspected.

It should be noted that incomplete ureteral opacification may at times be observed in the absence of any traumatic injury, due to the presence of an obstructive clot. This clot leads to increased pressure upstream of the obstruction, which may facilitate extravasation of urine. Retrograde ureteroscopy allows confirmation of the diagnosis and elimination of ureteral laceration.

7.2 CT Pitfalls

The most common pitfall is the lack of diagnosis of excretory tract injury. It is avoided by obtaining delayed images in the case of renal traumatic injury to allow for complete urinary tract injury screening.

The identification of renal active bleeding is a key point. Active bleeding may spread in a most delayed phase (e.g., portal versus arterial phase) or may be contained in cases of pseudoaneurysm. In this latter case, pseudoaneurysm may be differentiated from scattered renal parenchyma because they have different kinetics of enhancement (Fig. 23).

As for all the other organs, motion or beam hardening artifacts may produce false images of laceration or subcapsular hematoma. A cortical notch (either physiological or sequelar) or preexisting lesions should not be mistaken for traumatic lesions.

7.3 Impact on Management

Most patients are currently treated nonoperatively, with clinical and biological surveillance (diuresis, arterial pressure, etc.) and bed rest. No control CT scan is required except in cases where new clinical or

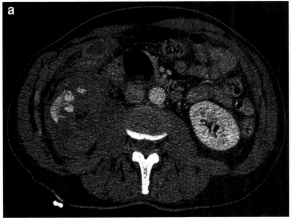 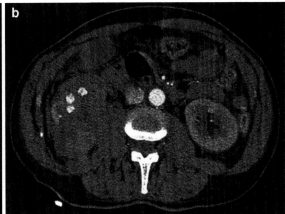

Fig. 23 Contained bleeding in the lower part of the right kidney. The three enhanced dots in the right kidney seen in the portal phase (**a**) have the same enhancement as right and left parenchyma and could correspond to fragments of renal parenchyma. However, in the arterial phase (**b**) their enhancement is greater than renal enhancement, meaning that they correspond to arterial bleeding

biological findings are observed. The evolution is usually favorable. In most cases, hematomas decrease in size and density (with at times persistence of peripheral parietal enhancement), and areas of contusion and laceration undergo fibrosis. Urinary or caliceal extravasations spontaneously stop in more than 80% of cases. For some patients, the possibility of urinary derivation by a JJ catheter or nephrostomy may be envisaged. Antibiotherapy may be proposed to prevent urinoma superinfection.

Emergency surgical treatment is reserved for patients with severe pyelic lesions (avulsion of the pyeloureteral junction), and those with active bleeding associated with hemodynamic instability (hemostatic nephrectomy). For patients with contained active arterial bleeding (pseudoaneurysm) and blood pressure stability, selective embolization via the femoral artery may be indicated (Fig. 21).

In "dumb kidneys" associated with dissection, revascularization techniques (either surgical or endovascular stenting) must be performed as soon as possible, within the first 4–6 h, as the loss of renal function begins 2 h after injury (hot ischemia of kidney). In clinical practice, these procedures are not often performed, as their results regarding renal function are still uncertain, and spontaneous renal revascularizations are possible. If more time has elapsed, and if renal injury is limited to one kidney, treatment usually consists of simple clinical surveillance.

Ureteral injuries are treated depending on the length and the severity of the lesions, with interventions ranging from simple ureteral stenting using a JJ catheter to surgical reparation (ureteroureterostomy, transposition of injured ureter on the contralateral ureter, etc.).

8 Adrenal Gland Injury

Adrenal injury is not a frequent complication of blunt abdominal trauma, as the adrenal glands are small, located at depth, and well protected by surroundings tissues and organs. Adrenal injury is caused by a violent mechanism, as shown in 25% of autopsy series.

The lesion mechanisms are still equivocal (Mehrazin et al. 2007):

- Direct compression shock with crushing of the adrenal gland between the liver and the spine, which accounts for the right adrenal gland being more frequently injured.
- Deceleration with laceration of the multiple small vessels crossing the adrenal capsule, accounting for the often voluminous hematomas.
- Rapid pressure increase in the venous system of the adrenal gland due to compression of the inferior vena cava, resulting in an intravascular blast phenomenon associated with rupture. The right adrenal gland, which lies closer to the inferior vena cava, appears to be more exposed to the wave of increased venous pressure propagating from the inferior vena cava to the blood sinusoids of the gland.

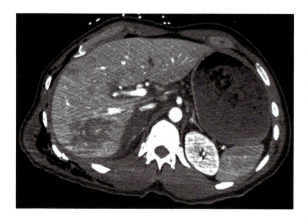

Fig. 24 Right adrenal gland injury associated with hepatic contusion

8.1 CT Findings

The right adrenal gland is more commonly injured than the left one (in approximately 75% of cases of adrenal injury) and is often associated with liver lesions (Sinelnikov et al. 2007; Pinto et al. 2006; Ikeda et al. 2007) (Fig. 24).

Commonly, CT signs of adrenal gland injury include morphological changes of the adrenal gland, along with anomalies of adrenal enhancement and periglandular fat. In patients with adrenal gland injury, there is a high correlation with injuries to adjacent solid viscera, such as the liver, kidney, and spleen, but also ipsilateral hemithorax, and these must be investigated further.

8.1.1 Periadrenal Abnormalities

CT findings typically include increased density of periadrenal fat (infiltrated aspect), hematic fluid collection in the periphery of the gland, or a real hematoma of the adrenal fossa. As the adrenal gland is located in the perirenal space, the fluid collection may extend around the kidney and, if it is abundant, to other retroperitoneal spaces. Active bleeding must be systematically examined for.

8.1.2 Adrenal Gland Abnormalities

In most cases, the CT appearance of the adrenal gland is enlarged by an intraglandular, round or ovular, spontaneously hyperdense (40–60 HU) hematoma, which is not enhanced and is usually voluminous (2–5 cm), owing to the complexity and abundance of the adrenal vascular network.

Some hematomas are small and associated with very moderate gland hypertrophy, reflecting ecchymosis or contusion. The worst-case scenario is that of an adrenal gland fracture, which can no longer be recognized, as it is hidden within a voluminous hematoma of the adrenal loggia.

8.2 CT Pitfalls

The main diagnostic difficulties are false-positive diagnoses:
- An injury to the diaphragmatic crus causes a hematoma which may be mistaken for an adrenal gland hematoma. Coronal and sagittal reconstructions may be useful to differentiate these two entities. For each CT investigation of abdominal trauma, adrenal glands need to be visualized so as to ensure their integrity.
- An isolated adrenal mass, without surrounding fat infiltration (incidentaloma), makes a purely traumatic origin rather unlikely. The detection of such a mass should lead to a CT control examination in order to differentiate a benign (adenoma) from a malignant tumor. An adrenal adenoma is usually small (less than 4 cm), hypodense (spontaneous density less than 10 HU), with homogenous enhancement, usually maintaining a stable size over time, whereas a hematoma is larger, spontaneously hyperdense, nonenhanced, while decreasing in size and density over time, which may at times be associated with the appearance of calcifications.
- The CT appearance of adrenal glands in patients in hypovolemic shock is characterized by intense contrast enhancement, decreasing following appropriate vascular filling, which should not be confused with traumatic lesions.

8.3 Impact on Management

With unilateral injury, there is no acute adrenal insufficiency.

Although adrenal gland injury usually reflects a violent mechanism, it is not "serious" per se, and its prognosis depends on the associated lesions, which are common. Patients with adrenal gland injury are treated conservatively, with strict clinical and biological surveillance (hemoglobin level, renal function,

Table 17 Mechanisms and pattern of bladder rupture

Type of rupture	Intraperitoneal	Extraperitoneal
Frequency	1/3	2/3
Mechanisms	Direct compression on a fluid-filled bladder: Increase on the vesical pressure with rupture	Pelvic fracture with bladder lesion due to a bone fragment Shearing of the junction points between the bladder and the pelvis (pubic disjunction ++)
Topography	Dome	Anterolateral ++ or anterior closed to the bladder neck
Treatment	Surgical	Conservative

Table 18 Anatomic lesions encountered in bladder trauma

Contusion
Laceration
Intraperitoneal, extraperitoneal, or combined rupture

electrolytes, etc.), in association with symptomatic treatment (analgesics, transfusion, etc.).

With bilateral injury, acute adrenal insufficiency may result, which must be detected early so as to promptly initiate hormone replacement therapy.

In the case of active arterial bleeding, embolization may be performed. The evolution is favorable, and CT findings typically regress over time. Hematoma superinfection may lead to posttraumatic sepsis. In the case of concomitant serious renal injury requiring nephrectomy, the injured adrenal gland is usually removed with the kidney.

9 Vesical Traumas

Bladder injury is associated in more than 75% of cases with pelvic fracture, although bladder injury is observed in only 5–10% of patients presenting with pelvic fracture depending on the type of fracture (Paparel et al. 2003).

The bladder is an extraperitoneal organ. When empty, the bladder forms a tertrahedron, with its posteroinferior base being fixed and triangular, referred to as trigone. It is made up of the interureteral bar, joining the two ureteral orifices, which represents the base of the triangle, and the vesical neck, representing its top. The other parts are mobile and extensible, with two anterolateral faces and the bladder dome. The latter is separated from the abdominal cavity by the peritoneum. When the bladder is full, it has a capacity of 300–400 ml, which may reach 1.5 l at maximum distention.

The bladder is more frequently injured in blunt traumas than in open traumas. The lesion mechanisms involved account for the two main types of bladder rupture (Table 17), which impact therapeutic management.

Some centers integrate CT cystography (Vaccaro and Brody 2000), in which the bladder is filled via the vesical catheter, into routine trauma imaging of patients with pelvic fractures in order to optimize the detection of bladder rupture at an early stage without increasing the duration of the examination, but avoiding the need for subsequent cystography (less irradiation).

9.1 CT Findings

It is necessary to clamp the urinary catheter for the CT examination.

The most common lesion is extraperitoneal bladder rupture observed in patients with pelvic fracture, showing urine and thus contrast medium extravasation on late CT images. However, other lesion types may be found on CT (Table 18). Pelvic fluid collection and thickening of pelvic fascias are ancillary signs.

9.1.1 Vesical Rupture

This injury is characterized by urinary fluid collection, which may be visualized on late imaging or on CT cystography by extravesical extravasation of contrast medium (Fig. 1). Depending on the precise location of the rupture, the escape of urine will be inside the peritoneum, outside the peritoneum, or

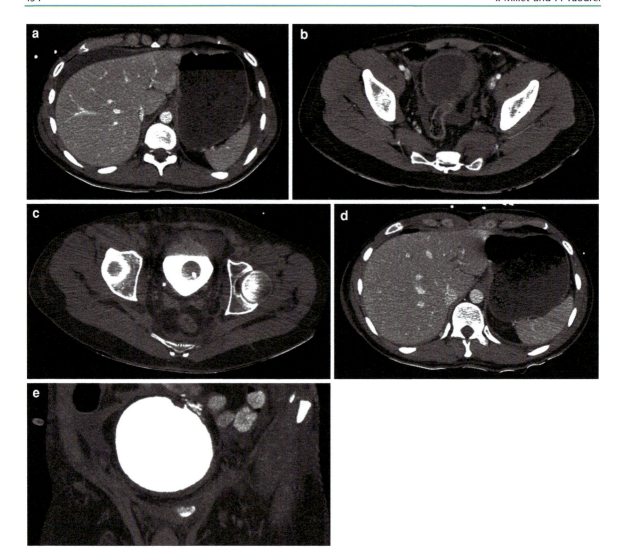

Fig. 25 Bladder perforation masked in the initial phase by a bladder hematoma. In the initial phase (**a–c**), axial slices show free peritoneal fluid (**a**) and a localized thickening of the left bladder wall (**b**) without rupture seen on a delayed phase image (**c**). One day later, there is a paradoxical appearance of a pneumoperitoneum with a decrease of the amount of the peritoneal fluid (**d**) which does not match the findings expected for a bowel injury. Coronal reformatting after CT cystography (**e**) revealed a bladder perforation

both. The exact location of pelvic fluid collection or urinary contrast medium orients the diagnosis toward one of the following hypotheses:
- Intraperitoneal rupture: In this case, there is intraperitoneal fluid collection of liquid density or that is slightly bloody, with extravasation of contrast medium at the level of the peritoneal recesses (Douglas pouch, parietocolic gutters, or between intestinal loops). The pelvic collections are separated from the bladder by a fatty border, corresponding to the perivesical and prevesical spaces (extraperitoneal).
 Intraperitoneal ruptures occur more often in children, owing to a higher frequency of bladder repletion and a more abdominal location of the bladder.
 Intraperitoneal rupture is a cause of pneumoperitoneum due to the passage of air from the vesical probe (Fig. 25).
- Extraperitoneal rupture: The fluid collection and extravesical contrast medium are localized in the

subperitoneal and preperitoneal spaces, thus in a perivesical (loss of the fatty perivesical border) and prevesical (Retzius space) location, resulting in a molar-tooth-shaped appearance. As these extraperitoneal spaces communicate with each other, fluid may diffuse to the anterior abdominal wall, along the thigh, the penis, or the scrotum if the urogenital diaphragm is ruptured; this fluid may even run across the orifices of the pelvis, namely, the obturator hole, and the sciatic notch. There is usually an important hematoma, due to the large perivesical venous plexus, which may compress the bladder and seal the breach, thus preventing its detection.
- Mixed rupture: This concerns approximately 10% of all ruptures and manifests itself intraperitoneal and extraperitoneal extravasation.

9.1.2 Vesical Contusion

Vesical contusion appears as a partial, incomplete tear of the vesical mucosa, manifesting itself as parietal edema and the presence of a blood clot. Generally, it is not visualized on CT images, but it may be suspected in the case of parietal focal wall thickening when the bladder is in repletion. Of note is that the thickness of the bladder wall cannot be evaluated in the case of an empty bladder cavity.

9.1.3 Interstitial Laceration

This is an intramural laceration, preserving the serosa, which may theoretically be visualized on CT as a strictly intramural extravasation of contrast medium. Yet, in practice, this observation is exceptional.

9.2 CT Pitfalls

A significant diagnostic difficulty is the differentiation between intraperitoneal from extraperitoneal rupture; however, a good understanding of the CT peritoneal radioanatomy along with a detailed analysis of fluid collection using multiplanar reconstructions may afford improved ability to differentiate between these injuries.

False-negative interpretation of bladder rupture may occur, with the bladder breach remaining undetected, in one of the following situations:

- Insufficient bladder filling after intravenous injection of contrast medium
- Presence of bladder spasm
- Presence of a breach sealed by perivesical hematoma (Fig. 25), peritoneal folds, or intestinal loops

In the case of a mural hematoma involving the bladder base and spreading under the pelvic floor, the differentiation between bladder injury and urethral injury may be difficult.

If there is a discrepancy between intraperitoneal air which appears or increases in volume and intraperitoneal fluid which decreases in volume, the possibility of a bladder perforation must be kept in mind.

9.3 Impact on Management

Mortality is mainly due to associated injuries, whereas morbidity is related to the risk of urinary incontinence and bladder instability.

Treatment is surgical (repair by suture) in the case of intraperitoneal bladder rupture in order to prevent the risk of urinary peritonitis. Other surgical indications include the presence of a bone splinter in the bladder fracture area, significant intravesical clotting, and associated injuries requiring surgery. In fact, in the case of complex pelvic fracture requiring internal surgical fixation, the presence of an associated intravesical injury, even if it is extraperitoneal in location, justifies surgical bladder reparation during the same operative intervention in order to prevent surgical materials becoming infected by urinary bacteria.

The treatment is conservative in the other types of injuries, and comprises mainly urine drainage via a suprapubic or intravesical catheter. In most cases, the breach dries up within approximately 10 days.

10 Urethral Injury

With the advent of multidetector CT using millimetric slices and image processing, the ensuing excellent spatial resolution allows a scanographic evaluation of urethral traumatic injuries. Yet, retrograde urthrography remains the reference examination and should be performed systematically to confirm urethral injury which was strongly suspected on the basis of CT findings, or to exclude such a lesion in the case of inconclusive CT signs.

The male urethra is divided into two segments. The posterior segment comprises the prostatic and membranous parts and is responsible for the vesicourethral sphincter function. The anterior segment is divided into the bulbar and penile parts.

The female urethra is relatively protected owing to is anatomical location, and therefore injury of it is exceptional (in association with vaginal lacerations).

In men, posterior urethral injuries are seen in approximately one patient in ten presenting with pelvic fracture. Urethral injury is due to a shearing mechanism, involving mainly the membranous part. For the most part, injury is due to fractures of the ischiopubic or iliopubic rami or is caused by pubic disjunction. Anterior urethral injuries are less common, and are mainly caused by a direct blow caused by falling astride. These injuries are not dealt with in this chapter, as their diagnosis is not based on CT imaging.

10.1 CT Findings

The elementary lesions are elongations, lacerations, and complete or partial urethral ruptures. CT scan findings can be divided into direct and indirect signs (Ali et al. 2003).

10.1.1 Direct Signs

The diagnosis is confirmed only in the case of extravasation of iodinated urinary contrast medium, subvesical in location, dissecting the genital fascias. An uplifting of the prostatic tissue of more than 2 cm above the urogenital diaphragm is considered by some authors to be a reliable sign indicative of puboprostatic ligament rupture.

10.1.2 Indirect Signs

Numerous indirect signs have been described, in decreasing degree of specificity, as follows:
- Infiltration or filling of the urogenital diaphragm with apical fat (highly specific)
- Hematoma of ischiocavernosus muscles (highly specific)
- Filling of preprostatic fat, loss of prostatic contours, or intraprostatic bleeding
- Hematoma of internal obturator muscle

10.2 Impact on Management

As an emergency procedure, simple urine drainage must be performed using a subpubic catheter. In a second step, retrograde urethrography must be carried out to allow precise injury screening to guide therapeutic management. Depending on the extent of injury, treatment will be conservative or surgical (immediate or delayed) so as to limit risks of subsequent fibrous cicatricial urethral stenosis, erectile dysfunction, and urinary incontinence.

11 Genital Organ Injury

A CT scan is not indicated for the exploration of genital organ injury.

In women, internal genital organ injury is exceptional, mainly occurring in the presence of preexisting lesions such as ovarian cysts. A CT scan allows the extent of pelvic hematoma to be determined and screening of associated lesions. Vaginal lacerations must be looked for in the case of any pelvic injury because of the risk of pelvic abscess.

In men, testicle injuries are investigated using echography to detect albugineous rupture, hematocele, scrotal hematoma, laceration, fragmentation, hematoma, or testicle infarction. Penile injury requires MRI or echography to confirm the integrity of the cavernous bodies, which guides the therapeutic strategy. The search for an associated urethral lesion requires retrograde urethrography if there is the slightest clinical doubt.

12 Abdominal Vessel Injury

Vascular injuries are a major source of morbidity and mortality in patients with blunt pelvic trauma. Sources of hemorrhage within the pelvis include injuries to major pelvic arterial and venous structures and vascular damage related to osseous fractures.

In contrast to pelvic vessels, injuries to the aorta or inferior vena cava are rare, and in more than 90% of cases are caused by penetrating traumas (firearms) or are of iatrogenic origin. The remaining cases are due to blunt traumas.

Large vessel trauma is a very serious injury, usually leading to death at the accident site. The very few patients reaching the intensive care unit are usually in

Abdominal Trauma

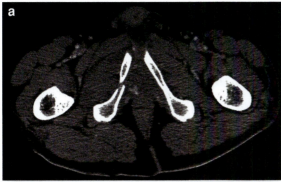

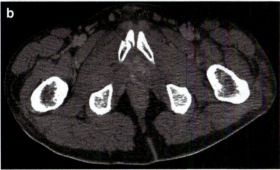

Fig. 26 Pelvic arterial bleeding. The axial slice in the arterial phase (**a**) shows bleeding which spreads out in the portal phase (**b**). Note also the contact between the bleeding and a fracture of the ischiopubic branch. The bleeding originates from the right pudendal artery

a critical state, with significant hypovolemic shock. In most cases, these patients are immediately sent for rescue laparotomy. Therefore, only very few lesions have been described using CT imaging.

12.1 Pelvic Vessels

Among patients with pelvic fractures, up to 20% require emergency transcatheter embolization, depending on the type of injury, and it is crucial to differentiate the different types. Arterial hemorrhage is one of the most serious problems associated with pelvic fractures, and it remains the leading cause of death attributable to pelvic fracture, with a mortality rate that is still high and more than 30% in patients who have hypotension attributable to pelvic fractures.

12.1.1 CT Findings

Pelvic CT angiography is useful in assessing vascular injuries. Arterial phase imaging provides optimal visualization of the arterial structures and, in combination with portal venous phase imaging, can help differentiate between arterial and venous hemorrhage.

12.1.1.1 Active Extravasation

Active arterial hemorrhage appears as extravascular regions of hyperattenuation; the attenuation is similar to or greater than that of the aorta on arterial phase images. Areas of active arterial extravasation should increase in size and have greater attenuation than the aorta on both portal venous and delayed phase images (Fig. 26). Moreover, the site of the fracture (Fig. 26) and the site of contrast medium extravasation can be an indicator of injury to a specific artery passing through the region of the pelvis where the extravasation is noted on CT scans with precise correlation between CT and angiographic extravasation (Fig. 27) (Yoon et al. 2004). The main sites of arterial bleeding are the iliolumbar, lateral sacral arteries dorsally, the obturator arteries ventrally, the superior and inferior gluteal arteries, and the internal pudendal arteries.

By contrast, foci of extravascular hyperattenuation that are identified only on portal venous phase images, without corresponding abnormalities on arterial phase images, likely represent areas of venous hemorrhage. Fracture-related hemorrhage appears similar to pelvic venous injuries.

A pseudoaneurysm must be differentiated from active extravasation. It occurs secondary to disruption of either the inner layers or the entire vessel wall, with blood contained by the adventitia or perivascular soft tissues. On portal venous and delayed phase images, arterial pseudoaneurysms have attenuation similar to that of the arterial structures and are stable in size. Pelvic arterial pseudoaneurysms may rupture and cause subsequent hemorrhage, or they may partially thrombose and cause distal emboli to form.

12.1.1.2 Arteriovenous Fistula

Arteriovenous fistula is exceptional in blunt trauma but is seldom seen in open trauma. It must be suspected in early and asymmetric enhancement of venous structures.

12.1.1.3 Arterial Obstruction

Occlusion may result from embolus or local injuries such as intimal disruption with subsequent thrombosis. Occlusion appears as an abrupt interruption in the flow of contrast-enhanced blood on pelvic CT

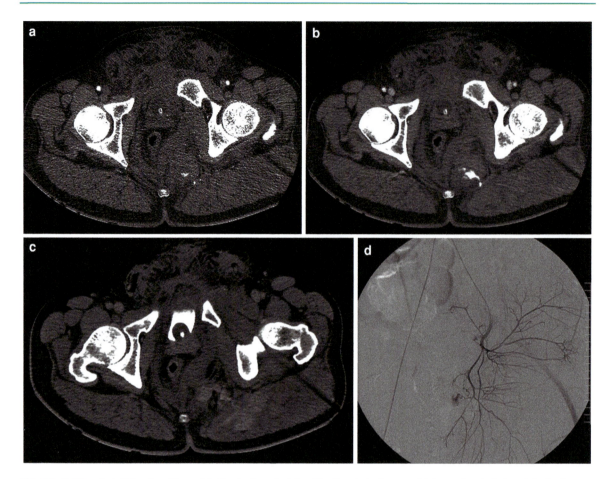

Fig. 27 Pelvic arterial bleeding. The axial slice in the arterial phase (**a**) shows bleeding which spreads out in the portal phase (**b**) and in a more delayed phase (**c**). The location of the bleeding is in favour of injury of an inferior gluteal artery, as confirmed by angiography (**d**)

angiographic images, whereas arterial dissection is characterized by direct depiction of the intimal flap, which is evidenced by a curvilinear filling defect within the lumen of the vessel. The main differential diagnosis of obstruction is spasm encountered in response to arterial injury.

12.1.2 CT Pitfalls

The most classic pitfall is the distinction between an active extravasation, a pseudoaneurysm, and a bone fragment. However, this is easily avoided since an area of active extravasation should increase in size with time, a small pseudoaneurysm should wash out, and a bone fragment should remain unchanged. The most tricky pitfall is the diagnosis of subtle arterial lesions with sometimes extravasation seen only in the portal phase, making impossible the diagnosis and the differentiation with venous injuries.

12.1.3 CT Impact

Although the treatment of a patient with a pelvic bleeding is chosen on a case-by-case basis depending on the clinical status, some key rules are given by CT results. Arterial bleeding is generally managed by endovascular embolization even if in some cases of injury of very small branch arteries and hemodynamically stable patients with no signs of significant blood loss, conservative management without embolization may be preferred. For managing venous hemorrhage, pelvic stabilization is usually successful (Kertesz et al. 2009).

12.2 Abdominal Aorta

Fewer than 100 cases of abdominal aorta injury have been reported in the scientific literature. Abdominal

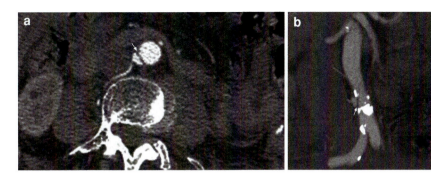

Fig. 28 Traumatic dissection of the aorta. The axial slice (**a**) as well as coronal reformatting (**b**) show well the intimal flap (*arrow*), diagnosing a limited dissection of the infrarenal aorta

aorta injury represents less than 5% of all aorta injuries.

These lesions are mainly caused by high-speed car accidents, with the passenger typically wearing a seat belt (two or three points). During a violent deceleration mechanism, the seat belt plays the role of a rotation center, around which the dorsolumbar spine bends. As a result, a direct compression of the aorta and viscera between the seat belt and the spine ensues, mostly facing L3 and the aortoiliac bifurcation, leading to digestive, vertebral (especially Chance fracture), and aortic lesions, the association of which is referred to as the seat belt syndrome. Indirect stretching and tearing forces also come into play.

The presence of atherosclerotic lesions is considered to be a predisposing factor of parietal wall fragility. The compressive object may be the steering wheel, seat belt, or any other object.

12.2.1 CT Findings

The CT findings are similar to those seen in the case of thoracic aorta injury. Lesions may include simple intimal laceration with intimal flap (Fig. 28), dissection with rather pronounced occlusive thrombosis, or partial transection with bleeding contained within a false aneurysm or presenting as massive hemoperitoneum (Choit et al. 2006).

The permeability and topography of the different visceral aortic branches must be defined to allow optimal therapeutic management.

12.2.2 Impact on Management

These injuries present a vital and functional prognostic value, with risk of peripheral embolism resulting in acute inferior limb injury, risk of paraplegia, anterior medullar ischemia (injury to the Adamkiewicz branch originating from an inferior intercostal artery or superior lumbar artery), or risk of peripheral nerve injury in the case of occlusive dissection (Meghoo et al. 2003) which may be reversible depending on the delay until effective reperfusion.

The treatment of aortic injury is either surgical with extra-anatomic bypass or endovascular with implementation of a covert stent, depending on the type of lesion, the experience of the surgical team, and the availability of technical equipment. The main long-term complications are the risks of developing aortocaval fistulas (Spencer et al. 2006).

12.3 Inferior Vena Cava

This injury is rare and often fatal, mostly due to a laceration phenomenon (deceleration mechanism), which preferentially occurs at bifurcation levels (atriocaval junction, hepaticocaval junction, renocaval junction, etc.) (Buckman et al. 2001).

Lesions mostly occur at the following levels in decreasing order of frequency: suprarenal part, then retrohepatic, infrarenal, and lastly, pararenal parts (2 cm above and below the renal veins).

12.3.1 CT Findings

Depending on the significance of the trauma, the CT findings include endothelial laceration along with spontaneous intraluminal hemostasis resulting in an endoluminal thrombus, or a rather complete wall rupture with parietal irregularities and extravasation of contrast medium, along with an extraluminal pericaval hematoma, in direct contact with the injured venous segment (Bersani et al. 1997). Of note is that bleeding is rapidly contained within the hematoma, thereby facilitating hemostasis via tamponade, which may lead to a pseudoaneurysm image. In light of these conditions, any surgical intervention may be dangerous with risk of massive hemorrhage and cardiac arrest, caused by sudden pressure increase within the hematoma.

The permeability of the afferent venous branches must be determined.

12.3.2 CT Pitfalls

Major diagnostic errors include flow artifacts (inhomogeneous vena cava opacification on early CT acquisitions) which may be mistaken for thrombi. CT diagnosis requires images to be obtained with several acquisition times, with ideally an acquisition in systemic venous time, obtained approximately 120 s after starting the injection (ideal time for confirming the presence of an endoluminal clot).

The other causes of retroperitoneal hematoma must be rejected prior to incriminating the inferior vena cava.

12.3.3 Impact on Management

The main risks include hemorrhagic shock and massive pulmonary embolism.

In the case of a simple thrombus, the treatment is medical and consists of efficacious anticoagulation, which, however, is often contraindicated owing to multiple concomitant visceral lesions. In some cases, surgical thrombectomy is performed (occlusive thrombus, renal vein injury, etc.) by specialized teams.

In the case of wall rupture, the treatment is usually surgical, consisting of suturing, venorrhaphy, bypass, etc. Endovascular techniques are being carried out with increasing frequency (Castelli et al. 2005), using a common femoral vein approach.

13 Parietal Injury

Injuries to the abdominal wall are found in two situations:
1. Penetrating traumas with substance loss all along the trajectory of the injuring object. In the case of firearm injury, great care should be taken in identifying the exit orifice.
2. Blunt traumas from a direct anterior parietal blow responsible for cutaneous and musculoaponeurotic lesions caused by crushing or compression.

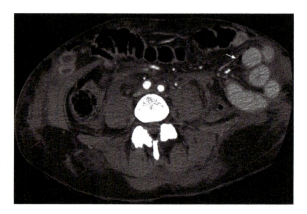

Fig. 29 Left abdominal wall rupture with small bowel perforation. Note the subcutaneous location of the small bowel loops with fluid and air bubbles (*arrows*) around these herniated loops

This abdominal compression results in increased intra-abdominal pressure responsible for traumatic hernia at fragility areas. With this type of mechanism, injury must occur at high velocity so as to interrupt the abdominal rather than the diaphragmatic muscle band. Abdominal wall lesions of the classic seat belt syndrome are due to a direct blow while wearing a seat belt.

13.1 CT Findings

Several lesions may be found on CT images and are described below. They essentially involve the anterior abdominal wall. However, soft tissues of the buttocks or lumbar regions may also be affected and the patient must be systematically examined for these.

13.1.1 Complete Wall Rupture

This lesion corresponds to evisceration. On the CT scan, the anterior parietal peritoneum and the musculoaponeurotic band are ruptured, with visualization of a fluid level, along with significant muscle diastasis. The intestinal loops may be visualized subcutaneously or may be exteriorized. This is a surgical emergency because of the risk of digestive necrosis (Fig. 29).

13.1.2 Posttraumatic Hernia

This lesion is secondary to an increase in intra-abdominal pressure, with aggravation of a preexisting wall dehiscence. As a result, there is a hernia of intestinal loops through a preexisting physiological orifice, with intestinal loops covered by the parietal peritoneum. This type of lesion is rarely diagnosed on initial presentation, but rather months or even years after the trauma.

The CT scan should define the exact location of the hernia (generally umbilical or lumbar), its content, and possible signs of digestive injury, as well as associated intra-abdominal lesions, which are present in more than 60% of cases (Aguirre et al. 2005).

13.1.3 Abdominal Muscle Disinsertion

This lesion is one of the most frequent parietal injuries and is characterized by musculotendinous disinsertion. When it occurs in adults, it appears as muscle retraction, with a focal hematoma in the area where disinsertion occurred; in children, it appear as an avulsion fracture. Elective locations include the rectus abdominis muscle at the level of its pubic insertion, and the oblic and transverse muscles at the level of their iliac insertion (iliac crest), and more rarely, at the level of their insertion on the ribs.

13.1.4 Wall Hematoma

Wall hematoma may be subcutaneous or intramuscular. In the latter case, it may be due to an intrinsic (muscle rupture) or extrinsic (direct shock) mechanism. On the CT scan, it appears as a hyperdense, intramuscular or subcutaneous, blood collection. It is essential to screen for active bleeding at this site (small arteries or muscular veins) as this may require specific treatment.

13.1.5 Ecchymosis (Parietal Contusion)

The CT scan shows simple subcutaneous tissue infiltration, appearing as subcutaneous fat opacification.

13.2 Impact on Management

Ecchymoses do not require any specific treatment, besides analgesics as necessary.

The evolution of hematomas is often benign, resulting in the formation of a retractile scar and a fibrous granuloma, which is, however, associated with a risk of superinfection. Voluminous hematomas may be surgically removed, and the presence of active bleeding may require embolization.

In other cases including abdominal wall disruption, the management is surgical (Brenneman et al. 1995). Evisceration, which is associated with risk of necrosis, is a surgical emergency.

In the case of an isolated and uncomplicated digestive hernia, treatment is usually deferred and consists of closing the orifice of the hernia via the interposition of a prosthetic plaque (Dacron prosthesis). However, if there is an associated intra-abdominal lesion requiring surgical intervention, hernia repair may be performed at the same time, depending on the severity of the patient's status. Muscle disinsertions are repaired surgically.

14 Diaphragmatic Injury

Blunt injuries to the diaphragm are uncommon in blunt trauma patients and are more often encountered in open trauma.

In blunt trauma, injuries are caused by a sudden increase in intra-abdominal or intrathoracic pressure against a fixed diaphragm. The tears are typically large and involve the posterolateral surface of the hemidiaphragm. Injuries may occur at the central portion of the diaphragm or at the site of diaphragmatic attachments. In open trauma, the tears are small, less than 2 cm.

The right hemidiaphragm is less frequently injured than the left, which may be explained by the greater strength of the right hemidiaphragm and the protective effect of the liver. The type of herniated contents depends on the size and location of the injury. The liver, small bowel, or large bowel may herniate through a right-sided diaphragmatic defect; the stomach, small bowel, large bowel, or spleen may herniate through a left-sided defect. Rare locations of traumatic diaphragmatic herniation include the pericardium and the esophageal hiatus.

14.1 CT Findings

The CT findings of diaphragmatic injury include four cardinal signs (Iochum et al. 2002) (Fig. 30):
1. Direct discontinuity of the hemidiaphragm, better seen with coronal and sagittal reformation (Chen et al. 2010).

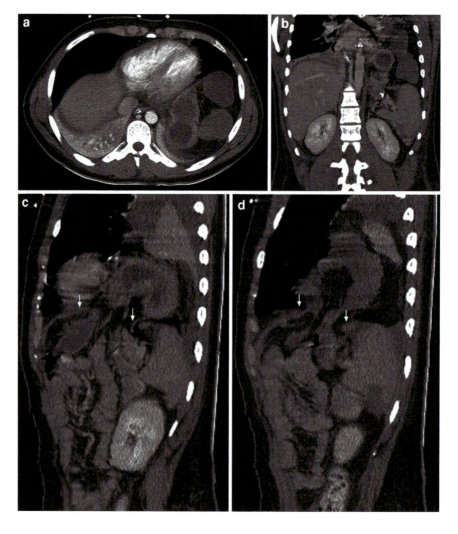

Fig. 30 Left-sided diaphragmatic rupture. The axial slice (a) shows an intrathoracic herniation of the stomach and the descending colon with a dependent stomach sign, with these bowel segments located above the left hemidiaphragm on coronal reformatting (b) whereas sagittal reformatting show the discontinuity of the left hemidiaphragm (*arrow*) at the level of the passage of the stomach (c) and of the colon (d)

2. Intrathoracic herniation of abdominal contents, with the stomach and colon, the most common viscera to herniate on the left side, and the liver the most common viscus to herniate on the right side.
3. The collar sign is produced by a waistlike constriction of herniated viscera at the site of herniation.
4. The dependent viscera sign results from the abdominal viscera falling dependently against the posterior chest wall through the diaphragmatic tear.

There are two other findings that are less specific but that are sometimes useful for the diagnosis of diaphragmatic injury:

1. Localized thickening of the diaphragm which may indicate a hematoma caused by a rupture
2. The presence of both a hemothorax and a hemoperitoneum without obvious intra-abdominal injury

14.2 CT Pitfalls

They are less numerous since the development of multislice CT with sagittal and coronal reformatting, which allows one to individualize even a small diaphragmatic hiatus.

False negatives are due to the absence of herniation of intra-abdominal viscera, especially when pleural effusion or lung condensation masks the diaphragm. False positives may be due to a diaphragmatic defect, which may be congenital, such as Bochdalek hernia, or

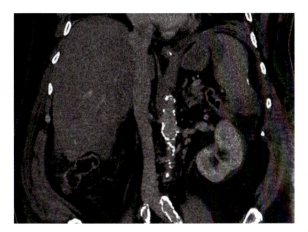

Fig. 31 Thickening of the left crus of the diaphragm in a patient with a splenic trauma. CT follow-up did not show any findings of diaphragmatic rupture

acquired and more commonly seen in women, in patients with emphysema, and with increasing age. Diaphragmatic eventration with isolated elevation of the diaphragm was a cause of false positives before the availability of multiplanar reformatting, which shows the continuity of the diaphragm.

An isolated thickening of the diaphragm must be interpreted with caution and may be the consequence of the diffusion of a thoracic or abdominal effusion or may be due to a contusion without diaphragmatic rupture (Fig. 31).

14.3 CT Impact

Injuries to the diaphragm pose a risk of visceral organ herniation through the defect, which can occur acutely at the time of injury or may be delayed. Visceral organ herniation may result in organ incarceration, strangulation, or perforation. Consequently diaphragmatic rupture may be repaired.

References

Aguirre DA, Santosa AC, Casola G, Sirlin CB (2005) Abdominal wall hernias: imaging features, complications, and diagnostic pitfalls at multi-detector row CT. Radiographics 25(6):1501–1520

Ali M, Safriel Y, Sclafani SJ, Schulze R (2003) CT signs of urethral injury. Radiographics 23(4):951–963; discussion 63–66

Anderson SW, Varghese JC, Lucey BC, Burke PA, Hirsch EF, Soto JA (2007) Blunt splenic trauma: delayed-phase CT for differentiation of active hemorrhage from contained vascular injury in patients. Radiology 243(1):88–95

Arvieux C, Letoublon C (2005) Traumatic pancreatic injuries. Ann Chir 130(3):190–198

Asayama Y, Matsumoto S, Isoda T, Kunitake N, Nakashima H (2005) A case of traumatic mesenteric bleeding controlled by only transcatheter arterial embolization. Cardiovasc Intervent Radiol 28(2):256–258

Atri M, Hanson JM, Grinblat L, Brofman N, Chughtai T, Tomlinson G (2008) Surgically important bowel and/or mesenteric injury in blunt trauma: accuracy of multidetector CT for evaluation. Radiology 249(2):524–533

Bersani D, Montaudon M, Borocco A, Parent Y, Barrère JP (1997) Traumatisme de la veine cave inférieure, aspect tomodensitométrique et angiographique. J Radiol 78:1163–1165

Blayac PM, Kessler N, Lesnik A, Lopez FM, Bruel JP, Taourel P (2002) Traumatismes du tube digestif. Encycl Méd Chir (Editions Scientifiques et Médicales Elsevier SAS, Paris, tous droits réservés), Radiodiagnostic-Appareil Digestif, 33-016-A-40, 7p

Brenneman FD, Boulanger BR, Antonyshyn O (1995) Surgical management of abdominal wall disruption after blunt trauma. J Trauma 39(3):539–544

Brofman N, Atri M, Hanson JM, Grinblat L, Chughtai T, Brenneman F (2006) Evaluation of bowel and mesenteric blunt trauma with multidetector CT. Radiographics 26(4):1119–1131

Buckman RF, Pathak AS, Badellino MM, Bradley KM (2001) Injuries of the inferior vena cava. Surg Clin N Am 81(6): 1431–1447

Castelli P, Caronno R, Piffaretti G, Tozzi M (2005) Emergency endovascular repair for traumatic injury of the inferior vena cava. Eur J Cardiothorac Surg 28(6):906–908

Chen HW et al (2010) Computed tomography in left-sided and right-sided blunt diaphragmatic rupture: experience with 43 patients. Clin Radiol 65:206–212

Choit RL, Tredwell SJ, Leblanc JG, Reilly CW, Mulpuri K (2006) Abdominal aortic injuries associated with chance fractures in pediatric patients. J Pediatr Surg 41(6):1184–1190

Drasin TE, Anderson SW, Asandra A, Rhea JT, Soto JA (2008) MDCT evaluation of blunt abdominal trauma: clinical significance of free intraperitoneal fluid in males with absence of identifiable injury. AJR Am J Roentgenol 191(6):1821–1826

Duchesne JC, Schmieg R, Islam S, Olivier J, McSwain N (2008) Selective nonoperative management of low-grade blunt pancreatic injury: are we there yet? J Trauma 65(1):49–53

Ekeh AP, Saxe J, Walusimbi M, Tchorz KM, Woods RJ, Anderson HL 3rd et al (2008) Diagnosis of blunt intestinal and mesenteric injury in the era of multidetector CT technology—are results better? J Trauma 65(2):354–359

Harris AC, Zwirewich CV, Lyburn ID, Torreggiani WC, Marchinkow LO (2001) CT findings in blunt renal trauma. Radiographics 21(Spec No):S201–S214

Hunter JD, Damani Z (2004) Intra-abdominal hypertension and the abdominal compartment syndrome. Anaesthesia 59(9):899–907

Ikeda O, Urata J, Araki Y, Yoshimatsu S, Kume S, Torigoe Y et al (2007) Acute adrenal hemorrhage after blunt trauma. Abdom Imaging 32(2):248–252

Iochum S et al (2002) Imaging of diaphragmatic injury: a diagnostic challenge? Radiographics 22(Spec No):S103–S116; discussion S116–S118

Kaseje N, Agarwal S, Burch M, Glantz A, Emhoff T, Burke P et al (2008) Short-term outcomes of splenectomy avoidance in trauma patients. Am J Surg 196(2):213–217

Kawashima A, Sandler CM, Corl FM, West OC, Tamm EP, Fishman EK et al (2001) Imaging of renal trauma: a comprehensive review. Radiographics 21(3):557–574

Kertesz JL et al (2009) Detection of vascular injuries in patients with blunt pelvic trauma by using 64-channel multidetector CT. Radiographics 29:151–164

Lee YJ, Oh SN, Rha SE, Byun JY (2007) Renal trauma. Radiol Clin N Am 45(3):581–592 ix

Linsenmaier U, Wirth S, Reiser M, Korner M (2008) Diagnosis and classification of pancreatic and duodenal injuries in emergency radiology. Radiographics 28(6):1591–1602

Liu PP, Chen CL, Cheng YF, Hsieh PM, Tan BL, Jawan B et al (2005) Use of a refined operative strategy in combination with the multidisciplinary approach to manage blunt juxtahepatic venous injuries. J Trauma 59(4):940–945

Lubner M, Menias C, Rucker C, Bhalla S, Peterson CM, Wang L et al (2007) Blood in the belly: CT findings of hemoperitoneum. Radiographics 27(1):109–125

Marmery H, Shanmuganathan K (2006) Multidetector-row computed tomography imaging of splenic trauma. Semin Ultrasound CT MR 27(5):404–419

Marmery H, Shanmuganathan K, Mirvis SE, Richard H 3rd, Sliker C, Miller LA et al (2008) Correlation of multidetector CT findings with splenic arteriography and surgery: prospective study in 392 patients. J Am Coll Surg 206(4):685–693

Mattei-Gazagnes M, Taourel P, Thiebaut C, Vivens F, Bruel JM, Lopez FM (2001) Contusions hépatiques: diagnostic et traitement conservateur. Encycl Méd Chir (Editions Scientifiques et Médicales Elsevier SAS, Paris), Radiodiagnostic-Appareil digestif, 33-515-A-60, 7p

Meghoo CA, Gonzalez EA, Tyroch AH, Wohltmann CD (2003) Complete occlusion after blunt injury to the abdominal aorta. J Trauma 55(4):795–799

Mehrazin R, Derweesh IH, Kincade MC, Thomas AC, Gold R, Wake RW (2007) Adrenal trauma: Elvis Presley Memorial Trauma Center experience. Urology 70(5):851–855

Mirvis SE, Whitley NO, Vainwright JR, Gens DR (1989) Blunt hepatic trauma in adults: CT-based classification and correlation with prognosis and treatment. Radiology 171:27–32

Pal JD, Victorino GP (2002) Defining the role of computed tomography in blunt abdominal trauma: use in the hemodynamically stable patient with a depressed level of consciousness. Arch Surg 137(9):1029–1032; discussion 32–33

Paparel P, Badet L, Tayot O, Fessy MH, Bejui J, Martin X (2003) Mécanismes et fréquence des complications urologiques de 73 fractures instables du bassin. Prog Urol 13:54–59

Pinto A, Scaglione M, Guidi G, Farina R, Acampora C, Romano L (2006) Role of multidetector row computed tomography in the assessment of adrenal gland injuries. Eur J Radiol 59(3):355–358

Poletti PA, Mirvis SE, Shanmuganathan K, Killeen KL, Coldwell D (2000) CT criteria for management of blunt liver trauma: correlation with angiographic and surgical findings. Radiology 216(2):418–427

Romano L, Giovine S, Guidi G, Tortora G, Cinque T, Romano S (2004) Hepatic trauma: CT findings and considerations based on our experience in emergency diagnostic imaging. Eur J Radiol 50(1):59–66

Romano S, Scaglione M, Tortora G, Martino A, Di Pietto F, Romano L et al (2006) MDCT in blunt intestinal trauma. Eur J Radiol 59(3):359–366

Santucci RA et al (2004) Evaluation and management of renal injuries: consensus statement of the renal trauma subcommittee. BJU Int 93:937–954

Savage SA, Zarzaur BL, Magnotti LJ, Weinberg JA, Maish GO, Bee TK et al (2008) The evolution of blunt splenic injury: resolution and progression. J Trauma 64(4):1085–1091; discussion 91–92

Shuman WP (1997) CT of blunt abdominal trauma in adults. Radiology 205(2):297–306

Sinelnikov AO, Abujudeh HH, Chan D, Novelline RA (2007) CT manifestations of adrenal trauma: experience with 73 cases. Emerg Radiol 13(6):313–318

Spencer TA, Smyth SH, Wittich G, Hunter GC (2006) Delayed presentation of traumatic aortocaval fistula: a report of two cases and a review of the associated compensatory hemodynamic and structural changes. J Vasc Surg 43(4):836–840

Stafford RE, McGonigal MD, Weigelt JA, Johnson TJ (1999) Oral contrast solution and computed tomography for blunt abdominal trauma: a randomized study. Arch Surg 134(6):622–626; discussion 6–7

Strouse PJ, Close BJ, Marshall KW, Cywes R (1999) CT of bowel and mesenteric trauma in children. Radiographics 19(5):1237–1250

Stuhlfaut JW, Anderson SW, Soto JA (2007) Blunt abdominal trauma: current imaging techniques and CT findings in patients with solid organ, bowel, and mesenteric injury. Semin Ultrasound CT MR 28(2):115–129

Taourel P, Camus C, Lesnik A, Mattei-Gazagnes M, Gallix B, Pujol J, Lopez FM, Bruel JM (1999) Imagerie du péritoine normal et pathologique. Encycl Méd Chir (Elsevier, Paris), Radiodiagnostic-Appareil digestif, 33-482-A-10, 29p

Taourel P, Vernhet H, Suau A, Granier C, Lopez FM, Aufort S (2007) Vascular emergencies in liver trauma. Eur J Radiol 64(1):73–82

Taourel P, Merigeaud S, Millet I, Devaux Hoquet M, Lopez FM, Sebane M (2008) Traumatisme thoraco-abdominal: stratégie en imagerie. J Radiol 11(2):1833–1854

Tezval H, Tezval M, von Klot C, Herrmann TR, Dresing K, Jonas U et al (2007) Urinary tract injuries in patients with multiple trauma. World J Urol 25(2):177–184

Uriot C, Hoa D, Leguen V, Lesnik A, Lopez FM, Pujol J, Taourel P (2005) Traumatismes du rein et de l'uretère. EMC Radiol 2:637–652

Vaccaro JP, Brody JM (2000) CT cystography in the evaluation of major bladder trauma. Radiographics 20(5):1373–1381

Wei B, Hemmila MR, Arbabi S, Taheri PA, Wahl WL (2008) Angioembolization reduces operative intervention for blunt splenic injury. J Trauma 64(6):1472–1477

Yoon W et al (2004) Pelvic arterial hemorrhage in patients with pelvic fractures: detection with contrast-enhanced CT. Radiographics 24:1591–1605

Yoon W, Jeong YY, Kim JK, Seo JJ, Lim HS, Shin SS et al (2005) CT in blunt liver trauma. Radiographics 25(1):87–104

Index

A

"Acalculous" cholecystitis, 96
AAST classification of hepatic injuries, 423
AAST classification of pancreatic injuries, 423–424
AAST classification of renal injury, 424
AAST classification of splenic injuries, 423
Abbreviated injury score, 21
Abdominal aorta, 458
Abdominal aortic aneurysms, 7, 9–10, 348–349
Abdominal cocoon, 290
Abdominal compartment syndrome, 22
Abdominal muscle desinsertion, 461
Abdominal wall hematomas, 407, 413
Abscess, 156, 159, 164, 226, 232, 408
Accordion sign, 33, 230
Actinomyces israelii, 379
Actinomycosis, 227, 301, 379
Active arterial bleeding, 37
Active extravasation, 334, 457
Acute adrenal insufficiency, 453
Acute appendicitis, 5, 39, 45, 68, 380
Acute bacterial nephritis, 364
Acute bacterial pyelonephritis, 363
Acute BCS, 86
Acute cholecystitis, 8, 93, 96
Acute colonic diverticulitis, 200
Acute coronary syndrome, 10
Acute degeneration, 386
Acute diverticulitis of the right colon, 168
Acute diverticulitis, 39, 45
Acute duodenitis and enteritis, 250
Acute fatty liver, 91
Acute gastric volvulus, 276
Acute gastritis, 239
Acute hemoperitoneum, 84
Acute hepatitis, 47, 88, 99
Acute ischemia of the mesentery, 317
Acute necrotic hemmorrhagic pancreatitis, 11
Acute pancreatitis, 4–6, 8, 10, 45, 126, 247, 251
Acute proctitis, 234
Acute pyeloneophritis, 366, 446
Acute radiation enteritis, 263
Acute renal infarction, 368
Acute splenic sequestration crisis, 121
Acute torsion of a wandering spleen, 118, 120
Acute variceal hemorrhage, 337
Acute-disseminated lupus erythematosus, 261
Adénocortical carcinoma, 354
Adenoma, 345–347
Adenomyomatosis, 99
Adhesions, 34, 282–283, 287, 412
Adhesive bands, 41, 77, 283, 287
Adhesive small bowel obstruction, 6
Adnexal torsion, 9, 10, 381
Adrenal adenoma, 353
Adrenal gland injuries, 446, 452
Adrenal hematoma, 353
Adrenal hemorrhage, 352
Adrenal injury, 451
Adult congenital pyloric stenosis, 275
Adult idiopathic hypertrophic pyloric stenosis, 275
Adynamic ileus, 55
Aerobilia, 100
Air in the portal venous system, 442
Alcohol, 126
Alcoholic etiology, 133
Alvarado score, 146
Amanita phalloides, 89
Amyloidosis, 122
Aneurysm of a pancreaticoduodenal artery, 355
Aneurysm of the intrarenal arteries, 372
Angiodysplasia, 331
Angiomyolipoma, 350–352, 370, 372
Angioneurotic oedema of the small intestine, 263
Anikiasis, 241
Anisakis, 253
Annular pancreas, 275–276
Aortic aneurysm rupture, 138
Aortic aneurysm, 8, 40
Aortic dissection, 362
Aortic injury, 459
Apache II, 128
Appendiceal abscess, 165
Appendiceal adenocarcinomas, 172
Appendiceal carcinoid tumor, 172
Appendiceal diverticulitis, 171
Appendiceal lymphoma, 173
Appendiceal perforation, 156, 313, 315, 323–324

A (cont.)

Appendiceal tumor, 145
Appendicitis, 4–5, 7, 9, 282–283, 291, 370
Appendicoliths, 153, 156–158, 164
Appendix, 68, 144–145, 147, 161
Arrowhead sign, 154, 202
Arterial dissection, 449
Arterial pedicle injury, 447
Arterial-venous fistulas, 432, 437
Arteriovenous fistula, 457
Arteriovenous malformation, 370
Artery-ureteral fistula, 371
Ascaris lumbricoides, 253
Aspergillosis, 259
Aspergillus, 117
Atlanta definition, 128
Auto immune pancreatitis, 134
Avulsion of the right hepatic vein, 435

B

Bacterial gastritis, 240
Bacterial or fungal enteritis, 48
Balthazar score, 131
Band, 311
Beak sign, 33, 288, 294
Behcet syndrome, 37, 318
Behcet's disease, 287
Bezoar, 252, 275, 285
Bile duct traumas, 436
Bile leakage, 94
Bile peritonitis, 414
Biliary ileus, 282
Biliary obstruction, 73
Biliary stones, 94
Biliary-enteric anastomosis, 49
Bilomas, 113, 414, 436
Bladder hematoma, 454
Bladder injury, 453
Bladder perforation, 373, 454
Bladder rupture
Blunt abdominal trauma, 23, 43, 51, 53
Blunt bowel trauma, 48
Blunt hepatic trauma, 47
Blunt retroperitoneal trauma, 43
Blunt traumas, 17, 18, 42, 422, 432
Bochdalek hernia, 462
Boerhaave syndrome, 310
Bone marrow transplants, 47
Bouveret syndrome, 275–276
Bowel halo sign, 34
Bowel ischemia syndrome, 443
Bowel ischemia, 34, 51, 54
Bowel metastases, 286
Bowel obstruction, 51, 167, 205, 317, 380
Bowel perforation, 138, 157, 390, 415, 443, 445
Breast cancer, 90
Budd–Chiari syndrome(BCS), 86
Buerger's disease, 264

C

C. difficile, 233
Calculous acute cholecystitis, 101
Campylobacter jejuni, 256
Campylobacter, 228
Cancer cytoreductive therapy, 19
Candida, 117
Carcinoma, 232
Carcinomatosis, 290
Cardiac failure, 48
Catarrhal appendicitis, 145
Cecal adenocarcinoma, 168
Cecal bar, 154
Cecal
  cancer, 164
  ischemia, 164
Cecal diastatic perforations, 319
Cecal diverticulitis, 157, 207
Cecal neoplasm, 208
Cecal pneumatosis, 304
Cecal volvulus, 34, 299–300
Cervicitis, 378
Chance fracture, 443, 459
Chemoembolisation, 100
Chemotheraphy-related mucositis, 258
Chlamydia trachomatis, 228, 378
Chlamydiae, 228
Cholangitis, 109, 157
Cholecystitis, 4–5, 7–8
Choledocolithiasis, 110
Choledocuduodenal or hepatico-jejunal anastomosis, 109
Cholelithiasis, 126
Choleperitoneum, 436
Choriocarcinoma, 85–86, 388
Chronic appendicitis, 162
Chronic BCS, 86
Chronic cholecystitis, 99
Chronic enteritis after cytoreductive therapy, 41
Chronic mesentric ischemia, 287
Chronic pancreatitis, 134
Chronic radiation enteritis, 41
Churg–strauss syndrome, 260–261
Cirrhosis, 109
Clofazimine, 265
Closed-loop construction, 34, 54, 278, 293, 406, 412
Clostridium difficile, 229
CMV gastritis, 241
CMV infections, 257
CMV intestinal infections, 257
Cocaine, 89
Coeliac disease, 249
Coffee bean sign, 35
Colic carcinoma, 204
Colic pain, 360
Colitides
  infectious, 33
  inflammatory, 33
  ischemic, 33
Colitis, 204

Index
467

Collagen vascular disease, 287
Collagenous colitis, 249
Collar sign, 36, 462
Colon cancer, 232, 299, 302, 304
Colon diverticular bleed, 334
Colonic carcinoma, 204–205, 214, 217
Colonic diverticulitis, 157
Colonic ischemia, 191
Colonic obstructions, 6
Colonic pathology, 9
Colonic pseudoobstruction, 296–297
Colonic tuberculosis, 298
Colonic volvulus, 298
Colonoscopy, 51
Colovesical fistulas, 212
Comb sign, 36
Common bile duct stone, 110–111
Common bile duct stone migration, 134
Common bile duct, 436
Complicated acute diverticulitis, 51
    pylephlebitis, 51
Complicated diverticular disease, 5
Complications of ovarian cyst, 207
Congestion of mesenteric vessels, 294
Congestive heart failure, 46
Constrictive pericarditis, 46
Contusions, 438–439, 446
Corpus luteum cyst, 384–385
Cortial rim sign, 447
Corticosurrenaloma, 370
Crescent sign, 350
Crohn disease, 34, 36, 41, 282–283, 286, 292, 365
Crohn's disease, 157, 161, 167, 207, 223–224, 266–268, 311, 316–317
Cryptococcus, 117
Cryptosporidiosis, 231, 257
CT severity, 131
    index, 138
    perisigmoid abscess, 51
Cystic fibrosis, 280
Cystitis, 363
Cytomegalovirus colitis, 10
Cytomegalovirus, 228
Cytomegalovirus E. coli, 229

D
Dependent viscera sign, 38, 462
Desmoid tumors, 290
Diaphragmatic eventration, 463
Diaphragmatic injury, 461
Diaphragmatic rupture, 36
Diaphragmatic tear, 36
Digestive hematoma, 441
Digestive ischemia, 442
Digestive lymphoma, 317
Digestive perforation, 440
Digestive tract perforation, 426
Digestive tuberculosis, 317
Disproportionate fat stranding, 38
Dissection of the celiac trunk, 428, 431

Dissection of the renal artery, 369
Dissection of the splenic artery, 429
Dissection, 447, 459
Diverticular abscesses, 210
Diverticular disease of the colon and sigmoid volvulus of the elderly, 6
Diverticular hemorrhage, 200, 337
Diverticular sigmoiditis, 315
Diverticulitis, 68, 167, 282, 299, 319, 370, 390
Diverticulosis, 203
Diverticulum, 331
Draped aorta sign, 39, 349
Drop gallstones, 159
Dropped (or retained) appendicolith, 158
Dropped gallstones, 414
Drug-induced enterocolitis, 264
Dumb kidneys, 451
Dumb, 447
Duodenal bezoar, 277
Duodenal hematoma, 442
Duodenal perforation, 50
Duodenoduodenal intussusception, 277
Durg-induced hepatitis, 88

E
Ecstasy, 89
Ectopic pregnancy, 42, 348, 384–385
Embolization, 457
Emphysematous
    pyelitis, 364
    pyelonephritis, 364
Emphysematous cholecystitis, 100
Emphysematous cystitis, 49, 363, 365
Emphysematous gastritis, 243
Endocarditis, 117
Endometriosis of the appendix, 172
Endometriosis, 283, 303, 380
Endometritis, 378, 388
Endoscopic sphincterotomy, 109
Enterovesical fistula, 365
Eosinophilic gastroenteritis, 242, 253, 275
EPIC score, 133, 139
Epiploic appedagitis, 39, 168, 204, 205, 393
    primary, 205, 395
    secondary, 205
Escherischia coli, 116, 146
Excretory tract injury, 449
External hernias, 283, 285
Extraperitoneal rupture, 454
Extra-peritoneal, 453
Extra-uterine pregnancy, 173

F
False aneurysm, 437
FAST ultrasound, 22
Fat halo sign, 40, 250
Fat notch sign, 41, 288
Fatty halo sign, 227
Fecal impactions, 285, 299, 302

F (cont.)

Fecal peritonitis, 204, 211
Feces sign, 279
Femoral hernias, 403
Fibrofatty changes, 287
Fistulas, 227
Fitz–hugh–curtis syndrome, 378
Flat vena cava sign, 42
Focal nodular hyperplasia, 86
Foramen of Winslow hernia, 290
Foreign bodies, 283, 299
Foreign body, 313–314, 317
Fournier gangrene, 367
Fracture shattering of the kidney, 446
Free artery rupture, 434
Free intra- or retroperitoneal air, 440
Free perforation into the retroperitoneum, 209
Fullen's classification of gastrointestinal injuries, 424
Functional colonic disorders, 204–205
Fungal splenic abscesses, 117–118

G

Gallbladder cancer, 3, 104, 106
Gallbladder haemorrhage, 109
Gallbladder stones, 96
Gallbladder, 436
Gallstone ileus, 49, 281, 285
Gallstones, 99, 285, 299
Gangrenous appendicitis, 146
Gangrenous cholecystitis, 98, 102–103
Gas in the mesentericoportal, 213
Gastric abscess, 241
Gastric emphysema, 245
Gastric inflammatory pseudotumour, 251
Gastric neoplasia, 274
Gastric outlet obstruction, 274
Gastric pneumatosis, 277
Gastric trichophytobezoar, 249
Gastric tuberculosis, 242
Gastric tumor perforations, 310
Gastric ulcers, 6, 51
Gastric volvulus, 277, 311
Gastrinoma, 253–254
Gastro-colic fistula, 316
Gastroduodenal ulcer, 310
    perforations, 315, 323
Gastroenteritis, 8, 275
Gastrointestinal anastomosis leakage, 50
Gastrointestinal bleeding, 2, 53
Gastrointestinal perforation, 50, 167
Gastro-intestinal tract, 25
Gaucher disease, 346
Generalized peritonitis, 213
Genital organ injury, 456
Gestational trophoblastic neoplasia, 388
GI tract tumor, 334
GI ulcer, 334
Giardia lamblia, 252
Graded compression US technique, 147

Graft-versus-host disease, 41, 235
Graft-versus-host reaction, 259, 261, 267
Granulomatous colitis, 205
Grynflett-Lesshaft, 404

H

H. pylori gastritis, 249
Haematoma, 267
Halo sign, 225
HELLP syndrome, 90, 347
Hemangioma, 86, 122, 347
Hematoma, 443, 446
Hematomas of the rectus sheath, 407
Hemobilia, 436
Hemoperitoneum, 9–10, 18, 42, 52, 90, 123, 344–345, 384, 425, 428, 432
Hemoretroperitoneum, 43, 427, 447
Hemoritoneum, 109
Hemorrhage of an ovarian cyst, 383
Hemorrhagic cystitis, 370–371
Hemorrhagic hepatocellular carcinoma, 84
Hemorrhoidal rectal bleeding, 336
Hemorroid bleeding, 334
Henoch–Schönlien purpura, 259, 287
Hernias
    inguinal, 289
    femoral, 288–289
    umbilical, 289
    spigelian, 289
    incisional, 289
    external, 289
    obturator, 290
    richter, 290
    paraduodenal, 290
    transmesenteric, 290
    internal, 290–291
Hepatic abscesses, 214
Hepatic artery embolization, 91
Hepatic contusion, 452
Hepatic infarction, 87
Hepatic traumas, 20
Hepatitis viruses, 89
Hepatitis, 47
Hepatocellular adenomas, 85
Hepatocellular carcinoma(HCC), 84, 344–345
Hernia, 56, 311
Herpes virus, 228
High-attenuating crescent sign, 44
Hinchey classification, 323
Hinchey grading system, 319
Hinchey's scheme, 208
Hinchey's surgical scheme, 211
Hinchey, 211
Histoplasmosis, 257
Hodgkin lymphoma, 90
Horseshoe kidney, 445
Hypoperfusion complex, 42
Hypovolemic shock, 449
Hypoxic hepatitis, 88

Index

I

Ileal diverticulitis, 170
Ileal melanosis, 265
Ileocecal lymphoma, 317
Impending abdominal aortic rupture aneurysm, 44
Incarceration, 405
Incisional hernias, 283, 404, 413
Incompetence of the sphincter of oddi, 49
Indinavir stone, 361
Infarction of the greater omentum, 207
Infarction, 184
Infection of necrosis, 136
Infectious colitis, 205, 227
Infectious enteritis, 267, 286
Infectious enterocolitis, 34
Infectious rectitis, 234
Inflamed jejunal diverticulum, 338
Inflammatory bowel disease, 157
Inflammatory pseudotumour, 249
Ingested foreign bodies, 285
Inguinal hernias, 403
    direct type, 403
    indirect type, 403
Injuries to the abdominal wall, 460
Injury severity score, 21
Intense contrast enhancement, 452
Internal hernias, 285
Interstitial laceration, 455
Intestinal obstruction, 6, 8
Intestinal and mesenteric traumas, 440
Intestinal hematoma, 35
Intestinal perforation, 135
Intra cystic haemorrhage, 138
Intraabdominal hemorrhage, 67
Intraabdominal hemorrhagic tumors, 38, 43
Intraductal papillary mucinous tumors, 134
Intrahepatic bile ducts, 436
Intramural gas, 153
Intramural hemorrhage, 190
Intraparenchymal hematoma, 90, 439
    intra-peritoneal, 453
Intraperitoneal hemorrhage, 343
Intrasplenic hemorrhage, 122
Intrauterine device, 379
Intussusception, 275, 283, 285, 292, 299
Irritable bowel syndrome, 11
Ischaemia, 267
Ischaemic necrosis of the stomach, 246
Ischemia, 184, 293–295, 304, 406, 443
Ischemic bowel, 48
Ischemic cholangitis, 112–113
Ischemic cholecystitis, 96, 100
Ischemic colitis, 205, 231, 298, 300, 321
Ischemic digestive strangulation, 311
Ischemic necrosis of the cecum, 169
Isosporal belli, 257

J

Jejunal hematoma, 292
Jejunal ulcer, 312, 317
Junction syndrome, 446

K

Kaposi sarcoma, 283, 286
Kayexalate, 265
Kidney fracture, 446

L

Laceration, 446
Laparoscopic, 283
Leiomyomas, 385–386
Lesion of the small intestine, 19
Leukemia, 117
Leukemic spleen, 122
Lipoma, 286, 299
Little rose, 192
    sign, 192
Littre hernias, 405
Liver abscess, 104, 212
Liver biliary abscesses, 113
Liver metastases, 85, 347
Liver packing, 437
Liver rupture, 90
Liver transplantation, 51
Liver transplants, 47
Liver traumas, 24
Low-grade obstruction, 282
Lumbar hernias, 404
Lung carcinoma, 85
Lupus erythematosus, 35
Lupus mesenteric vasculitis, 37
Lupus vasculitis, 231
Lymphedema, 45
    radiation therapy, 45
Lymph node enlargement, 154
Lymphocytic colitis, 249
Lymphocytic gastritis, 249
Lymphoid hyperplasia, 286
Lymphoma, 118, 311, 372
Malignant melanoma, 286
Malignant tumour, 111
Mallory–Weiss syndrome, 310
Mallory–Weiss tear, 330
Matted adhesions, 280
Matted obstruction, 292
Mcburney's point, 144, 146
McBurney sign, 147
Mechanical obstruction, 442
    bowel, 445
Mechanical small bowel obstruction, 55
Meckel diverticulitis, 157, 170, 207, 282–283, 312, 317

L (cont.)

Mediastinitis, 310, 316
Melanoma, 85, 90, 283
Ménétrier's disease, 249, 254
Mesenteric
    panniculitis, 395
    lipodystrophia, 396
Mesenteric adenitis, 167
Mesenteric edema, 44
    hypoalbuminemia, 44
    heart failure, 45
    tricuspid disease, 45
    portal hypertension, 45
    nephrosis, 45
    constrictive pericarditis, 45
    mesenteric artery, 45
    vein thrombosis, 45
    vasculitis, 45
    budd-chiari syndrome, 45
    vena cava obstruction, 45
Mesenteric hematoma, 443
Mesenteric ischemia, 11, 67, 138
Mesenteric panniculitis, 45, 235, 445
Mesenteric pseudoaneurysm, 443
Mesenteric thromboembolism, 37
Metastases, 118
Microscopic polyangiitis, 37, 260
Midgut volvulus, 56
Mild pancreatitis, 127, 133, 139
Mirizzi syndrome, 103, 107, 109
Misty mesentery, 44
Mononucleosis, 122
Mosaic pattern, 45
Mucocele, 172, 286, 299
Mucormycosis, 259
Mucosal sloughing, 99
Multiple organ failure, 19
Mural hemorrhage, 188
Murphy's sign, 4, 97
Mycobacterium avium intracellulare, 117
Myelolipoma, 370
Myeloproliferative diseases, 86–87
Myeloproliferative syndromes, 118
Myositis, 406, 408

N

Necrosis, 129
Necrotizing cholecystitis, 97
Necrotizing fasciitis, 160
Necrotizing pancreatitis, 44, 51, 127
Neisseria gonorrhoeae, 378
Neoplasm, 330
Neutropenic colitis, 204–205
Neutropenic enterocolitis, 45, 47, 90, 233, 258,
        283, 286
Nodular hyperplasia, 347
Non-occlusive ischemia, 185
Non-hodgkin lymphoma, 47, 90, 283, 286
Northern exposure sign, 46
Nutcracker syndrome, 371

O

Obstructing colonic stenoses, 213
Obstruction, 7
Obturator hernias, 405
Oesophagitis, 330
Omental infarction, 168
Oophoritis, 378
Open abdominal trauma, 18, 426
Open trauma, 422, 445, 461
Ovarian carcinoma, 290
Ovarian cyst, 173
Ovarian hyperstimulation syndrome, 384
Ovarian malignancies, 379
Ovarian torsion, 390
Ovarian vein thrombosis, 388

P

Pancreas, 25
Pancreatitis, 348, 354–355
Pancreatic abscess, 131
Pancreatic adenocarcinoma, 118
Pancreatic cancer, 274
Pancreatic duct injury, 438
Pancreatic enzymes, 439
Pancreatic laceration, 438
Pancreatic necrosis, 127, 131
Pancreatic pseudocysts, 338
Pancreatic traumas, 437
Pancreatitis, 7, 118, 157, 167, 249–250, 275–276, 301, 338
Paracetamol overdose, 89
Parastomial hernias, 283
Parenchymal contusion, 429, 432
Parenchymal laceration, 429, 432
Parietal haematoma, 268
Parietal pneumatosis of the stomach, 246
Parietal pneumatosis, 192, 195, 442
Peliosis, 122, 348
Pelvic abscess, 379, 388
Pelvic hematomas, 389
Pelvic infection, 157
Pelvic inflammatory condition, 8
Pelvic inflammatory disease, 207, 378, 385, 388, 390
Pelvic peritonitis, 282
Pelvic vessels, 457
Penetrating abdominal traumas, 23, 25
Penetrating peritoneal trauma, 50
Penetrating traumas, 18, 432, 450, 460
Penile injury, 456
Peptic ulcer, 330, 348
Peptic ulcer bleeding, 331
Peptic ulcer disease, 274–275
Peptic ulceration, 337
Percutaneous drainage of the gallbladder, 103
Percutaneous drainage, 157
Perforated appendicitis, 6
Perforated cholecystitis, 107
Perforated diverticulitis, 21
Perforated sigmoid cancer, 390
Perforated ulcer, 7
Perforation complicating IUD placement, 387

Index

Perforation of a duodenal diverticulum, 318
Perforation of sigmoid diverticulitis, 320, 323
Perforation of the gallbladder, 100
Perforation, 146, 227, 304, 310
Periappendiceal abscess, 157
Periappendiceal phlegmon, 156
Periarteritis nodosa, 260, 350
Periportal collar sign, 47
Periportal edema, 47, 434, 436–437
Periportal halo, 47
Perirenal edema, 361
Perirenal hematoma, 447
Perirenal urinoma, 449
Peritoneal carcinomatosis, 274, 283, 292, 379
Peritoneal endometriosis, 290
Peritoneal mesenteric lesions, 442
Peritonis, 9
Peritonitis, 146, 157, 209, 211, 282, 304, 313, 411
Peutz–Jeghers syndrome, 286
Pheochromocytoma, 354, 370–371
Phleboliths, 361
Phlegmon, 156–157, 164
Phlegmonous cholecystitis, 107–108
Phlegmonous gastritis, 243
Pneumatosis cystoides coli, 48
Pneumatosis intestinalis, 48, 226, 229
Pneumatosis, 48, 156, 194, 233, 285, 292, 294, 304
Pneumocystis carinii, 117
Pneumomediastinum, 50, 316, 426
Pneumoperitoneum, 49, 68, 216, 315–317, 319, 321,
          325–326, 410, 426
Pneumoretroperitoneum, 50
Pneumothorax, 426
Polyarteritis nodosa, 37, 318, 368, 370
Polycystic kidney disease, 371
Portal enteritis, 256
Portal hypertension, 35, 99, 190
Portal hypertensive gastritis, 248
Portal hypertensive gastropathy, 247
Portal pneumatosis, 277
Portal septic thrombosis, 206
Portal vein thrombosis, 86–87, 136
Portal venous thrombosis, 191
Portomesenteric veins septic thrombosis, 212, 214–215
Portomesenteric venous gas, 51
Post-colonoscopy perforation, 325
Postoperative abscesses, 441
Postpolypectomy bleeding, 331
Primary carcinoid, 286
Primary ischemia, 311
Primary malignant tumors
Proliferation of mesenteric fat, 226
Proximal dissection, 429
Pseudoaneurysm, 135, 137, 338
Pseudo-aneurysm, 430, 432, 435, 449, 451, 457
Pseudocyst, 129, 131, 136
Pseudomembranous colitis, 33, 227, 229, 258
Pseudomyxoma peritonei, 173
Pseudo-pneumoperitoneum, 320
Purulent peritonitis, 204, 211
Pyelonephritis, 205, 363, 366

Pyeloureteral junction lesions, 450
Pylephlebitis, 148, 157
Pyogenic abscesses, 118
Pyogenic cholangitis, 49
Pyogenic splenic abscess, 116–117
Pyonephrosis, 362, 366–367
Pyosal-pinx, 157

R

Radiation colitis, 227, 300
Radiation enteritis, 267, 292
Radiation enteropathy, 287
Radiation induced colitis, 235
Ranson, 128
    score, 127
Rapunzel's syndrome, 249
Rectal perforation, 50
Rectal ulcer, 334
Rectal varices, 331
Recurrent appendicitis, 162
Renal artery aneurysm, 350–351
Renal artery dissection, 368
Renal carcinoma, 85
Renal cell carcinoma, 350, 370
Renal colic, 7, 9, 71, 205
Renal failure, 109
Renal infarct, 369
Renal infarction, 350
Renal injury, 445
Renal or ureteric colic, 4
Renal polykystosis, 446
Renal vein thrombosis, 350, 368–369
Reperfusion damage, 194
Reperfusion process, 184
Retained product of concept, 388
Retroperitoneal air, 192
Retroperitoneal hemorrhage, 343, 348–349
Retroperitoneum, 317
Retropneumoperitoneum, 427–428
Revised trauma score, 21
Reye syndrome, 89
Rheumatoid vasculitis, 262
Richter, 405
Right colon acute diverticulitis, 157
Right hepatic vein avulsion, 433
Right-sided colonic diverticulitis, 207
Rotavirus, 228
Round belly sign, 51
Rupture of a uterine leimyoma, 386
Rupture of an abdominal
          aortic aneurysm, 43
Rupture of the uterus, 386
Rupture, 447
Ruptured abdominal aortic aneurysm, 363
Ruptured aneurysm, 11
Ruptured corpus luteum, 384
Ruptured ectopic pregnancy, 10–11
Ruptured HCC, 84
Ruptured ovarian cysts, 348, 383
Ruptured splenic artery aneurysm, 43

S

Salmonella, 116, 228–229, 235
  typhi, 256
Salpingitis, 173
Sarcoidosis, 118
Scattered renal parenchyma, 450
Scattered spleen, 429
Schistomiasis, 229
Sclerolipomaatous, 167
Seat belt syndrome
Seat belt, 459
Segmental dissection, 434
Segmental infact, 447
Segmental omental infarction, 39
Sentinel blood clot, 428
Sentinel clot sign, 52, 123, 425
Sentinel clot, 443
Serous cystadenoma, 382
Severe acute pancreatitis, 127
Severe pancreatitis, 132
Severity index score, 132
Shigella, 228–229, 253
Shock bowel, 442
Shock liver, 88, 434, 436
Shock spleen, 431
Shock, 42
Sickle cell anemia, 8
Sickle-cell disease, 116, 118, 121
Sigmoid colon, 301
Sigmoid diverticulitis, 313, 365
Sigmoid volvulus, 34, 36, 46, 56, 301–302
Simple prognostic score, 133
Simplified acute physiology score, 22
Small bowel diverticulitis, 317, 334
Small bowel feces finding, 282
Small bowel feces sign, 53
Small bowel obstruction, 9, 41, 53
  strangulated, 37
Small bowel perforation, 317
Small bowel volvulus, 34, 54, 56, 283, 288
Small intestine diverticulitis, 312
Small stone of the common bile duct, 111
Sorbitol, 265
Sphincterotomy, 49
Spiegel hernia, 404
Spleen, 23
Splenectomy, 23, 25, 431–432
Splenia infarct, 117
Splenic abscess, 119
Splenic angiosarcoma, 122
Splenic artery aneurysm, 118, 348
Splenic artery embolization, 24
Splenic fracture, 431
Splenic indentation, 430–431
Splenic infarction, 118
Splenic laceration, 119
Splenic rupture, 121
Splenic traumas, 20, 428
Spoke wheel sign, 54
Spontaneous bowel hematomas, 66
Spontaneous hematoma, 287
Spontaneous intramural hematoma, 287
Spontaneous retroperitoneal hemorrhage, 44
Spontaneous spleen rupture, 38, 43, 53, 122
Spontaneous splenic rupture, 347
Spotted spleen, 430
Staphylococcus aureus, 112
Staphylococus, 228
Steatotic, 85
Stercoral colitis, 314
Strangulating construction, 412
Strangulating obstruction, 296
Strangulation, 6, 280, 282, 293, 295, 406
Striated nephrogramc, 364
String of pearls sign, 54
Strongyloides stercoralis, 253
Stump appendicitis, 162
Sub acute cholecystitis, 108
Subcapsular hematoma, 84, 90, 429, 431, 433, 447
Subcutaneous emphysema, 367
Submucosal fatty metaplasia, 250
Submucosal pseudolipomatosis, 267
Superior mesenteric artery syndrome, 275, 277
Suppurative appendicitis, 146
Suppurative cholecystitis, 97
Systemic lupus erythematosus, 368

T

Target or halo sign, 294, 304
Target sign, 194, 225
Telangiectatic, 85
Teratoma, 382
Testile injuries, 456
The normal appendix, 151
Thrombophlebitis, 157
Thrombosed right ovarian, 173
Thrombosis of superior mesentric artery, 190–191
Thrombosis, 165
Tip appendicitis, 163
Tissue rim sign, 55
Torsion of the uterus, 386
Toxic hepatitis, 89
Toxic megacolon, 226
Transcatheter arterial embolization, 84, 415
Transition point, 281
Transmesenteric hernias, 283, 412
Tuberculosis colitis, 231
Tuberculosis, 227, 257, 287, 311, 379
Tuberculous peritonitis, 290
Tubo-ovarian abscess, 157, 378–379
Tumoral colic perforation, 313
Type 1 glycogen storage disease, 346
Typhlitis, 157, 169–170, 207, 233, 235, 258

U

Ulcer perforations, 321
Ulcerative colitis, 34, 41, 51, 205, 223–224, 226
Ulceronecrotic acute gastritis, 242
Umbilical hernias, 404
Ureteral injury, 450–451

Index

473

Ureterolithiasis, 55
Uretheral injury, 455–456
Urinary calculi, 68
Urinary leakage, 416
Urinary stone, 360
Urinary tract lesions, 445
Urinoma/Urohematoma, 447
Uterine rupture, 389
Uterine torsion, 387
  leiomyoma, 387

V

Vaginal lacerations, 456
Varices, 330
Vascularitis, 318
Vasculitis linked to cocaine, 264
Vasculitis, 259, 267, 312, 368, 370
Vein pedicle injury, 449
Venous ischemia, 158
Venous occlusions, 188
  mesenteric, 189
Venous traumas, 435
Vesical contusion, 455
Vesical rupture, 453

Viral hepatitis, 88
Vittel criteria, 21
Volvulus of the sigmoid or cecum, 77
Volvulus, 6, 278, 283

W

Wall hematoma, 461
Wall thinning, 294
Wandering spleen, 120
Wegener's granulomatosis, 260
Whipple's disease, 257
Whirl sign, 56, 294
  primary volvulus of the small bowel, 288
Wilson disease, 89

Y

Yersinia, 228–229
Yersiniosis, 256

Z

Zollinger–Ellison syndrome, 249, 312, 317

9783540892311